Advances in epilepsy research are occurring at a rapid rate, aided particularly by new technologies that permit the study of cell activity at a molecular level. As a result, a bewildering wealth of data is available and the implications of this new knowledge for future research and clinical practice can be confusing. This volume therefore concentrates on the concepts and models of epilepsy that have been developed as a result of this research. Within the framework of such models, further progress in understanding can be made and new clinical approaches to treatment can be developed.

Written by prominent researchers in the field, this book presents a number of major concepts and hypotheses through which epilepsy research is currently being advanced. It describes three different levels of approach to the study of epileptic mechanisms: individual cellular responses and activity, the local interaction of neurons within a regional focus, and the spread of epileptic activity throughout wider regions of the brain. Both in-vivo and in-vitro techniques are evaluated in chapters that focus on special features of epileptogenesis in the immature brain, work on human epileptic tissue, and models such as kindling. These discussions elucidate the pathways and mechanisms through which seizure activity is initiated and spread, and illustrate how an appreciation of differences between the normal and abnormal brain can advance understanding of the pathological mechanisms.

In a field in which rapid advances lead to constant update of empirical data, this book takes a conceptual approach to the subject and provides a solid framework within which to understand the emerging issues. It provides a broad review of current concepts in the field of epilepsy research and will be a valuable source of reference and knowledge for basic neuroscientists, as well as for neurologists and neurosurgeons with a special interest in the epilepsies.

EPILEPSY: MODELS, MECHANISMS, AND CONCEPTS

EPILEPSY: MODELS, MECHANISMS, AND CONCEPTS

Edited by

PHILIP A. SCHWARTZKROIN
Professor of Neurological Surgery and Physiology and Biophysics, University of Washington

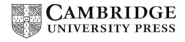

Published by the Press Syndicate of the University of Cambridge
The Pitt Building, Trumpington Street, Cambridge CB2 1RP
40 West 20th Street, New York, NY 10011-4211, USA
10 Stamford Road, Oakleigh, Melbourne 3166, Australia

First published 1993

Printed in Great Britain at the University Press, Cambridge

A catalogue record for this book is available from the British Library

Library of Congress cataloguing in publication data

Epilepsy : models, mechanisms, and concepts / edited by Philip A.
    Schwartzkroin.
        p.   cm.
    Includes index.
    ISBN 0–521–39298–5 (hc)
    1. Epilepsy – Pathophysiology.   2. Epilepsy – Animal models.
    I. Schwartzkroin, P. A. (Philip A.)
        [DNLM: 1. Brain – metabolism.   2. Disease Models, Animal.
    3. Epilepsy – etiology.   4. Seizures – etiology.   WL 385 E6433]
    RC372.5.E66   1993
    616.8′5307 – dc20   92-49037 CIP

ISBN 0 521 39298 5   hardback

KW

This volume is dedicated to the memory of JoAnn E. Franck, Ph.D. (15 February 1950 to 2 September 1992). In a prematurely curtailed career devoted to basic research on the neuropathology of the epilepsies, JoAnn established herself as a first-class scientist. She was a generous colleague and friend, and we will miss her.

Contents

Contributors

Dr Yael Amitai
Department of Physiology, Faculty of Medicine, Ben-Gurion University of the Negev, Beersheva, Israel

Dr Massimo Avoli
Montreal Neurological Institute, 3801 University, Montreal, QC, Canada H3A 2B4

Dr Edward H. Bertram
Department of Neurology, University of Virginia Medical Center, Charlottesville, VA 22908, USA

Dr Douglas W. Bonhaus
Epilepsy Research Laboratory, Department of Veteran Affairs Medical Center, Durham, NC 27705, USA.
Present address: *Department of Neuroscience, Syntex, Palo Alto, CA 94304, USA*

Dr Robert J Brady
Wadsworth Center for Laboratories and Research, New York State Department of Health, Empire State Plaza, Albany, NY 12201, USA

Dr Andrew Bragdon
Department of Neurology, State University of New York at Syracuse, NY 13210, USA

Dr Barry W. Connors
Section of Neurobiology, Division of Biology and Medicine, Brown University, Providence, RI 02912, USA

Dr John W. Dailey
Department of Basic Sciences, University of Illinois College of Medicine, Peoria, IL 61656, USA

Dr Raymond Dingledine
Department of Pharmacology, University of North Carolina at Chapel Hill, Chapel Hill, NC 27599, USA
Present address: *Department of Pharmacology, Emory University, Atlanta, GA 30322, USA*

Dr JoAnn E. Franck
Department of Neurological Surgery, University of Washington, Seattle, WA 98195, USA

Dr Karen Gale
Department of Pharmacology, Georgetown University Medical Center, Washington, DC 20007, USA

Dr Phillip C. Jobe
Department of Basic Sciences, University of Illinois College of Medicine, Peoria, IL 61656, USA

Dr Olle Lindvall
Department of Neurology, University Hospital, S-221 85 Lund, Sweden

Dr Eric W. Lothman
Department of Neurology, University of Virginia Medical Center, Charlottesville, VA 22908, USA

Dr Nandor Ludvig
Department of Basic Sciences, University of Illinois College of Medicine, Peoria, IL 61656, USA

Dr Christopher J. McBain
Department of Pharmacology, University of North Carolina at Chapel Hill, Chapel Hill, NC 27599, USA
Present address: *Unit for Cellular and Synaptic Physiology, National Institutes of Health, Bethesda, MD 20892, USA*

Dr James O. McNamara
Department of Medicine (Neurology), Duke University Medical Center, Durham, NC 27705, USA

Dr Richard Miles
Laboratoire de Neurobiologie Cellulaire, Institut Pasteur, 28 rue de Dr Roux, 75264 Paris Cédex 15, France

Dr Pravin K. Mishra
Department of Basic Sciences, University of Illinois College of Medicine, Peoria, IL 61656, USA

Dr Solomon L. Moshé
Department of Neuroscience, Laboratory of Developmental Epilepsy, Albert Einstein College of Medicine and Montefiore Medical Center, Bronx, NY 10461, USA

Dr Martha G. Pierson
Wadsworth Center for Laboratories and Research, New York State Department of Health, Empire State Plaza, Albany, NY 12201, USA
Present address: *Cain Foundation Laboratories for Epilepsy Research, Baylor College of Medicine, Houston, TX 77030, USA*

Dr Philip A. Schwartzkroin
Department of Neurological Surgery, University of Washington, Seattle, WA 98195, USA

Dr Cheolsu Shin
Department of Medicine (Neurology), Duke University Medical Center, Durham, NC 27705, USA

Dr Karen L. Smith
Wadsworth Center for Laboratories and Research, New York State Department of Health, Empire State Plaza, Albany, NY 12201, USA
Present address: *Cain Foundation Laboratories for Epilepsy Research, Baylor College of Medicine, Houston, TX 77030, USA*

Dr Erwin-Joseph Speckmann
Institut für Physiologie, Universität Münster, D-4400 Münster, Germany

Dr Ellen F. Sperber
Department of Neuroscience, Laboratory of Developmental Epilepsy, Albert Einstein College of Medicine, Bronx, NY 10461, USA

Dr Patric K. Stanton
Department of Neuroscience, Laboratory of Developmental Epilepsy, Albert Einstein College of Medicine, Bronx, NY 10461, USA

Dr Janet L. Stringer
Department of Neurology, University of Virginia Medical Center, Charlottesville, VA 22908, USA
Present address: *Department of Pharmacology, Baylor College of Medicine, Houston, TX 77030, USA*

Dr Thomas P. Sutula
Department of Neurology, University of Wisconsin, Madison, WI 53792, USA

Dr John W. Swann
Wadsworth Center for Laboratories and Research, New York State Department of Health, Empire State Plaza, Albany, NY 12201, USA
Present address: *Cain Foundation Laboratories for Epilepsy Research, Baylor College of Medicine, Houston, TX 77030, USA*

Dr Stephen F. Traynelis
Department of Pharmacology, University of North Carolina at Chapel Hill, Chapel Hill, NC 27599, USA
Present address: *Molecular Neurobiology Laboratory, Salk Institute, San Diego, CA 92138, USA*

Dr Jörg Walden
Institut für Physiologie, Universität Münster, D-4400 Münster, Germany

Dr Wilkie A. Wilson
Department of Pharmacology and Medicine, Veterans Administration Medical Center, Durham, NC 27705, USA

Dr Robert K. S. Wong
Department of Pharmacology, State University of New York, Health Science Center, Brooklyn, NY 11203, USA

General introduction

PHILIP A. SCHWARTZKROIN

Concepts and models

There is little doubt that advances in epilepsy research are occurring at a rapid rate. For those of us who are interested in understanding the mechanisms underlying epileptiform activities – whether because of a basic interest in how the brain works, or driven by a concern for more effective treatments for the epilepsies – progress in the laboratory has been almost bewildering. It seems that in each new issue of each neuroscience publication there are new insights and possibilities that we must integrate into our old frameworks. Much of the 'progress' has been propelled by advances in technology. For example, at the electrophysiological level, new recording techniques such as patch-clamping have allowed investigators to gain much greater detailed understanding of single-cell properties. New antibodies and tract-tracing techniques have provided information about specific cell populations and about plasticity in neuronal interconnections. Molecular neurobiology is beginning to make a considerable impact on epilepsy research, providing techniques for studying the genetics of inherited epilepsies, as well as for examining the structure and expression of channels and receptors. Pharmacological and neurochemical methods now provide highly sensitive means for analyzing receptor populations, and for assaying transmitter systems (e.g., with microdialysis). Clearly, a single volume cannot hope to deal with all this information, not even were we to focus exclusively on 'new' data. This explosion of information undoubtedly accounts for the many new books, published within the last few years, with a focus on the epilepsies. Each stakes out its own particular area of interest, and attempts to develop that part of the grand picture. Each volume inevitably reflects the interest and expertise of the participating authors. This volume is no exception.

1

The primary goal of this volume is not simply to review current information. Indeed, the particular areas of interest and technical approaches taken by the authors are secondary. Rather, the authors' major task has been to develop a discussion about key hypotheses that they feel are particularly important in the field of modern epilepsy, to write chapters that focus primarily on concepts and ideas, rather than on results and data. Our hope is that these ideas and concepts will not be outdated in six months, but will continue to be relevant to our studies of the basic mechanisms of the epilepsies.

In some important ways, the development of conceptual frameworks within which to fit experimental data is much more difficult than producing laboratory results. If we survey the current literature on epilepsy, we find an incredible wealth of experimental data – details about how and why cells discharge, how that activity is modulated, what factors influence cell reorganization, etc. It is becoming increasingly clear that virtually anything we learn about normal neuronal activity helps us to understand the basis of epileptogenesis and epileptiform activities. Thus, studies ranging from micro-analysis of channel currents to macro-analysis of lesions to large brain regions have proven to be 'relevant' to epilepsy research. Given such a wealth of data, how does one decide which factors are salient with respect to the various forms of epileptiform activity? We have known for many years that innumerable features of the brain change during development and maintenance of hyperexcitability. How do we tell which features are *causally* related to seizure development, which are *required* for seizure maintenance, and which are simply results of seizure activity? To begin to approach such questions, the investigator must generate conceptual frameworks within which to test specific hypotheses. Then, to translate these ideas to the laboratory, it is necessary to develop 'appropriate' experimental models. The choice of model with which we work, and its connection to the hypotheses developed to explain epileptiform activity, is critical. In fact, the choice of model inevitably influences the conceptual frameworks within which our ideas develop; it is only by developing models that we can test hypotheses.

Twenty years ago, the book *Experimental Models of Epilepsy – A Manual for the Laboratory Worker* (Purpura *et al.*, 1972) was published. Many models were described by investigators who were pioneers in epilepsy research. It is interesting to note that then, as now, the number of available models was impressive. One can only speculate about the drive to develop such a multitude of experimental approaches. One rationale is that there are so many different forms of epilepsy that no one model is sufficient. A rather different view is that these models multiply at random, as though they have a life of their own. Indeed, one of the revelations about possible underlying mechanisms of the epilepsies (and ways to model them) is that epileptiform activity can be produced as a result of many types of experimental intervention. The brain appears to have a rather limited repertoire of behaviors by which to respond to trauma/insult, or to deal with inborn errors. One of the most common responses is for the abnormal region to become hyperexcitable. The activity that we call epilepsy, then, may reflect a basic underlying propensity of the central nervous system.

These two general views of model generation are, I think, less than optimal. The implication of the first line of reasoning is that one develops models to mimic particular clinical phenomena. To do so successfully requires that we can clearly define the salient features of the epileptic brain that should be mimicked in the model. However, it takes only a short time, sitting in a conference of 'epileptologists', to discover that there is little agreement about the defining feature of epilepsy. Each investigator has a slightly different, and rather individual, definition – implicit or explicit. We should expect no less, scientific investigation being a human enterprise. The implication of the second approach is that the specific model does not really matter, since similar phenomenology can be reproduced in so many ways.

My own bias is that models are most successful when they are used as a means by which specific problems and questions related to the epilepsies may be approached. Therefore, different models are appropriate for studying different issues. For example, to answer the question 'Is hyperexcitability always associated with loss of inhibition?', one would like to examine a number of models in which inhibition was not blocked a priori. A model in which GABAergic inhibition (GABA is γ-aminobutyric acid) was completely blocked, e.g., by bicuculline, would be inappropriate to the question – although not necessarily irrelevant to studies of the epilepsies.

The range of ideas relevant to the generation of epileptiform activity is indeed broad. In this volume, the work reported ranges from the level of receptor molecules and cell membranes to the interaction of long-loop neuronal pathways, and from naturally occurring genetic determinants of epileptiform activity to artificially produced epilepsy models in vitro. Throughout, there is an implicit understanding that abnormal activities can be understood at a variety of levels, each building upon the other as one would build an elaborate castle out of simple building blocks. What constitutes the various blocks contributing to the epilepsy 'castle' is the focus of this volume. For the present discussion, I will divide the issue into three major levels of complexity: (a) intrinsic cellular properties, including channel and receptor expression; (b) the interaction of neurons with each other, and with their extracellular environment within a limited region which one defines as the 'focus'; and (c) the involvement of larger populations of neurons, and hence the spread of epileptiform activity from a localized region to broader areas of the brain.

Basic building blocks

Intrinsic cell properties

To think of a neuron as the most basic building block is in some ways misleading, given the apparently endless means by which the activity of a given neuron can be modified. For example, the list of voltage-gated (and ligand-gated) channels that determine cellular properties is continually growing. Each cell type appears to have a unique complement and distribution of these channels, although many of the channels are common across virtually all cell groups. An outline of voltage-gated channels is inevitably incomplete, but gives some hint about how the interaction of even these 'simple' elements can modulate the excitability of a given neuron in a complex manner (Crill & Schwindt, 1983).

The basic Hodgkin–Huxley sodium channel (Hodgkin & Huxley, 1952) is an important component of most neurons, with its rapid voltage-dependent activation and inactivation properties. Recent molecular studies have found, however, that sodium channel subunit construction may divide the channels into at least two subgroups with specific preferential cellular localizations (axon versus soma/dendrite) (Westenbroek *et al.*, 1989). This differential localization of sodium channel subtypes may parallel the distinction between the rapidly inactivating and 'persistent' sodium channels. The latter (Stafstrom *et al.*, 1984), although similar to the Hodgkin–Huxley-type channels in their tetrodotoxin sensitivity, do not inactivate quickly, and are largely activated at membrane potentials just subthreshold for spike discharge. The persistent sodium current can therefore contribute substantially to the efficacy of excitatory postsynaptic potentials in triggering action potentials, or can modulate postsynaptic potential amplitude when those synaptic inputs are subthreshold.

A number of different calcium channels have been described, and an attempt has been made to divide them into three (or four) major types (Nowycky *et al.*, 1985): (a) L-type, with a high activation threshold and slow (if any) inactivation, probably the major contributor to calcium 'spikes' in many cells (Hess, 1990); (b) T-type, with low threshold and rapid inactivation (indeed, normally inactivated at or near resting potential), involved in the generation of rhythmic activities (e.g., in thalamic contribution to absence spike-and-wave activity) (Mogul & Fox, 1991); and (c) N-type, often thought to constitute the major presynaptic terminal population of calcium channels (Tsien *et al.*, 1988). These different calcium channels are distinguishable on the basis of their kinetics, as well as their differential drug antagonist sensitivity: L-type specifically blocked by dihydropyridines (Seagar *et al.*, 1988); T-type blocked by ethosuximide-like drugs (Coulter *et al.*, 1989); and N-type blocked by ω-conotoxin (Plummer *et al.*, 1989). It is clear that the density and distribution of these channels profoundly influence the discharge properties of neurons in the central nervous system (CNS).

The list of potassium-channel-mediated currents is ever-growing; one might well wonder why so many different potassium currents are needed by CNS neurons. Most of the potassium currents are turned on by membrane depolarization, and are hyperpolarizing in function – contributing to spike repolarization, interspike interval, or intervals between bursts of cell activity (Crill & Schwindt, 1983; Storm, 1987). Such currents may be voltage sensitive, e.g., A-currents and delayed rectifier currents (for which there is now molecular evidence of a large variety, although their various functions are by no means clear; Connor & Stevens, 1971; Wei *et al.*, 1990). Another group of potassium currents appears to be modulated by intracellular ion concentrations: calcium dependent (Schwartzkroin & Stafstrom, 1980; producing either long-lasting or brief hyperpolarizing effects) and sodium dependent (Schwindt *et al.*, 1989; which may also contribute long-lasting hyperpolarizations, and apparently reflect cellular discharge during which sodium enters the cell). Finally, there is a voltage-sensitive potassium conductance (I_H) that is generally depolarizing. These anomalous rectifier I_H channels open when the cell is hyperpolarized, and tend to resist further hyperpolarizing drive (Spain *et al.*, 1987).

Interference, blockade, or modulation of any one of these channels could have dramatic effects on the discharge properties of CNS neurons, and thus on the population responses in various parts of the brain. Given that these channels are composed of protein subunits, coded for by specific genetic sequences, alterations/mutations in the genetic machinery could selectively affect one or more of these channels (Wei *et al.*, 1990). More typically, however, neurotransmitter systems (e.g., using cholinergic, noradrenergic, and serotonergic agents) potently and selectively modulate these channels. The growing complexity of these neurotransmitter systems complicates an understanding of these interactions. For example: there are at least two separate receptors for GABA ($GABA_A$ and $GABA_B$) (Hill & Bowery, 1981; Olsen, 1981; Bormann, 1988; Schofield, 1989); a large number of receptors for excitatory amino acids, including N-methyl-D-aspartate (NMDA) and 'non-NMDA' (quisqualate/kainate) ionotropic receptors (Mayer & Westbrook, 1987; Collingridge & Lester, 1989), as well as metabotropic glutamate receptors (Houamed *et al.*, 1991); a variety of noradrenergic (Kobilka, 1992), serotonergic (Peroutka, 1988), and cholinergic (North, 1986) receptors; and 'innumerable' peptide–receptor interactions (Lundberg & Hökfelt, 1983). A detailed listing would be almost impossible, and certainly inappropriate, in this General introduction.

General issues relevant to the interaction between voltage-gated and ligand-gated channels include the following: (a) the function of at least some of the ligand-gated receptors is voltage dependent (Mayer *et al.*, 1984); therefore, voltage-gated channels can influence directly the operation of the neurotransmitter-gated channels; (b) most receptors are coupled, directly or indirectly, to channels which allow ions to enter into and/or exit from the cell. Since some of the voltage-gated channels are ion dependent, neurotransmitters can gate not only the channels to which they are coupled, but also influence other, related, ion-sensitive systems. (c) Many of the transmitter-gated systems engage intracellular second (and even third) messenger systems (e.g., G-proteins) (Andrade *et al.*, 1986), which often involve kinase activation and protein phosphorylation (Chen *et al.*, 1990). It seems quite likely that phosphorylation affects not only the ion channels to which these receptors are coupled, but also receptor molecules (e.g., GABA) or ion channels (e.g., voltage-dependent sodium channels) (Catteral *et al.*, 1990) that are not coupled to receptors. We know relatively little about how the various phosphorylation steps modulate cell excitability; however, phosphorylation of specific membrane-associated proteins does appear to be critical in the development of normal synaptic plasticity – at least as modeled by long-term potentiation.

Since the complexity of these voltage-, ion-, and transmitter-sensitive channels in the membrane of each neuron has become so difficult to comprehend at an intuitive level, their function is now often approached within the context of computer models of single neurons. When considered as units of epileptiform activity – i.e., as basic building blocks of a more elaborate system – this single-cell complexity is quite impressive. It is therefore not surprising that some investigators have described 'epileptic' neurons', and posed hypotheses regarding single-cell 'seizure' generation (Segal, 1991). This focus on single neurons is reminiscent of analyses traditionally carried out by neurobiologists interested in pacemaker activity in invertebrates (Connor, 1982). Clearly one can elicit bursting activity in single isolated neurons via a variety of manipulations. Even within this simplified single-cell context, however, it is difficult to determine which cell features are salient in the generation of epileptiform activity. The critical question remains: can a single neuron really be epileptic?

Local interactions

Further insight into issues of epileptogenicity necessarily involves the study of populations of neurons. This second step in building the epilepsy 'castle' deals with how the blocks fit together. Within a local environment, how do the cells interact? What is the nature of the connectivity and how is it modified and/or influenced by the extracellular environment? Much of the current investigation into mechanisms of epileptogenesis falls within this category. For example, an investigator may ask, 'How do neurotransmitter substances affect the excitability of a given neuronal population?' This question is certainly related to the issue of how a drug might affect an individual neuronal building block. However, as we consider the role of transmitters/modulators in 'circuitry', the issue is not only how a given transmitter gates channels *within* single-cell membranes, but also how it changes the likelihood of *output* from a given neuron – and thus increases or decreases cellular interaction within the population. A given transmitter may give rise to a number of different such effects. For example, GABA can produce inhibition or 'excitation', depending on where and how much of the drug is released, the maturity of the system in which it is tested, and the types of receptor upon which it acts (Alger & Nicoll, 1982; Mueller *et al.*, 1982; Michelson & Wong, 1991). Effects of other transmitters, acting on diverse sets of receptors, can be even more complex. For example, the net effect of norepinephrine on individual cortical building blocks often appears to be excitation, mediated through beta-receptors (Madison & Nicoll, 1986). Beta-receptor activation leads to a loss of cell afterhyperpolarizations and a decrease in cell accommodative properties – which increases the cell's responsiveness to incoming excitatory stimuli. However, when analyzed within the context of the intact CNS, noradrenergic action is more often inhibitory than excitatory. For example, lesions of the noradrenergic system generally produce animals that are significantly more prone to seizure than is the norm (McIntyre & Edson, 1981).

Perhaps the most excitement in this area of neurotransmitter effects on cell excitability has come from recent investigations of the NMDA receptor. Studies suggest that, at least in some models such as kindling, NMDA receptor function is significantly enhanced (Mody *et al.*, 1988). Since NMDA receptor function is modulated by a number of different binding sites on the NMDA receptor/ionophore molecule (Williams *et al.*, 1990), modulation of this important receptor may occur through a variety of cellular pathways. The relationship between NMDA and non-NMDA receptors, their respective roles in various hyperexcitability phenomena, and the possibility that non-NMDA receptors are potentiated via NMDA-mediated mechanisms during stimulation (Muller & Lynch, 1988) (or as a result of discharging seizure foci) are issues of critical importance that involve an understanding of cellular interactions.

Other recent studies of cell–cell interactions focus on circuitry requirements for producing synchronized discharge activity (one of the characteristics of epileptiform discharge). Modeling work started in the early 1980s (Traub & Wong, 1981) suggested that even a small degree of recurrent excitatory interconnection within a local cell group (for example, in the CA3 region of hippocampus) was sufficient to mediate synchronized discharge. Occurrence of such discharge was based, in part, on the intrinsic properties of the participating neurons, and mediated by the excitatory interactions among the cells. Although it is unclear how common the functional recurrent excitatory interactions normally are within cortical areas of the CNS, both hippocampal and neocortical regions show significant excitatory interactions when inhibition is reduced (Christian & Dudek, 1988). Further, even in the absence of normal excitatory interconnections, it is possible that emergent recurrent excitatory collaterals – i.e., sprouting fibers – may be important contributors to the development of synchronized hyperexcitability (Cronin & Dudek, 1988). Synchronized excitatory drive may result either from potentiation of already-existing synaptic contacts, or the development of new contacts through 'plastic' mechanisms.

Perhaps the oldest of the hypotheses developed to 'explain' epilepsy focuses on inhibitory control (mediated via GABA receptors) within neuronal populations, with the loss of inhibition seen as the critical step in development of hyperexcitability (Schwartzkroin & Prince, 1980;

Schwartzkroin & Wyler, 1980). The inhibition story has, however, become exceedingly complex. The nature of the inhibition within any given brain region depends on the existence of inhibitory (often GABAergic) interneurons (Lacaille *et al.*, 1989) that make divergent connections to the principal cells in each region, and that receive convergent inputs from principal cells. The function of these interneurons – i.e., their modulation of principal cell output – depends on their patterns of connectivity with other cells in the local region. Inhibitory inter-neuron connections with other inhibitory interneurons, as well as with excitatory cells, endow the system with innumerable points of control. The recent interest in the role of GABA receptors on presynaptic terminals now adds even more complexity to the system (Thompson & Gähwiler, 1989).

We can delineate many ways of producing inhibition or excitation by manipulating the interneuronal inhibitory circuit. For example, if inhibition were produced only by postsynaptic contacts of interneurons onto pyramidal cells, then loss of those interneurons – or diminished effectiveness of the pathway by which the interneurons are excited – would yield net excitation in the system. If, on the other hand, interneurons also made strong connections with other inhibitory interneurons, then loss of drive onto the initial interneuron population might yield greater net inhibition onto pyramidal cells, as a result of the 'release' of the second inhibitory population. If we then add the effects of presynaptic GABA receptors on either excitatory or inhibitory terminals (or both), the various scenarios multiply exponentially. Finally, and realistically, the investigator must face the likelihood that changes in inhibitory (or excitatory) circuitry are not all-or-none, and thus must be evaluated quantitatively. How much inhibition must be lost to produce hyperexcitability (Chagnac-Amitai & Connors, 1989)? How much excitatory interaction is necessary to synchronize a cell population?

CNS plasticity is another important factor that influences how interaction among neurons may give rise to epileptiform phenomena. One question that highlights the critical nature of this plasticity is 'What happens to tissue excitability when a part of the nervous system is damaged (Meldrum & Corsellis, 1984), as seems often to be the case in epileptic brain?'In building a castle of wooden blocks, if we remove a number of critically located individual blocks, the entire castle is likely to collapse. Such a collapse does not occur often in the CNS, perhaps because there is so much 'redundancy'. It is clear, however, that the CNS also displays a strong capacity for replacing lost elements with newly grown processes (sprouting). Can new processes replace lost elements in a functionally adaptive manner, or is the plasticity likely to be dysfunctional? How do these changes bias the general excitability of the region?

Cell–cell interaction is significantly impacted by contributions from the extracellular environment. Experimenters have long known that tissue excitability is dramatically affected by changes in extracellular ionic concentrations. Increases in potassium concentration (which may result from prolonged cell discharge) may produce further hyperexcitability (Rutecki *et al.*, 1985). Lowering of the extracellular calcium concentration leads to a loss of synaptic drive (since transmitter release is dependent on calcium influx), but may also (at least in some tissues) result in spontaneous synchronized cell discharge (presumably via non-synaptic mechanisms) (Konnerth *et al.*, 1986). Both this calcium effect and the effects of extracellular potassium are probably modulated by changes in the extracellular space (Traynellis & Dingledine, 1989). Decreased extracellular space, as might occur when cells swell (e.g., as a result of prolonged discharge and the subsequent entry of sodium and water into neurons), significantly magnifies changes in extracellular ion concentrations. Potassium release into a decreased extracellular space is even more likely to increase excitability, thus contributing to a 'positive feedback' cycle. A small extracellular space, in addition, magnifies the effects of extracellular current flow. The effects of this current, the basis of so-called ephaptic interactions among cells (Taylor & Dudek, 1984), is to help to synchronize discharge in cell populations, and to excite cells that are only marginally depolarized by direct synaptic interactions. In addition to these extracellular factors, one must consider glial contributions. Glia have traditionally been thought to be important in the uptake of extracellular potassium (Dietzel *et al.*, 1989). The infiltration of glia into damaged tissue may impact directly on the excitability of the region – from the mechanical effects of interposed glial elements between neuronal processes, or by altering the normal potassium distribution. The function of glia, based on their active ionic conductances, has also been hypothesized; for example, calcium conductances have been demonstrated in glia (MacVicar, 1984), and waves of calcium flux investigated with optical imaging techniques. Given the importance of calcium function in controlling normal neuronal excitability, the occurrence of such calcium activity in glia suggests an important coupling between neurons and glia in normal CNS function. Loss of appropriate glial controls may give rise to regions of abnormal neuronal activity.

Spread of epileptiform activity

These various means of cell–cell interaction provide countless pathways for development of an epileptic aggregate – an interaction of elements giving rise to hyperexcitability and hypersynchrony. The third level of investigation relevant for our studies of epileptogenicity is at this aggregate level. Understanding the communication/interaction between neuronal aggregates – often via long fiber tracts – remains as critical today as it was 50 years ago when such studies were started. Today, however, questions have become more complex. For example, why is one region of the brain, as opposed to any other, more likely to develop into an epileptic 'focus'? Even more intriguing, why is it that the discharge from a focus is sometimes 'benign', but sometimes develops into a drive of sufficient magnitude to become a behavioral/medical problem? How does such a focus involve other regions of the brain, and under what conditions? When we study epilepsy, these questions translate into two major areas of inquiry: why and where does seizure discharge start (i.e., does it require some kind of extrinsic drive)? and how does it spread (i.e., how does focal hyperexcitability become a seizure that engulfs the rest of the brain)? To answer these questions, we must understand not only the factors that increase the excitability of single cells and modulate the interaction among small groups of neurons, but also how various regions of the brain interact. Are there low threshold brain regions that are most likely to be affected, whatever the brain trauma, wherever the insult? Are the pathways of communication for epileptic activity the same pathways that mediate normal communication from cell population to cell population? These questions have not been as popular as single cell issues in the research literature in recent years, primarily because so many investigators have forsaken intact animal preparations to use in-vitro approaches. Yet, we do have a growing basis of knowledge about these issues.

Clinically, it has long been clear that temporal lobe structures are particularly prone to seizure, with regions in and around the hippocampus apparently initiating epileptic activity. Can we identify which of these regions is most likely to be the primary generator of abnormal activity (i.e., the site of the focus) – or is the epileptic activity the product of a relatively random discharge of large populations of neurons? In trying to answer such questions, most of the in-vitro work, and many of the in-vivo studies, have concentrated on the hippocampus proper. However, recent data suggest that other parts of the temporal limbic system may be even more critical. Studies have implicated the dentate region as an important control site for the development and dissemination of hyperexcitability through the hippocampus and beyond (Stringer & Lothman, 1989). Other investigators have suggested that entorhinal (Jones & Heinemann, 1988; Wilson *et al.*, 1988) and/or pyriform cortices (Piredda & Gale, 1985; Hoffman & Haberly, 1991) are particularly low threshold regions for seizure induction. The development of the kindling model has also shifted the emphasis to other limbic structures which have kindling thresholds lower than that of the hippocampus. Kindling is more easily induced by stimulation in the amygdala than that in the hippocampus (Racine, 1978), and in-vitro studies have suggested that amygdala regions, even in the non-stimulated brain, tend to be very excitable (McIntyre & Wong, 1986). The low kindling threshold of rather discrete regions in the deep pyriform cortex (Morimoto *et al.*, 1986), coupled with detailed in-vitro cellular studies of pyriform cortex and surrounding regions, suggests that these regions may often be trigger zones for the development of limbic seizure activity.

The literature on kindling suggests that repetitive discharge emanating from a given region (often one of the low threshold limbic regions) can have long-term potentiating effects on other sites; transmission through the pathways involved in the kindling-induced afterdischarge then becomes more efficacious. This aspect of kindling appears to have important clinical implications. The slow development of some seizure foci – e.g., after traumatic head injury, or in the developing nervous system exposed to early trauma and/or lesion – suggests subtle incremental processes at work that take time to reach a threshold for pathological expression. Mechanisms underlying this kindling effect have been studied intensively. Investigators have examined: mechanisms of synaptic facilitation (is kindling based on the same mechanisms that underlie long-term potentiation?; Oliver & Miller, 1985; Mody *et al.*, 1990); changes in transmitter release, and/or receptor density localization and function (Valdes *et al.*, 1982; Yeh *et al.*, 1989); regulation of cell proteins and immediate early genes (Baimbridge *et al.*, 1984; Dragunow & Robertson, 1987); and sprouting of additional afferents as a result of stimulation-induced cell death (Sutula *et al.*, 1988). Of particular interest is the question 'Is the cell damage that is often associated with epileptic foci a result of abnormal excitatory activity within a region that is particularly sensitive to high levels of input, or is some non-excitatory event the cause of cell death (e.g., an ischemic insult), which in turn leads to hyperexcitability?' These alternatives are important not only in laboratory search for underlying mechanisms, but also in determining how best to treat particular conditions. For example, is it important to stop febrile seizure activity in a child? Such seizure events could cause cell damage, which in turn might produce sprouting of recurrent collaterals and elaboration of circuits that would support epileptiform activity in later life. Is it important to take aggressive actions to minimize cell damage due to hypoxic (or ischemic or traumatic) insult, even when no seizures occur? Such action would be important if the resulting cell damage is likely to lead to hyperexcitability and epileptiform activity at a later date.

The above discussion is predicated on the proposition that a discrete area initially forms a 'focus' and then projects abnormal discharge to distant, relatively normal sites. There is some evidence, however, that supports the hypothesis that reverberatory interaction between quite separate brain regions may be a basis for seizure activity. The hypothesized existence of such an interaction provides the rationale for carrying out the split-brain procedure in epileptic patients – a technique that has been quite successful in many cases (Spencer *et al.*, 1988). Separating the cortical hemispheres results in a significant drop in seizure incidence, suggesting that seizure maintenance may involve pathways connecting the two sides of the brain. Studies using imaging techniques have shown that there are often multiple foci in the epileptic brain (Engel *et al.*, 1982). Yet, in practice, it is not necessary to remove all the foci to reduce seizure activity. Is it sufficient simply to isolate them so that they do not interact with each other?

Conclusion

Given the wealth of information already available, one might ask how much more we really need to know to be able to understand and/or make reasonable hypotheses about generation of epileptiform activity. Is it possible that we want to know too much? Clearly, the suggestion of this General introduction is that almost everything we can find out about how the normal brain works will give us some important information about how and/or why epileptiform activity develops. Yet, no single research program has a sufficiently wide scope to pursue all the possibilities. Each researcher concentrates on what he or she believes to be the most interesting or most salient features of epileptiform activity, and seeks a way to understand them as completely as possible. Models develop as a consequence of trying to address specific questions. The following chapters perhaps reflect the conflict between wanting to know as much as possible about everything, and needing to restrict one's investigative focus. This volume is neither a textbook nor a comprehensive review for the epilepsy expert. It is, rather, an exploration of both recent and long-standing issues in epilepsy research – an opportunity to speculate about them and discuss data within the context of models that have provided insights into the underlying bases of the epilepsies.

References

Alger, B. E. & Nicoll, R. A. (1982). Pharmacological evidence for two kinds of GABA receptor on rat hippocampal pyramidal cells studied *in vitro*. *Journal of Physiology*, **328**: 125–41.

Andrade, R., Malenka, R. C. & Nicoll, R. A. (1986). A G-protein couples serotonin and $GABA_B$ receptors to the same channels in hippocampus. *Science*, **234**: 1261–5.

Baimbridge, K. G., Mody, I. & Miller, J. J. (1984). Reduction of rat hippocampal calcium-binding protein following commissural, amygdala, septal, perforant path, and olfactory bulb kindling. *Epilepsia*, **26**: 460–5.

Bormann, J. (1988). Electrophysiology of $GABA_A$ and $GABA_B$ receptor subtypes. *Trends in Neurosciences*, **11**: 112–16.

Catteral, W. A., Nunoki, K., Lai, Y., DeJongh, K., Thomsen, W. & Rossie, S. (1990). Structure and modulation of voltage-sensitive sodium and calcium channels. In *The Biology and Medicine of Signal Transduction*, ed. Y. Nishizuka, J. Endo & C. Tanaka, pp. 30–4. New York: Raven Press.

Chagnac-Amitai, Y. & Connors, B. W. (1989). Horizontal spread of synchronized activity in neocortex and its control by GABA-mediated inhibition. *Journal of Neurophysiology*, **61**: 747–58.

Chen, Q. X., Stelzer, A., Kay, A. R. & Wong, R. K. S. (1990). $GABA_A$ receptor function is regulated by phosphorylation in acutely dissociated guinea-pig hippocampal neurones. *Journal of Physiology*, **420**: 207–21.

Christian, E. P. & Dudek, F. E. (1988). Electrophysiological evidence from glutamate microapplications for local excitatory circuits in the CA1 area of rat hippocampal slices. *Journal of Neurophysiology*, **59**: 110–23.

Collingridge, G. L. & Lester, R. A. J. (1989). Excitatory amino acid receptors in the vertebrate central nervous system. *Pharmacological Review*, **40**: 143–210.

Connor, J. A. (1982). Mechanisms of pacemaker discharge in invertebrate neurons. In *Cellular Pacemakers*, vol. 1, *Mechanisms of Pacemaker Generation*, ed. D. O. Carpenter, pp. 187–217. New York: John Wiley & Sons.

Connor, J. A. & Stevens, C. F. (1971). Voltage clamp studies of a transient outward membrane current in gastropod neural somata. *Journal of Physiology*, **213**: 21–30.

Coulter, D. A., Huguenard, J. R. & Prince, D. A. (1989). Characterization of ethosuximide reduction of low-threshold calcium current in thalamic neurons. *Annals of Neurology*, **25**: 582–93.

Crill, W. E. & Schwindt, P. C. (1983). Active currents in mammalian central neurons. *Trends in Neurosciences*, **6**: 236–46.

Cronin, J. & Dudek, F. E. (1988). Chronic seizures and collateral sprouting of dentate mossy fibers after kainic acid treatment in rats. *Brain Research*, **474**: 181–4.

Dietzel, I., Heinemann, U. & Lux, H. D. (1989). Relations between slow extracellular potential changes, glial potassium buffering, and electrolyte and cellular volume changes during neuronal hyperactivity in cat brain. *Glia*, **2**: 25–44.

Dragunow, M. & Robertson, H. A. (1987). Kindling stimulation induces *c-fos* protein(s) in granule cells of the rat dentate gyrus. *Nature*, **329**: 441–2.

Engel, J., Jr, Kuhl, D. E. & Phelps, M. E. (1982). Comparative localization of epileptic foci in partial epilepsy by PCT and EEG. *Annals of Neurology*, **12**: 529–37.

Hess, P. (1990). Calcium channels in vertebrate cells. *Annual Review of Neuroscience*, **13**: 337–56.

Hill, D. R. & Bowery, N. G. (1981). ^{3}H-Baclofen and ^{3}H-GABA bind to bicuculline-insensitive $GABA_B$ sites in rat brain. *Nature*, **290**: 149–52.

Hodgkin, A. L. & Huxley, A. F. (1952). Currents carried by sodium and potassium ions through the membrane of the giant axon of *Loligo*. *Journal of Physiology*, **116**, 449–71.

Hoffman, W. H. & Haberly, L. B. (1991). Bursting-induced epileptiform EPSPs in slices of piriform cortex are generated by deep cells. *Journal of Neuroscience*, **11**: 2021–31.

Houamed, K. M., Kuijper, J. L., Gilbert, T. L., Haldeman, B. A., O'Hara, P. J., Mulvihill, E. R., Almers, W. & Hagen, F. S. (1991). Cloning, expression, and gene structure of a G protein-coupled glutamate receptor from rat brain. *Science*, **252**: 1318–21.

Jones, R. S. G. & Heinemann, U. (1988). Synaptic and intrinsic responses of medial entorhinal cortical cells in normal and magnesium-free medium in vitro. *Journal of Neurophysiology*, **59**: 1476–96.

Kobilka, B. (1992). Adrenergic receptors as models for G protein-coupled receptors. *Annual Review of Neuroscience*, **15**: 87–114.

Konnerth, A., Heinemann, U. & Yaari, Y. (1986). Nonsynaptic epileptogenesis in the mammalian hippocampus in vitro. I. Development of seizure-like activity in low extracellular calcium. *Journal of Neurophysiology*, **56**: 409–423.

Lacaille, J.-C., Kunkel, D. D. & Schwartzkroin, P. A. (1989). Electrophysiological and morphological characterization of hippocampal interneurons. In *The Hippocampus: New Vistas*, ed. V. Chan-Palay & C. Köhler, pp. 287–305. New York: Alan R. Liss.

Lundberg, J. M. & Hökfelt, T. (1983). Coexistence of peptides and classical transmitters. *Trends in Neuroscience*, **6**: 325–33.

MacVicar, B. A. (1984). Voltage-dependent calcium channels in glial cells. *Science*, **226**: 1345–7.

Madison, D. V. & Nicoll, R. A. (1986). Actions of noradrenaline recorded intracellularly in rat hippocampal CA1 pyramidal neurons, *in vitro*. *Journal of Physiology*, **372**: 221–44.

Mayer, M. L. & Westbrook, G. L. (1987). The physiology of excitatory amino acids in the vertebrate central nervous system. *Progress in Neurobiology*, **28**: 197–276.

Mayer, M. L., Westbrook, G. L. & Guthrie, P. B. (1984). Voltage-dependent block by Mg^{++} of NMDA responses in spinal cord neurones. *Nature*, **309**: 261–3.

McIntyre, D. C. & Edson, N. (1981). Facilitation of amygdala kindling after norepinephrine depletion with 6-hydroxydopamine in rats. *Experimental Neurology*, **74**: 748–57.

McIntyre, D. C. & Wong, R. K. S. (1986). Cellular and synaptic properties of amygdala-kindled pyriform cortex in vitro. *Journal of Neurophysiology*, **55**: 1295–307.

Meldrum, B. S. & Corsellis, J. A. N. (1984). Epilepsy. In *Greenfield's Neuropathology*, ed. J. A. N. Corsellis & L. W. Duchen, pp. 921–50. New York: John Wiley & Sons.

Michelson, H. B. & Wong, R. K. S. (1991). Excitatory synaptic responses mediated by GABA$_A$ receptors in the hippocampus. *Science*, **253**: 1420–3.

Mody, I., Stanton, P. K. & Heinemann, U. (1988). Activation of N-methyl-D-aspartate receptors parallels changes in cellular and synaptic properties of dentate granule cells after kindling. *Journal of Neurophysiology*, **59**: 1033–54.

Mody, I., Reynolds, J. N., Salter, M. W., Carlen, P. L. & McDonald, J. F. (1990). Kindling-induced epilepsy alters calcium currents in granule cells of rat hippocampal slices. *Brain Research*, **531**: 88–94.

Mogul, D. J. & Fox, A. P. (1991). Evidence for multiple types of Ca^{2+} channels in acutely isolated hippocampal CA3 neurones of the guinea pig. *Journal of Physiology*, **433**: 259–81.

Morimoto, K., Dragunow, M. & Goddard, G. V. (1986). Deep prepiriform cortex kindling and its relation to amygdala kindling. *Experimental Neurology*, **94**: 637–48.

Mueller, A. L., Taube, J. S. & Schwartzkroin, P. A. (1982). Development of hyperpolarizing inhibitory postsynaptic potentials and hyperpolarizing response to GABA in rabbit hippocampus in vitro. *Journal of Neuroscience*, **4**: 860–7.

Muller, D. & Lynch, G. (1988). Long-term potentiation differentially affects two components of synaptic responses in hippocampus. *Proceedings of the National Academy of Sciences, USA*, **85**: 9346–50.

North, R. A. (1986). Receptors on individual neurons. *Neuroscience*, **17**: 899–907.

Nowycky, M. C., Fox, S. P. & Tsien, R. W. (1985). Three types of neuronal calcium channel with different calcium agonist sensitivity. *Nature*, **316**: 440–3.

Oliver, M. W. & Miller, J. J. (1985). Alterations of inhibitory processes in the dentate gyrus following kindling-induced epilepsy. *Experimental Brain Research*, **57**: 443–7.

Olsen, R. W. (1981). The GABA postsynaptic membrane receptor-ionophore complex. *Molecular and Cellular Biochemistry*, **39**: 261–79.

Peroutka, S. J. (1988). 5-Hydroxytryptamine receptor subtypes. *Annual Review of Neuroscience*, **11**: 45–60.

Piredda, S. & Gale, K. (1985). A crucial epileptogenic site in the deep prepiriform cortex. *Nature*, **317**: 623–5.

Plummer, M. R., Logothetis, D. E. & Hess, P. (1989). Elementary properties and pharmacological sensitivities of calcium channels in mammalian peripheral neurons. *Neuron*, **2**: 1453–63.

Purpura, D. P., Penry, J. K., Tower, D., Woodbury, D. M. & Walter, R. (1972). *Experimental Models of Epilepsy – A Manual for the Laboratory Worker.* New York: Raven Press.

Racine, R. J. (1978). Kindling: the first decade. *Neurosurgery*, **3**: 234–52.

Rutecki, P. A., Lebeda, F. J. & Johnston, D. (1985). Epileptiform activity induced by changes in extracellular potassium in hippocampus. *Journal of Neurophysiology*, **54**: 1363–74.

Schofield, P. R. (1989). The $GABA_A$ receptor: molecular biology reveals a complex picture. *Trends in Pharmacological Science*, **10**: 476–8.

Schwartzkroin, P. A. & Prince, D. A. (1980). Changes in excitatory and inhibitory synaptic potentials leading to epileptogenic activity. *Brain Research*, **183**: 61–76.

Schwartzkroin, P. A. & Stafstrom, C. E. (1980). Effects of EGTA on the calcium-activated afterhyperpolarization in hippocampal CA3 pyramidal cells. *Science*, **210**: 1125–6.

Schwartzkroin, P. A. & Wyler, A. R. (1980). Mechanisms underlying epileptiform burst discharge. *Annals of Neurology*, **7**: 95–107.

Schwindt, P. C., Spain, W. J. & Crill, W. E. (1989). Long-lasting reduction in excitability by a sodium-dependent potassium current in neocortical neurons. *Journal of Neurophysiology*, **61**: 233–44.

Seagar, M. J., Takahashi, M. & Catterall, W. A. (1988). Molecular properties of dihydropyridine-sensitive calcium channels. *Annals of the New York Academy of Science*, **522**: 162–75.

Segal, M. M. (1991). Epileptiform activity in microcultures containing one excitatory hippocampal neuron. *Journal of Neurophysiology*, **65**: 761–70.

Spain, W. J., Schwindt, P. C. & Crill, W. E. (1987). Anomalous rectification in neurons from cat sensorimotor cortex in vitro. *Journal of Neurophysiology*, **57**: 1555–76.

Spencer, S. S., Spencer, D. D., Williamson, P. D., Sass, K., Novelly, R. A. & Mattson, R. H. (1988). Corpus callostomy for epilepsy. I. Seizure effects. *Neurology*, **38**: 19–24.

Stafstrom, C. E., Schwindt, P. C., Chubb, M. C. & Crill, W. E. (1984). Properties of persistent sodium conductance and calcium conductance of layer V neurons from cat sensorimotor cortex in vitro. *Journal of Neurophysiology*, **52**: 244–63.

Storm, J. F. (1987). Action potential repolarization and a fast after-hyperpolarization in rat hippocampal pyramidal cell. *Journal of Physiology*, **385**: 733–59.

Stringer, J. L. & Lothman, E. W. (1989). Maximal dentate gyrus activation. Characteristics and alterations after repeated seizures. *Journal of Neurophysiology*, **63**: 225–39.

Sutula, T., Xiao-Xian, H., Cavazos, J. & Scott, G. (1988). Synaptic reorganization in the hippocampus induced by abnormal functional activity. *Science*, **239**: 1147–50.

Taylor, C. P. & Dudek, F. E. (1984). Excitation of hippocampal pyramidal cells by an electrical field effect. *Journal of Neurophysiology*, **52**: 126–42.

Thompson, S. M. & Gähwiler, B. E. (1989). Activity-dependent disinhibition. III. Desensitization and $GABA_B$ receptor-mediated presynaptic inhibition in the hippocampus in vitro. *Journal of Neurophysiology*, **61**: 524–32.

Traub, R. D. & Wong, R. K. S. (1981). Penicillin-induced epileptiform activity in the hippocampal slice: a model of synchronization of CA_3 pyramidal cell bursting. *Neuroscience*, **6**: 223–30.

Traynellis, S. F. & Dingledine, R. (1989). Role of extracellular space in hyperosmotic suppression of potassium-induced electrographic seizures. *Journal of Neurophysiology*, **61**: 927–38.

Tsien, R. W., Lipscombe, D., Madison, D. V., Bley, K. R. & Fox, A. P. (1988). Multiple types of neuronal calcium channels and their selective modulation. *Trends in Neurosciences*, **11**: 431–8.

Valdes, F., Dashieff, R. M., Birmingham, F., Crutcher, K. A. & McNamara, J. O. (1982). Benzodiazepine receptor increases after repeated seizures: evidence for localization to dentate granule cells. *Proceedings of the National Academy of Sciences, USA*, **79**: 193–7.

Wei, A., Covarrubias, M., Butler, A., Baker, K., Pak, M. & Salkoff, L. (1990). K^+ current diversity is produced by an extended gene family conserved in *Drosophila* and mouse. *Science*, **248**: 599–603.

Westenbroek, R. W., Merrick, D. K. & Catteral, W. A. (1989). Differential subcellular localization of the RI and RII sodium channel subtypes in central neurons. *Neuron*, **3**: 695–704.

Williams, K., Dawson, V. L., Komano, C., Dichter, M. A. & Molinoff, P. B. (1990). Characterization of polyamines having agonist, antagonist, and inverse agonist effects at the polyamine recognition site of the NMDA receptor. *Neuron*, **5**: 199–208.

Wilson, W. A., Swartzwelder, H. S., Anderson, W. W. & Lewis, D. V. (1988). Seizure activity in vitro: a dual focus model. *Epilepsy Research*, **2**: 289–93.

Yeh, G.-C., Bonhaus, D. W., Nadler, J. V. & McNamara, J. O. (1989). N-Methyl-D-aspartate receptor plasticity in kindling: quantitative and qualitative alterations in the N-methyl-D-aspartate receptor–channel complex. *Proceedings of the National Academy of Sciences, USA*, **86**: 8157–60.

Section 1

Chronic models in intact animals – concepts and questions

Introduction

Models of the epilepsies have been developed to address a variety of different issues. Although much of the current focus in epilepsy research is on the cellular and molecular mechanisms underlying abnormal activities of the central nervous system (CNS), the usefulness of such information becomes clear only within a larger context that is provided most valuably by intact-animal models of the epilepsies. Chapters 1 to 5 provide an introduction to some of the issues that can be addressed effectively using intact-animal models. The discussions concerning these models make it clear that we can learn a great deal simply from careful examination of the intact animal – from characterization of behavioral seizures, as well as from electroencephalographic (EEG) phenomenology. These discussions also illustrate a major advantage of studying 'epilepsy' in animal models, as opposed to examining the epilepsies directly in human clinical material – the ability to control what appear to be a large number of relevant variables.

Control of the stimuli that initiate the epileptogenic process is a feature of kindling that has made this model perhaps the most widely used of all the current intact animal approaches to studies of the epilepsies. McNamara, one of the leaders in investigation of the kindling model (McNamara et al., 1985), lays out a number of salient features of this model – both technical and conceptual (Chapter 1, this volume). Using the kindling approach, we can differentiate between two critical states: the process of epileptogenesis, during which the stimuli induce changes such that the brain becomes more sensitive to seizure-precipitating factors; and the kindled state itself, which is in many respects like the condition faced by clinicians – an already achieved state of hyperexcitability, with the 'changes' laid down permanently in brain 'engrams'. That these states differ significantly can be demonstrated in a variety of ways. Investigators

20

have shown, for example, that a given anti-epileptic drug may block the kindling process but not affect seizure activity once the kindled state has been reached (Anderson *et al.*, 1987; McNamara, 1989). Other studies have demonstrated changes at the receptor level during kindling; these changes disappear when the animal is fully kindled, despite the fact that the animal has attained a high level of seizure sensitivity (Savage *et al.*, 1984).

The epileptogenic process gives us an opportunity to investigate what factors are critical in inducing a relatively normal brain to become abnormal. Several key factors have been identified. The site at which stimulation occurs (or drug is injected, as in chemical kindling) is clearly of significance (Racine, 1978). Regions of the limbic system tend to be especially sensitive; that is, the fully kindled state is achieved with relatively fewer stimulations in these structures than in neocortical sites. It is of interest, then, to determine what it is about these particular regions that endows them with such low thresholds. As argued by Gale (Chapter 2, this volume), there may be complex relationships between seizure 'trigger' zones, regions that show low threshold for seizure generation, and structures that are critical to the generalization and maintenance of seizure activity. The critical concepts – which are sometimes overlooked – are that these regions may be physically separated, and that these functions may involve rather different underlying mechanisms. Although amygdala kindling is by far the most commonly used procedure (yielding the shortest time to establishment of a full-blown kindled state), there appear to be other key regions that participate in the initiation and development of these seizures. Studies by Gale and coworkers have implicated a region of pyriform cortex as a critical zone (Piredda & Gale, 1985). The low threshold nature of pyriform cortex discharge has recently been supported by the work of Hoffman & Haberly (1991) in cellular studies on slices of pyriform cortex, and by Burchfiel & Applegate (1991) in kindling transfer studies. The latter work identifies the pyriform region as a site whose activation appears to be central to the kindling process initiated from a variety of stimulation sites; once the pyriform cortex is activated, kindling transfers rapidly to other brain stimulation sites.

The kindling model introduces another important issue which has significant clinical implications. The kindling process depends on the occurrence of afterdischarge activity – i.e., short seizure-like events – within specific brain circuits. Stimulation without afterdischarge induction does not produce kindling. This observation suggests that the seizure itself, the afterdischarge, is a critical factor in inducing an epileptic state; the seizure induces brain changes which are conducive to, or required for, further seizures. In kindling, the repetition of afterdischarge activity can enhance brain circuits to the point at which they support *spontaneous* (Pinel & Rovner, 1978) and repeated seizure activity.

The hypothesis that seizures are essential to the induction of the epileptic state is quite different from the starting point of studies on animals that are genetically prone to epilepsy. In such animals, as described by Jobe *et al.* (Chapter 3, this volume), seizures apparently develop as a result of some genetically determined inborn error. Such being the case, prevention of seizures in the young animal would not (in theory) alter the likelihood that the animal will be seizure prone when it grows to maturity. This difference in point of view is of considerable concern to the pediatric epileptologist. Even in the normal animal, features of the developing nervous system yield a particularly seizure-prone brain (see Chapter 5 (Moshé *et al.*) and Chapter 6 (Swann *et al.*), this volume). In fact, seizures are relatively common in children, but do not necessarily presage epilepsy in adolescence or adulthood (Nelson & Ellenberg, 1981). There is some indication, however, that the genetic predisposition toward febrile seizures yields a statistically significant higher percentage of adults with epilepsy (Falconer, 1971). In some models of genetically epilepsy-prone animals, seizure activation during a critical window of development appears to be necessary to switch on the machinery encoded in the animals' genes (Pierson & Swann, 1991). Given these data, it seems likely that early seizures may act as trigger elements under special conditions. It is important now to determine under what conditions seizures in the immature brain can kindle the epileptic state.

The kindling process involves a variety of brain changes, and it is still unclear which are salient – or even how to determine which are critical. The data can be quite confusing. Indeed, results from different models are apparently contradictory. For example, norepinephrine provides a potent modulatory effect on kindling, and in a number of other models; loss of norepinephrine input to the limbic system and cortex, via lesioning of the dorsal noradrenergic pathway or destroying the cells of origin in locus coeruleus, yields a brain that tends to be hyperexcitable and is easily triggered to an epileptiform state (Corcoran & Mason, 1980; see also Chapter 4 (Lindvall), this volume). These results are generally consistent with data that show a noradrenergic deficit in the genetically epilepsy prone rats (see Chapter 3, this volume), but rather different from observations on the *tottering* mouse model (Noebels, 1984), in which spike-and-wave activity appears to be dependent on a hyperinnervation of noradrenergic fibers into the cortex and hippocampus. The key role of norepinephrine in the hyperexcitability of hippocampal tissue has been confirmed at the cellular level by the work of Noebels & Rutecki (1990).

There are a number of ways in which we can approach this set of apparently contradictory data. First, the nature of the epileptiform abnormality is quite different across the models in question. In the *tottering* mouse (with noradrenergic hyperinnervation), the spike-and-wave discharge is similar to generalized absence epilepsy. In contrast, more convulsive epileptiform activities are seen in the kindled and genetically epilepsy prone rat. Second, in the kindling model, there appears to be an epileptic focus, whereas the abnormality in *tottering* is generalized. It is unclear if such differences in seizure phenotype are associated with the difference in noradrenergic innervation, but they illustrate how many and complex variables must be considered when we are analyzing the bases of epileptiform activity in intact-animal models.

Perhaps one of the most important messages in Chapters 1 to 5 is that various forms of seizure activity are really different – not only phenomenologically but also in their underlying pathways, processes, and mechanisms. The mechanisms underlying seizures generated by kindling and those seen in the genetically epilepsy-prone animal may have nothing to do with each other. Similarly, status epilepticus, as described in the Lothman *et al.* model (see Chapter 10, this volume), may be quite different from the periodic seizure activity (i.e., epileptiform activity) seen in kindled or genetically epilepsy-prone rats. Spontaneous repeated seizures, in turn, may have properties different from those of an isolated seizure episode (i.e., 'epilepsy' is not the same as 'seizure'). The variability among seizure states, and the danger in assuming common underlying mechanisms, are seen particularly clearly in comparing epileptiform activities in mature and immature brains. As Moshé *et al.* (Chapter 5) so clearly argue, seizures seen in the immature nervous system are quite distinct from those in the adult. Such differences are reflected in differential anti-epileptic drug sensitivities of animals of different ages. An effective drug against focal temporal lobe seizures in the mature brain (e.g., phenytoin) is not effective against spike-and-wave absence epilepsy in the still maturing CNS; in fact, drugs used in adults may be proconvulsive in children. In theory, identification of effective drugs could provide clues about the underlying mechanisms responsible for the abnormal discharge associated with a given form of epilepsy. Unfortunately, such backward reasoning has yet to provide profitable insights. Rather, it is by virtue of understanding basic seizure mechanisms in these models that more effective drugs are now being designed.

These chapters in Section 1 serve to illustrate the differences between normal and epileptic brain, and between the epileptogenic process and the epileptic state. Unfortunately, our understanding is complicated by the fact that the mechanisms and pathways that support seizure activity in the normal brain may be quite different from those that are involved in seizure production in the epileptic brain. Different transmitters may be used, and different cell–cell interactions are almost certainly critical. Therefore, it is important to examine how, once seizures are induced in the normal brain and changes are initiated, the epileptic state is structurally encoded. Much recent work has focused on gene-mediated events that may modulate a variety of relevant targets that could encode structural changes. Immediate early genes (IEGs) such as c-*fos*, c-*jun*, and *zif-268* have been examined in a number of laboratories (Dragunow *et al.*, 1988; Saffen *et al.*, 1988; Simonato *et al.*, 1991; see also Chapter 2 of this volume). The mRNA transcripts of these IEGs show dramatic increases associated with seizure activity. However, the target genes of immediate early gene proteins are still a mystery. Some speculation has centered on IEG regulation of, for example, the *N*-methyl-D-aspartate (NMDA) receptor and its modulating sites. Other hypotheses have suggested a possible link between IEGs and the various neurotrophic factors, such as nerve growth factor (NGF), since NGF mRNA levels also rise dramatically in epileptic foci (at least in some models; Gall & Isackson, 1989). Such trophic factors might directly affect the structure of cells participating in seizure activity. Identification of activity-dependent factors that are modulated by IEG products will undoubtedly provide a set of new insights into the establishment of the epileptic state.

It seems likely that genetic factors are not only involved in structural solidification of seizure state, but also in initial seizure susceptibility. Although many of the models that we use do not have an obvious genetic component, there is a compeling reason for seeking inborn seizure propensities. All individuals do not respond to potentially epileptogenic stimuli in the same way. Genetic factors may determine seizure suscepti-bility indirectly by modulating such common factors as sensitivity to norepinephrine (e.g., in the *tottering* mouse). Or the genetic action may be quite direct, affecting inhibitory mechanisms (e.g., determining the number or the subunit arrangement of γ-aminobutyric acid receptors; Peterson *et al.*, 1985) or excitatory elements (e.g., the glycine modula-tion site on the NMDA receptor; Yeh *et al.*, 1989). Subtle differences between individual elements in apparently homogeneous populations may give us clues about important differences that have thus far been neglected.

To be sure, the intact animal models do not, at least at present, offer solutions to the multitude of issues that have been raised regarding seizure mechanisms. These models tend rather to generate key questions and hypotheses, to be pursued at more reductionist levels. These approaches provide a clearly relevant context within which we can begin to examine which basic phenomena are relevant to epilepsy. The following chapters illustrate the importance of such approaches.

References

Anderson, W. W., Swartzwelder, H. S. & Wilson, W. A. (1987). The NMDA receptor antagonist 2-amino-5-phosphonovalerate blocks stimulus train-induced epileptogenesis but not epileptiform bursting in the rat hippocampal slice. *Journal of Neurophysiology*, **57**: 1–21.

Burchfiel, J. L. & Applegate, C. D. (1991). The pyriform cortex and kindling: behavioral and physiological evidence for a common substrate. *Epilepsia*, **32** (Suppl. 3): 41.

Corcoran, M. E. & Mason, S. T. (1980). Role of forebrain catecholamines in amygdaloid kindling. *Brain Research*, **190**: 473–84.

Dragunow, M., Robertson, H. A. & Robertson, G. S. (1988). Amygdala kindling and c-*fos* protein(s). *Neuroscience Letters*, **102**: 261–3.

Falconer, M. A. (1971). Genetic and related aetiological factors in temporal lobe epilepsy: a review. *Epilepsia*, **12**: 13–31.

Gall, C. M. & Isackson, P. J. (1989). Limbic seizures increase neuronal production of messenger RNA for nerve growth factor. *Science*, **245**: 758–61.

Hoffman, W. H. & Haberly, J. B. (1991). Bursting-induced epileptiform EPSPs in slices of piriform cortex are generated by deep cells. *Journal of Neuroscience*, **11**: 2021–31.

McNamara, J. O. (1989). Development of new pharmacological agents for epilepsy: lessons from the kindling model. *Epilepsia*, **30** (Suppl. 1): S13–S18.

McNamara, J. O., Bonhaus, D. W., Shin, C., Crain, B. J., Gellman, R. L. & Giacchino, J. L. (1985). The kindling model of epilepsy: a critical review. *CRC Critical Reviews of Neurobiology*, **1**: 341–92.

Nelson, K. B. & Ellenberg, J. H. (1981). *Febrile Seizures*. New York: Raven Press.

Noebels, J. L. (1984). A single gene error in noradrenergic axon growth synchronizes central neurons. *Nature*, **310**: 409–11.

Noebels, J. L. & Rutecki, P. A. (1990). Altered hippocampal network excitability in the hypernoradrenergic mutant mouse *tottering*. *Brain Research*, **524**: 225–30.

Peterson, G. M., Ribak, C. E. & Oertel, W. H. (1985). A regional increase in the number of hippocampal GABAergic neurons and terminals in the seizure-sensitive gerbil. *Brain Research*, **340**: 384–9.

Pierson, M. G. & Swann, J. (1991). Ontogenetic features of audiogenic seizure susceptibility induced in immature rats by noise. *Epilepsia*, **32**: 1–9.

Pinel, J. P. J. & Rovner, L. I. (1978). Electrode placement and kindling-induced experimental epilepsy. *Experimental Neurology*, **58**: 335–46.

Piredda, S. & Gale, K. (1985). A crucial epileptogenic site in the deep prepiriform cortex. *Nature*, **317**: 623–5.

Racine, R. (1978). Kindling: the first decade. *Neurosurgery*, **3**: 234–52.

Saffen, D. W., Cole, A. J., Worley, P. F., Christy, B. A., Ryder, K. A. & Baraban, J. M. (1988). Convulsant-induced increase in transcription factor mRNAs in rat brain. *Proceedings of the National Academy of Sciences, USA*, **85**: 7795–9.

Savage, D. D., Werling, L. L., Nadler, J. V. & McNamara, J. O. (1984). Selective and reversible increase in the number of quisqualate-sensitive glutamate binding sites on hippocampal synaptic membranes after angular bundle kindling. *Brain Research*, **307**: 332–5.

Simonato, M., Hosford, D. A., Labiner, D. M., Shin, C., Mansbach, H. H. & McNamara, J. O. (1991). Differential expression of immediate early genes in the hippocampus in the kindling model of epilepsy. *Molecular Brain Research*, **11**: 115–24.

Yeh, G.-C., Bonhaus, D. W., Nadler, J. V. & McNamara, J. O. (1989). N-Methyl-D-aspartate receptor plasticity in kindling: quantitative and qualitative alterations in the N-methyl-D-aspartate receptor–channel complex. *Proceedings of the National Academy of Sciences, USA*, **86**: 8157–60.

1

The kindling model of epilepsy

JAMES O. McNAMARA, DOUGLAS W. BONHAUS, and CHEOLSU SHIN

Introduction

The epilepsies represent a heterogeneous group of disorders with diverse etiologies, electrographical and behavioral seizure patterns, and pharmacological sensitivities. The subtype termed complex partial epilepsy (Commission on Classification and Terminology of the ILAE, 1981) is one of the most devastating forms of human epilepsy. Complex partial seizures (CPSs) constitute the single most common seizure type, accounting for approximately 40% of all cases in adults (Hauser & Kurland, 1975). CPSs are often quite resistant to available anticonvulsant drugs; only 25% of adults with CPS experience complete seizure control despite optimal contemporaneous treatment (Mattson et al., 1985). CPSs induce impairment of consciousness, thereby limiting performance of many tasks, such as driving a motor vehicle; as a result, finding and maintaining employment is difficult for sufferers. Complex partial epilepsy is a major public health problem affecting at least 800 000 people in the United States alone.

Insight into the mechanisms underlying this disorder is limited. Three main questions arise. (a) What is(are) the mechanism(s) underlying the expression of the hyperexcitability? (b) How does hyperexcitability develop? (c) Why does hyperexcitability persist? Developing answers to these questions in cellular and molecular terms may lead to more effective therapy, prevention, or even cure of this disorder.

One approach to these questions is to study an animal model. For the past 15 years, we have studied a model of CPSs produced by a phenomenon termed kindling. The goals of this chapter are: (a) to describe the kindling phenomenon; (b) to examine whether kindling might actually contribute to some forms of human complex partial epilepsy; (c) to consider which questions related to human complex partial epilepsy may

27

be approached with this model, and to outline some assets and limitations of the model in addressing these questions; (d) to provide a brief review of current hypotheses and data regarding the anatomical frame-work of kindling and the mechanisms underlying the expression of the hyperexcitability.

The kindling model

Several features of kindling and kindled animals are mentioned briefly below; the reader can consult primary references for more detailed information.

Kindling refers to a process whereby repeated, focal application of initially subconvulsive electrical stimulations to a brain structure eventually results in intense limbic and clonic motor seizures (Goddard *et al.*, 1969). Once established, this enhanced sensitivity may persist, in the absence of additional stimulations, for the life of the animal. The initial stimulus ordinarily elicits minimal or no change in behavior or brain electrical activity measured with an electroencephalograph (EEG). Subsequent stimulations evoke electrographic seizures or afterdischarge, mainly localized initially to the stimulated structure. Repeated stimu-lations produce progressive lengthening and propagation of afterdischarge coinciding with expression of behavioral seizures as classified by Racine (1972*b*): class 1, facial clonus; class 2, head nodding; class 3, contra-lateral forelimb clonus; class 4, rearing; class 5, rearing and falling. In addition to the enhanced propagation of an afterdischarge, kindled animals exhibit a lowering of the afterdischarge threshold, i.e. the minimum amount of current required to elicit an afterdischarge (Racine, 1972*a*).

Repeated elicitation of afterdischarge is the necessary and sufficient stimulus to induce kindling (Racine, 1972*b*). Periodic application of electrical current that does not elicit an afterdischarge does not result in kindling (Goddard *et al.*, 1969). Moreover, periodic induction of an afterdischarge by microinjection of the muscarinic cholinergic agonist carbachol is sufficient to produce kindling (Vosu & Wise, 1975; Wasterlain & Jonec, 1983). Electrical stimulations are simply the most convenient means of triggering an afterdischarge and, therefore, kindling. Thus, the essence of kindling development is that seizures (afterdischarges) beget a lasting propensity for longer and more widely propagated electrographic seizures paralleled by more intense behavioral seizures and a lowered afterdischarge threshold.

Kindling can be induced by stimulation of many, but not all, sites in the brain. Stimulation of multiple limbic (including the hippocampus, entorhinal cortex, pyriform cortex, and others), neocortical, and basal ganglia (caudate, putamen, globus pallidus) structures results in kindling (Goddard *et al.*, 1969; Racine, 1972*b*, 1975). The amygdala is the most commonly used structure, in part because of the relatively few (approximately 13) stimulations required to produce kindling. The progressive intensification of stimulus-evoked seizures does not occur with stimulation of the superior colliculus, reticular formation, or cerebellum (Goddard *et al.*, 1969; Racine, 1972*a*).

Important differences exist in the electrographic and behavioral patterns of the seizures evoked by initial stimulation of the amygdala, hippocampus, and anterior neocortex. In contrast to the brief after-discharge (approximately 10–15 s) evoked by amygdala stimulation, dorsal hippocampal stimulation evokes a much longer afterdischarge (25–60 s) accompanied by subtle behavioral changes, the most prominent of which are frequent 'wet dog shakes' (Lerner Natoli *et al.*, 1984). Stimulation of the anterior neocortex evokes brief (5–15 s) mouth move-ments and myoclonic contractions of the forelimbs (Racine, 1975); repeated application of this stimulation eventually evokes brief tonic–clonic seizures followed by propagation of the afterdischarge into the hippocampus, amygdala, and other structures, with accompanying clonic motor seizure with rearing and falling typical of the stimulation of limbic sites. This latter pattern is reminiscent of the behavior observed in some complex partial seizures originating outside the hippocampus in humans (Commission on Classification and Terminology of the ILAE, 1989).

In rats, the rate of development of kindling varies as a function of age and interstimulus interval. Compared to young adult rats, young (18 day old) animals require fewer stimulations to produce clonic motor seizures (Moshé *et al.*, 1983). By contrast, aged (at least one year old) rats require more stimulations to produce clonic motor seizures in comparison to young adults (Fanelli & McNamara, 1986). Interstimulus intervals ranging from 30 min (Racine *et al.*, 1973) to as long as seven days (Goddard *et al.*, 1969) can be used to establish kindling. Greater numbers of stimulations are required with interstimulus intervals of 30 min compared to intervals of 60 min or longer. Kindling cannot be reliably induced in adult rats with interstimulus intervals as brief as 15 min (Racine *et al.*, 1973).

Actual epilepsy or spontaneous (not simply stimulation-induced) seizures can be reliably induced if kindled animals are subjected to hundreds of stimulation-induced kindled seizures (Pinel & Rovner, 1978*a*). Moreover, spontaneous seizures persist for as long as seven months following termination of the stimulations, suggesting that epilepsy itself is long lasting and perhaps permanent in this condition (Pinel & Rovner, 1978*b*).

Does the kindling phenomenon contribute to epileptogenesis in humans?

While stimulus-evoked afterdischarge in kindled animals, like electro-shock or chemoconvulsant evoked seizures, can be used to screen potential anticonvulsants without regard to the underlying mechanisms of seizure generation, the relevance of mechanistic investigations of kindling will be greatest if kindling-like processes contribute to the development (i.e., epileptogenesis) or expression of human complex partial epilepsy.

Similarities in basic features of kindled and human complex partial seizures have led to speculation that kindling or kindling-like processes may contribute to epileptogenesis in humans. These include: similar EEG activity recorded from intracerebral electrodes during kindled seizures and human CPSs; strikingly analogous behaviors in kindled seizures and in human CPSs with secondary generalization; and similar sensitivities to conventional anticonvulsants. This last point is striking in that carbamazepine, phenobarbital, phenytoin, and valproic acid are effective, whereas ethosuximide and trimethadione are ineffective against both human complex partial and kindled seizures (Albright & Burnham, 1980; Albertson *et al.*, 1980; McNamara *et al.*, 1989).

Given these similarities in the basic properties of kindled seizures and human CPSs, it seems worthwhile to consider exactly what aspects of human epilepsy may be the consequence of kindling mechanisms. This may lead to optimal utilization of the model and to specific tests of hypotheses on the pathophysiology of the human condition.

One group in which kindling might contribute to epileptogenesis consists of patients with a defined lesion such as a low grade glioma or a hamartoma (e.g., a vascular malformation). These patients exhibit a modest loss (approximately 20–25%) of pyramidal neurons in the hippocampus compared to autopsy controls without epilepsy (de Lanerolle *et al.*, 1989; Kim *et al.*, 1990). Quite clearly none of these patients has an intracerebral electrode periodically triggering afterdischarges. However, it seems plausible that a lesion such as a focal vascular malformation that undergoes microhemorrhages could deposit iron in the form of hemosiderin in the brain (Russell & Rubinstein, 1977; Bruton, 1988) and serve to induce focal electrical seizure activity (Reid & Sypert, 1984), thereby mimicking the effects of the stimulating electrode. Likewise, focal hyperexcitability related to a tumor could have the same net effect. The idea is that the lesions induce focal hyperexcitability, which in turn induces focal afterdischarge, a lowering of seizure threshold, and kindling of synaptically connected structures.

Apart from patients with a definable lesion, kindling might contribute to epileptogenesis in other settings. For example, among patients suffering prolonged and intense febrile seizures, it seems plausible that the seizures themselves could cause neuronal death within the hippocampus (Ammon's horn sclerosis) and that focal hyperexcitability could result from the ensuing neuronal rearrangements (Tauck & Nadler, 1985; Schwartzkroin & Franck, 1986). This sclerotic hippocampus could then serve to kindle target pathways and epileptogenesis could evolve. A similar hypothesis has been advanced for the delayed onset of epilepsy occurring after head injury; that is, a focal lesion created by the injury somehow kindles target pathways and leads to the delayed onset of epilepsy months to years after the injury.

Despite the seeming reasonableness of such schemes for kindling in humans, there is little direct evidence to support such a hypothesis. Apart from a single case report of putative kindling in a patient receiving thalamic stimulation for the treatment of chronic pain (Sramka *et al.*, 1977), there are no reported instances of electrical kindling in humans. Moreover, several long-standing arguments against this hypothesis must be addressed.

One frequently made argument against kindling is that there is no overt neuronal loss in the brains of kindled rats whereas such loss is detectable in the hippocampus of many human epileptic patients. Recent studies by Sutula and his colleagues have shed light on this issue (see e.g., Cavazos & Sutula, 1990; Chapter 9, this volume). In animals stimulated to the point of three class 5 seizures, small but significant loss of neurons is detectable in the hippocampus. Increasing the number of stimulus-evoked seizures to approximately 30 class 4 or 5 kindled seizures results in striking losses of neurons in the hilar (CA4) region of the hippocampus. This result is important because it demonstrates that isolated, periodic seizures (in contrast to status epilepticus) are sufficient to cause neuron death and provides an explanation for the neuron loss seen in the human condition. Moreover, it shows a clear parallel between kindling and at least one form of severe complex partial seizure in humans.

Another argument against the hypothetical role of kindling in the pathogenesis of human epilepsy is that complex partial seizures in humans are relatively insensitive to conventional anticonvulsants whereas kindled seizures themselves are sensitive to the drugs. This paradox can be explained by examining the results of different measurements of anticonvulsant effectiveness against kindled seizures together with the seizure types most resistant to these drugs in humans. A complex partial seizure refers to a seizure localized to *parts* of the brain, the parts consisting mainly of limbic system structures such as the amygdala and hippocampus. The seizure may become a secondarily generalized tonic and/or clonic motor seizure; i.e., the seizure propagates out of the limbic system into motor system structures. Afterdischarge localized to limbic structures is a model of complex partial seizures and is associated with classes 1 and 2 behavioral seizures (Racine, 1972*b*); the seizure may become a secondarily generalized tonic and clonic motor seizure (classes 3–5). Complex partial seizures are much more resistant to conventional anticonvulsants than are secondarily generalized seizures (Mattson *et al.*, 1985). Likewise, focal afterdischarge is much more resistant to anti-convulsants than are class 4 or 5 seizures (Albright & Burnham, 1980; McNamara *et al.*, 1989). Thus, while kindled seizures are inhibited by phenobarbital, carbamazepine, phenytoin, and valproic acid, the focal afterdischarge is much more resistant to drug therapy than the class 4 and 5 behavioral components of the seizures (Albright & Burnham, 1980).

The other critical factor lies in how anticonvulsant efficacy is measured. For example, measurements of efficacy of carbamazepine (10 mg/kg) against afterdischarge threshold (ADT) (i.e., the lowest intensity of current required to elicit an afterdischarge) disclosed a 30% elevation of threshold; the average seizure rank was 1.6 and afterdischarge duration only 21.6 s when evoked by a stimulus with a current intensity that barely exceeds the threshold (Albertson *et al.*, 1984). By contrast, measurement of efficacy of the same dose of carbamazepine in the same study with current intensity exceeding ADT by approximately 100% disclosed an average seizure rank of 3.5 and afterdischarge duration of 61 s. Kindled seizures could therefore be used to model medically refractory complex partial seizure if high current intensity relative to the ADT is used. These findings suggest that a progressive lowering of the seizure threshold by a focal lesion in humans could contribute to the emergence of refractoriness to anticonvulsant medication.

A third argument against the idea that kindling occurs in humans has come from studies in primates. This argument is based on the observation that, in Rhesus monkeys, administration of electrical stimulations to the amygdala quite readily induced complex partial but not clonic motor seizures typical of other animals such as rats or cats (Goddard *et al.*, 1969; Wada *et al.*, 1978). In fact, this result cannot be generalized to all primates, as convulsive seizures can be readily produced by electrical stimulations of the amygdala in the seizure-sensitive Senegalese baboon, *Papio papio* (see Chapter 3, this volume); this suggests that differences in genetic susceptibility within primates might determine the extent to which seizures propagate and thus the behavioral manifestations of kindling. Importantly, the behavioral patterns of kindled seizures in Rhesus monkeys are strikingly reminiscent of the human condition in that 25% of humans with complex partial seizures (similar to class 1 and 2 seizures) never experience a secondarily generalized tonic–clonic seizure (similar to class 4 and 5 seizures) (Gibbs & Gibbs, 1952). In the remaining 75%, the frequency of complex partial seizures is far greater than the frequency of secondarily generalized seizures. Perhaps differences in the organization of the nervous system between rodents and non-seizure-susceptible primates explains the reduced propensity of primates to exhibit robust seizure propagation. In any case, the results of the Rhesus monkey experiments do not argue convincingly against the possibility that kindling contributes to human epileptogenesis.

A final argument for the presence of kindling-like processes in humans is the occasional finding of secondary foci in a subset of human epileptic patients. Some patients with epilepsy due to a localized lesion such as a tumor or hamartoma develop evidence of two sites of seizure initiation (or foci), one in the vicinity of the lesion and another in the contralateral hemisphere (Falconer & Kennedy, 1961; Falconer *et al.*, 1962). The evidence for a secondary focus in some instances consists of epileptiform abnormalities recorded in the EEG between seizures but in other instances consists of behavioral and EEG seizure patterns distinct from those of the primary focus and indicative of a focus in the opposite hemisphere (Morrell, 1979). Interestingly, in kindled animals stimulated to the point of exhibiting spontaneous seizures, at least some of these seizures are initiated at sites remote from the stimulating electrode (Pinel & Rovner, 1978a). This suggests that the primary focus kindled the secondary focus to the extent that an independent seizure initiation site has developed, a scenario similar to that likely occurring in the above-mentioned group of patients.

These considerations raise the question of whether one can prove that kindling contributes to epileptogenesis in humans. The first step is to establish a series of correlations between kindling and human epilepsy with respect to anatomical, biochemical, and electrophysiological measures as a mechanistic understanding of kindling emerges. A subsequent step would arise if a means of reversing kindling could be developed and then successfully applied to human epilepsy. However, barring such a 'proof in the cure', the issue remains unresolved. Clearly, however, there is no compelling evidence against the hypothesis that kindling contributes to the expression of human epilepsy.

Experimental questions approachable with the kindling model

One question approachable with the kindling model is whether a putative anticonvulsant is efficacious against partial and secondary generalized seizures. The advantages of kindling as a tool for quantifying anticonvulsant drug efficacy reside in two key features of the model. First, in comparison to other in-vivo models of focal epilepsy such as those induced by iron, cobalt, alumina, freezing, etc., the seizures are evoked at the convenience of the investigator, thereby facilitating design and execution of experiments. By contrast, establishing such control and reproducibility using models such as alumina focus, is problematic at best. Second, in contrast to seizures evoked in a naive or normal animal, the kindled animal contains within its brain permanent elements of hyperexcitability. Thus seizures evoked in the kindled animal are propagating through an abnormal, hyperexcitable brain. This key difference may well modify drug efficacy, producing findings unanticipated on the basis of acute models. Importantly, drugs such as the α_2-adrenergic receptor agonist, clonidine, or the N-methyl-D-aspartate receptor antagonist, MK-801, inhibit focal afterdischarge more effectively in a naive than in a kindled brain, indicating that the mechanisms responsible for seizures in the normal and kindled brain are at least partly different (Gellman *et al.*, 1987; McNamara *et al.*, 1988; Williamson & Lothman, 1989). The ease of inexpensive screening of large numbers of compounds is an enormous advantage of the electroshock and pentylenetetrazol models, but the kindling model can provide additional valuable information. In our opinion, demonstrating anticonvulsant effectiveness with an adequate therapeutic index against kindled seizures would seem to be a judicious step prior to clinical trials of anticonvulsant drugs for partial or secondarily generalized seizures.

Another question approachable with the kindling model is whether a given agent exhibits anti-epileptogenic properties. The high incidence of epilepsy arising months to years after certain kinds of head injury provides an opportunity for pharmacological intervention aimed at preventing development of epilepsy (i.e., anti-epileptogenesis). No drug with anti-epileptogenic efficacy has been identified in human studies (Temkin *et al.*, 1990). Availability of an animal model would facilitate identification of effective drugs for clinical trials. At present, kindling is the leading model for identification of such drugs. The highly reproducible and graded development of kindling produced at the convenience of the investigator provides a simple means for quantifying epileptogenesis. The direction and magnitude of the effect of a drug on epileptogenesis can be determined by comparing the number of stimulation-induced afterdischarges required to produce kindling in the presence of a drug or vehicle. This approach has been used to quantify the anti-epileptogenic properties of conventional anticonvulsants (Wise & Chinerman, 1974; Racine *et al.*, 1975; Wada *et al.*, 1976; Leviel & Naquet, 1977; Albertson *et al.*, 1984; Silver *et al.*, 1990), which has facilitated selection of drugs for ongoing clinical trials examining agents for efficacy in prophylaxis against post-traumatic epilepsy. The effects of a diversity of experimental drugs with known mechanisms of action on specific neurotransmitter systems have also been examined (McNamara *et al.*, 1985; McNamara, 1989).

Beyond the screening of anticonvulsants and anti-epileptogenic agents, kindling provides a convenient tool for addressing a host of questions related to epileptogenesis. The development of kindling permits analysis of mechanisms of epileptogenesis, i.e., the process by which a lasting hyperexcitability can develop. Studies of development of kindling also permit investigation of intrinsic brain mechanisms that inhibit epileptogenesis. Animals kindled to the point of class 5 seizures permit analysis of the mechanisms underlying expression of the hyperexcitability itself. The long duration of the hyperexcitability permits analysis of mechanisms responsible for its permanence. Comparison of animals kindled to the point of class 5 seizures with animals receiving hundreds of stimulation-evoked kindled seizures permits the study of mechanisms underlying the emergence of spontaneous seizures. The mechanisms underlying the initiation and propagation of seizures in an epileptic (as distinct from naive) brain can be addressed with this model. Apart from these questions related to epilepsy per se, insights into the mechanisms underlying kindling may shed light on the mechanisms of physiological processes, including learning and memory, neuronal rearrangements in vivo, and others.

Importantly, a number of limitations confront the investigator addressing the questions above. The chronic nature of the model limits the number of experiments possible and the long time required to answer experimental questions slows the rate of progress. The in-vivo nature of the model renders mechanistic analyses far more difficult than with an in-vitro system in which many variables are subject to rigorous experimental control; this problem can be circumvented to some extent by ex-vivo analyses with biochemical and electrophysiological methods of brain slices from kindled and control animals (King *et al.*, 1985; Morrisett *et al.*, 1989). The greatest difficulty lies in the enormous complexity of the mammalian brain simply in terms of the diversity of cell types and the heterogeneity of members of each cell type. The organization of these cells into discrete nuclei, interacting with one another to regulate the expression of a kindled seizure (McNamara *et al.*, 1984) provides an added level of complexity. Uncertainty about the anatomical network containing the abnormal hyperexcitability or responsible for its development is yet another difficulty; this issue is considered in greater detail below.

These limitations notwithstanding, we believe that kindling is the best in-vivo model available for elucidating mechanisms of epileptogenesis, mechanisms underlying certain forms of hyperexcitability, and mechanisms responsible for the persistence of hyperexcitability. The chronic nature of the model is a necessity for addressing these questions. The investigator can control for the presence of the electrode (using electrode-implanted, unstimulated animals) and even of the electrical current (using low frequency stimulations that do not trigger afterdischarge). This simplifies interpreting biochemical studies and thus facilitates the correlative biochemical, anatomical, and electrophysiological studies needed to elucidate the biology of the process. The highly reproducible and graded development of kindling permits analysis of epileptogenesis at defined stages.

The ability to elucidate the network underlying the development of kindling and the expression of a kindled seizure and to analyze mechanisms in distinct components of the network permits mutually reinforcing interpretation of data from each line of investigation. By contrast, the time and effort required to produce animals with spontaneous seizures diminishes the attractiveness of this model for study of such animals. The in-vivo nature of the model renders analysis of mechanisms underlying the initiation and propagation of kindled seizures difficult. Given the fragmentary information available, such questions are probably best studied with several recently developed models of inducing seizures in hippocampal slices in vitro; the model of stimulus-train-induced seizures (Stasheff *et al.*, 1989; Chapter 11, this volume) in hippocampal slices seems especially well suited to address questions related to epileptic seizures.

The anatomical network of kindling

Limited insight into the precise anatomical distribution of the brain nuclei containing the abnormal hyperexcitability or responsible for its development hampers investigation of the mechanisms. Stated simply, how does one know that the neurons or glia one is studying by whatever technique contribute to the development or expression of the hyper-excitability defined in situ as kindling? As a first step, some investigators determined which structures exhibit electrical seizure activity or altered metabolism during a kindled seizure (Engel *et al.*, 1978; Lothman *et al.*, 1985); this led to hypotheses on the functional significance of a given nucleus or pathway in the development or expression of kindling. This in turn led to experiments in which specific nuclei or pathways were destroyed and the effects of these treatments on the threshold or propagation of a kindled seizure or on the rate of kindling development were determined (Messenheimer *et al.*, 1979; Corcoran & Mason, 1980; McNamara *et al.*, 1984; Savage *et al.*, 1985; Frush *et al.*, 1986; Sutula *et al.*, 1986; Shin *et al.*, 1987). These approaches have been followed by experiments examining a diversity of electrophysiological properties of discrete neuronal populations in slices isolated from kindled animals (King *et al.*, 1985; Mody & Heinemann, 1987; Bragdon *et al.*, 1988; Mody *et al.*, 1988; Traynelis *et al.*, 1989). The results of these approaches have been reviewed in detail (McNamara, 1988; McNamara *et al.*, 1988).

A number of conclusions can be drawn from these studies.

(1) Changes intrinsic to targets of the stimulated structure (i.e., the structure containing the kindling electrode) alone are sufficient to account for the expression of kindling (Messenheimer *et al.*, 1979).

(2) No single nucleus or pathway has been demonstrated to be critical for either the development or expressions of kindling.

(3) Nuclei regulating the development of kindling differ at least in part from those regulating the expression of kindling; that is, lesions of the noradrenergic projection from the locus coeruleus facilitate the development of kindling but do not modify the threshold or propagation of a kindled seizure (Corcoran & Mason, 1980; Westerberg *et al.*, 1984).

(4) The pars reticulata of the substantia nigra, a subcortical nucleus, serves a pivotal role in regulating the expression of kindled seizures (McNamara *et al.*, 1984). It can regulate seizure activity expressed locally in multiple forebrain sites and also the propagation of clonic motor seizure activity initiated by stimulation of a diversity of forebrain structures.

(5) The hippocampus, a structure which appears to mediate the initiation and propagation in the majority of cases of complex partial seizures in humans, facilitates kindling development initiated from multiple limbic sites because treatments that destroy dentate granule cells or transect entorhinal projections to the hippocampus inhibit kindling development (Savage *et al.*, 1985; Frush *et al.*, 1986; Sutula *et al.*, 1986).

(6) Abnormal hyperexcitability has been defined as being intrinsic to multiple neuronal populations and/or their synapses, by in-vitro studies of slices removed from kindled rats; sites include the three principal neuronal populations of the hippocampus (dentate granule cells, CA3 and CA1 pyramidal neurons; King *et al.*, 1985; Mody & Heinemann, 1987; Bragdon *et al.*, 1988; Mody *et al.*, 1988; Traynelis *et al.*, 1989), pyramidal neurons of the pyriform cortex (McIntyre & Wong, 1986), and neurons in the basolateral nucleus of the amygdala (Gean *et al.*, 1989).

These data suggest that there is a multitude of sites containing abnormal hyperexcitability in a kindled brain; that is, the expression of kindling is likely due to pathological hyperexcitability intrinsic to multiple synaptic stations within a synaptically related network. Moreover, the distribution of these sites is probably highly specific and determined by the site of the kindling electrode; the involvement of some structures (e.g., the hippocampus, pyriform cortex, substantia nigra) will be common to kindling initiated from multiple sites, whereas other structures will be involved only with kindling initiated from one site. It seems likely that these sites somehow interact to promote the enhanced seizure propagation typical of a kindled animal. We and others have used the convergent results of the lesion and electrophysiological studies as the justification for study of the hippocampus as a model structure that is causally involved in the development of kindling. The hippocampus exhibits many experimental advantages for in-vivo and in-vitro study with anatomical, biochemical, and electrophysiological methods. The hope is that changes identified in this structure will provide a clue to abnormalities elsewhere in the kindled brain. Whether the cellular and molecular basis of the abnormal hyperexcitability is identical at multiple synaptic stations within the kindled brain is a key unresolved question.

Mechanisms underlying the hyperexcitability of kindling

Extensive work has sought to elucidate the mechanisms underlying the expression of the hyperexcitability. In theory, the increased excitability could be due to a large number of possibilities, three of which are a reduction of synaptic inhibition, an enhancement of synaptic excitation, or a combination of the two. Analyses of synaptic inhibition disclosed a paradoxical *increase* in some synapses (King *et al.*, 1985; Maru & Goddard, 1987) and a small decrease in one neuronal population, the CA1 pyramidal neurons of the hippocampus (King *et al.*, 1985; de Jonge & Racine, 1987; Kapur *et al.*, 1989; Michelson *et al.*, 1989). The lack of robust and consistent evidence of disinhibition led to a recent focus on the role of excitatory synapses in the kindled brain.

Analyses of synaptic excitation have centered on excitatory amino acids (EAA) such as glutamic acid or aspartic acid because EAAs constitute the principal excitatory neurotransmitters in pathways commonly used for kindling. Among the receptors with which synaptically released EAAs might interact to produce a biological response, the *N*-methyl-D-aspartate (NMDA) subtype is a particularly attractive candidate for a causal role in kindling. The reasons are three-fold: (1) the distinctive voltage dependence of NMDA receptor-mediated synaptic transmission is associated with regenerative properties, which results in burst firing similar to that observed in epileptiform discharge (Mayer *et al.*, 1984; Nowak *et al.*, 1984; Dingledine *et al.*, 1986; Herron *et al.*, 1986); (2) NMDA receptor antagonists exhibit anticonvulsant properties in several seizure models (Croucher *et al.*, 1982; Czuczwar & Meldrum, 1982); and (3) NMDA receptor activation has been linked to a number of plastic processes such as long-term potentiation of synaptic trans-mission (Harris *et al.*, 1984), learning and memory (Morris *et al.*, 1986), and formation and stabilization of synaptic connections (Cline *et al.*, 1987). These findings have led to a series of studies, the results of which are reviewed briefly below.

Pharmacological studies with both competitive and uncompetitive antagonists of the NMDA receptor have demonstrated that these com-pounds inhibit kindled seizures (McNamara *et al.*, 1990). Although these drugs more effectively inhibit the development of kindling than the expression of kindled seizures, the drugs nonetheless clearly exhibit anticonvulsant properties in this model. Thus, enhancement of transmission at synapses using NMDA receptors could contribute to the expression of the hyperexcitability of kindling. A selective and long-lasting enhancement of NMDA receptor-mediated synaptic activation of the dentate granule cells by entorhinal cortical afferents was demonstrated in hippocampal slices isolated from kindled animals (Mody & Heinemann, 1987; Mody *et al.*, 1988). Biochemical evidence of a selective and long-lasting enhanced sensitivity of hippocampal neurons to NMDA-evoked depolarization was found in slices isolated from kindled animals (Martin *et al.*, 1988; Morrisett *et al.*, 1989). This was subsequently localized to CA3 but not to CA1 neurons. The molecular basis of some of these findings appears to be emerging. Increases in the number of NMDA receptors (detected with a radiolabeled antagonist (Yeh *et al.*, 1989) but not with agonist (Okazaki *et al.*, 1989)) and the allosterically linked glycine receptor were recently identified in membranes isolated from the hippocampus of kindled animals one month after the last seizure. An increase in calcium-dependent, potassium-evoked release of endogenous glutamate has been found in slices of CA3 but not those of CA1 or dentate isolated from kindled animals one month after the last kindled seizure (Jarvie *et al.*, 1990).

Together with the pharmacological evidence, the data emerging from these electrophysiological and biochemical studies suggest that an enhancement of transmission at excitatory synapses using NMDA receptors may contribute to the hyperexcitability underlying the expression of kindling. Moreover, both presynaptic (i.e., release) and postsynaptic (i.e., sensitivity and receptors) components appear to be up-regulated. Important unanswered questions emerge.

(1) Do the biochemical findings provide part or all of the explanation of the electrophysiological findings?

(2) Are the alterations in NMDA receptor sensitivity, EAA release, and NMDA-receptor-mediated synaptic transmission causally related to the lasting enhancement of seizure propagation in a kindled animal?

(3) What is the anatomical distribution of these electrophysiological and biochemical findings in structures outside the hippocampus? Related questions include: on what neurons do the increased numbers of NMDA receptors reside within and outside the hippocampus? Do the discrepant findings between agonist and antagonist binding to the NMDA receptor reflect regulation of a discrete subtype of the NMDA

receptor? If so, is this subtype particularly important in mediating the enhanced seizure propagation in a kindled brain?

(4) How do these biochemical and electrophysiological abnormalities develop and how are they maintained for such a long duration? Answers to these and related questions will almost certainly emerge in the near future.

Closing remarks

The quickening pace of discovery in neuroscience has impacted on epilepsy in general and on the kindling model in particular. Given the enormous complexity of the mammalian brain and the equally enormous number of possible explanations of the hyperexcitability underlying this model, it is remarkable that some insight into the underlying mechanisms seems to be emerging. With the rapid pace of technical advances in so many areas of fundamental neuroscience and the advancement of knowledge that results, it seems possible that the mechanisms underlying the development, expression, and persistence of the hyperexcitability in this model will soon be elucidated. If so, it is to be hoped that this will provide novel therapeutic approaches for patients afflicted with complex partial epilepsy.

Acknowledgments

Work presented here was in part supported by grants from NIH (NS17771, NS27311, NS24448) and the Department of Veterans Affairs and Epilepsy Foundation of America.

Appendix: A protocol for kindling

Surgery

Male Sprague-Dawley rats (Charles River, Wilmington, DE) weighing 300–325 g are used. Under pentobarbital anesthesia (50 mg/kg intraperitoneally), an animal is placed on a stereotaxic apparatus (David Kopf). A bipolar electrode (twisted nichrome wire, 254 µm diameter) is implanted using stereotaxic coordinates: for the right amygdala; 0.8 mm posterior from the bregma, 4.8 mm lateral (from mid line), 8.5 mm ventral from the dura. Skull screws serve as reference electrodes and as anchor points; the assembly is attached to the skull with dental acrylic. Animals are then allowed at least seven days to recover postoperatively. Once the experiments are completed and the animal killed, histological confirmation is necessary to verify that the electrode tips are located in the intended target. Frozen sections stained for Nissl are usually sufficient to localize the electrode tips without making electrolytic lesions.

Stimulation set-up and parameters

Kindling stimulations can be delivered through two Grass PSIU-6 constant current stimulation isolation units driven by a Grass S-88 stimulator. The system is configured to generate biphasic rectangular pulses. The amount of current to be delivered is predetermined by measuring the voltage drop across a resistor (e.g., 1 kΩ) with an oscilloscope. Actual current during stimulation is also monitored on the oscilloscope with a resistor in series with the animal. A mechanical relay is used to switch the electrical leads between the EEG machine and the stimulation set-up. A 1 s train of 1 ms biphasic pulses at 60 Hz is frequently used for kindling; trains can be repeated as frequently as every 90 min but once- or twice-daily stimulations provide for optimum rates of kindling.

Determination of seizure threshold

Initial afterdischarge threshold (ADT) is determined by administering a series of stimulations at 1 min intervals beginning at 100 µA and increasing in 100 µA steps, until an afterdischarge is recorded by EEG. Stimulations can then be delivered at ADT to kindle the animal.

Once the animals are fully kindled, generalized seizure threshold (GST) can be measured by observing the daily responses to specified current intensities on four consecutive days. A stable GST is defined as a current intensity at which stimulations 20 µA above this value evoke class 4 or 5 seizures, while stimulations 20 µA below do not. A current intensity for testing a given treatment paradigm can then be chosen; for example, current can be set to be 40 µA over the GST or 20% over the GST.

References

Albertson, T. E., Joy, R. M. & Stark, L. G. (1984). Carbamazepine: a pharmacological study in the kindling model of epilepsy. *Neuropharmacology*, **23**: 1117–23.

Albertson, T. E., Peterson, S. L. & Stark, L. G. (1980). Anticonvulsant drugs and their antagonism of kindled amygdaloid seizures in rats. *Neuropharmacology*, **19**: 643–52.

Albright, P. S. & Burnham, W. M. (1980). Development of a new pharmacological seizure model: effects of anticonvulsants on cortical- and amygdala-kindled seizures in the rat. *Epilepsia*, **21**: 681–9.

Bragdon, A. C., Taylor, D. M., McNamara, J. O. & Wilson, W. A. (1988). Abnormal hyperexcitability of hippocampal slices from kindled rats is transient. *Brain Research*, **453**: 257–64.

Bruton, C. J. (1988). *The Neuropathology of Temporal Lobe Epilepsy*. New York: Oxford University Press.

Cavazos, J. E. & Sutula, T. P. (1990). Progressive neuronal loss induced by kindling: a possible mechanism for mossy fiber synaptic reorganization and hippocampal sclerosis. *Brain Research*, **527**: 1–6.

Cline, H. T., Debski, E. A. & Constantine-Paton, M. (1987) N-Methyl-D-aspartate receptor antagonist desegregates eye-specific stripes. *Proceedings of the National Academy of Sciences, USA*, **84**: 4342–5.

Commission on Classification and Terminology of the International League
Against Epilepsy (ILAE) (1981). Proposal for revised clinical and
electroencephalographic classification of epileptic seizures. *Epilepsia*, **22**:
489–501.

Commission on Classification and Terminology of the International
League Against Epilepsy (ILAE) (1989). Proposal for revised
classification of epilepsies and epileptic syndromes. *Epilepsia*, **30**:
389–99.

Corcoran, M. E. & Mason, S. T. (1980). Role of forebrain catecholamines in
amygdaloid kindling. *Brain Research*, **190**: 473–84.

Croucher, M. J., Collins, J. F. & Meldrum, B. S. (1982). Anticonvulsant action
of excitatory amino acid antagonists. *Science*, **216**: 899–901.

Czuczwar, S. J. & Meldrum, B. S. (1982). Protection against chemically induced
seizures by 2-amino-7-phosphonoheptanoic acid. *European Journal of
Pharmacology*, **83**: 335–8.

de Jonge, M. & Racine, R. J. (1987). The development and decay of
kindling-induced increases in paired-pulse depression in the dentate gyrus.
Brain Research, **412**: 318–28.

de Lanerolle, N. C., Kim, J. H., Robbins, R. J. & Spencer, D. D. (1989).
Hippocampal interneuron loss and plasticity in human temporal lobe
epilepsy. *Brain Research*, **495**: 387–95.

Dingledine, R., Hynes, M. A. & King, G. L. (1986). Involvement of
N-methyl-D-aspartate receptors in epileptiform bursting in the rat
hippocampal slice. *Journal of Physiology*, **380**: 175–89.

Engel, J., Wolfson, L. & Brown, L. (1978). Anatomical correlates of electrical
behavioral events related to amygdaloid kindling. *Annals of Neurology*, **3**:
538–44.

Falconer, M. A., Driver, M. V. & Serefetinides, E. A. (1962). Temporal lobe
epilepsy due to distant lesions: two cases relieved by operation. *Brain*, **85**:
521–34.

Falconer, M. A. & Kennedy, W. A. (1961). Epilepsy due to small focal temporal
lesions with bilateral independent spike-discharging foci. *Journal of
Neurology, Neurosurgery and Psychiatry*, **24**: 205–12.

Fanelli, R. J. & McNamara, J. O. (1986). Effects of age on kindling and kindled
seizure-induced increase of benzodiazepine receptor binding. *Brain
Research*, **362**: 17–22.

Frush, D. P., Giacchino, J. L. & McNamara, J. O. (1986). Evidence implicating
dentate granule cells in development of entorhinal kindling. *Experimental
Neurology*, **92**: 92–101.

Gean, P. W., Shinnick Gallagher, P. & Anderson, A. C. (1989). Spontaneous
epileptiform activity and alteration of GABA- and of NMDA-mediated
neurotransmission in amygdala neurons kindled in vivo. *Brain Research*,
494: 177–81.

Gellman, R. L., Kallianos, J. A. & McNamara, J. O. (1987). Alpha-2 receptors
mediate an endogenous noradrenergic suppression of kindling
development. *Journal of Pharmacology and Experimental Therapeutics*, **241**:
891–8.

Gibbs, F. A. & Gibbs, E. L. (1952). *Atlas of Electroencephalography*, 2nd edn,
vol. 2. Cambridge, MA: Addison-Wesley.

Goddard, G. V., McIntyre, D. C. & Leech, C. K. (1969). A permanent change
in brain function resulting from daily electrical stimulation. *Experimental
Neurology*, **25**: 295–330.

Harris, E. W., Ganong, A. H. & Cotman, C. W. (1984). Long-term potentiation in the hippocampus involves activation of N-methyl-D-aspartate receptors. *Brain Research*, **323**: 132–7.

Hauser, W. A. & Kurland, L. T. (1975). The epidemiology of epilepsy in Rochester, Minnesota, 1935 through 1967. *Epilepsia*, **16**: 1–66.

Herron, C. E., Lester, R. A. J., Coan, E. J. & Collingridge, G. L. (1986). Frequency-dependent involvement of NMDA receptors in the hippocampus: a novel synaptic mechanism. *Nature*, **322**: 265–8.

Jarvie, P. A., Logan, T. C., Geula, C. & Slevin, J. T. (1990). Entorhinal kindling permanently enhances Ca^{2+}-dependent L-glutamate release in regio inferior of rat hippocampus. *Brain Research*, **508**: 188–93.

Kapur, J., Michelson, H. B., Buterbaugh, G. G. & Lothman, E. W. (1989). Evidence for a chronic loss of inhibition in the hippocampus after kindling: electrophysiological studies. *Epilepsy Research*, **4**: 90–9.

Kim, J. H., Guimaraes, P. O., Shen, M. Y., Masukawa, L. M. & Spencer, D. D. (1990). Hippocampal neuronal density in temporal lobe epilepsy with and without gliomas. *Acta Neuropathologica*, **80**: 41–5.

King, G. L., Dingledine, R., Giacchino, J. L. & McNamara, J. O. (1985). Abnormal neuronal excitability in hippocampal slices from kindled rats. *Journal of Neurophysiology*, **54**: 1295–304.

Lerner Natoli, M., Rondouin, G. & Baldy Moulinier, M. (1984). Evolution of wet dog shakes during kindling in rats: comparison between hippocampal and amygdala kindling. *Experimental Neurology*, **83**: 1–12.

Leviel, V. & Naquet, R. (1977). A study of the actions of valproic acid on the kindling effect. *Epilepsia*, **18**: 229–34.

Lothman, E. W., Hatlelid, J. M. & Zorumski, C. F. (1985). Functional mapping of limbic seizures originating in the hippocampus: a combined 2-deoxyglucose and electrophysiologic study. *Brain Research*, **360**: 92–100.

Martin, D., Bowe, M. A., McNamara, J. O. & Nadler, J. V. (1988). Kindling depresses magnesium regulation of depolarizing responses to amino acid excitants. *Society for Neuroscience Abstracts*, **14**: 865.

Maru, E. & Goddard, G. V. (1987). Alteration in dentate neuronal activities associated with perforant path kindling. III. Enhancement of synaptic inhibition. *Experimental Neurology*, **96**: 46–60.

Mattson, R. H., Cramer, J. A., Collins, J. F., Smith, D. B., Delgado-Escueta, A. V., Browne, T. R., Williamson, P. D., Treiman, D. M., McNamara, J. O., McCutchen, C. B., Homan, R. W., Crill, W. E., Lubozynski, M. F., Rosenthal, N. P. & Mayersdorf, A. (1985). Comparison of carbamazepine, phenobarbital, phenytoin, and primidone in partial and secondary generalized tonic–clonic seizures. *New England Journal of Medicine*, **313**: 145–51.

Mayer, M. L., Westbrook, G. L. & Guthrie, P. B. (1984). Voltage-dependent block by Mg^{2+} of NMDA responses in spinal cord neurones. *Nature*, **309**: 261–3.

McIntyre, D. C. & Wong, R. K. (1986). Cellular and synaptic properties of amygdala-kindled pyriform cortex in vitro. *Journal of Neurophysiology*, **55**: 1295–307.

McNamara, J. O. (1988). Pursuit of the mechanisms of kindling. *Trends in Neurosciences*, **11**: 33–6.

McNamara, J. O. (1989). Development of new pharmacological agents for epilepsy: lessons from the kindling model. *Epilepsia*, **30**: S13–S18.

McNamara, J. O., Bonhaus, D. W., Nadler, J. V. & Yeh, G. C. (1990).
N-Methyl-D-aspartate (NMDA) receptors and the kindling model. In
Kindling 4, ed. J. A. Wada, pp. 197–208. New York: Plenum Press.

McNamara, J. O., Bonhaus, D. W. & Shin, C. (1988). Mechanisms of kindling:
a speculative hypothesis. In *Mechanisms of Epileptogenesis*, ed. M. A.
Dichter, pp. 85–99. New York: Plenum Press.

McNamara, J. O., Bonhaus, D. W., Shin, C., Crain, B. J., Gellman, R. L. &
Giacchino, J. L. (1985). The kindling model of epilepsy: a critical review.
CRC Critical Reviews in Clinical Neurobiology, **1**: 341–91.

McNamara, J. O., Galloway, M. T., Rigsbee, L. C. & Shin, C. (1984). Evidence
implicating substantia nigra in regulation of kindled seizure threshold.
Journal of Neuroscience, **4**: 2410–17.

McNamara, J. O., Rigsbee, L. C., Butler, L. S. & Shin, C. (1989). Intravenous
phenytoin is an effective anticonvulsant in the kindling model. *Annals of
Neurology*, **26**: 675–8.

McNamara, J. O., Russell, R. D., Rigsbee, L. & Bonhaus, D. W. (1988).
Anticonvulsant and antiepileptogenic actions of MK-801 in the kindling
and electroshock models. *Neuropharmacology*, **27**: 563–8.

Messenheimer, J., Harris, E. & Steward, O. (1979). Sprouting fibers gain access
to circuitry transsynaptically altered by kindling. *Experimental Neurology*,
64: 469–81.

Michelson, H. B., Kapur, J. & Lothman, E. W. (1989). Reduction of paired
pulse inhibition in the CA1 region of the hippocampus by pilocarpine in
naive and in amygdala-kindled rats. *Experimental Neurology*, **104**: 264–71.

Mody, I. & Heinemann, U. (1987). NMDA receptors of dentate gyrus granule
cells participate in synaptic transmission following kindling. *Nature*, **326**:
701–4.

Mody, I., Stanton, P. K. & Heinemann, U. (1988). Activation of N-methyl-D-
aspartate receptors parallels changes in cellular and synaptic properties of
dentate gyrus granule cells after kindling. *Journal of Neurophysiology*, **59**:
1033–54.

Morrell, F. (1979). Human secondary epileptogenic lesions. *Neurology*, **29**:
558.

Morris, R. G. M., Anderson, E., Lynch, G. & Baudry, M. (1986). Selective
impairment of learning and blockade of long-term potentiation by an
N-methyl-D-aspartate receptor antagonist, AP5. *Nature*, **319**: 774–6.

Morrisett, R. A., Chow, C., Nadler, J. V. & McNamara, J. O. (1989).
Biochemical evidence for enhanced sensitivity to N-methyl-D-aspartate in
the hippocampal formation of kindled rats. *Brain Research*, **496**: 25–8.

Moshé, S. L., Albala, B. J., Ackermann, R. F. & Engel, J. Jr (1983). Increased
seizure susceptibility of the immature brain. *Brain Research*, **283**: 81–5.

Nowak, L., Bregestovski, P., Ascher, P., Herbet, A. & Prochiantz, A. (1984).
Magnesium gates glutamate-activated channels in mouse central neurones.
Nature, **307**, 462–5.

Okazaki, M. M., McNamara, J. O. & Nadler, J. V. (1989). N-Methyl-D-
aspartate receptor autoradiography in rat brain after angular bundle
kindling. *Brain Research*, **482**: 359–64.

Pinel, J. P. J. & Rovner, L. I. (1978a). Experimental epileptogenesis:
kindling-induced epilepsy in rats. *Experimental Neurology*, **58**: 190–202.

Pinel, J. P. J. & Rovner, L. I. (1978b). Electrode placement and
kindling-induced experimental epilepsy. *Experimental Neurology*, **58**:
335–46.

Racine, R. J. (1972*a*). Modification of seizure activity by electrical stimulation. I. After-discharge threshold. *Electroencephalography and Clinical Neurophysiology*, **32**: 269–79.

Racine, R. J. (1972*b*). Modification of seizure activity by electrical stimulation. II. Motor seizure. *Electroencephalography and Clinical Neurophysiology*, **32**: 281–94.

Racine, R. J. (1975). Modification of seizure activity by electrical stimulation: cortical areas. *Electroencephalography and Clinical Neurophysiology*, **38**: 1–2.

Racine, R. J., Burnham, W., Gartner, J. & Levitan, D. (1973). Rates of motor seizure development in rats subjected to electrical brain stimulation, strain and interstimulation interval effects. *Electroencephalography and Clinical Neurophysiology*, **35**: 553–6.

Racine, R. J., Livingston, K. & Joaquin, A. (1975). Effects of procaine hydrochloride, diazepam and diphenylhydantoin on seizure development in cortical and subcortical structures in rats. *Electroencephalography and Clinical Neurophysiology*, **38**: 355–65.

Reid, S. A. & Sypert, G. W. (1984). Chronic models of epilepsy. In *Electrophysiology of Epilepsy*, ed. P. A. Schwartzkroin & H. V. Wheal, pp. 137–51. London: Academic Press.

Russell, D. S. & Rubinstein, L. J. (1977). *Pathology of Tumours of the Nervous System*, 4th edn. London: Edward Arnold.

Savage, D. D., Rigsbee, L. C. & McNamara, J. O. (1985). Knife cuts of entorhinal cortex: effects on development of amygdaloid kindling and seizure-induced decrease of muscarinic cholinergic receptors. *Journal of Neuroscience*, **5**: 408–13.

Schwartzkroin, P. A. & Franck, J. E. (1986). Electrophysiology of epileptic tissue: what pathologies are epileptogenic. *Advances in Experimental Medicine and Biology*, **203**: 157–72.

Shin, C., Silver, J. M., Bonhaus, D. W. & McNamara, J. O. (1987). The role of substantia nigra in the development of kindling: pharmacologic and lesion studies. *Brain Research*, **412**: 311–17.

Silver, J. M., Shin, C. & McNamara, J. O. (1990). Antiepileptogenic effects of conventional anticonvulsants in the kindling model of epilepsy. *Annals of Neurology*, **29**: 356–63.

Sramka, M., Sedlak, P. & Nadvornik, P. (1977). Observation of kindling phenomenon in treatment of pain by stimulation in thalamus. In *Neurosurgical Treatment in Psychiatry, Pain, and Epilepsy*, ed. W. H. Sweet, pp. 651–4. Baltimore, MD: University Park Press.

Stasheff, S. F., Anderson, W. W., Clark, S. & Wilson, W. A. (1989). NMDA antagonists differentiate epileptogenesis from seizure expression in an in vitro model. *Science*, **245**: 648–51.

Sutula, T., Harrison, C. & Steward, O. (1986). Chronic epileptogenesis induced by kindling of the entorhinal cortex: the role of the dentate gyrus. *Brain Research*, **385**: 291–9.

Tauck, D. L. & Nadler, J. V. (1985). Evidence of functional mossy fiber sprouting in hippocampal formation of kainic acid-treated rats. *Journal of Neuroscience*, **5**: 1016–22.

Temkin, N. R., Dikmen, S. S., Wilensky, A. J., Keihm, J., Chabal, S. & Winn, H. R. (1990). A randomized, double-blind study of phenytoin for the prevention of post-traumatic seizures. *New England Journal of Medicine*, **323**: 497–502.

Traynelis, S. F., Dingledine, R., McNamara, J. O., Butler, L. & Rigsbee, L. (1989). Effect of kindling on potassium-induced electrographic seizures in vitro. *Neuroscience Letters*, **105**: 326–32.

Vosu, H. & Wise, R. A. (1975). Cholinergic kindling in rats: comparison of caudate, amygdala and hippocampus. *Behavioral Biology*, **13**: 491–5.

Wada, J. A., Mizoguchi, T. & Osawa, T. (1978). Secondarily generalized convulsive seizures induced by daily amygdaloid stimulation in rhesus monkeys. *Neurology*, **28**: 1026–36.

Wada, J. A., Sato, M., Wake, A., Green, J. R. & Troupin, A. S. (1976). Prophylactic effects of phenytoin, phenobarbital, and carbamazepine examined in kindling cat preparations. *Archives of Neurology*, **33**: 426–34.

Wasterlain, C. G. & Jonec, V. (1983). Chemical kindling by muscarinic amygdaloid stimulation in the rat. *Brain Research*, **271**: 311–23.

Westerberg, V., Lewis, J. & Corcoran, M. E. (1984). Depletion of noradrenaline fails to affect kindled seizures. *Experimental Neurology*, **84**: 237–40.

Williamson, J. M. & Lothman, E. W. (1989). The effect of MK-801 on kindled seizures: implications for use and limitations as an antiepileptic drug. *Annals of Neurology*, **26**: 85–90.

Wise, R. A. & Chinerman, J. (1974). Effects of diazepam and phenobarbital on electrically-induced amygdaloid seizure development. *Experimental Neurology*, **45**: 355–63.

Yeh, G. C., Bonhaus, D. W., Nadler, J. V. & McNamara, J. O. (1989). N-Methyl-D-aspartate receptor plasticity in kindling: quantitative and qualitative alterations in the N-methyl-D-aspartate receptor–channel complex. *Proceedings of the National Academy of Sciences, USA*, **86**: 8157–60.

2

Focal trigger zones and pathways of propagation in seizure generation

KAREN GALE

Introduction

It is becoming increasingly evident that epileptogenic processes derive in part from an imbalance between excitatory and inhibitory controls in selected brain regions. Determining the nature of such imbalances, where and how they relate to convulsive seizure generation, and how they may be corrected, requires an understanding of neural mechanisms of propagated seizure development in the brain. Presently, there is a large gap between our knowledge of synaptic mechanisms involved in local epileptiform discharge in vitro and our observations in vivo of the convulsant and anticonvulsant actions of systemically administered drugs. Within this gap are the myriad of neural pathways connecting brain regions and forming complex circuits that can both propagate seizures and act to prevent them.

The neural circuitry involved in the initiation and propagation of seizures is extensive, intricate and variable with seizure type. It is clear that there are no neural circuits unique to seizures, but that seizure activity represents abnormal neuronal discharge conducted along circuits that are normally utilized for physiological processes. Moreover, several constellations of brain circuits exist that are potential substrates for propagated seizures. Thus, much in the same way that there is no single 'memory' circuit in the brain, seizures may be generated and propagated within any of several functionally distinct circuits. In considering experimental models of seizures, it is important to understand the particular circuitry associated with each model; unfortunately, in most cases, this information is lacking. However, we can make some crude distinctions between seizures that are dependent upon forebrain (particularly limbic) circuits and those for which the hindbrain is necessary and sufficient.

The distinctions between 'forebrain' and 'hindbrain' seizures are discussed below; a region of the prepiriform cortex, and its target areas in the limbic system, will be used to exemplify an epileptogenic network in the forebrain.

Features of brain regions participating in epileptogenesis

In discussing processes of seizure initiation and propagation, it is useful to define several features that participate in the epileptogenic process.

(1) *Epileptogenic 'trigger' area*: a site in the brain which is capable of evoking propagated seizure activity upon focal electrical or chemical stimulation. The trigger area is not necessarily one of the first areas to exhibit ictal activity during seizure development.

(2) *Epileptogenic 'target' area*: a site in the brain that is especially vulnerable to the development of ictal activity, either by virtue of its anatomical inputs (e.g., from a trigger area) and/or by virtue of its intrinsic circuitry. This area would be one of the first areas to exhibit a pattern of ictal discharge during the initial development of a seizure.

(3) *Pathways involved in the propagation of the seizure*: these include pathways connecting trigger and target areas, pathways creating positive and/or negative feedback circuits, pathways allowing the seizure to spread to additional brain loci, and commissural pathways allowing bilateral spread.

(4) *Gating inputs*: neural inputs to the trigger and/or target areas that modulate the excitability of these regions. Changes in the activity of the gating inputs would alter seizure threshold in a predictable fashion. These inputs alone are not necessarily capable of inducing seizures.

(5) *Anticonvulsant sites*: sites at which drugs can be placed to alter seizure susceptibility or seizure progression. These would include all of the areas included in (1) through (4) above. In addition there may be sites in the brain where endogenous processes do not normally regulate seizure threshold or susceptibility but which nevertheless can be made to impede seizure propagation when artificially manipulated by exogenous drug application.

In the following discussion, examples are provided for each of the above categories. It should be noted that the areas in the first three categories are likely to be specific for a given seizure type, whereas the last two categories are likely to involve areas or pathways that may influence several different circuits and, consequently, a variety of different seizure types.

Methods used for identifying anatomical sites and circuits involved in seizure generation

In general, two different approaches to this issue have been taken. The first is to inactivate or activate specific brain regions by localized lesions or focally applied drugs, and then to examine the effect on the susceptibility to, and severity of, seizures. The second is to generate a 'map' of brain regions that show alterations of electrical, metabolic or gene transcriptional activity in association with seizures. The first approach involves anatomically site-specific interventions and manipulations and can therefore establish causal relationships between the activity of selected regions and seizure susceptibility. However, only one site at a time can be examined with this procedure. In contrast, the second approach, which is strictly correlational and by itself cannot discriminate between cause and effect, has the advantage of allowing a survey of the entire brain in a single experimental animal. Ideally, both approaches should be used together, so as to optimize the yield of interpretable information. Some of the specific methods used in these approaches are described briefly below.

Lesions

A large literature exists on the effects of unilateral or bilateral lesions of various brain regions on susceptibility to seizures in several different seizure models. From the results of the lesion studies, it would appear that there are only a few brain regions whose integrity is necessary for normal seizure susceptibility. Among these are the cerebellum (and cerebellar peduncles) and the nucleus reticularis pontis oralis, the integrity of which are necessary for normal tonic convulsive seizures (Gabreels, 1972; Raines & Anderson, 1976; Browning et al., 1981a), and the substantia nigra, which is necessary for normal susceptibility to seizures induced by amygdala kindling (McNamara et al., 1984), electroshock, and intravenous bicuculline (Garant & Gale, 1983). The substantia innominata appears to be necessary for the expression of motor components of amygdala-kindled seizures (Imura et al., 1981) and the inferior colliculus is required for the induction of seizures of audiogenic origin (Browning, 1986).

There is a far longer list of brain regions that have been destroyed without any measurable effect on seizure severity or threshold. One is tempted to conclude that such regions do not play a crucial role in seizure initiation or propagation. This conclusion is likely to be incorrect in many instances because of the limitations of the lesion approach. The ability of the brain to compensate for damage to circumscribed regions is well documented. In many cases, surrounding tissue may take over the function of the lesioned area. In addition, regions receiving inputs from the lesioned area may alter their responsivity to compensate for the loss of these inputs. It is possible that even a locus several synaptic links downstream from the lesion site could take on some of the functions of the damaged tissue. Consequently, the fact that a given seizure is unaffected by the lesion of a particular locus in the brain does not necessarily mean that the locus is not a crucial component of a seizure-generating circuit. One way to minimize the problem of compensation resulting from neural plasticity is to use focal drug injections in order to suppress, rapidly and reversibly, neural activity in the area. Anticonvulsant effects can then be evaluated before many of the adaptive and compensatory changes set in. Presently, however, relatively few brain regions have been examined in this fashion; it would certainly be worth while to re-evaluate the role played by various brain areas using focal drug injections in place of lesions.

Focal drug injections

In order to identify brain regions from which seizures may be initiated, drugs can be microinjected locally into specific sites in awake animals while electrographic and behavioral activity is monitored. In general, local excitatory responses can be reliably achieved using glutamate receptor agonists, cholinergic agonists, or γ-aminobutyric acid (GABA) receptor antagonists. Depending upon the brain area involved, various other agents may also elicit excitatory responses. In some regions, it is possible to evoke seizure activity localized to the structure within which the drug is injected. In many instances the localized seizure activity does not evoke a propagated seizure. In contrast, there are other areas from which propagated seizure activity can be evoked without a localized seizure discharge necessarily being induced first. In order to ascertain that the drug is evoking a seizure by an action specifically at the site of injection, one must demonstrate that the same dose of drug placed into adjacent brain regions fails to evoke a comparable effect.

Identifying brain regions that may regulate and/or conduct propagated seizures requires an evaluation of the effects of both excitatory and inhibitory agents applied to the area. If neural activity within the region is required for seizure initiation or propagation in a given seizure model, then inhibition of activity by administration of a GABA agonist (e.g., muscimol) or anesthetic agent (e.g., lidocaine) would be expected to attenuate seizure activity or raise seizure threshold in that model. Conversely, stimulation of the area by applying excitatory agents (e.g., glutamate agonists) or by blocking inhibition (e.g., using a GABA antagonist such as bicuculline) would be expected to potentiate seizure activity or lower seizure threshold.

Functional anatomical mapping studies

Techniques useful for monitoring the involvement of various brain regions in the seizure process include (a) electroencephalography (EEG), (b) autoradiographic analysis of ^{14}C-2-deoxyglucose (2DG) accumulation, and (c) evaluation of in-situ expression of immediate early genes (IEG) such as c-*fos*. Of these, the most sensitive monitor is the EEG recording, and only this technique allows for continuous registration of temporal changes in the pattern of activity. The 2DG and IEG techniques provide more detailed and comprehensive information on spatial patterns of activity, with in-situ IEG expression providing the highest degree of spatial resolution. IEG expression as evaluated by in-situ hybridization will be manifest in cell bodies of neurons. On the basis of evidence to date, increased expression of IEGs such as c-*fos*, c-*jun*, *jun-B*, *zif-268*, and *nur-77* occurs in neurons in response to enhanced excitatory stimulation (Greenberg *et al.*, 1986; Morgan & Curran, 1986; Cole *et al.*, 1989; Sheng & Greenberg, 1990). Thus, neuronal populations showing increased expression of mRNA for the IEGs in association with seizure activity are likely to be responding to excitatory inputs activated by the seizure.

In contrast, increases in 2DG accumulation result largely from ion fluxes associated with the opening of ligand- and voltage-dependent membrane channels of nerve terminals (Mata *et al.*, 1980; Kadekaro *et al.*, 1985; Nudo & Masterton, 1986). Consequently, in an area of increased 2DG accumulation during a seizure, it is likely that nerve terminals afferent to that area have been activated. Since these afferent terminals may produce either excitatory or inhibitory synaptic potentials (or both), the pattern of increased 2DG accumulation does not reveal whether the neurons intrinsic to the area have been excited or inhibited.

Characteristics that distinguish forebrain seizures from hindbrain seizures

While forebrain and hindbrain regions normally interact with each other via an abundant array of neural pathways, they are not strictly interdependent when it comes to generating seizures. In experimental animals, it can be demonstrated that some convulsive behavior depends upon the forebrain for its manifestation whereas there are other convulsive behaviors for which the hindbrain is sufficient (Gale & Browning, 1988; Gale, 1990).

A convulsive pattern typically associated with forebrain seizures in the rat involves facial and forelimb clonus with rearing (and often falling). This motor pattern is seen with seizures evoked by kindling of limbic system structures (Racine, 1972), systemic or intraventricular administration of kainic acid (Lothman & Collins, 1981; Ben Ari, 1985), systemic administration of pilocarpine (Turski *et al.*, 1983), and focal injection of GABA antagonists and muscarinic or glutamic acid agonists into area tempestas (AT), an epileptogenic trigger site within the deep prepiriform cortex (Piredda & Gale, 1985). In addition, by careful selection of the dose administered, this type of convulsion can be obtained with systemic injections of chemoconvulsants such as pentylenetetrazol and bicuculline (Gale, 1990). Similarly, with careful adjustment of current intensity, these seizures can be evoked using electroshock administered via corneal electrodes (Swinyard, 1972). If the doses of systemically administered chemoconvulsants are too high or if the electroshock current is too intense, then a tonic extensor convulsion is produced; in such circumstances, the appearance of facial and forelimb clonus is usually precluded. Tonic convulsions and the closely related explosive running–bouncing convulsions are dependent only upon brainstem circuits for their organization and expression (Browning *et al.*, 1981*b*; Browning, 1985; Browning & Nelson, 1986).

Since, by varying the stimulus intensity or dose, electroshock and systemically administered chemoconvulsants can produce facial and forelimb clonus with rearing, as well as running–bouncing and tonic seizures, these models have been employed to dissociate different convulsive patterns. Complete surgical transections that disconnect the forebrain from the hindbrain eliminate the ability to elicit the type of convulsion characterized by facial and forelimb clonus, but do not prevent the expression of running–bouncing clonus or tonic seizures (Browning *et al.*, 1981*b*; Browning, 1985; Browning & Nelson, 1986). If the seizure activity is recorded electrographically, it can be demonstrated that the severed forebrain is fully capable of generating propagated seizure activity of the kind typically associated with facial and forelimb clonus (Browning *et al.*, 1993). These observations indicate that, whereas circuits within the hindbrain are sufficient for the development and manifestation of running–bouncing clonus and tonic convulsions, the forebrain is required for convulsions characterized by facial and forelimb clonus. Moreover, it appears that circuitry intrinsic to the forebrain is sufficient for sustaining propagated electrographic seizure discharge.

In agreement with the above concepts, different types of convulsions are elicited by stimulation confined to forebrain or hindbrain regions. Acute drug stimulation of the AT (Piredda & Gale, 1985) or certain sites within the ventral hippocampus (Lee *et al.*, 1988; Thai *et al.*, 1990) evokes facial and forelimb clonus with rearing but does not evoke running–bouncing clonus or tonus. Conversely, in naive animals, a single application of drug (e.g., bicuculline) or electrical stimulation in the inferior colliculus elicits running–bouncing clonus (Frye *et al.*, 1986; Millan *et al.*, 1986*a*; Faingold *et al.*, 1988) and under certain circumstances can evoke tonic convulsions (Browning *et al.*, 1991) but never evokes facial and forelimb clonus or forebrain electrographic seizure activity (McCown *et al.*, 1984). Electroshock applied via ear clip electrodes rather than corneal electrodes fails to evoke facial and forelimb clonus at any stimulus intensity (Browning & Nelson, 1985) but is highly effective for evoking running–bouncing and tonic convulsions with relatively low stimulus intensities (Browning & Nelson, 1985). Evidently, the placement of electrodes on the ears preferentially routes the current through the brainstem, thereby precluding forebrain convulsive manifestations (Browning & Nelson, 1985).

Epileptogenic 'trigger' area

The brain site that is discussed here as an example of a trigger area, the AT, evokes forebrain seizures in association with limbic system circuits (Piredda & Gale, 1985; see Fig. 2.1).

Inhibitory and excitatory amino acid neurotransmitters are crucial for the regulation of output from the AT. Blockade of inhibitory neurotransmission (mediated by GABA) or augmentation of excitatory neurotransmission (mediated by glutamate or aspartate) within this site in one hemisphere initiates bilaterally synchronous motor and electrographic seizures that resemble those evoked by kindling of limbic structures (Piredda & Gale, 1985, 1986*b*). Picomole amounts of bicuculline (GABA antagonist) or kainic acid (glutamate agonist) in AT evoke convulsions characterized by facial and forelimb clonus with rearing and falling (Piredda & Gale, 1985). In addition, glutamate, aspartate, homocysteate, and *N*-methyl-D-aspartate (NMDA) evoke convulsive seizures from this

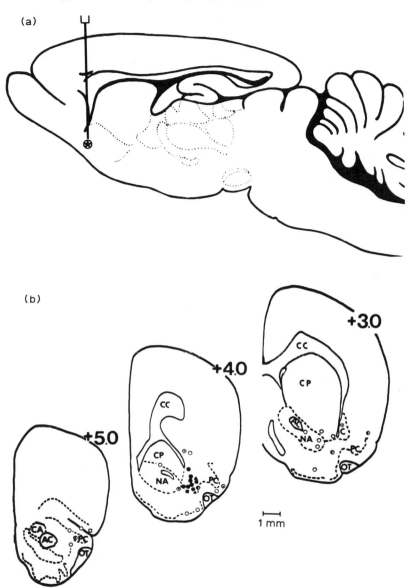

Fig. 2.1. Location of the area tempestas (a) in a schematic parasagittal drawing of the rat brain (cannula tip is located in the AT) and (b) on coronal drawings of rat brain in which solid symbols represent sites at which infusions of bicuculline (49 pmol), kainic acid (117 pmol) or carbachol (136 pmol) evoked convulsive seizures; open symbols represent sites ineffective for evoking seizures. CC, corpus callosum; CP, caudate-putamen; C, claustrum; PC, piriform cortex; OT, olfactory tract; NA, nucleus accumbens; CA, anterior pole of caudate nucleus; AC, anterior commissure. (From Piredda & Gale, 1985.).

site (Piredda & Gale, 1986*b*; Zrebeet & Gale, 1988), and stimulation of muscarinic receptors with carbachol, or opiate receptors with morphine, is also convulsant in the AT. As increasing doses of these drugs are applied to the AT, the frequency and duration of seizure activity become greater, culminating in status epilepticus. In all cases, the maximal intensity seizure corresponds to bilateral forelimb clonus, facial and mouth clonus, with rearing and falling. Under no circumstances does running–bouncing clonus or tonic extension emerge.

The seizure manifestations evoked from the AT are characteristic of limbic motor seizures, the type of seizure that has been proposed as an animal analogue of human complex partial seizures (with secondary generalization) (Turski *et al.*, 1983; Ben Ari, 1985; McNamara, 1986; Olney *et al.*, 1986). Consistent with this, AT-evoked seizures are sensitive to phenytoin and carbamazepine but not to ethosuximide (Zhong *et al.*, 1988; Gale, 1990). It is also interesting that limbic motor seizures induced in the systemic pilocarpine model are very sensitive to blockade by inhibition of excitatory transmission selectively within the AT (Millan *et al.*, 1986*b*).

On the basis of pharmacological characterization of the AT, it appears that excitatory mechanisms mediated by NMDA receptors are required for the genesis of seizures from the AT. Blockade of NMDA receptors by application of 2-amino-7-phosphonoheptanoic acid (2-APH, 100 pmol) into the AT attenuated the convulsant actions of bicuculline, carbachol, and kainic acid (Table 2.1); other competitive antagonists of NMDA receptors, such as CPP, exerted a similar effect. Moreover, interference with NMDA transmission due to blockade of the glycine recognition site on the NMDA receptor, using 7-chlorokynurenic acid or HA-966 in the AT, prevented seizures evoked by bicuculline, carbachol or kainic acid applied to the AT (Wardas *et al.*, 1990). These observations indicate that the removal of GABA-mediated inhibition in the AT (i.e., by bicuculline) is not sufficient to induce seizures in the absence of NMDA receptor-mediated activity. Seizures induced by muscarinic agonist in the AT also require NMDA receptor activation, as 2-APH prevented carbachol-induced seizures (Piredda & Gale, 1986*b*). Thus, glutamate-mediated transmission in the AT appears to be both necessary and sufficient for evoking seizures from this site. This is in contrast to muscarinic transmission, which does not appear to be necessary for evoking seizures from the AT, according to studies with focally applied atropine (Piredda & Gale, 1985). A diagrammatic portrayal summarizing some of the proposed neurotransmitter interactions in the AT is presented in Fig. 2.2.

Table 2.1. *Effect of an NMDA antagonist in rat on seizures evoked by bicuculline, carbachol, or kainic acid in the area tempestas*

Convulsant treatment	Pretreatment	Distribution of seizure scores[a] Score	0	1	2	3	4	5	Mean seizure score
Bicuculline	Control						5	3	4.4
(49 pmol)	2-APH		5				3		1.5[b]
Carbachol	Control						7	1	4.1
(272 pmol)	2-APH		4		1	1	2		1.6[b]
Kainic acid	Control						4	4	4.5
(117 pmol)	2-APH		6				2		1.0[b]

APH, 2-amino-7-phosphonoheptanoic acid.
[a] Below each seizure score, the number of rats reaching that score are shown.
[b] Significantly different from the control group (Mann–Whitney U-test for non-parametric grouped data; $P < 0.05$).
(From Piredda & Gale, 1986*b*.)

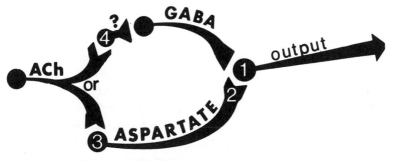

Fig. 2.2. Hypothetical interrelationship between neurotransmitter pathways, in the AT, for triggering seizures. GABA-mediated inhibition and aspartate (or glutamate)-mediated excitation control the seizure-triggering output. Bicuculline triggers seizures by removing the GABAergic inhibition of this output; glutamate, aspartate, and NMDA trigger seizures by directly activating the output. Kainic acid triggers seizures by evoking aspartate or glutamate release (from site 2), which in turn activates NMDA receptors on the output. Activation of muscarinic cholinergic receptors (e.g., with carbachol) can either stimulate glutamate or aspartate release or stimulate an inhibitory interneuron (site 4), which in turn suppresses GABAergic inhibitory activity. Atropine, by blocking muscarinic receptors at site 3 or 4 prevents carbachol-evoked seizures, but does not interfere with seizures evoked by bicuculline. NMDA receptor antagonists, by blocking the action of endogenous glutamate or aspartate at site 1, prevent seizures evoked by either GABA blockade, kainic acid, or muscarinic stimulation. Ach, acetylcholine. (From Piredda & Gale, 1986*b*.)

The evidence summarized above suggests that excitation of AT outputs is sufficient for the induction of generalized seizures of the limbic motor type. The next logical question is whether this site is an important participant in seizures evoked in systemic convulsant models. To answer this question, we need to know whether inhibition of neural activity in AT can interfere with seizure expression in such models. To date, this issue has been explored in three different chemoconvulsant models: (1) intravenous bicuculline; (2) subcutaneous isoniazid; and (3) intraperitoneal pilocarpine. Blockade of NMDA receptors or activation of GABA receptors in the AT, bilaterally, blocks clonic convulsions evoked by intravenous bicuculline (Piredda & Gale, 1986a). Blockade of NMDA receptors in the AT has also been shown to block seizures induced by intraperitoneal pilocarpine (Millan et al., 1986b), and elevation of GABA by application of γ-vinyl-GABA in the AT blocks clonic but not tonic convulsions evoked by subcutaneous isoniazid (Gale, 1992). These observations indicate that activity of AT outputs is required for the normal susceptibility to limbic motor seizures as produced in these models.

Only a few studies have explored the effects of lesions of the AT on seizures in systemic convulsant models. As discussed earlier (see p. 51), there are special problems connected with the lesion approach. Most noteworthy is the observation that, following a neurotoxin-induced lesion of the area, it is still possible to evoke convulsions in response to focal application of drugs in the vicinity of the lesion in many animals (H. A. Zrebeet and K. Gale, unpublished results). This suggested that, in the lesioned animals, intact tissue adjacent to the lesion may be responsible for triggering seizures in response to the focally applied drug, even though that tissue lies outside the immediate boundaries of the AT. It is conceivable that lesions of the AT cause changes in the surrounding tissue so that it takes on epileptogenic properties not normally expressed in the intact animal. To explore this possibility, we have implanted cannulae into the prepiriform cortex lateral and caudal to the AT, an area relatively insensitive to the convulsant effect of bicuculline application in the intact rat. Pilot studies suggest that, in some animals with neurotoxin-induced lesions of the AT, convulsive seizures can be triggered from the adjacent prepiriform area with low doses of bicuculline. Studies are now in progress to define the nature and extent of lesioning required to eliminate completely the potential substrate for generating seizures from the prepiriform cortex, if possible. Only then could the impact of such lesions on systemically evoked seizures be evaluated.

In terms of electrographic features, AT activity characteristically shows a high frequency and low amplitude pattern under baseline conditions (Massotti & Gale, 1989). When recordings are made from the AT during the process of initiating seizures from the same site (by microinjection of bicuculline methiodide), isolated spikes are registered. Not until bilateral generalization of seizure discharge is evident on the cortical EEG is paroxysmal seizure discharge registered from the AT (R. Fariello and K. Gale, unpublished results). This indicates that the area itself is not especially prone to seizure discharge, although it is particularly effective for triggering seizure activity in regions to which it projects. Thus, whereas changes in neural activity within the AT may start a seizure, the actual seizure discharge does not appear to start in the AT. This has important implications in the interpretation of EEG data.

When several brain regions are examined electrographically by depth recording during the onset of a seizure, certain regions can be identified that exhibit the earliest signs of seizure discharge. These regions are often assumed to be responsible for initiating the seizure process. However, it may be the case that the earliest signs of seizure discharge occur in regions that are especially seizure prone and that these regions are being recruited by a trigger area (e.g., the area tempestas) that eludes detection on the basis of EEG seizure criteria. The recognition that seizures may be triggered or organized by groups of neurons that would not readily be detected with EEG analysis prompts us to consider additional criteria or measurement techniques that might reveal such trigger regions. Moreover, it raises the possibility that there may be brain regions in which pathology could influence seizure susceptibility without creating obvious changes in the electrographic characteristics of the region(s).

While this discussion has focused on the AT, it should be recognized that this is not the only epileptogenic trigger region for initiating limbic motor seizures. The ventral hippocampus, when stimulated with opioid agonists or glutamate agonists (Lee *et al.*, 1988; Thai *et al.*, 1990), evokes limbic motor seizures resembling those evoked from the AT. Interestingly, this region is not especially sensitive to either bicuculline or carbachol in terms of inducing convulsive seizures (R. Maggio and K. Gale, unpublished results). Additional sites of convulsant action of bicuculline must be presumed to exist in view of the fact that convulsions evoked by systemic bicuculline can be elicited by increasing the dose of bicuculline in animals with focal bilateral inhibition (using muscimol or γ-vinyl-GABA) of the AT. Thus, whereas the AT may be especially sensitive to bicuculline in terms of triggering seizures, other forebrain regions may be capable of evoking a similar action in response to higher concentrations of this drug. Presently, we do not have good candidate sites for this. Doses of bicuculline more than 10–20-fold higher than those effective for evoking seizures from the AT have been placed into the striatum (K. Gale, unpublished results), substantia nigra (Olianas *et al.*, 1978; Gunne *et al.*, 1988; Maggio *et al.*, 1990*a*), amygdala (Turski *et al.*, 1985; Uemura & Kimura, 1988), and hippocampus (K. Gale and R. Maggio, unpublished results) without inducing convulsive seizures.

It is possible that the AT is unique in its ability to trigger limbic motor seizures in response to low doses of bicuculline applied focally to a single brain locus. However, other areas that do not trigger seizures in response to focally injected bicuculline may trigger seizures if the GABA antagonist is concurrently present at one or more other loci. In other words, systemically administered bicuculline, by antagonizing GABA transmission throughout the brain, may trigger seizures due to synergistic actions involving two or more loci. For example, suppose that bicuculline application into the amygdala could trigger seizures, but only under circumstances in which bicuculline is also present in the hippocampus. A requirement for the involvement of three (or more) sites could further complicate the picture. To date, there has been no exploration of such interactive processes between brain regions for the initiation of chemically evoked convulsive seizures.

In considering the interaction between brain regions in the process of seizure initiation, we also must recognize the fact that there are sites in the brain in which *excitatory* synaptic activity may be *anticonvulsant*. So, for example, electrical stimulation, or application, of a glutamate receptor agonist or a GABA antagonist (bicuculline) into the striatum (La Grutta *et al.*, 1971; Cavalhiero *et al.*, 1987; Turski *et al.*, 1987) or the superior colliculus (Redgrave *et al.*, 1988; Dean & Gale, 1989; Gale *et al.*, 1992) can block seizures in several models (pp. 76–7). Consequently, if a trigger area were located adjacent to such an 'anticonvulsant' site, it might be difficult to evoke seizures with a focal microinjection in the trigger area because spread of the drug to the adjacent tissue could mask any convulsant effect.

Anticonvulsant actions of focally applied bicuculline have also been used to argue against the seizure-triggering role of bicuculline in the AT. Turski *et al.* (1989) observed that very low doses (1 pmol or less) of intrastriatal bicuculline could block seizures induced by either systemic bicuculline or bicuculline applied into the AT. These authors therefore concluded that systemic bicuculline, by acting within the striatum, would exert an anticonvulsant action, in addition to its seizure-triggering actions

Table 2.2. *Effect of bilateral intrastriatal infusions of muscimol (5 ng) on seizures elicited by bicuculline (1.5 mg/kg subcutaneously)*

Muscimol-treated group data were not significantly different from saline-treated group; Mann–Whitney U-test for non-parametric data; $P > 0.05$)

Treatment in striatum	n	Score			Number of rats showing clonic seizures ($\geqslant$ score 3)
		Mean	Median	Mode	
Saline	10	1.0	0.75	1.0	1
Muscimol	10	0.9	0.75	1.0	1

From Maggio *et al.*, 1991.

at other loci. Since the dose required in the striatum for anticonvulsant effects is several fold lower than that required for convulsant effects in the AT, Turski *et al.* argued that the AT could not be a convulsant site of action of systemically administered bicuculline and that there must be some other trigger area sensitive to considerably lower doses of bicuculline. However, this argument is contradicted by the experimental findings discussed below.

First, the fact that muscimol application within the AT significantly attenuates convulsions evoked by systemic bicuculline (Piredda & Gale, 1986*a*) indicates that this area does in fact participate in seizure generation in this model. Second, if an anticonvulsant action in the striatum were a significant component of the effect of systemic bicuculline, then the application of muscimol to this region (i.e., intrastriatally) should remove this component and thereby significantly potentiate the convulsant action of bicuculline. This is not the case; as shown in Table 2.2, intrastriatal muscimol was without effect on the convulsant response to a subthreshold dose of systemically administered bicuculline (Maggio *et al.*, 1991). It should be noted that the dose of muscimol (5 ng) used here is more than an order of magnitude greater than that necessary to block bicuculline at the dose found to be effective by Turski *et al.* (1989). Thus, since neither the threshold nor the severity of the convulsive response to systemic bicuculline is limited by a lack of GABA transmission in the striatum, it must be concluded that the striatum is not a significant site of action of systemic bicuculline for influencing seizure susceptibility.

The foregoing discussion raises an important issue concerning the degree to which we can extrapolate from the results of focal microinjection studies. The fact that an effect can be obtained from the focal application of a drug into a specific brain region does not allow us to assume that the same drug administered systemically will evoke that effect by acting in that site. This is because, when given systemically, the drug exerts actions in multiple brain regions. These may interact so as to cancel out some effects and augment others. Such interactions cannot be readily reproduced using isolated individual microinjections. The best way to evaluate the importance of a given region for the response to a systemic drug treatment is to *block* the drug action in that specific brain region and determine the effect on the systemic drug response. In the example discussed above, blockade of the action of bicuculline in the AT by the focal application of muscimol did alter the response to bicuculline, whereas a similar manipulation in the striatum did not. These results are consistent with the conclusion that the AT participates in the convulsive action of systemic bicuculline and that this action is not compromised by an effect exerted in the striatum.

Epileptogenic target areas

To continue with this example of AT-evoked seizures, target areas responding to epileptogenic stimulation of the AT will be considered. This model has special advantages for use with either the 2DG or in-situ hybridization mapping techniques. First, since the drug treatment is limited to the AT, the results are not confounded by direct effects of the convulsant agents on the target areas of interest, as would occur in systemic chemoconvulsant models. Second, the seizures evoked from the AT recur continually over a 45 min period, so that seizure activity is the dominant feature during the period between microinjection into the AT and killing of the rat 30 to 45 min later. This is an advantage over kindled seizures evoked by electrical stimulation, as these seizures generally last for only tens of seconds. Since the 2DG procedure requires an interval of tens of minutes in order to allow washout of free 2DG, an experiment with kindled seizures generally includes a large proportion of postictal activity. However, in the course of this discussion it will become evident that the target areas of interest in the AT model also participate in epileptogenesis in several models of seizures involving forebrain circuits.

2-Deoxyglucose autoradiography

In order to obtain an indication of those regions in which neural activity is markedly altered during the seizure process, metabolic mapping using 2DG autoradiography is effective. Figure 2.3 shows autoradiographs

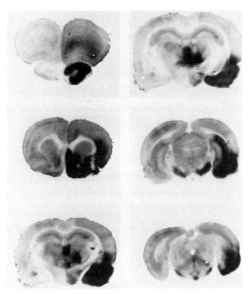

Fig. 2.3. ^{14}C-2-deoxyglucose autoradiography in coronal sections of the brain of a rat in which seizures were evoked by microinjection of bicuculline in the AT. Dark areas are regions of high density labeling, representing increases in accumulation of [14]C-2DG. Upper left panel: olfactory bulb and prefrontal cortex. Middle left panel: septum, nucleus accumbens and prepiriform cortex containing the injection site and cannula tract. Lower left panel: dorsal hippocampus, perirhinal and piriform cortex, amygdala, mediodorsal and ventroposterior thalamic nuclei. Upper right panel: dorsal hippocampus, piriform/entorhinal cortex, midline, parafascicular and ventroposterior thalamic nuclei. Middle right panel: substantia nigra, ventral hippocampus, entorhinal cortex. Lower right panel: substantia nigra, entorhinal cortex.

indicating patterns of accumulation of 2DG during the 45 min period of recurrent convulsive seizure episodes triggered by unilateral stimulation of the AT. In the hemisphere containing the stimulated AT, marked increases in labeling can be seen in the olfactory bulb, piriform cortex, entorhinal cortex, subiculum, and throughout the hippocampal formation. Also, the substantia nigra, entopeduncular nucleus, and selected regions of thalamus show strong increased activity. In the contralateral hemisphere, the substantia nigra, a few discrete regions of thalamus, and dorsal hippocampus show obvious increases in labeling.

This procedure has also been used to analyze seizures evoked by electrical stimulation of structures within the limbic system. In this case, the pattern of 2DG uptake depends upon the stage to which the animal has been kindled, i.e., the severity of the seizure. Partial seizures tended to be associated with increased 2DG uptake in the closest target regions to which the stimulated brain region directly projects (Engel *et al.*, 1978; R. C. Collins *et al.*, 1983). During full seizures, in which a complete pattern of convulsive seizure activity is manifest bilaterally, increased 2DG accumulation has been documented in the piriform cortex, hippocampus, amygdala, olfactory bulbs, nucleus accumbens, substantia nigra, entorhinal cortex, substantia innominata, and the anterior and periventricular nuclei of the thalamus (Engel *et al.*, 1978; Blackwood *et al.*, 1981; R. C. Collins *et al.*, 1983; Ackerman *et al.*, 1986).

Attempts to associate 2DG uptake patterns with behavioral manifestations of seizures have indicated that both the behavioral and 2DG patterns depend upon the area of the brain from which the seizure is generated. Stimulation that evokes both EEG seizures and activation of 2DG accumulation limited to the hippocampus is associated with staring and with behavioral arrest (R. C. Collins *et al.*, 1983). When bilateral activation of the amygdala, substantia nigra and thalamic nuclei occur, strong facial and forelimb clonus with rearing is usually evident (R. C. Collins *et al.*, 1983). This pattern is characteristic of propagated seizures evoked from limbic system structures.

In contrast to limbic-evoked seizures, focal motor seizures evoked by stimulation of discrete regions of neocortex are associated with increased 2DG labeling in the caudate–putamen and globus pallidus (Collins *et al.*, 1976). In addition, increased accumulation is found in the substantia nigra, and in the paraventricular and ventral thalamic nuclei, even with mild and unilateral seizure activity. With more severe seizures, larger areas of thalamus and contralateral frontal cortex become involved, and activation of medial thalamic nuclei is associated with bilateral seizure spread (Collins *et al.*, 1976).

In-situ hybridization for detecting immediate early gene expression

A group of recent reports suggest that convulsive seizures can provoke an increase in c-*fos* gene expression (Morgan *et al.*, 1987; Le Gal La Salle, 1988; Cole *et al.*, 1990) and that certain other immediate early genes (IEGs) are induced concurrently (Saffen *et al.*, 1988; Cole *et al.*, 1990). While these observations are intriguing, it must be realized that they do not establish whether certain features of the induction of IEG expression are in any way dependent upon seizure activity per se (as distinct from physiological stimulation). Nevertheless, it is clear that, at least for certain neuronal populations, induction of IEG expression can be used as a marker for increased activation of neuronal cells.

With seizures evoked from the AT, the most pronounced increases in

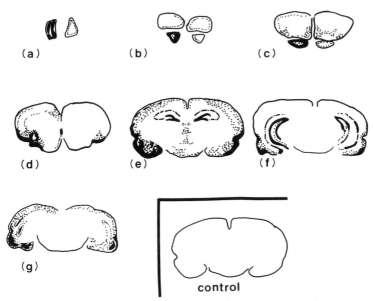

Fig. 2.4. Diagrammatic representation of c-*fos* mRNA levels 30 min following seizures evoked from the AT. Coronal sections are shown rostrocaudal (a) to (g) from an animal experiencing seizures evoked from the left AT. Control rats received saline into the AT; the control section shown is at a rostrocaudal level equivalent to (e). Black regions and heavy black lines (not including the outline of the brain section) represent highest density of autoradiographic grains (i.e., highest level of c-*fos* mRNA). Stippled regions represent moderately high density of grains; white areas are background activity. Most noteworthy increases occur in the hemisphere ipsilateral to the injected AT (injection artifact visible in (d)) and include olfactory bulb ((a), (b), (c)), prepiriform (d), piriform and perirhinal cortex (e), amygdala (e), hippocampus ((e), (f)), and entorhinal cortex ((f), (g)). (From Maggio *et al.*, 1993.)

mRNA for c-*fos* can be seen in the homolateral piriform cortex, entorhinal cortex, olfactory bulb, ventral hippocampus, and bilaterally in the dentate gyrus as well as CA1, CA3, and CA4 regions of the hippocampus (Fig. 2.4; see also Maggio *et al.*, 1993). Marked increases are also observed in the contralateral entorhinal cortex and ventral hippocampus, but these are less than the increases seen in these same regions on the side homolateral to the stimulated AT. A similar pattern of increase is evident with mRNAs for *zif-268*, c-*jun*, and *jun-B* (Maggio *et al.*, 1993). None of these changes occurs in response to either saline infusions into the AT or with infusions of bicuculline into areas adjacent to the AT that do not evoke convulsions. The increases in IEG expression reached a peak at 30 min after seizure initiation and started to decline after one hour; by three hours, mRNA levels for c-*fos* and *zif-268* returned to baseline, while that for c-*jun* and *jun-B* still showed slight elevation. In a separate experiment, the increase in mRNA levels was quantified by densitometric analysis of Northern blots of RNA extracted from several brain regions and found to be elevated several fold when compared to saline-injected controls (Lanaud *et al.*, 1993).

Enhanced expression of c-*fos* in the hippocampus has also been demonstrated to occur following convulsions induced by electroshock (Daval *et al.*, 1989; Cole *et al.*, 1990; Zawia & Bondy, 1990), systemically administered pentylenetetrazol (Morgan *et al.*, 1987; Dragunow & Robertson, 1988*a,b*; Saffen *et al.*, 1988), kainic acid (Le Gal La Salle, 1988), and picrotoxin (Saffen *et al.*, 1988), electrical stimulation of the hippocampus in both naive and kindled animals (Dragunow & Robertson, 1987; Shin *et al.*, 1990), and seizures induced by small lesions of the hilus in the hippocampus (White & Gall, 1987). In all cases, the dentate granule cells exhibit the most rapid and intense increase in Fos protein. These cells also exhibit an increase in Fos protein in response to high frequency electrical stimulation of neural inputs from the contralateral dentate gyrus via the commissural pathway or from entorhinal cortex via the perforant pathway (Douglas *et al.*, 1988; Cole *et al.*, 1989; Jeffrey *et al.*, 1990; Wisden *et al.*, 1990). To obtain increased expression of c-*fos* in dentate granule cells in response to perforant path stimulation, it is not necessary to evoke seizure discharge, but only multiple population spikes (Douglas *et al.*, 1988; Jeffrey *et al.*, 1990). Less intense stimulation of this pathway, such as that used for inducing long-term potentiation (LTP), can also induce c-*fos*, *zif-268*, and *jun-B* in the dentate granule cells, according to studies using in-situ hybridization (Cole *et al.*, 1989; Jeffrey *et al.*, 1990). A major difference between stimulation conditions evoking seizure activity and those that cause less severe activation of hippocampal neurons is that IEG expression increases *bilaterally* in the former case and only *unilaterally* (on the side of stimulation) in the latter.

Only a few studies have surveyed a large number of brain areas following seizures, and, in general, these have examined Fos-related proteins using immunocytochemistry (Dragunow & Robertson, 1988*a,b*; Le Gal La Salle, 1988). In addition to the hippocampus, the piriform cortex, entorhinal cortex, cingulate cortex, amygdala, and olfactory bulbs have been reported to exhibit increases in Fos protein immunoreactivity following convulsive seizures evoked by systemic kainic acid or metrazol (Morgan *et al.*, 1987; Le Gal La Salle, 1988). In-situ hybridization experiments have shown increased mRNA levels for c-*fos*, *zif-268*, *jun-B*, and c-*jun* in most of these same areas as early as 15 min after convulsant doses of metrazol or picrotoxin are systemically administered (Saffen *et al.*, 1988). A lack of detectable increase in IEG expression in superior and inferior colliculus, geniculate bodies, substantia nigra and cerebellar cortex has been consistently reported in the above studies. The anatomical pattern of IEG activation following convulsions evoked by systemic administration of chemoconvulsants appears to be quite similar to those evoked focally from the AT.

One major difference between the results obtained with systemic chemoconvulsants and those obtained with focal electrical or chemical stimulation concerns the time course of increased IEG expression relative to the onset of seizure activity. After seizures evoked from the AT, an increase in c-*fos* mRNA is just barely noticeable, beginning at 7–8 min after the first seizure. The onset of increase in Fos protein would be expected to follow this. With electrically induced seizures in the hippocampus produced by direct focal stimulation in kindled rats, no increase in Fos protein was evident at 10 min after the seizure, whereas a clear-cut increase was seen by 30 min (Dragunow & Robertson, 1987). In contrast, following systemic injection of kainic acid, evidence of increased Fos immunoreactivity was seen in the dentate gyrus and entorhinal cortex *coincident* with the time of onset of the first signs of electrographic seizure activity, which occur at approximately 30 min following the convulsant injection (Le Gal La Salle, 1988). This indicates that an initial increase in c-*fos* expression must have been triggered by direct effects of the kainic acid, prior to seizure onset. Such an effect would not be surprising in view of the fact that kainic acid stimulates glutamate receptors directly and can also induce glutamate release (Ferkany *et al.*, 1982; G. G. S. Collins *et al.*, 1983), which in turn may evoke increased c-*fos* expression (Szekely *et al.*, 1989, 1990). After seizure activity begins, there is a further increase in c-*fos* expression (Le Gal La Salle, 1988); this increase is probably related to the seizure activity superimposed upon the effects of direct stimulation by the kainic acid. Interestingly, the convulsant drugs isoniazid and thiosemicarbazide, which do not exert their action via direct receptor stimulation, do not appear to cause an increase in c-*fos* mRNA in animals killed at the time of onset of convulsions (at least 30 min after drug administration) (Mizuno *et al.*, 1989).

An important issue that needs to be addressed is the degree to which the anatomical pattern of induction of IEGs is specifically related to a particular type of seizure. Hyperactivity, stress, respiratory alterations, and other sequelae of seizures could contribute to the enhanced IEG expression associated with seizures. For example, even in the absence of seizures, moderate increases in brain c-*fos* expression have been observed in mice in response to the application of ear-clip electrodes, presumably due to the noxious stimulation of the ear clips (Daval *et al.*, 1989; Nakajima *et al.*, 1989). If clear differences in the anatomical pattern of IEG expression can be achieved by distinct types of seizure, then this would suggest that at least certain aspects of the pattern of IEG induction are not a result of non-specific physiological stress.

From the electrographic and behavioral characterization of convulsive seizures evoked from the inferior colliculus, we would not expect to see marked activation of IEG expression in forebrain areas in association with these seizures. Stimulation of inferior colliculus by focal application of bicuculline evokes explosive running–bouncing convulsions in the absence of forebrain electrographic seizure activity (McCown *et al.*, 1984) and this type of convulsion, as discussed earlier, is dependent upon hindbrain, but not forebrain, circuitry for its expression (Gale & Browning, 1988). Examination of brain sections for expression of c-*fos*, *zif-268*, c-*jun*, and *jun-B*, using in-situ hybridization in rats killed 30 min after initiation of convulsions from the inferior colliculus, revealed little or no elevation of the mRNAs of these IEGs in the hippocampus, entorhinal cortex, or piriform cortex. In general, there were no marked increases in IEG expression in any forebrain area surveyed (Maggio *et al.*, 1993). Similarly, increases in Fos protein in forebrain regions do not appear in response to audiogenic seizures (Le Gal La Salle & Naquet, 1990), another seizure model that is predominantly associated with hindbrain mechanisms (Browning, 1986). Interestingly, in the audiogenic seizure model, several subcortical auditory nuclei including inferior colliculus, exhibited marked increases in Fos immunoreactivity (Le Gal La Salle & Naquet, 1990). As these nuclei did not appear to have increased c-*fos* expression in association with seizures that were evoked from microinjections into inferior colliculus, it is likely that they reflect processing of the seizure-eliciting sensory (i.e., auditory) input and are not substrates involved in seizure propagation or expression. These observations allow us to conclude that seizure-evoked increases in IEG expression in forebrain limbic structures are not solely a result of non-specific factors associated with the convulsive state, regardless of seizure type, but most likely reflect the anatomical specificity of seizure propagation mechanisms.

At this point, it is interesting to compare the results obtained with 2DG accumulation and IEG expression (Table 2.3). With seizures evoked from the AT, both techniques reveal marked activation of the ipsilateral

Table 2.3. *Areas (ipsilateral to the stimulated area tempestas) showing marked increases during AT-evoked seizures*

	c-*fos*	2DG
Olfactory bulb	+ + +	+ + +
Prefrontal cortex	+	+
Prepiriform cortex	+ +	+
Piriform cortex	+ + +	+ + +
Neocortex	+	−
Amygdala	+ +	+ + +
Entorhinal cortex	+ +	+ + +
Hippocampus		
Pyramidal cells	+ +	+
Dentate granule cells	+ + +	−
Habenula	+	−
Mediodorsal, parafascicular, and ventromedial thalamus	±	+ + +
Globus pallidus, entopeduncular nucleus	−	+ + +
Substantia nigra	−	+ + +

2DG, 2-deoxyglucose; +, increase; −, no increase.

olfactory bulb, ipsilateral piriform and entorhinal cortex, ipsilateral ventral hippocampus, and bilateral dorsal hippocampus (Maggio *et al.*, 1990*b*). These target areas are interconnected via excitatory synaptic links that, on the basis of these mapping studies, appear to be activated by the seizures evoked from AT. With both procedures, regions in the hemisphere homolateral to the stimulated AT show more pronounced activation than those on the contralateral side (Maggio *et al.*, 1990*b*). This asymmetry may indicate that the seizure activity spreads first through homolateral structures before crossing into the contralateral hemisphere and that some decrement in the strength of activation takes place after the midline has been crossed. Interestingly, there is less extreme asymmetry with IEG expression than with 2DG accumulation. This is perhaps a reflection of differences in sensitivity between the two techniques; IEG expression, as a more sensitive technique, will be more likely to detect changes in regions which are less than maximally activated by the seizure activity. That significant seizure activity is present in the contralateral hemisphere is evidenced by EEG recordings (Piredda & Gale, 1985; M. Massotti, R. Fariello & K. Gale, unpublished results).

Several regions exhibit marked seizure-evoked increases in 2DG accumulation without showing obvious changes in IEG expression. In particular, the substantia nigra and selected thalamic nuclei have dramatic increases in the 2DG signal associated with AT-evoked seizures (Maggio *et al.*, 1990*b*), as well as with seizures evoked by kindling (Engel *et al.*, 1978; Blackwood *et al.*, 1981; R. C. Collins *et al.*, 1983; Ackerman *et al.*, 1986) and various chemoconvulsants (Pazdernik *et al.*, 1985). However, these same regions appear unchanged when examined for expression of c-*fos* or other IEGs following AT-evoked seizures (Maggio *et al.*, 1993) or systemic chemoconvulsant seizures (Dragunow & Robertson, 1988*a,b*; Le Gal La Salle, 1988). It is likely that, in these instances, increased 2DG accumulation is associated to a large extent with the activation of inhibitory inputs into these structures. This would be consistent with the high density of inhibitory GABA-containing terminals innervating the substantia nigra and the fact that 2DG accumulation largely reflects nerve-terminal activity, irrespective of whether that activity has an excitatory or inhibitory influence postsynaptically. However, increased inhibitory afferent input to a region would not necessarily evoke an increase in IEG expression in the postsynaptic cells, thus accounting for the discrepant patterns with the two techniques. While clear-cut increases in 2DG or in IEG mRNA signals indicate that a population of neurons in a given brain area has been affected by the seizure activity, no conclusions can be drawn from a lack of increase in any given area. With the 2DG technique, an absence of effect merely indicates that, if a change occurred, it was below detectability. This is illustrated by the notable lack of 2DG activation in the hemisphere contralateral to the stimulated AT (Maggio *et al.*, 1990), despite the fact that recurrent and prolonged paroxysmal discharge can be recorded from all deep structures in this hemisphere following AT-evoked seizures (R. Fariello, M. Massotti and K. Gale, unpublished results). With IEG expression, a lack of change in any given area may reflect either a relative lack of stimulation of neurons in that area, or the relative unresponsiveness of the IEG system in that area. Presently, it is not known whether all neurons in all brain regions have equivalent susceptibility and capacity to induce IEG expression upon stimulation. It is likely that certain neuronal populations may be more responsive than others. Thus, there may be areas that are involved in the active propagation of seizure activity but are resistant to showing changes in IEG expression. Conversely, the most marked changes in IEG expression following seizures may occur in brain areas with the most labile IEG transcription, not necessarily areas that are especially prone to seizure generation. Consequently, it is important to interpret the results obtained with metabolic or molecular mapping studies in the context of studies with EEG recordings.

Electroencephalographic recording

When depth electrodes were placed in limbic regions in order to record EEG activity during initiation of seizures evoked from the AT, the basolateral amygdala, entorhinal cortex, and dorsal hippocampus exhibited trains of spikes prior to any signs of epileptiform activity on the cortical EEG. The limbic structures in the hemisphere containing the stimulated AT showed seizure activity several seconds before the equivalent structures in the contralateral hemisphere became involved. Following the appearance of bilateral trains of spikes in limbic regions, leads on the cortical surface bilaterally and near the AT itself detected seizure activity (R. Fariello and K. Gale, unpublished results). Prior to spread of epileptic discharge to the cortex, isolated spikes were observed in the AT and no evidence of convulsive behavior was present. These observations corroborate certain features of the patterns of activation seen in the mapping studies. It appears that limbic targets such as the entorhinal cortex, piriform cortex, hippocampus and amygdala contain populations of neurons that are especially vulnerable to the seizure-triggering influence of the AT. These regions are also among the first to exhibit seizure activity during initiation of kindled seizures evoked by stimulation of various forebrain sites. It is likely that the propensity of these limbic targets for developing seizure discharge is determined by their intrinsic circuitry as well as by their mutual interconnections (see Fig. 2.5). Perhaps it is the ability to control the discharge pattern of these limbic targets that accounts for the seizure-triggering action of the AT.

Propagation pathways

While it is possible to construct a map of brain regions involved in seizure initiation and propagation using the various manipulations and mapping techniques described above, the actual *routes* utilized for propagation of seizures are usually inferred from known anatomical projections between these areas. However, defining the sequential links between the structures necessary for evoking a propagated seizure is far more complex.

Some indication of the sequence of activation of various structures can be obtained by examining the temporal pattern in studies with depth EEG recording. However, such studies do not define which areas are activated as a prerequisite for the activation of other structures and/or which regions constitute an *essential* link in seizure propagation. To make this determination, it is necessary to manipulate focally a selected brain region

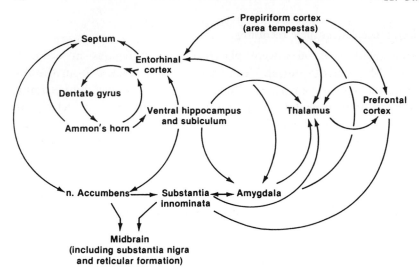

Fig. 2.5. Schematic representation of some anatomical connections between various limbic system regions and related structures in the forebrain and midbrain. (From Gale, 1991.)

presumed to be a crucial relay in a seizure-propagating circuit and concurrently monitor seizure activity as well as some index of activation of interconnected structures.

For example, let us suppose that, on the basis of the mapping studies discussed above, the entorhinal cortex is a primary target of the AT for evoking seizures and that, from this region, seizure activity propagates via the perforant pathway projecting to the dentate gyrus of the hippocampus. In approaching this hypothesis, three questions must be addressed. (a) Will inhibition of neural activity in entorhinal cortex prevent the activation of IEG expression or enhanced 2DG accumulation in this region following AT-evoked seizures? (b) Will inhibition of neural activity in entorhinal cortex prevent the activation of IEG expression and enhanced 2DG accumulation in the dentate gyrus and/or other regions of hippocampus following AT-evoked seizures? (c) Will inhibition of neural activity in entorhinal cortex interfere with the expression of convulsive seizures? While the answer to the first question should be 'yes' if the inhibitory manipulation is effective for suppressing local neural activity, the answer to the second question will be positive only if activation of entorhinal cortex is obligatory for activation of dentate and/or other hippocampal neurons. Even if this were to be the case, it would not necessarily follow that activation of the entorhinal–hippocampal pathway is necessary for motor expression of the seizure, as addressed by the third question.

Surprisingly little research has addressed these issues in the intact animal. Consequently, there is a list of brain regions and pathways that are potentially crucial for seizure propagation in certain models, but involvement of which remains to be tested experimentally. Not only must the neural projections that propagate and amplify seizure discharge be determined, but it is essential that the neurotransmitters and neuro-modulators utilized by these pathways be identified. This information will be especially helpful in the development of therapeutic drug strategies, and should also help in the identification of potential substrates involved in the etiology and pathophysiology of the epilepsies.

Gating mechanisms

In general, systems that diffusely influence seizure susceptibility, or seizure threshold, without actually inducing or propagating seizure discharge per se, tend to influence many different types of seizure. Two such systems will be described here as examples of mechanisms by which the probability of seizure occurrence may be regulated: (a) the ascending noradrenergic projection system, and (b) the substantia nigra and its associated circuits in the basal ganglia.

The ascending noradrenergic projection system

The noradrenergic system that arises from brainstem neurons that are located predominantly in the locus coeruleus has been repeatedly demonstrated to influence seizure susceptibility in animal models (Ferren-delli, 1984; Jobe *et al.*, 1986; Corcoran, 1988). In general, lesions that destroy the ascending noradrenergic projections from the locus coeruleus to the forebrain cause a decrease in seizure threshold. This suggests that these noradrenergic projection pathways normally confer some degree of seizure resistance. It is important to note that, whereas depletion of norepinephrine can lower seizure threshold, this manipulation by itself does not evoke seizures without a seizure-inducing stimulus.

One of the best-studied models with respect to the influence of norepi-nephrine is the genetically epilepsy-prone rat (GEPR). The GEPR has a lower than normal threshold for seizures induced by chemoconvulsants (Dailey *et al.*, 1989), shows unusually rapid seizure development during the process of limbic system kindling (Savage et al., 1986), and exhibits susceptibility to audiogenic seizures (Reigel et al., 1986). Two GEPR colonies have been established: one exhibiting severe, tonic, convulsions (GEPR-9), and the other exhibiting only clonic convulsions (GEPR-3). In the GEPR, several studies have documented a noradrenergic modulation of seizure response. Depletion of norepinephrine or neurotoxin-induced lesions of the ascending noradrenergic pathways increase the severity of audiogenic seizures in these rats (Jobe et al., 1986). Moreover, the GEPR-9 rat, which normally exhibits tonic audiogenic convulsions, has a lower concentration of norepinephrine in several brain areas when compared to the GEPR-3, and both colonies have significantly lower norepinephrine concentrations (compared to control animals that are not prone to epilepsy) in most brain regions examined (Jobe et al., 1986). When the GEPR-3 is treated with an agent causing norepinephrine depletion, tonic audiogenic convulsions are obtained. Interestingly, norepinephrine depletion also predisposes to tonic convulsions in normal animals in which seizures are evoked by microinjections of drugs into the inferior colliculus (Browning et al., 1991). As depletion of norepinephrine in normal rats does not render them susceptible to audiogenic seizures, it has been concluded that a noradrenergic deficiency is not itself sufficient to account for the full extent of the seizure-prone profile of the GEPR and that other non-monoaminergic determinants must also play a role (Jobe et al., 1986).

The substantia nigra and its associated circuits in the basal ganglia

The major components of the basal ganglia, i.e., the caudate–putamen (striatum), globus pallidus (in particular, entopeduncular nucleus), and substantia nigra, have all been demonstrated to influence seizure susceptibility in numerous experimental seizure models. The best studied of these structures is the substantia nigra, the only region that has been examined in connection with as many as ten different experimental seizure models. Treatments that either increase inhibitory transmission (mediated by the neurotransmitter GABA) in substantia nigra, or block excitatory transmission (mediated by glutamate or certain neuropeptides such as substance P) in this nucleus in both hemispheres, prevent or attenuate convulsive seizures induced by several chemoconvulsants (pilocarpine, kainic acid, bicuculline, and flurothyl, among others (Iadarola & Gale, 1982; Le Gal La Salle et al., 1984; Moshé & Albala, 1984; Turski et al., 1986a,b; Garant & Gale, 1986), by maximal electroshock (Iadarola & Gale,

1982), by kindling of amygdala (Le Gal La Salle *et al.*, 1983; McNamara *et al.*, 1984), by drug application into the AT (Maggio & Gale, 1989), and by acoustic stimulation in rats susceptible to audiogenic seizures due to either ethanol withdrawal (Frye *et al.*, 1983; Gonzales & Hettinger, 1984) or genetic determinants (Millan *et al.*, 1988). In addition, inhibition within the substantia nigra decreases susceptibility to non-convulsive electrographic seizures that occur either spontaneously (in genetically predisposed strains of animals; Depaulis *et al.*, 1988) or as a consequence of treatment with drugs such as pentylenetetrazol in low doses (Depaulis *et al.*, 1989).

The integrity of the substantia nigra is not required for seizure induction (Garant & Gale, 1983; McNamara *et al.*, 1984), indicating that this structure is not part of a crucial seizure-conducting pathway. Instead, the substantia nigra is probably part of a seizure-suppressing circuit that may become engaged by seizure discharge. Viewed in this way, the substantia nigra and associated nuclei of the basal ganglia act to maintain a homeostatic balance of brain excitability by creating a resistance to seizure spread and generalization.

Certain key structures of the forebrain and midbrain may work in concert with the substantia nigra in this seizure-resisting capacity. The striatum is one major source of neural input to the substantia nigra, whereas the superior colliculus (deep layers) is one important target of neural projections coming from the nigra. One of the most prominent pathways connecting the striatum and the substantia nigra is inhibitory and utilizes GABA as its transmitter (Hattori *et al.*, 1973; Fonnum *et al.*, 1978). Likewise, the substantia nigra sends an inhibitory GABA-containing projection to the superior colliculus (Vincent *et al.*, 1978; DiChiara *et al.*, 1979). Consequently, it might be expected that the stimulation of the neurons in the striatum that give rise to the GABA inputs to the substantia nigra would be anticonvulsant (see Fig. 2.6) because this would enhance GABA transmission in the substantia nigra. The experimental evidence supports this proposal: electrical or drug-induced excitatory stimulation in striatum tends to exert an anticonvulsant action in the few experimental seizure models that have been examined so far (La Grutta *et al.*, 1971, 1986; Amato *et al.*, 1982; Cavalheiro *et al.*, 1987; Turski *et al.*, 1987).

Within the substantia nigra, inhibitory GABAergic transmission acts to suppress the activity of output projections to the superior colliculus (Fig. 2.6). This relationship predicts that blockade of GABA transmission in the nigral projection target area of the superior colliculus should be anticonvulsant. Again, the experimental evidence is consistent with

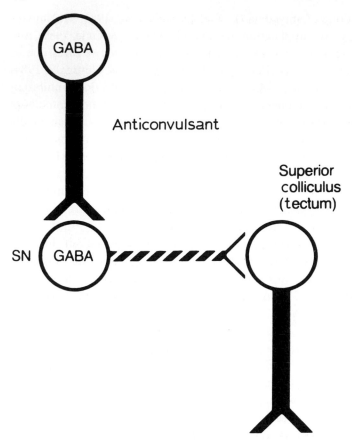

Fig. 2.6. Proposed relationship between serial GABAergic neuronal links involving substantia nigra (SN) and superior colliculus (SC). The first GABA pathway represents inputs to the SN; this innervates a GABA output to the SC. Increasing the GABAergic input to the SN (heavy black line) results in a suppression of nigrotectal GABA neuronal activity (broken line) and a net disinhibition of target neurons in tectum; this condition is anticonvulsant. (From Dean & Gale, 1989.)

expectations. Blockade of GABA receptor-mediated transmission in the deep layers of the superior colliculus is anticonvulsant against both clonic and tonic forms of convulsive seizure activity (Dean & Gale, 1989; Gale *et al.*, 1992) as well as against non-convulsive spike-and-wave electrographic seizure discharge (Redgrave *et al.*, 1988). This illustrates a fundamental principle of central nervous system organization – disinhibition. Inhibitory transmission from the substantia nigra acts to reduce the activity of the nigral outputs to the colliculi (which are themselves inhibitory) resulting in the withdrawal of inhibition, or disinhibition of neuronal targets in the superior colliculus. Presently, it is not understood how neuronal activity within the superior colliculus acts to impede seizure progression. Some of the colliculus neurons that are activated by nigral disinhibition may be those that project to the brainstem reticular formation, where they can relay with both ascending and descending neural pathways. Stimulation of certain regions of the reticular formation is capable of interfering with the development of a synchronized pattern of neuronal discharge in cortex (Testa & Gloor, 1974). By engaging these desynchronizing influences of the reticular formation, the superior colliculus could disrupt the generation of seizures, which require synchronized neuronal bursting.

The entopeduncular nucleus, also known as the medial segment of the globus pallidus, is similar to the substantia nigra in terms of function, morphology, and neuroanatomical connections. Together with the substantia nigra, this nucleus relays neuronal outputs from the striatum. It is therefore not surprising that the same treatments that suppress seizure propagation when placed in the substantia nigra exert a similar action in the entopeduncular nucleus (De Sarro *et al.*, 1986; Patel *et al.*, 1986). However, unlike the substantia nigra, the entopeduncular nucleus does not appear to exert an influence on brainstem seizure substrates. Whereas blockade of glutamate transmission in the substantia nigra attenuated audiogenic seizures in the GEPR, this manipulation in the entopeduncular nucleus did not reduce audiogenic seizure activity (Millan *et al.*, 1988) under the same conditions in which it blocked pilocarpine-induced limbic motor seizures (Patel *et al.*, 1986). Moreover, GABA agonist application in the entopeduncular nucleus did not prevent maximal electroshock-induced tonic convulsions under conditions in which it prevented pilocarpine-induced limbic motor seizures (Hosford & McNamara, 1988). Thus, it appears that the influence of the entopeduncular nucleus may be preferentially directed at forebrain seizure circuitry, perhaps via its close connections with the habenula and other limbic structures.

The influence of the basal ganglia on seizure generalization is not confined to the motor manifestations of the seizures. In instances in which electrographic signs of seizures have been monitored, anticonvulsant manipulations of basal ganglia structures induce a corresponding suppression of electrographic seizure discharge in cortical and subcortical structures (Le Gal La Salle *et al.*, 1983, 1984; McNamara *et al.*, 1984;

Garant & Gale, 1986; Turski *et al.*, 1986*a,b*). This is consistent with a role of basal ganglia circuits in the control of cortical excitability and the regulation of synchronization of neuronal discharge in widespread regions of the forebrain.

It is noteworthy, however, that impairment of GABA transmission in the substantia nigra does not potentiate seizures in most seizure models. Depletion of nigral GABA by the bilateral focal injection of isoniazid (Gale & Iadarola, 1980) did not affect either the threshold or the severity of seizures induced by systemic bicuculline, systemic kainic acid, bicuculline in the AT (Maggio *et al.*, 1991) or amygdala kindling (Löscher *et al.*, 1987); blockade of GABA receptors bilaterally in the substantia nigra also failed to potentiate non-convulsive spike-and-wave discharge in a selected strain of Wistar rat (Depaulis *et al.*, 1988). These seizure models have all been shown to be highly sensitive to the anticonvulsant effect of GABA agonist application in the substantia nigra.

This raises a crucial question: why is a decrease of nigral GABA-mediated inhibition not proconvulsant in the very same models in which an increase in nigral GABA transmission is anticonvulsant? One possibility is that in these seizure models, GABAergic transmission in substantia nigra is relatively inactive. Accordingly, when augmented by exogenous GABA agonists or GABA-elevating agents, an anticonvulsant action is obtained, but there is little or no impact of a decrease in endogenous nigral GABA transmission. Another possibility is that very early in the development of a seizure, GABA inputs to the nigra may be highly activated to the point of GABA depletion. If such a depletion occurs very rapidly, then the presence of a GABA synthesis inhibitor or a GABA receptor antagonist would have little additional effect. In either case, we are forced to conclude that tonic endogenous GABA transmission in the substantia nigra is not normally playing an active role in restraining seizure propagation in most of the seizure models studied. Perhaps the nigral circuitry is not physiologically utilized to control seizure propagation, despite the fact that it represents a site of action for anticonvulsant effects of exogenous treatments.

The only model in which GABA depletion in the substantia nigra has been shown to have a profound proconvulsant action is the pilocarpine seizure model (Turski *et al.*, 1986*a*). In this situation, intranigral isoniazid shifts the threshold dose to less than half of the normal threshold (Turski *et al.*, 1986*a*). This would suggest that endogenous GABA tone in nigra must be relatively high during these seizures. Perhaps the activity of the GABAergic projections to the nigra is altered as a secondary consequence of the stimulation of muscarinic receptors in the striatum and/or globus pallidus by pilocarpine. We can conclude from this that, under special circumstances, endogenous GABA transmission in the substantia nigra acts to restrain or limit seizure susceptibility. It is conceivable that nigral GABA transmission may also serve this function in response to chronic neuropathological alterations, but there are presently no data that address this speculation.

In conclusion, the substantia nigra may be viewed as an important site of action for anticonvulsant drugs that work via augmentation of GABA transmission or blockade of glutamatergic transmission. However, the nigral outflow cannot be considered to function in a generally seizure facilitating manner, as many investigators have assumed or implied. It appears that, in the case of the nigra, there may be a gating mechanism that works only in a unidirectional (i.e., seizure-suppressing) fashion; this mechanism depends upon exogenous drug treatments, or perhaps pathological insults, in order to exert a seizure-suppressing influence.

Anticonvulsant sites

It should be clear from the foregoing discussion that all regions participating in the initiation, propagation, and gating of convulsant seizure activity are potential sites at which pharmacological interventions may prove to be anticonvulsant. Since the sites involved in seizure initiation and the targets of these sites are often selectively related to a particular type of seizure, it stands to reason that the spectrum of anticonvulsant actions obtained from such sites will be likewise selective. So, for example, reduced excitation or enhanced inhibition in the AT (bilaterally) that is anticonvulsant against clonic seizures evoked by systemic bicuculline (Piredda & Gale, 1986a), pilocarpine (Millan *et al.*, 1986b) or isoniazid (S. Piredda and K. Gale, unpublished results) has no anticonvulsant action against the tonic convulsions evoked by either electroshock (Piredda *et al.*, 1987) or isoniazid (Gale, 1992). This is consistent with the fact that the AT is a site from which it is possible to evoke limbic motor (clonic) seizures but not seizures involving tonic extension (see Table 2.4 and Fig. 2.7).

Another example of selective anticonvulsant effects of focal inhibition involves the inferior colliculus. As this nucleus is part of the auditory sensory projection system, it is probably a crucial afferent relay station for converting acoustic stimulation into convulsive discharge. Accordingly, bilateral focal inhibition of neural activity in the inferior colliculus

Table 2.4. *Focal drug applications: comparison of effect in the substantia nigra (SN) and area tempestas (AT)*

Focal application of	Effect obtained from SN	Effect obtained from AT
GABA agonist	Anticonvulsant	Anticonvulsant (except *vs* MES)[a]
GABA antagonist	None or proconvulsant	Convulsant
Excitatory amino acid agonist	None or proconvulsant	Convulsant
Excitatory amino acid antagonist	Anticonvulsant	Anticonvulsant (except *vs* MES)[a]
Opioid agonist (morphine)	Anticonvulsant[b]	Convulsant

MES, maximal electroshock seizure.
[a] Anticonvulsant actions do not extend to tonic convulsions as evoked by MES or chemoconvulsant agents.
[b] Morphine in SN is anticonvulsant against MES convulsions.

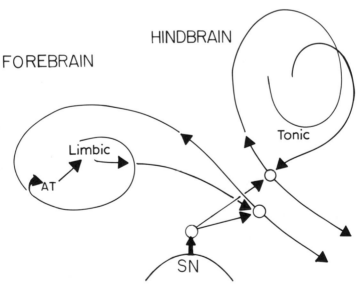

Fig. 2.7. Forebrain circuitry involving limbic structures and the area tempestas (AT) is required for generating limbic motor seizures with clonic manifestations, whereas hindbrain circuits are necessary and sufficient for generating tonic extensor convulsions in rodents. Although both types of seizure-generating substrate are subject to common control by the substantia nigra (SN) and other systems which influence seizure susceptibility (e.g., noradrenergic), they are experimentally separable and independent in normal animals (see the text).

can protect against audiogenic seizures (Faingold *et al.*, 1988); this effect is selective for these seizures and does not extend to seizures induced by other mechanisms.

In contrast to the anticonvulsant substrates that are related selectively to specific seizure-generating circuits, there are those that can protect against a wide variety of seizure types and seizure components. The 'gating' systems involved in determining seizure susceptibility can typically influence seizure threshold in several different models. As discussed earlier, the substantia nigra is an especially good example of a region from which protection against a wide range of seizure types can be elicited (see Table 2.4 and Fig. 2.7). Limbic afterdischarge, limbic motor seizures, tonic extension, running–bouncing convulsions, as well as electrographic activity associated with convulsive (Garant & Gale, 1986) and non-convulsive seizures (Depaulis *et al.*, 1988), are subject to blockade by inhibition of neural activity in the substantia nigra. In fact, for tonic convulsions evoked by maximal electroshock, it appears that the substantia nigra is the *only* region in which elevation of GABA (with γ-vinyl-GABA) is anticonvulsant (Iadarola & Gale, 1982). Regions such as the substantia nigra that have the capacity to protect against seizures generated from a variety of brain circuits are likely to be important as targets of broad-spectrum anticonvulsant therapeutic interventions. In analyzing the anticonvulsant influence of a brain region it is therefore critical to evaluate experimentally the selectivity and specificity of the influence. For example, let us assume that inhibition in site X has been found to protect against convulsive seizures evoked by amygdala stimulation in kindled animals. We then need to know: (a) is this specific for amygdala-evoked seizures or does it extend to other models of limbic seizures and (b) is it selectively related to limbic seizures or does it extend to running–bouncing and/or tonic convulsive seizures, or to non-convulsive electrographic seizures? The answers to these questions tell us the extent to which the anticonvulsant substrate in question is model specific and/or selective for seizure type. The greater the number of seizure models evaluated in this context, the greater will be the precision of the analysis.

Seizures and epilepsy

This chapter has confined itself to a discussion of anatomical substrates of propagated seizures. While seizures are the hallmark symptom of epilepsy, an understanding of how seizures can be triggered and controlled is not equivalent to an understanding of how an epileptic disorder originates or can be cured. A seizure is an acute phenomenon that can be induced in the normal brain by a variety of stimuli, such as those used in most experimental animal models. Epilepsy, on the other hand, is a disorder of the brain that results in the occurrence of repeated seizure episodes. This disorder, which often occurs in response to a traumatic brain injury, is indicative of an underlying pathophysiology that is not well defined and most certainly takes on a variety of characteristics. Because of this uncertain and variable nature of the pathophysiology of epilepsy, it is far more difficult to develop valid models for epilepsy than it is to develop valid seizure models. Accordingly, we know considerably more about the substrates involved in seizure generation than we know about the mechanisms underlying the development of epilepsy.

Because the anatomical substrates of seizures have been explored largely in otherwise normal brains, it is not known whether all of the experimental observations would also hold true in an individual with epilepsy. In addition to the presence of an underlying pathology is the consideration that the individual with epilepsy is experiencing seizures *chronically*.

From experimental animal studies, it is known that a history of repeated seizure episodes can alter molecular, morphological, and electro-physiological characteristics of particular populations of neurons in the brain. Furthermore, repeated seizure episodes can influence subsequent seizure susceptibility. In general, intense or prolonged convulsive seizures tend to reduce susceptibility to subsequent convulsant stimuli. This phenomenon, which may be considered a form of 'tolerance', can be seen after as few as three days of daily maximal electroshock seizures and persists for at least one week after cessation of seizure stimuli (Boschulte & Gale, 1985). Furthermore, cross-tolerance to other types of convulsive seizures also occurs (Boschulte & Gale, 1985). In contrast, repeated exposure to a threshold or subthreshold convulsant stimulus causes a progressive *sensitization* to that stimulus. In this case seizure susceptiblity is increased, and previously subconvulsant or threshold stimuli come to elicit full convulsive responses (Ramer & Pinel, 1976; Majkowski, 1986). Again, in this situation, there is cross-sensitization to a wide variety of chemical and electrical stimuli (Cain, 1982, 1985, 1987). Kindling of specific brain areas is one form of seizure sensitization that has the additional attribute of being irreversible (Racine, 1972).

From the perspective of understanding neural circuitry involved in the generation and control of seizures, it is especially interesting to note that disparate types of convulsive seizures can markedly influence one another in circumstances of chronic recurrence. For example, in rats that have been kindled by repeated stimulation of the amygdala, the threshold for obtaining tonic hindlimb extension with electroshock was found to be significantly reduced (Applegate *et al.*, 1991). Thus, even though the amygdala-kindled seizures do not themselves engage the brainstem circuits responsible for running–bouncing and tonic convulsions, the kindling *process* must affect a substrate that influences the seizure-susceptibility of those brainstem circuits. Consequently, in addition to the brain areas involved in the initiation and propagation of a given type of seizure, there may be additional regions and circuits that can be altered as a *consequence* of the seizure. These latter regions, while not participating in the development or expression of the seizure itself, may regulate *susceptibility* to convulsant stimuli and this regulation need not be limited to any specific seizure type. These regions or circuits would most likely belong to the category of gating mechanisms: systems that can simultaneously influence the threshold for a variety of seizure types and seizure components.

Conclusion

Convulsive seizures that depend upon limbic forebrain circuits for their initiation and propagation can be distinguished anatomically from those types of convulsion that depend only upon hindbrain circuits (Fig. 2.7). The former, in rodent models, are characterized by facial and forelimb clonus with rearing and falling. The latter are characterized by explosive running and bouncing and/or tonic extension of the limbs. A variety of seizure-inducing stimuli (including electrical kindling, electrical or chemical stimulation of the AT, low doses of systemic chemoconvulsants, and low currents of electroshock administered via corneal electrodes) can be used to induce limbic motor seizures. Some of these same stimuli (i.e., systemic chemoconvulsants or electroshock) at higher doses (or current strengths) can be used to provoke convulsions characterized by running–bouncing and tonic extension (for detailed discussion of several animal seizure models and types of seizure components, see Gale, 1990). In general, focal stimulation of specific brain regions can selectively evoke either the limbic seizure pattern or the hindbrain seizure pattern: e.g., stimulation of the AT, or kindling of the amygdala, selectively evokes limbic motor seizures, whereas stimulation of the inferior colliculus selectively evokes running–bouncing convulsions. Studies of regional

IEG expression support this neuroanatomical dissociation: limbic motor seizures evoked by various means cause a pattern of increased IEG expression associated with prominent limbic areas (olfactory bulb, piriform cortex, amygdala, entorhinal cortex, and hippocampal formation) whereas convulsions evoked from the inferior colliculus are not associated with changes in IEG expression in these regions.

By using focal intracerebral injections of drugs, particularly those that stimulate or block neurotransmission mediated by glutamate or GABA, we can begin to dissect the circuitry responsible for generating each of the various types of seizures. In doing so, it is advisable to select seizure models that are behaviorally well defined and selective for a particular seizure type. Focally evoked seizures have the advantage of having a defined and limited site of seizure initiation. Once a site is identified from which seizures can be triggered, the target regions recruited by stimulation of the trigger site can be explored. Crucial target regions, i.e., those necessary for the development and maintenance of the convulsive response, can be identified by examining the influence of focal drug injections on the ability to evoke seizures. It stands to reason that various seizure models that evoke a similar seizure type, e.g., limbic motor seizures, will for the most part engage a common set of target regions, and that these will be differentiated from the target regions engaged by seizure models that evoke a different type of seizure, e.g., involving tonic extension of the limbs.

In addition to the specific circuits that are responsible for triggering and conducting propagated seizures of various types, there are circuits that are responsible for determining seizure susceptibility, or seizure threshold. In this category are brain regions and pathways (e.g., the substantia nigra and its associated basal ganglia circuits) that are capable of simultaneously influencing susceptibility to many types of seizure. This relatively non-selective influence on seizure propagation derives from what are termed gating mechanisms. It is especially important to identify the anatomical substrates responsible for gating seizure sensitivity because these substrates can be powerful targets of therapeutic drug action. Moreover, it is likely that the functional state of these gating mechanisms becomes altered as a result of repeated seizure episodes, accounting for the progressive increases or decreases in seizure susceptibility observed in conditions of recurrent seizures.

The knowledge of cellular mechanisms that give rise to paroxysmal firing of neurons within a given brain region or within a given population of neurons provides an understanding of the ways in which those specific groups of neurons may be provoked into participating in propagated seizures. This information cannot, however, explain how propagated seizures develop in the brain. In fact, the ability to evoke local seizure discharge within a structure is unrelated to the ability to provoke a propagated seizure. Focal drug stimulation in certain brain areas (e.g., the dorsal hippocampus) can evoke local electrographic seizure discharge without evoking a propagated seizure, whereas in other regions (e.g., the AT) focal drug stimulation can evoke propagated seizures without first evoking local seizure discharge. Because a propagated seizure is an emergent property of interconnected neural circuits throughout the brain, we cannot expect to understand its development by examining regions of the brain, or groups of neurons, in isolation. Only by exploring the ways in which various distant brain regions interact during the process of seizure generation can we begin to gain insight into the complex dynamics that contribute to this process. In so doing, we can reveal important fundamental aspects of normal neural processes in brain at the same time as we attempt to unravel the functional neuroanatomical basis for epileptogenesis.

References

Ackermann, R. F., Chugani, H. T., Handforth, A., Moshé, S., Caldecott-Hazard, S. & Engel, J., Jr (1986). Autoradiographic studies of cerebral metabolism and blood flow in rat amygdala kindling. In *Kindling 3*, ed. J. A. Wada, pp. 78–87. New York: Raven Press.

Amato, G., Crescimanno, G., Sorbera, F. & La Grutta, V. (1982). Relationship between the striatal system and amygdaloid paroxysmal activity. *Experimental Neurology*, 77: 492–504.

Applegate, C. D., Samoriski, G. M. & Burchfiel, J. L. (1991). Evidence for the interaction of brainstem systems mediating seizure expression in kindling and electroconvulsive shock seizure model. *Epilepsy Research*, 10: 142–7.

Ben Ari, Y. (1985). Limbic seizure and brain damage produced by kainic acid: mechanisms and relevance to human temporal lobe epilepsy. *Neuroscience*, 14: 375–403.

Blackwood, D. H. R., Kapoor, V. & Martin, M. J. (1981). Regional changes in cerebral glucose utilization associated with amygdaloid kindling and electroshock in the rat. *Brain Research*, 204: 204–8.

Boschulte, J. & Gale, K. (1985). Decreased seizure response to electroshock and bicuculline in rats after one week of daily maximal electroshock treatment. *Society for Neuroscience Abstracts*, 11: 636.

Browning, R. (1985). Role of the brainstem reticular formation in tonic–clonic seizures: lesion and pharmacological studies. *Federation Proceedings*, 44: 2425–31.

Browning, R. A. (1986). Neuroanatomical localization of structures responsible for seizures in the GEPR: lesion studies. *Life Sciences*, 39: 857–67.

Browning, R., Maggio, R., Sahibzada, N. & Gale, K. (1993). Role of brainstem structures in seizures initiated from the deep prepiriform cortex of rats. *Epilepsia*, in press.

Browning, R. & Nelson, D. (1985). Variation in threshold and pattern of electroshock-induced seizures in rats depending on site of stimulation. *Life Sciences*, **37**: 2205–11.

Browning, R. & Nelson, D. (1986). Modification of electroshock and PTZ seizure patterns in rats after precollicular transections. *Experimental Neurology*, **93**: 546–56.

Browning, R. A., Simonton, R. L. & Turner, F. J. (1981a). Antagonism of experimentally-induced tonic seizures following a lesion of the midbrain tegmentum. *Epilepsia*, **22**: 595–601.

Browning, R., Turner, F., Simonton, R. & Bundman, M. (1981b). Effect of midbrain and pontine tegmental lesions on the maximal electroshock seizure pattern in rats. *Epilepsia*, **26**: 175–83.

Browning, R. A., Wang, C. & Faingold, C. L. (1991). Effect of norepinephrine depletion on audiogenic-like seizures elicited by microinfusion of an excitant amino acid into the inferior colliculus of normal rats. *Experimental Neurology*, **112**: 200–5.

Cain, D. P. (1982). Bidirectional transfer of intracerebrally administered pentylenetetrazol and electrical kindling. *Pharmacology, Biochemistry and Behavior*, **17**: 1111–13.

Cain, D. P. (1985). Transfer of kindling: clinical relevance and a hypothesis of its mechanism. *Progress in Neuropsychopharmacology, Biology and Psychiatry*, **9**: 467–72.

Cain, D. P. (1987). Kindling by repeated intraperitoneal or intracerebral injection of picrotoxin transfers to electrical kindling. *Experimental Neurology*, **97**: 243–54.

Cavalheiro, E. A., Bortolotto, Z. A. & Turski, L. (1987). Microinjections of the γ-aminobutyrate antagonist, bicuculline methiodide, into the caudate-putamen prevent amygdala-kindled seizures in rats. *Brain Research*, **411**: 370–2.

Cole, A. J., Abu-Shaka, S., Saffen, D. W., Baraban, J. M. & Worley, P. F. (1990). Rapid rise in transcription factor mRNAs in rat brain after electroshock-induced seizures. *Journal of Neurochemistry*, **55**: 1920–7.

Cole, A. J., Saffen, D. W., Baraban, J. M. & Worley, P. F. (1989). Rapid increase of an immediate early gene messenger RNA in hippocampal neurons by synaptic NMDA receptor activation. *Nature*, **340**: 474–6.

Collins, G. G. S., Ansou, J. & Surtes, L. (1983). Presynaptic kainate and N-methyl-D-aspartate receptors regulate excitatory amino acid release in the olfactory cortex. *Brain Research*, **265**: 157–9.

Collins, R. C., Kennedy, C., Sokoloff, L. & Plum, F. (1976). Metabolic anatomy of focal motor seizures. *Archives of Neurology*, **33**: 536–42.

Collins, R. C., Tearse, R. G. & Lothman, E. W. (1983). Functional anatomy of limbic seizures: focal discharges from medial entorhinal cortex in rat. *Brain Research*, **280**: 25–40.

Corcoran, M. E. (1988). Characteristics of accelerated kindling after depletion of noradrenaline in adult rat. *Neuropharmacology*, **27**: 1081–4.

Dailey, J. W., Reigel, C. E., Mishra, P. K. & Jobe, P. C. (1989). Neurobiology of seizure predisposition in the genetically epilepsy-prone rat. *Epilepsy Research*, **3**: 3–17.

Daval, J. L., Nakajima, J., Gleiter, C. H., Post, R. M. & Marangos, P. J. (1989). Mouse brain c-*fos* mRNA distribution following a single electroconvulsive shock. *Journal of Neurochemistry*, **52**: 1954–7.

Dean, P. & Gale, K. (1989). Anticonvulsant action of GABA receptor blockade in the nigrotectal target region. *Brain Research*, **477**: 391–5.

Depaulis, A., Snead, O. C., Marescaux, C. & Vergnes, M. (1989). Suppressive effects of intranigral injection of muscimol in three models of generalized non-convulsive epilepsy induced by chemical agents. *Brain Research*, **498**: 64–72.

Depaulis, A., Vergnes, M. & Marescaux, C., Lannes, B. & Warter, J. M. (1988). Evidence that activation of GABA receptors in the substantia nigra suppresses spontaneous spike-and-wave discharges in the rat. *Brain Research*, **448**: 20–9.

De Sarro, G. D., Meldrum, B. S. & Reavill, C. (1986). Anticonvulsant action of 2-amino-7-phosphonoheptanoic acid in the substantia nigra. *European Journal of Pharmacology*, **106**: 175–9.

DiChiara, G., Porceddu, M. L., Morelli, M., Mulas, M. L. & Gessa, G. L. (1979). Evidence for a GABAergic projection from the substantia nigra to the ventromedial thalamus and to the superior colliculus of the rat. *Brain Research*, **272**: 368–72.

Douglas, R. M., Dragunow, M. & Robertson, H. A. (1988). High frequency discharge of dentate granule cells, but not long term potentiation induce c-fos protein. *Molecular Brain Research*, **4**: 259–62.

Dragunow, M. & Robertson, H. A. (1987). Kindling stimulation induces c-fos protein(s) in granule cells of dentate gyrus. *Nature*, **328**: 441–2.

Dragunow, M. & Robertson, H. A. (1988*a*). Generalized seizures induce c-fos protein(s) in mammalian neurons. *Neuroscience Letters*, **82**: 157–61.

Dragunow, M. & Robertson, H. A. (1988*b*). Localization and induction of c-fos protein-like immunoreactive material in the nuclei of adult mammalian neurons. *Brain Research*, **440**: 252–60.

Engel, J., Jr, Wolfson, L. & Brown, L. (1978). Anatomical correlates of electrical and behavioral events related to amygdala kindling. *Annals of Neurology*, **3**: 538–44.

Faingold, C. L., Millan, M. H., Boersma, C. A. & Meldrum, B. S. (1988). Excitant amino acids and audiogenic seizures in the genetically epilepsy-prone rat. I. Afferent seizure initiation pathways. *Experimental Neurology*, **99**: 678–86.

Ferkany, J. W., Zaczek, R. & Coyle, J. T. (1982). Kainic acid stimulates excitatory amino acid neurotransmitter release at presynaptic receptors. *Nature*, **298**: 757–9.

Ferrendelli, J. A. (1984). Roles of biogenic amines and cyclic nucleotides in seizure mechanisms. *Annals of Neurology*, **16** (suppl.): S98–S103.

Fonnum, F., Gottesfeld, Z. & Grofova, I. (1978). Distribution of glutamate decarboxylase, choline acetyl-transferase and aromatic amino acid decarboxylase in the basal ganglia of normal and operated rats. Evidence for striatopallidal, striatoentopallidal, striatoentopeduncular and striatonigral GABAergic fibers. *Brain Research*, **143**: 125–38.

Frye, G., McCown, T. & Breese, G. (1983). Characterization of susceptibility to audiogenic seizures in ethanol-dependent rats after microinjection of GABA agonists into the inferior colliculus, substantia nigra or medial septum. *Journal of Pharmacology and Experimental Therapeutics*, **227**: 663–70.

Frye, G. D., McCown, T. J., Breese, G. R. & Peterson, S. L. (1986). GABAergic modulation of inferior colliculus excitability: role in ethanol withdrawal audiogenic seizures. *Journal of Pharmacology and Experimental Therapeutics*, **237**: 478–85.

Gabreels, F. (1972). De involved van phenytoine op de Purkinjecell van de rat. Doctoral dissertation, Catholic University of the Netherlands, Nijmegen.

Gale, K. (1990). Animal models of generalized convulsive seizures: some neuroanatomical differentiation of seizure types. In *Generalized Epilepsy, Neurobiological Approaches*, ed. M. Avoli, P. Gloor, G. Kostopoulos & R. Naquet, pp. 329–343. Boston: Birkhäuser.

Gale, K. (1991). Seizure generation, subcortical mechanisms. In *Encyclopedia of Human Biology*, vol. 6, ed. R. Dulbecco, pp. 329–43. San Diego: Academic Press.

Gale, K. (1992). Role of GABA in the genesis of chemoconvulsant seizures. *Proceedings of the VI International Congress of Toxicology*, ed. P. Preziosi. Amsterdam: Elsevier, in press.

Gale, K. & Browning, R. A. (1988). Anatomical and neurochemical substrates of clonic and tonic seizures. In *Mechanisms of Epileptogenesis from Membranes to Man*, ed. M. Dichter, pp. 111–52. New York: Plenum Press.

Gale, K. & Iadarola, M. J. (1980). GABAergic denervation of rat substantia nigra: functional and pharmacological properties. *Brain Research*, **183**: 217–23.

Gale, K., Pazos, A., Maggio, R., Japikse, K. & Pritchard, P. (1992). GABA-receptor blockade in superior colliculus blocks limbic-motor seizures evoked from area tempestas. *Brain Research*, in press.

Garant, D. S. & Gale, K. (1983). Lesions of substantia nigra protect against experimentally induced seizures. *Brain Research*, **273**: 156–61.

Garant, D. & Gale, K. (1986). Intranigral muscimol attentuates electrographic signs of seizure activity induced by intravenous bicuculline in rats. *European Journal of Pharmacology*, **124**: 365–9.

Gonzales, L. & Hettinger, M. (1984). Intranigral muscimol suppresses ethanol withdrawal seizures. *Brain Research*, **298**: 163–6.

Greenberg, M. E., Ziff, E. B. & Greene, L. A. (1986). Stimulation of neuronal acetylcholine receptors induces rapid gene transcription. *Science*, **234**: 80–3.

Gunne, L. M., Bachus, S. E. & Gale, K. (1988). Oral movements induced by interference with nigral GABA neurotransmission: relationship to tardive dyskinesias. *Experimental Neurology*, **100**: 459–69.

Hattori, T., McGeer, P. L., Fibiger, H. C. & McGeer, E. G. (1973). On the source of GABA-containing terminals in the substantia nigra. Electron microscopic, autoradiographic and biochemical studies. *Brain Research*, **54**: 103–14.

Hosford, D. A. & McNamara, J. O. (1988). Microinjection of muscimol into entopeduncular nucleus suppresses pilocarpine but not maximal electroshock seizures in rats. *Brain Research*, **462**: 205–10.

Iadarola, M. J. & Gale, K. (1982). Substantia nigra: site of anticonvulsant activity mediated by gamma-aminobutyric acid. *Science*, **218**: 1237–40.

Imura, J., Kaneko, Y. & Wada, J. A. (1981). Catecholamine and cholinergic systems and amygdaloid kindling. In *Kindling 2*, ed. J. A. Wada, pp. 265–87. New York: Raven Press.

Jeffrey, K. J., Abraham, W. C., Dragunow, M. & Mason, S. E. (1990). Induction of Fos like immunoreactivity and the maintenance of long-term potentiation in the dentate gyrus of unanesthetized rats. *Molecular Brain Research*, **8**: 267–74.

Jobe, P. C., Dailey, J. W. & Reigel, C. E. (1986). Noradrenergic and serotonergic determinants of seizure susceptibility and severity in genetically epilepsy-prone rats. *Life Science*, **39**: 775–82.

Kadekaro, M., Crane, A. M. & Sokoloff, L. (1985). Differential effects of electrical stimulation of sciatic nerve on metabolic activity in spinal cord and dorsal root ganglion in the rat. *Proceedings of the National Academy of Sciences, USA*, **82**: 6010–13.

La Grutta, V., Amato, G. & Zigami, M. T. (1971). The importance of caudate nucleus on paroxysmal activity in hippocampus of the cat. *Electroencephalography and Clinical Neurophysiology*, **31**: 57–59.

La Grutta, V., Sabatino, M., Ferraro, G., Liberti, G. & La Grutta, G. (1986). Modulation of paroxysmal activity in the hippocampus by caudate stimulation in the chronic cat. *Neuroscience Letters*, **67**: 251–6.

Lanaud, P., Maggio, R., Gale, K. & Grayson, D. (1993). Temporal and spatial pattern of expression of c-*fos*, *zif–268*, c-*jun* and *jun-B* mRNAs in rat brain following seizures evoked focally from the deep prepiriform cortex. *Experimental Neurology*, in press.

Le Gal La Salle, G. (1988). Long-lasting and sequential increase of c-fos oncoprotein expression in kainic acid-induced status epilepticus. *Neuroscience Letters*, **88**: 127–30.

Le Gal La Salle, G., Kijima, M. & Feldblum, S. (1983). Abortive amygdaloid kindled seizures following microinjection of gamma-vinyl-GABA in the vicinity of substantia nigra in rats. *Neuroscience Letters*, **36**: 69–74.

Le Gal La Salle, G. & Naquet, R. (1990). Audiogenic seizures evoked in DBA/2 mice induce c-*fos* oncogene expression in subcortical auditory nuclei. *Brain Research*, **158**: 308–12.

Le Gal La Salle, G., Shen, K. F. & Feldblum, S. (1984). Role of the hippocampus, amygdala and the substantia nigra in the evolution of status epilepticus induced by systemic injection of kainic acid in the rat. *Electroencephalography and Clinical Neurophysiology*, **14**: 235–40.

Lee, P. H., Obie, J. & Hong, J. S. (1988). Intrahippocampal injections of a specific mu-receptor ligand PL017 produce generalized convulsions in rats. *Brain Research*, **441**: 381–5.

Löscher, W., Czuczwar, S. J., Jäckel, R. & Schwartz, M. (1987). Effect of microinjections of gamma-vinyl-GABA or isoniazid into substantia nigra on the development of amygdala kindling in rats. *Experimental Neurology*, **95**: 622–38.

Lothman, E. W. & Collins, R. C. (1981). Kainic acid induced limbic seizures; metabolic, behavioral, electroencephalographic and neuropathological correlates. *Brain Research*, **218**: 299–318.

Maggio, R. & Gale, K. (1989). Seizures evoked from area tempestas are subject to control by GABA and glutamate receptors in substantia nigra. *Experimental Neurology*, **105**: 184–8.

Maggio, R., Lanaud, P., Grayson, D. R. & Gale, K. (1993). Expression of c-*fos* mRNA following seizures evoked from an epileptogenic site in the deep pyriform cortex: regional distribution in brain as shown by *in situ* hybridization. *Experimental Neurology*, in press.

Maggio, R., Liminga, U. & Gale, K. (1990*a*). Selective stimulation of kainate but not quisqualate or NMDA receptors in substantia nigra evokes limbic motor seizures. *Brain Research*, **528**: 223–30.

Maggio, R., Pazos, A. J., Ackermann, R. F. & Gale, K. (1990*b*). Anatomical characterization of the functional interrelation between area tempestas and substantia nigra in seizure propagation. *Society for Neuroscience, Abstracts*, **16**: 155.

Maggio, R., Sohn, E. & Gale, K. (1991). Lack of proconvulsant action of GABA depletion in substantia nigra in several seizure models. *Brain Research*, **547**: 1–6.

Majkowski, J. (1986). Kindling: a model for epilepsy and memory. *Acta Neurologica Scandinavica*, **109** (suppl.): 97–108.

Massotti, M. & Gale, K. (1989). Electroencephalographic evidence for a dose-related biphasic effect of morphine on bicuculline-induced seizures in the rat. *Epilepsy Research*, **4**: 81–9.

Mata, M., Fink, D. J., Gainer, H., Smith, C. B., Davidsen, L., Savaki, H., Schwartz, W. J. & Sokoloff, L. (1980). Activity dependent energy metabolism in rat posterior pituitary primarily reflects sodium pump activity. *Journal of Neurochemistry*, **34**: 213–15.

McCown, T. J., Greenwood, R. S., Frye, G. & Breese, G. R. (1984). Electrically-elicited seizures from the inferior colliculus: a potential site for the genesis of epilepsy? *Experimental Neurology*, **86**: 527–42.

McNamara, J. O. (1986). Kindling model of epilepsy. *Advances in Neurology*, **44**: 857–77.

McNamara, J. O., Galloway, M. T., Rigsbee, L. C. & Shin, C. (1984). Evidence implicating substantia nigra in regulation of kindled seizure threshold. *Journal of Neuroscience*, **4**: 2410–17.

Millan, M. H., Meldrum, B. S., Boersma, C. A. & Faingold, C. L. (1988). Excitant amino acids and audiogenic seizures in the genetically epilepsy prone rat. II. Efferent seizure propagating pathways. *Experimental Neurology*, **99**: 687–98.

Millan, M. H., Meldrum, B. S. & Faingold, C. S. (1986*a*). Induction of audiogenic seizure susceptibility by focal infusion of excitant amino acid or bicuculline into the inferior colliculus of normal rats. *Experimental Neurology*, **91**: 634–9.

Millan, M., Patel, S., Mello, L. & Meldrum, B. (1986*b*). Focal injection of 2-amino-7-phosphonoheptanoic acid into prepiriform cortex protects against pilocarpine-induced limbic seizures in rats. *Neuroscience Letters*, **70**: 69–74.

Mizuno, A., Mizobuchi, T., Ishibashi, Y. & Matsuda, M. (1989). c-*fos* mRNA induction under vitamin B_6 antagonist-induced seizure. *Neuroscience Letters*, **98**: 272–5.

Morgan, J. I., Cohen, D. R., Hempstead, J. L. & Curran, T. (1987). Mapping patterns of c-*fos* expression in the central nervous system after seizure. *Science*, **237**: 192–7.

Morgan, J. I. & Curran, T. (1986). The role of ion flux in the control of c-*fos* expression. *Nature*, **322**: 552–5.

Moshé, S. & Albala, B. (1984). Nigral muscimol infusions facilitate the development of seizures in immature rats. *Developmental Brain Research*, **13**: 305–8.

Nakajima, T., Daval, J. L., Gleiter, C. H., Deckert, J., Post, R. M. & Marangos, P. J. (1989). c-*fos* mRNA expression following electrically induced seizure and acute nociceptive stress in mouse brain. *Epilepsy Research*, **4**: 156–9.

Nudo, R. J. & Masterton, R. B. (1986). Stimulation-induced ^{14}C-2-deoxyglucose labeling of synaptic activity in the central auditory system. *Journal of Comparative Neurology*, **245**: 553–65.

Olianas, M. C., De Montis, G. M., Mulas, G. & Tagliamonte, A. (1978). The striatal dopaminergic function is mediated by the inhibition of a nigral, non-dopaminergic neuronal system via a striatonigral gabaergic pathway. *European Journal of Pharmacology*, **49**: 233–41.

Olney, J. W., Collins, R. C. & Sloviter, R. S. (1986). Excitotoxic mechanisms of epileptic brain damage. *Advances in Neurology*, **44**: 857–77.

Patel, S., Millan, M., Mello, L. & Meldrum, B. (1986). 2-Amino-7-phosphonoheptanoic acid (2APH) infusion into entopeduncular nucleus protects against limbic seizures in rats. *Neuroscience Letters*, **64**: 226–30.

Pazdernik, T. L., Cross, R. S., Giesler, M., Samson, F. E. & Nelson, S. R. (1985). Changes in local cerebral glucose utilization induced by convulsants. *Neuroscience*, **14**: 823–35.

Piredda, S. & Gale, K. (1985). A crucial epileptogenic site in the deep prepiriform cortex. *Nature*, **317**: 623–5.

Piredda, S. & Gale, K. (1986a). Anticonvulsant action of 2-amino-7-phosphonoheptanoic acid and muscimol in the deep prepiriform cortex. *European Journal of Pharmacology*, **120**: 115–18.

Piredda, S. & Gale, K. (1986b). Role of excitatory amino acid transmission in the genesis of seizures elicited from the deep prepiriform cortex. *Brain Research*, **377**: 205–10.

Piredda, S., Pavlick, M. & Gale, K. (1987). Anticonvulsant effects of GABA elevation in the deep prepiriform cortex. *Epilepsy Research*, **1**: 102–6.

Racine, R. (1972). Modification of seizure activity by electrical stimulation. II. Motor seizures. *Electroencephalography and Clinical Neurophysiology*, **32**: 281–94.

Raines, A. & Anderson, R. J. (1976). The effects of acute cerebellectomy on maximal electroshock seizures and the anticonvulsant efficacy of diazepam in the rat. *Epilepsia*, **17**: 177–82.

Ramer, D. & Pinel, J. P. J. (1976). Progressive intensification of motor seizures produced by periodic electroconvulsive shock. *Experimental Neurology*, **51**: 421–33.

Redgrave, P., Dean, P. & Simkins, M. (1988). Intratectal glutamate suppresses pentylenetetrazol-induced spike-and-wave discharge. *European Journal of Pharmacology*, **158**: 283–7.

Reigel, C. E., Dailey, J. W. & Jobe, P. C. (1986). The genetically epilepsy-prone rat: an overview of seizure prone characteristics and responsiveness to anticonvulsant drugs. *Life Sciences*, **39**: 763–74.

Saffen, D. W., Cole, A. J., Worley, P. F., Christy, B. A., Ryder, K. & Baraban, J. M. (1988). Convulsant-induced increase in transcription factor messenger mRNAs in rat brain. *Proceedings of the National Academy of Sciences, USA*, **85**: 7795–9.

Savage, D. D., Reigel, C. E. & Jobe, P. C. (1986). Angular bundle kindling is accelerated in rats with a genetic predisposition to acoustic stimulus-induced seizures. *Brain Research*, **376**: 412–15.

Sheng, M. & Greenberg, M. E. (1990). The regulation and function of c-*fos* and other immediate early genes in the nervous system. *Neuron*, **4**: 447–85.

Shin, C., McNamara, J. O., Morgan, J. I., Curran, T. & Cohen, D. R. (1990). Induction of c-*fos* mRNA expression by afterdischarge in the hippocampus of naive and kindled rats. *Journal of Neurochemistry*, **55**: 1050–5.

Swinyard, E. (1972). Electrically induced convulsions. In *Experimental Models of Epilepsy*, ed. D. Purpura, J. Penry, D. Tower, D. Woodbury & R. Walters, pp. 433–58. New York: Raven Press.

Szekely, A. M., Barbaccia, M. L., Alho, H. & Costa, E. (1989). In primary cultures of cerebellar granule cells the activation of N-methyl-D-aspartate-sensitive glutamate receptors induces c-*fos* mRNA expression. *Molecular Pharmacology*, **35**:, 401–8.

Szekely, A. M., Costa, E. & Grayson, D. R. (1990). Transcriptional program coordination by NMDA-sensitive glutamate receptor stimulation in primary cultures of cerebellar neurons. *Molecular Pharmacology*, **38**: 624–33.

Testa, G. & Gloor, P. (1974). Generalized penicillin epilepsy in the cat: effect of midbrain cooling. *Electroencephalography and Clinical Neurophysiology*, **36**: 517–24.

Thai, L., He, X. P., Zhang, W. Q. & Hong, J. S. (1990). Synergistic effects of co-injection of mu and glutamate receptor agonists into the ventral hippocampus in producing seizure activity. *Society for Neuroscience Abstracts*, **16**: 22.

Turski, L., Cavalheiro, E. A., Calderazzo-Filho, L. S., Bortolotto, Z. A., Klockgether, T., Ikonomidou, C. & Turski, W. A. (1989). The basal ganglia, the deep prepyriform cortex, and seizure spread: bicuculline is anticonvulsant in the rat striatum. *Proceedings of the National Academy of Sciences, USA*, **86**: 1694–7.

Turski, W. A., Cavalheiro, E. A., Calderazzo-Filho, L. S., Kleinrok, Z., Czuczwar, S. J. & Turski, L. (1985). Injections of picrotoxin and bicuculline into the amygdaloid complex of the rat: an electroencephalographic, behavioral and morphological analysis. *Neuroscience*, **14**: 37–53.

Turski, W. A., Cavalheiro, E. A., Schwartz, M., Czuczwar, S. J., Kleinrok, Z. & Turski, L. (1983). Limbic seizures produced by pilocarpine in rats: behavioral, electroencephalographic and neuropathological study. *Behavioral Brain Research*, **9**: 315–36.

Turski, L., Cavalheiro, E. A., Schwartz, M., Turski, F. W. A., DeMorales Mello, L. E. A., Bortolotto, Z. A., Klockgether, T. & Sonntag, K. H. (1986*a*). Susceptibility to seizures produced by pilocarpine in rats after microinjections of isoniazid or gamma-vinyl-GABA into the substantia nigra. *Brain Research*, **370**: 294–309.

Turski, L., Cavalheiro, E., Turski, W. & Meldrum, B. (1986*b*). Excitatory neurotransmission within substantia nigra pars reticulata regulates threshold for seizures produced by pilocarpine in rats: effects of intranigral 2-amino-7-phosphonoheptanoate and N-methyl-D-aspartate. *Neuroscience*, **18**: 61–77.

Turski, L., Meldrum, B. S., Cavalheiro, E. A., Calderazzo-Filho, L. S., Bortolotto, Z. A., Ikonomidou-Turski, C. & Turski, W. A. (1987). Paradoxical anticonvulsant activity of the excitatory amino acid N-methyl-D-aspartate in the rat caudate-putamen. *Proceedings of the National Academy of Sciences, USA*, **84**: 1689–93.

Uemura, S. & Kimura, H. (1988). Amygdaloid kindling with bicuculline methiodide in rats. *Experimental Neurology*, **102**: 346–53.

Vincent, S. R., Hattori, T. & McGeer, E. G. (1978). The nigrotectal projection: a biochemical and ultrastructural characterization. *Brain Research*, **151**: 159–64.

Wardas, J., Graham, J. & Gale, K. (1990). Evidence for a role of glycine in area tempestas for triggering convulsive seizures. *European Journal of Pharmacology*, **187**: 59–66.

White, J. D. & Gall, C. M. (1987). Differential regulation of neuropeptide and protooncogene mRNA content in the hippocampus following recurrent seizures. *Molecular Brain Research*, **3**: 21–9.

Wisden, W., Errington, M. L., Williams, S., Dunnett, S. B., Waters, C., Hitchcock, D., Evan, G., Bliss, T. V. & Hunt, S. P. (1990). Differential expression of immediate early genes in hippocampus and spinal cord. *Neuron*, **4**: 603–14.

Zawia, N. H. & Bondy, S. C. (1990). Electrically stimulated rapid gene expression in the brain: ornithine decarboxylase and c-*fos*. *Molecular Brain Research*, **7**: 243–7.

Zhong, P., Schlichting, J. & Gale, K. (1988). Effects of ethosuximide and phenytoin on convulsions induced by focal injection of bicuculline in area tempestas: comparison with effects on systemic pentylenetetrazol-induced convulsions. Poster presented at Generalized Epilepsy Symposium, Montreal.

Zrebeet, H. A. & Gale, K. (1988). Convulsant actions of putative endogenous ligands for excitatory amino acid receptors upon focal injection in area tempestas. *Society for Neuroscience Abstracts*, **14**: 864.

3

Genetic models of the epilepsies

PHILLIP C. JOBE, PRAVIN K. MISHRA,
NANDOR LUDVIG, and JOHN W. DAILEY

Introduction

The normal human brain can produce seizures upon stimulation with a convulsant drug or an electrical current. This capacity of intact brain is not, however, tantamount to epilepsy. Rather, the disease occurs in response to a multifaceted etiology in which genetically determined 'seizure susceptibility factors' play a crucial role. Therefore, seizure-triggering mechanisms may be activated in epileptic patients by potentially unrecognized variations in intrinsic neuronal activity or by input from environmental stimuli that do not cause seizures in normal people. The complex pathophysiological interplay between combinations of these various factors determines the seizure disorder that will be exhibited by a given patient.

The genetic animal models of the epilepsies fill a special niche in epileptology because they provide the means for examining questions relating to the fundamental mechanisms of seizure predisposition. They can also be used to investigate the mechanisms by which seizures occur, as can neurologically normal animals. Seizures can be initiated in almost all mammals, including neurologically normal humans. Humans with epilepsy, however, are neurologically distinctive: they exhibit seizures in response to stimuli that do not cause such episodes in normal human subjects. Since the genetic models share this trait, they provide an opportunity to elucidate the underlying neurological dysfunctions that distinguish epilepsy from normal neurological activity, especially from the mechanisms that lead to seizures when the normal brain is subjected to a seizure-provoking stimulus. The genetic models cannot circumvent the need for continued investigations of seizure mechanisms and other pertinent biological processes in neurologically normal subjects. Only by comparison of phenomena in the genetic models with normal subjects can the mechanisms of seizure predisposition be judged.

Experimentation with the genetic models has progressed significantly in the past 20 years. The results partly clarify the fundamental property of seizure predisposition. Some of the insights have emerged from studies designed to determine the overt manifestations of this trait. The results of these experiments enabled and prompted neuroanatomical, biochemical and electrophysiological inquiries. Also, scientific interest has developed in the role of seizure predisposition in the appearance of genetically determined seizure-triggering mechanisms and in other related issues. These areas of inquiry are summarized below. Each broad research category offers opportunities for future investigation. Space limitations here prohibit an exhaustive description of the contributions derived from studies of each of the different genetic models. In lieu of a more comprehensive approach, we have chosen to highlight and clarify the areas of inquiry by presentation of data only from selected models. We have relied often on observations made with genetically epilepsy prone rats (GEPRs) because they are models of convulsive epilepsy and because they are the chief models associated with our laboratory. The genetically absence epilepsy rat (GAER) has been emphasized because it is a model of non-convulsive epilepsy. The photosensitive epileptic baboon is accorded special attention because it is a primate. Studies with genetically epileptic mice and gerbils are highlighted for comparative purposes and because some elements of their seizure predisposition contrast with those of the other models. Genetic models of the epilepsies have been derived also in chickens, other mice and rats, rabbits and dogs (see multispecies reviews by Jobe & Laird, 1981, 1987; Löscher, 1984). They, too, could have been relied upon for exemplification. Their exclusion does not stem from a judgment that they are less potentially valuable to the field of epileptology.

Overt characteristics of seizure predisposition

Seizure predisposition in the genetic models is striking. This predilection apparently exists also in the case of the human epilepsies. For example, small doses of pentylenetetrazol cause seizure discharges in some epileptic patients, but not in humans without neurological disorder (Kaufman *et al.*, 1947). Also, epileptic humans have spontaneous seizures and some exhibit seizures in response to externally encountered stimuli that fail to cause seizures in neurologically normal subjects.

Predisposition in genetically epilepsy prone rats

A non-epileptic control colony and a moderate seizure (GEPR-3) and a severe seizure (GEPR-9) strain of the GEPR have been developed (Reigel *et al.*, 1986). The non-epileptic control colony was initiated because the population of unselected Sprague-Dawley rats carries the genetic material that is responsible for seizure predisposition in GEPRs. In normal Sprague-Dawley rats, somewhat fewer than 4% exhibit evidence of seizure activity in response to sound. Selective breeding of these animals for seizure traits has resulted in the present GEPR colonies.

GEPR-3s and GEPR-9s share all three types of seizure predisposition described above for human epilepsies. First, some exhibit spontaneous seizures (Dailey *et al.*, 1989). Second, both colonies exhibit exaggerated responsiveness to seizures induced by many modalities that in larger doses or magnitudes also produce seizures in non-epileptic rats (Dailey *et al.*, 1988; Jobe *et al.*, 1988; Browning *et al.*, 1990; Savage *et al.*, 1986). Third, almost all GEPRs are susceptible to the induction of seizures by stimuli such as sound, which fail to induce seizures in non-epileptic adult controls (Jobe *et al.*, 1973a; Mishra *et al.*, 1988b, 1989; Faingold & Naritoku, 1992). Handling-induced convulsions have been noted occasionally in GEPR-9s (P. C. Jobe and P. K. Mishra, unpublished results). Generally speaking, all three types of seizure predisposition are more pronounced in GEPR-9s than in GEPR-3s (Savage *et al.*, 1986; Jobe *et al.*, 1988; Browning *et al.*, 1990).

Seizure predisposition is represented broadly throughout the GEPR brain, including circuitry of the brainstem and the forebrain (Jobe *et al.*, 1992). The relatively mild audiogenic seizures of the GEPR-3 and the more severe audiogenic seizures of the GEPR-9 are expressions of brainstem predisposition (Browning, 1987; Burnham, 1987; Jobe, 1987; Browning *et al.*, 1990; Jobe *et al.*, 1992). Also, several other types of brainstem seizure predilection have been documented in GEPRs (Dailey *et al.*, 1988; Jobe *et al.*, 1988, 1992; Browning *et al.*, 1990). In contrast, seizures characterized by facial and forelimb clonus with or without rearing and falling occur in response to activation of forebrain seizure circuitry. Convulsions produced by intracerebral limbic kindling and by minimal electroshock from corneal electrodes are expressions of forebrain seizures. In this context, GEPRs exhibit an exaggerated responsiveness to forebrain seizures elicited by either technique (Savage *et al.*, 1986; Browning *et al.*, 1990).

Ontogenetic evaluations have contributed to a better understanding of seizure predisposition in GEPRs (Jobe *et al.*, 1980; Hjeresen *et al.*, 1987; Ribak *et al.*, 1988*b*; Franck *et al.*, 1989; Reigel *et al.*, 1989*a*). For example, we now know that audiogenic seizures develop similarly in GEPR-3s and GEPR-9s until divergence appears in the fourth postnatal week. At this latest point of equivalence, audiogenic seizure severity of GEPR-3s has exceeded its adult phenotype, whereas that of the GEPR-9 has not yet escalated to the adult level. Past this point, GEPR-3s exhibit a decline in mean seizure severity, achieving their adult phenotype by 45 days of age. In contrast, GEPR-9s experience a final period of escalation, achieving the characteristic maximal severity equivalent to that of adulthood around postnatal day 45.

Also, the generalized aspects of seizure predisposition in GEPRs do not appear to depend on the presence of audiogenic seizure susceptibility. Observations by Franck *et al.* (1989) suggested that the condition of generalized seizure predisposition in the GEPR occurs independently of the specific abnormalities underlying audiogenic seizure susceptibility. Experimentally, animals from the GEPR-9 colony were divided into two groups, those with audiogenic seizure susceptibility and litter mates without susceptibility. Both groups of GEPRs were characterized by abnormally low thresholds to flurothyl-induced clonic and tonic extensor convulsions.

Unlike in adult animals, forebrain-like seizures occur as a secondary event in response to brainstem convulsions in developing GEPR-3s (Reigel *et al.*, 1989*a*). On postnatal day 15, half of the GEPR-3s exhibiting generalized audiogenic clonus (typical of brainstem seizures) subsequently experience 10 to 15 s of quiescence followed by piloerection, tremor and a series of unilateral forelimb clonic episodes accompanied by rearing. These episodes of forelimb clonus and rearing are similar to limbic seizures. Secondary forelimb clonus and rearing are exhibited by 100% of the pups at 16 days of age. By day 45, however, such episodes no longer occur. Secondary forebrain-like seizures do not appear to occur in GEPR-3s that experience audiogenic seizures of class 4 (Jobe *et al.*, 1973*a*) or greater. Also, the secondary seizures do not seem to emerge in GEPR-9s. These observations support the hypothesis that, early in life, brainstem epileptic neuronal activity can activate seizures within the forebrain of GEPR-3s (Jobe *et al.*, 1992). Moreover, they are compatible with the concept that the forebrain seizure circuitry may have an especially low threshold in GEPR-3s during this period of maturation. Possibly, these GEPR-3s are characterized by a deficiency in the functional status of a crucial area of the brain that serves as an interface between the caudal and rostral seizure circuitries. Accordingly, this pivotal area might facilitate cross-activation during the vulnerable period of early development. Secondary forebrain seizures may disappear with increasing age because developmentally emergent anticonvulsant mechanisms appear within the interfacing area.

Predisposition in genetically absence epilepsy rats

Spontaneous, bilaterally synchronous spike-and-wave discharges in cortical electroencephalography (EEG), coupled with behavioral arrest, were noted in a colony of Wistar rats maintained in Strasbourg, France, by Vergnes *et al.* (1982). The original observations showed that approximately 38% of the animals tested exhibited this trait. Subsequent imposition of a selective inbreeding protocol led to an increase in the fraction of progeny with spike-and-wave discharges. By the third generation of inbreeding, all progeny were exhibiting spontaneous spike-and-wave discharges (Vergnes *et al.*, 1987*b*). These GAERs contrast clearly with other Wistar rats that do not appear to exhibit spike-and-wave discharges and may therefore be useful as control subjects in experimental paradigms.

Seizure predisposition in the GAER was documented with an additional finding. Relatively low doses of pro-γ-aminobutyric acid (GABA)-ergic drugs within specific relay nuclei of the medio-lateral thalamus activate spike-and-wave discharges in the GAER, whereas higher doses are required to produce these electrographic discharges in non-epileptic control rats (Liu *et al.*, 1991). These observations suggest that the GAER has an abnormally low threshold for GABAergic activation of spike-and-wave discharges. Experimental elucidation of the mechanism underlying the seizure predisposition of the GAER may provide an important insight into epileptogenesis. Conceptually, epilepsy might occur in a largely normal brain afflicted with a discrete focus caused by abnormally large amounts of endogenous seizure-producing transmitter being released onto relatively normal neurons. To investigate this contingency, one might determine the mechanism by which pro-GABAergic agents produce seizures in normal animals. The GAER and many humans with epilepsy are, however, seemingly predisposed to seizures caused by low doses of convulsant drugs or seizure-producing neurotransmitters. Since epilepsy probably derives from this type of seizure predisposition, experimental paradigms should be designed to determine the mechanisms that cause a predisposed subject to exhibit seizures when normal subjects do not. The

GAER provides an ideal model for such studies in the domain of non-convulsive seizures.

Predisposition in epileptic mice

Many strains of mice are predisposed to epilepsy. Predisposition is manifest as either spontaneous or environmentally induced seizures. The strains that experience environmentally induced seizures generally also have behavioral convulsions. These are induced by sensory input such as auditory stimulation, vestibular stimulation, or handling. The most prominent example of a mouse model that experiences audiogenic seizures is the DBA/2 mouse (Chapman & Meldrum, 1987). Seizures induced by vestibular stimulation are seen in the *el* (epilepsy like) mouse (Naruse *et al.*, 1960; Suzuki & Nakamoto, 1977; Mori, 1988). Handling-induced seizures occur in the *quaking* mouse (Chermat *et al.*, 1979).

Spontaneous seizures can be either convulsive or 'absence-like'. Absence-like spike-and-wave discharges and focal motor seizures are seen in the *tottering* mouse (Noebels & Sidman, 1979; Heller *et al.*, 1983) and the *spontaneous seizure* mutant (Maxson *et al.*, 1983). Spontaneous tonic seizures are displayed by the *lurcher* (Noebels, 1979); and *staggerer* (Sax *et al.*, 1968). Besides being susceptible to audiogenic seizures, DBA/2 mice have lower than normal seizure thresholds for maximal electroshock (Ludvig *et al.*, 1985a) and flurothyl (Davis & King, 1966; Marley *et al.*, 1986). Also, young DBA/2 mice occasionally experience tonic convulsions in response to handing (Chapman & Meldrum, 1987).

Predisposition in the epileptic Mongolian gerbil

In the late 1960s, Thiessen *et al.* (1968), Goldblatt (1968), and others observed that some of the Mongolian gerbils (*Meriones unguiculatus*) exhibited motor seizures in response to a variety of stimuli. Subsequently, epileptic seizure-sensitive and non-epileptic seizure-resistant strains were developed by Loskota *et al.* (1974). Seizures can be induced in the Mongolian gerbil by natural stimuli, many of which fail to cause seizures in the other genetic models. Exposure to a novel environment, falling from a height, or handling by the experimenter are occasionally effective convulsant modalities in susceptible subjects. Sometimes seizures occur in response to environments that are 'strange' (Kaplan, 1975) or difficult to explore (Ludvig *et al.*, 1991). Specific sensory stimuli are demonstrated to be ineffective in triggering seizures (Ludvig *et al.*, 1991). Debate surrounds the possibility that one or more undefined factors are common to the heterogeneous group of seizure-precipitating factors in the gerbils. Some authors emphasize the role of stress (Frey, 1987), while others underscore a unique role for exploratory behavior.

Predisposition in the epileptic baboons

Electrographic seizures can be elicited in the Senegalese baboon, *Papio papio*, by an intermittent light stimulus (ILS) (Killam *et al.*, 1967; Naquet, 1973; Naquet & Meldrum, 1972, 1986; Menini & Naquet, 1980). Convulsions may also become evident. Light-induced seizures in *Papio papio* were discovered by Killam *et al.* (1966*a,b,c*). Although susceptibility to ILS-induced seizures probably occurs in a small proportion of the general population of baboons, a remarkably high fraction of the Senegalese animals exhibit this trait.

ILS-induced convulsions in the epileptic baboons begin as a limited bilaterally synchronous myoclonus (Killam *et al.*, 1966*b*, 1967). Secondary generalization progressing to tonic convulsion may also occur (Meldrum *et al.*, 1970). Seizures have also been induced in *Papio papio* by hyperventilation, excessive exertion, stress and restraint, or perhaps the handling necessary for restraint (Killam *et al.*, 1967; Killam, 1976; Killam & Killam, 1984). Furthermore, the pentylenetetrazol threshold for seizures is thought to be abnormally low. *Papio papio* may also exhibit spontaneous seizures.

Electrophysiology of seizure predisposition

Electrophysiological evaluations are a cornerstone of epilepsy research. In studies with the genetic models, EEG has been used to verify the epileptic nature of convulsions and to clarify key questions related to seizure neuroanatomy.

GEPR electrophysiology

The inferior colliculus appears to play a critical role in audiogenic seizure initiation in the GEPR (Faingold & Naritoku, 1992). Paralyzed and behaving GEPR-9s exhibit acoustically induced epileptiform extracellular action potentials in the central nucleus of the inferior colliculus (Faingold *et al.*, 1986*b,c*; Faingold & Boersma-Anderson, 1988). These abnormalities consist of prominent peaks of firing at short latencies from both the onset and offset of the high intensity acoustic stimulus. The episodes of offset peaks seemingly represent afterdischarges similar to the poststimulus neural activity in other seizure models (see Faingold & Naritoku, 1992). Additional experiments indicate that binaurally induced inhibition of neuronal firing in the inferior colliculus is deficient in GEPRs (Faingold *et al.*, 1986*a*). The absence of this protective process may contribute to audiogenic seizure susceptibility.

With larger bipolar electrodes prepared for detecting localized electro-encephalographic field potentials within the central nucleus of the inferior colliculus, Ludvig & Moshé (1989) clearly demonstrated paroxysmal spikes and waves in unanesthetized freely moving GEPRs subjected to a seizure-inducing acoustic stimulus. These discharges are accompanied by the behavioral seizures defined by Jobe *et al.* (1973*a*). The GEPR-9s used in the experiment of Ludvig & Moshé (1989) exhibited spike discharges during the initial wild running episode and rhythmic spike-and-wave activity during the clonic–tonic convulsions. Non-epileptic control rats did not exhibit electrographic or behavioral seizures upon exposure to the acoustic stimulus. Holmes *et al.* (1990) also noted acoustically induced epileptic spiking in GEPR-9s that appears in the inferior colliculus before spreading to the medial geniculate and other brain areas.

The epileptic condition of the auditory system represents only one aspect of seizure predisposition in the GEPR. A predilection to seizures is clearly evident in the forebrain structures, including those of the limbic system. Yet, most electrophysiological studies have been orientated towards the auditory system. Outside this area, one preliminary and interesting electrophysiological finding has been pointed out by Schwartzkroin (1986). He detected a decrease in the efficacy and/or occurrence of inhibitory postsynaptic potentials in the hippocampus of the GEPR. The role that the abnormal hippocampus of the GEPR plays in forebrain seizure predisposition and the possible influence of this dysfunction on brainstem seizure circuitry remains to be elucidated. Electrophysiological studies designed to clarify such issues are essential for the synthesis of an accurate and complete concept of seizure predisposition in the GEPR.

GAER electrophysiology

The frequency within each episode of multiple spike-and-wave discharges in the GAER is approximately 7 to 8 Hz (Vergnes *et al.*, 1990). The amplitude of the spike-and-wave discharges varies from 300 to 1000 µV, approximately three to six times greater than the baseline. Individual episodes of spike-and-wave activity occur about once per minute. Typically, either the animals are already immobile or they become immobile at the onset of the episodes of spike-and-wave activity. Often, rhythmic twitching of the vibrissae and a head drop occur during the electrographic episodes. A sudden extension of the head has been reported to precede recovery of mobility (Vergnes *et al.*, 1990). Vergnes *et al.* are aware that the 7 to 8 Hz in the GAER exceeds the 3 Hz characteristic of human absence epilepsy. They have concluded, however, that the faster rate is compatible with a rodent model of human non-convulsive epilepsy.

Epileptic mice electrophysiology

The characteristics of audiogenic seizures exhibited by mice suggest that they are driven by brainstem seizure circuitry. The *tottering* mouse presents a marked contrast. This animal has been of considerable interest, in part because it was the first genetic rodent model of spontaneous non-convulsive seizures characterized by spike-and-wave discharges (Green & Sidman, 1962). This model also may exhibit ataxia and intermittent focal myoclonic convulsions (Noebels & Sidman, 1979). Arrest seizures begin to develop in the third postnatal week while ataxia and intermittent myoclonic seizures are seen by the fourth postnatal week (Noebels, 1986). Arrest seizures occur coincidentally with 6 to 7 Hz spike-and-wave discharges (Kaplan *et al.*, 1979; Noebels & Sidman, 1979; Noebels, 1984, 1986).

Epileptic gerbil electrophysiology

Six successive pathological EEG seizure patterns occur in response to novelty in the epileptic gerbil: the incipient seizure, four phases of generalized seizure, and one phase of postictal depression (Loskota & Lomax, 1975; Majkowski & Donadio, 1984). The incipient seizure is characterized by sporadic spikes and sharp waves, usually over the occipital areas of both hemispheres. This initial response has no convulsive concomitant. As the behavioral seizures emerge, abnormalities in the electroencephalogram progress. Generalized spikes and spike-and-wave complexes of gradually increasing amplitude dominate the cortical and hippocampal tracings. Subsequently, the intensity of the electrographic activity decays into a pattern of reduced amplitude and generalization, and the electroencephalographic seizure is terminated.

Epileptic baboon electrophysiology

ILS-induced seizures in the epileptic baboon are characterized by paroxysmal polyspikes, polyspikes and waves, and spikes and waves (Naquet & Meldrum, 1986; Naquet *et al.*, 1988). These discharges are bilateral and synchronous. The electrographic seizures are either focally contained or they are generalized (Naquet *et al.*, 1988). The electrographic abnormalities associated with either type of seizure appear to originate in the fronto-rolandic region. Although the initial responses to ILS are 'hardly appreciable,' they increase progressively in amplitude as the ILS continues (Naquet *et al.*, 1988). With progression of the seizure, focally contained bilateral spikes and waves or waves become slower and larger in amplitude. Spread of the discharges may occur so that the seizures become more neuroanatomically extensive. Maximally, the ILS-induced seizures encompass all areas of the brain with the exception of the limbic structures (Fischer-Williams *et al.*, 1968).

Biochemistry of seizure predisposition

GEPR neurochemistry

Monoaminergic regulation of seizure predisposition

Noradrenergic and serotonergic deficits appear to serve as determinants of forebrain and brainstem seizure predisposition in the GEPR. In contrast, evidence consistently indicates that dopaminergic systems have no role in the seizure regulatory processes of the GEPR brainstem. Evidence pertaining to these concepts has been summarized by Dailey *et al.* (1989) and Jobe *et al.* (1992). In general terms, experimentally induced changes in noradrenergic or serotonergic activity produce reciprocal changes in audiogenic seizure *severity* in the GEPR (Jobe *et al.*, 1973*a,b,c*; Ko *et al.*, 1982, 1984; Mishra *et al.*, 1988*a*; Yan *et al.*, 1990*a,b*). In contrast, alterations in dopaminergic activity are without effect (Jobe *et al.*, 1973*a*; Ko *et al.*, 1982). Moreover, noradrenergic deficits appear to contribute importantly (along with non-monoaminergic factors) to the appearance of *susceptibility* to audiogenic seizures (Jobe *et al.*, 1981; Reigel & Aldrich, 1990).

In addition to these pharmacological investigations, several studies have demonstrated innate noradrenergic and serotonergic deficits in GEPRs, but intrinsic dopaminergic influences appear to be normal in the GEPR. This finding, coupled with the absence of an effect on audiogenic seizures by pharmacologically induced changes in dopaminergic activity, provides a basis for rejecting the dopaminergic hypothesis of seizure predisposition in the GEPR.

Neurochemical investigations of innate serotonergic deficits have been more limited than those for noradrenergic deficiencies. With the exception of one examination of receptors (Booker *et al.*, 1986), studies of serotonergic neurons have been restricted to analyses of neurotransmitter concentration in discrete regions of the brain (Jobe *et al.*, 1982; Jobc *et al.*, 1986). Noradrenergic deficits have been further documented by assessments of other key indices of function: determinations of turnover rates and the fractional rate constants (Jobe *et al.*, 1984), dopamine β-hydroxylase activity (Browning *et al.*, 1989*b*), tyrosine hydroxylase activity (Dailey & Jobe, 1986), high affinity uptake into synaptosomes (Browning *et al.*, 1989*b*), the number of dopamine β-hydroxylase-immunoreactive processes per unit volume of brain tissue (Lauterborn & Ribak, 1989), and receptor binding and/or signal transduction (Ko *et al.*, 1984; Nicoletti *et al.*, 1986; Yourick *et al.*, 1990).

These studies all support the concept that the GEPR brain is characterized by deficits in the number of noradrenergic terminals and in the amount of norepinephrine released per terminal. Moreover, these presynaptic deficiencies are apparently not compensated for by postsynaptic increments. Serotonergic systems may be similarly characterized, but additional studies will be required to bring our understanding of the role of these neurons to the same level as that for norepinephrine. The possibility that postsynaptic compensatory processes are deficient for noradrenergic and serotonergic systems warrants elucidation.

The studies cited above, together with ontogenetic investigations (Hjeresen *et al.*, 1987; Reigel *et al.*, 1987*a,b*, 1989*b*; Ribak *et al.*, 1988*b*), provide a means for determining whether monoaminergic deficits in the GEPR occur as a consequence rather than as a probable cause of seizure predispositions. The observations clearly support the concept that monoaminergic deficits are determinants of seizure predisposition in the GEPR and that they do not occur as a result of seizure activity (see Jobe *et al.*, 1992).

Amino acid neurotransmitters

The existence of non-monoaminergic determinants of seizure predisposition in the GEPR is becoming increasingly clear (Jobe *et al.*, 1981; Faingold & Copley, 1988; Faingold *et al.*, 1988*a,b*; Faingold & Naritoku, 1992). The preponderance of evidence supports a GABAergic defect as an important cause of the seizure prone state of the GEPR (Duplisse *et al.*, 1974; Duplisse, 1976; Laird & Huxtable, 1976; Tacke & Braestrup, 1984; Faingold *et al.*, 1985, Roberts *et al.*, 1985*a,b*; Booker *et al.*, 1986; Browning *et al.*, 1989*a*; Roberts & Ribak, 1986; Waterhouse, 1986; Ribak *et al.*, 1988*a,b*; Lasley *et al.*, 1989). In our view, the results of these studies support the concept that GABAergic deficits characterize the GEPR brain and that the normal noradrenergic facilitation of GABAergic inhibition does not occur in the GEPRs.

Within the inferior colliculus itself, the functional GABAergic deficiency may contribute to the onset of electrographic seizure activity in response to ascending auditory impulses (Faingold & Naritoku, 1992). The conversion of the rostrally directed impulses into paroxysmal discharges may, however, depend on contributions from the excessive activity of neurons utilizing excitatory amino acids as neurotransmitters (Chapman *et al.*, 1986; Lehmann *et al.*, 1986; Millan *et al.*, 1986, 1988; Faingold & Boersma-Anderson, 1988; Faingold & Copley, 1988; Faingold *et al.*, 1988*a*, 1989; Meldrum *et al.*, 1988; Ribak *et al.*, 1988*a,b*; Lasley *et al.*, 1989; Riaz & Faingold, 1989). The inferor colliculus is included among the areas wherein excessive indices of excitatory amino acids have been detected.

Some of the excessive aspartatergic and glutamatergic indices cited above also exist in the forebrain. Perhaps the seizure predisposition in these more rostral structures also depends partially on circuitry activation by aspartic and glutamic acids. However, some evidence suggests that potassium-stimulated excessive release of excitatory amino acid in the GEPR hippocampus (Lehmann *et al.*, 1986) may be at least partially offset by abnormally low numbers of kainate receptor binding sites in this structure (Mills *et al.*, 1990).

Although all studies do not support the hypothesis, benzodiazepine receptors associated with the $GABA_A$ complex may be present in excessive numbers in the GEPR brain (Mimaki *et al.*, 1984; Tacke & Braestrup, 1984; Booker *et al.*, 1986). These increments are consistent with the documented existence of an excessive density of $GABA_A$ receptor complexes in the GEPR.

Recently, Ducis *et al.* (1990) reported deficits in the so-called 'peripheral-type' benzodiazepine receptor in cultured astrocytes derived from GEPR-9s. According to the evidence marshalled by these investigators, the reduced number of these receptors in GEPR-9s could represent an adaptive response to seizure predisposition, since fewer peripheral-type benzodiazepine receptors would decrease the amount of central excitation in the presence of elevated levels of an endogenous ligand. Other studies indicate that activation of peripheral-type benzodiazepine receptors produces convulsant effects in rodents (Benavides *et al.*, 1984; Pellow & File, 1984).

Taurine

An abnormality in taurine may contribute to the seizure prone condition of the GEPR. Pharmacological experiments show that intracerebroventricular injections of taurine suppress audiogenic seizures in GEPR-9s (Laird & Huxtable, 1976, 1978; Huxtable & Laird, 1978). Also, microinfusion of taurine into the inferior colliculus raises the electroshock seizure threshold in GEPR-9s but has no effect in control rats. Interestingly, this anticonvulsant effect in GEPRs lasts for 18 days. Lehmann (1989) reported that potassium-stimulated taurine release in the hippocampus is lower in GEPR-9s than in control rats. He noted also that striatal and cortical taurine concentrations are deficient in GEPR-9s.

Cyclic AMP

Ludvig *et al.* (1985*b*) and Ludvig & Moshé (1989) have observed that audiogenic seizure activity in the GEPR may stem from a malfunction of the cyclic AMP system within the inferior colliculus. In fact, these investigators could mimic the electrographic and behavioral manifestations of audiogenic seizures in GEPR-9s by microinjections of cyclic AMP analogs into the inferior colliculus.

Hypothyroidism

Deficient levels of serum thyroxine and triiodothyronine coupled with high concentrations of thyroid-stimulating hormone have been detected in GEPR-9s (Mills & Savage, 1988). These observations open the possibility that GEPR-9s are functionally hypothyroid from the second week of life and that this condition is also characteristic of adulthood. Partly because experimentally induced hypothyroidism by propylthiouracil causes the development of audiogenic seizure susceptibility and an abnormally low electroshock seizure threshold in normal rats, Mills & Savage (1988) have suggested that neonatal hypothyroidism could be one factor contributing to seizure predisposition in the GEPR.

The concept that hypothyroidism is insufficient to account totally for seizure predisposition in GEPRs is supported by several observations (Patrick & Faingold, 1989, 1990; Razani-Boroujerdi & Savage, 1990). Some of the data discount the notion that hypothyroidism functions as an etiologically significant factor. In general, we interpret the existing data to support the concept that hypothyroidism may serve as a minor mechanism for seizure predisposition in the GEPR-9. Moreover, it does not appear to be responsible for causing GEPR-9s to exhibit the severe convulsions characteristic of their phenotype. Whether hypothyroidism or other elements of the abnormal thyroid status of the GEPR-3 plays a role in audiogenic seizure susceptibility is questionable.

Trace elements

Abnormalities in trace element concentrations in GEPR-9s have been reported by Carl *et al.* (1990). Iron and manganese levels are deficient in GEPR-9 brain compared to non-epileptic control brain. Liver iron and copper, as well as heart manganese levels, are also low in the GEPR-9. Seizure experienced GEPR-9s exhibit blood manganese levels that are lower than the deficient concentrations of seizure naive GEPR-9s. Seizure episodes caused elevations in zinc concentrations in brain and heart.

Opioids

One manifestation of seizure predisposition in GEPR-9s is an exaggerated responsiveness to seizures induced by intracerebroventricularly administered morphine (Reigel *et al.*, 1988). Also, these epileptic animals are characterized by an increase in the number of mu receptors in the pyramidal cell layer of the CA3 and CA1 regions of the ventral hippocampus (Savage *et al.*, 1988). These observations coupled with other data support the concept that opioid abnormalities may be one of several determinants of seizure predisposition in the GEPR.

GAER neurochemistry

Catecholamines

Micheletti *et al.* (1987) have reported that a decrement in noradrenergic transmission is associated with increases in spike-and-wave discharges in the GAER. Analogous experimentation has also implicated dopaminergic deficits as facilitating spike-and-wave discharges (Warter *et al.*, 1988).

GABA

Pharmacological studies show that GABAergic effects aggravate spike-and-wave discharges in the GAER (Vergnes *et al.*, 1984; Micheletti *et al.*, 1985). Furthermore, increments in GABAergic transmission precipitate spike-and-wave discharges in non-epileptic control rats. These observations suggest a direct role of GABA in generating spike-and-wave discharges in the GAER (Vergnes *et al.*, 1990).

DBA/2 mice neurochemistry

Monoamines

Biochemical and pharmacological studies have evaluated the possibility that abnormalities in monoaminergic transmission may contribute to seizure susceptibility in DBA/2 mice (Schlesinger *et al.*, 1965, 1970; Lehmann, 1967; McGreer *et al.*, 1969; Boggan & Seiden, 1971; Boggan *et al.*, 1971; Kellogg, 1971, 1976; Anlezark & Meldrum, 1975; Alexander & Kopeloff, 1976; Anlezark *et al.*, 1976, 1978; Lints *et al.*, 1980; Dailey & Jobe, 1984; Chapman & Meldrum, 1987). The results suggest an important seizure inhibitory role for dopamine. The data pertaining to noradrenergic and serotonergic determination of seizure predisposition are open to multiple interpretations (see Jobe, 1981; Jobe & Laird, 1981) and do not consistently and firmly establish a determinant role for these two neurotransmitters in the DBA/2 mouse.

GABA

Several studies have evaluated GABAergic factors and benzodiazepine receptors in DBA/2 mice (Ticku, 1979; Robertson, 1980; Horton *et al.*, 1982, 1984; Toth *et al.*, 1983; Chapman *et al.*, 1985; Chapman & Meldrum, 1987). These results show convincingly that enhancing GABA-mediated inhibition is an effective means of suppressing seizures in DBA/2 mice. However, they do not persuasively demonstrate that innate deficiencies in the GABA system are of etiological significance.

Cellular biochemistry, hormones, enzymes, and cofactors

Prenatal antithyroid paradigms suppress audiogenic seizure susceptibility in DBA/2 mice (Seyfried *et al.*, 1979, 1981). Postnatal thyroxine treatment reverses this anticonvulsant effect. Excess thyroxine postnatally causes the appearance of audiogenic seizure susceptibility in a significant fraction of C57Bl/6j mice. Studies with several DBA × C57 recombinant inbred strains provide no support for thyroid abnormalities as a cause of seizure predisposition in DBA/2 mice (Seyfried *et al.*, 1984).

Studies of deficits in ATPase activities in DBA/2 mice are notable (Abood & Gerard, 1955; Rosenblatt *et al.*, 1976; Trams & Lauter, 1978; Palayoor & Seyfried, 1984a). Palayoor & Seyfried (1984b) demonstrated that, in DBA/2-derived recombinant inbred strains, the reduction in Ca^{2+}-ATPase in brainstem is inherited together with audiogenic seizure susceptibility.

El *mice neurochemistry*

GABA levels are lower in *el* mice than in their controls (Naruse *et al.*, 1960; Mori, 1988). Also, it has been reported (Mori, 1988) that *el* mice have decreased brain norepinephrine concentrations and elevated levels of dopamine and serotonin. Mori (1988) has concluded that a deficiency in serotonergic inhibition is etiologically important in susceptibility to seizures in *el* mice.

Tottering *mice neurochemistry*

A selective axonal overgrowth in noradrenergic neurons arising from the locus coeruleus is evident in *tottering* mice (Levitt & Noebels, 1981). The noradrenergic cell bodies in the locus coeruleus are not increased in number, but the increase in axonal projections corresponds to a 100–200% increase in norepinephrine levels within terminal fields (Noebels, 1986). If *tottering* mice are treated with the neurotoxin 6-hydroxydopamine to reduce noradrenergic function, the arrest seizures, spike-and-wave discharges, and ataxia are abolished (Noebels, 1984). Myoclonus is reduced in incidence and severity.

Epileptic gerbil neurochemistry

In epileptic gerbils, the density of benzodiazepine/GABA receptor binding sites is abnormally low in the midbrain (Olsen *et al.*, 1985) and GABA receptor stimulants block generalized seizures (Löscher, 1985). They also exhibit an abnormally high density of opioid (^{3}H-dihydromorphine) binding, especially in the periaqueductal gray, substantia nigra, and medial geniculate body (Lee *et al.*, 1986). Furthermore, agonists for mu, kappa, and sigma opiate receptors protect epileptic gerbils against seizures (Lee *et al.*, 1984). These observations were advanced by Lee *et al.* (1986) as indices of deficient opioid transmission.

Both apomorphine and L-dopa (in combination with carbidopa) were observed to exert a dose-related anticonvulsant effect (Löscher, 1985). These pharmacological data provide evidence that dopaminergic neurons have the capacity to regulate seizure intensity in the epileptic gerbil. However, whether innate abnormalities in dopaminergic transmission characterize the epileptic gerbils remains unanswered.

The GABAergic, opioidergic and dopaminergic studies suggest that seizure predisposition in the epileptic gerbil may result from multiple derangements in the inhibitory repertoire of the central nervous system. All three types of neurotransmitter system may be unable to control the development of epileptic events in these animals.

Other neurotransmitter and second-messenger systems have also been examined for a role in seizure processes in the epileptic gerbil. Some positive results have been obtained for somatostatin (Wolf-Dieter *et al.*, 1989), the prostaglandins (Seregi *et al.*, 1984, 1985) and the cyclic AMP/cyclic GMP second messenger system (Wolf-Dieter *et al.*, 1989).

Serotonergic, cholinergic and excitatory amino acid neurotransmission does not seem to play a significant role in the etiology of seizure predisposition in the epileptic gerbil (Löscher, 1985; Löscher & Czuczwar, 1985; Löscher *et al.*, 1988). A possible role for a noradrenergic determinant of epilepsy in these animals is unclear, the data being subject to conflicting interpretations (Philo, 1982; Champney, 1989; Löscher, 1985).

Epileptic baboon neurochemistry

GABAergic systems

Although all innate indices are not abnormal, we believe that existing evidence generally supports the concept that an innate GABAergic deficit contributes to seizure predisposition in the epileptic baboon (Hansen *et al.*, 1973; Lloyd *et al.*, 1986). This hypothesis is upheld by several studies of drugs known to influence GABAergic transmission (Killam *et al.*, 1966a, 1967; Meldrum *et al.*, 1970, 1975, 1977, 1979, 1988; Stark, Killam & Killam, 1970; Meldrum & Horton, 1971, 1978, 1979; Horton & Meldrum, 1973; Killam, 1976; Menini *et al.*, 1977; Cepeda *et al.*, 1981, 1982; Valin *et al.*, 1982, 1983; Killam & Killam, 1984; Meldrum, 1984;

Chambon *et al.*, 1985; Naquet & Meldrum, 1986; Brailowsky *et al.*, 1989, 1990). A few GABAergic agents, however, do not exert anticipated effects on ILS-induced seizures (Pedley *et al.*, 1979; Meldrum & Horton, 1980).

Excitatory amino acids

Some data suggest a possible role for excitatory amino acids in seizure mechanisms in the epileptic baboon (Meldrum *et al.*, 1983*a*,*b*; Pumain *et al.*, 1985; Pumain *et al.*, 1986). Other findings do not (Meldrum *et al.*, 1983b; Geddes *et al.*, 1989).

Monoaminergic systems

Evidence relative to a possible role for central monoaminergic systems as determinants of seizure predisposition in *Papio papio* has been reviewed by Killam & Killam (1984) and by Naquet & Meldrum (1986). Several investigations highlight the possible importance of dopamine, norepinephrine and serotonin (Meldrum & Naquet, 1971; Walter *et al.*, 1971; Meldrum *et al.*, 1972, 1975; Vuillon-Cacciuttolo & Balzano, 1972; Wada *et al.*, 1972; Vuillon-Cacciuttolo *et al.*, 1973; Altshuler *et al.*, 1976; Killam, 1976; Brailowsky & Naquet, 1976; Trimble, 1977; Anlezark & Meldrum, 1978; Anlezark *et al.*, 1978, 1981; Naquet & Meldrum, 1986). Presently, insufficient information prohibits a satisfactory conclusion regarding the individual contributions of the three monoaminergic systems.

Neuroanatomy of seizure predisposition

The anatomical localization of seizure predisposition within the brains of genetically epileptic animals is of increasing interest in epileptology. In some models, the neuroanatomical substrates responsible for the epileptic condition were thought initially to be confined within a highly restricted topography. This concept arose partly because these particular models were known to be susceptible to seizures caused by specific sensory stimuli. For example, animals susceptible to audiogenic seizures were thought to have etiologically significant abnormalities that were restricted to the auditory pathways.

During the last few years, the restricted topography concept has been challenged successfully. Emerging experimentation now shows that seizure predisposition is broadly represented within the brains of at least some genetic models, despite the fact that they are characterized by susceptibility to specific types of sensory-induced seizures. These findings form the basis for a useful caveat. Evidence demonstrating the possible etiological significance of a restricted group of neurons in epileptic disorders should not be set forth a priori as a demonstration that the seizure disorder is completely or even largely defined by pathophysiological mechanisms within this specific region.

GEPR neuroanatomy

Audiogenic seizures

Evidence summarized by Faingold & Naritoku (1992) supports the concept that the afferent pathway for audiogenic seizures transfers sensory impulses from the cochlea to the cochlear nucleus, then the superior olivary complex and to the inferior colliculus. The appearance of electrographic seizure activity occurs most readily in this latter structure, with output to the medial geniculate body and the reticular formation. Also, the cochlear nucleus and the superior olivary complex probably contribute to activation of the reticular formation. Afferent and efferent impulses are exchanged between the reticular formation and the substantia nigra. Convulsive behaviors (running, clonus, and tonus) result when impulses from within this circuitry are delivered at a sufficient rate to the spinal cord.

Acoustically induced paroxysmal discharges from the inferior colliculus are not always transferred to the cerebral cortex of the GEPR. What factors, then, cause the transfer? Naritoku *et al.* (1988) have shown that corticopetal pathways may begin to transfer seizure activity from the brainstem in response to repeated acoustically induced seizures. Accordingly, multiple audiogenic seizures in GEPR-9s lead to the appearance of polyspike and spike-and-wave activity in surface electroencephalographic recordings. Moreover, the multiplicity of seizures prolongs audiogenic convulsions and causes the appearance of clonus at the termination of tonic pelvic limb extension. Electroencephalographic evidence for seizure generalization from the brainstem to the cortex has also been obtained in audiogenic seizure-susceptible rats other than the GEPR (Marescaux *et al.*, 1987; Vergnes *et al.*, 1987*a*).

Studies by Mishra *et al.* (1988*b*, 1989) documented a type of audiogenic seizure kindling that occurs in response to repeated acoustically induced seizures in GEPR-3s and GEPR-9s. The mean seizure severity score (audiogenic response score, ARS) increases and the latency to the onset of convulsion decreases between the first- and third-weekly exposures to the stimulus. Interestingly, the generalization from brainstem to cerebral cortex reported by Naritoku *et al.* (1988) occurs in response to as few as three sound-induced seizures. The findings of Mishra *et al.* (1988*b*, 1989) and Naritoku *et al.* (1988) are compatible with the hypothesis that a decrease in seizure latency and an increase in severity, as well as the appearance of the post-tonic clonic phase, occur partly in response to a kindling-induced generalization of brainstem seizures to the cerebral cortex in the GEPR. Furthermore, these findings are in harmony with the concept that seizure severity is determined by the number of impulses per unit time delivered to the spinal cord. Maximal activation of the brainstem seizure circuitry coupled with parallel augmentation of impulse frequency from the forebrain would have the net effect of providing a larger number of impulses to the cord than would be delivered by the brainstem alone.

Preliminary studies designed to identify the corticopetal seizure-generalizing pathways of the GEPR have implicated the medial geniculate body and the amygdala (Faingold & Naritoku, 1992; Naritoku *et al.*, 1989*a,b*). The medial geniculate body appears to participate in generalization of electrographic seizure activity and in the exacerbation of seizure severity that occurs in response to repetitive seizure episodes. By comparison, the role of the amygdala seems to be more restricted in that it participates primarily in the exacerbation of behavioral seizures.

Noradrenergic neuroanatomy of seizure predisposition

Evidence implicating specific noradrenergic terminal fields as determinants of seizure predisposition in the GEPR has been summarized by Jobe *et al.* (1992). The midbrain excluding the inferior colliculus is particularly notable as a site wherein noradrenergic deficiencies may act to determine the magnitude of brainstem seizures in the GEPR (Jobe *et al.*, 1982, 1984; Dailey & Jobe, 1986; Browning *et al.*, 1989*b*; Mishra *et al.*, 1990; Dailey *et al.*, 1991). Defects in other noradrenergic terminal fields may also contribute to seizure prone condition of the GEPR (Dailey & Jobe, 1986; Dailey *et al.*, 1991). In general terms, forebrain noradrenergic terminals appear to be uninvolved in the regulation of brainstem seizure circuitry (Wang *et al.*, 1990). The identification of noradrenergic terminal fields that predispose GEPRs to forebrain seizures is a subject of current study (Mishra *et al.*, 1990; Wang *et al.*, 1990).

Serotonergic neuroanatomy of seizure predisposition

Serotonergic deficits in several areas of the brain may serve as determinants of audiogenic seizure susceptibility in the GEPR (see Dailey *et al.*, 1989). Since serotonergic influences may be less in the GEPR-9 striatum than in that of the GEPR-3, these particular terminals have become candidates for the regulation of audiogenic seizure severity as well as other types of seizure that are more severe in GEPR-9s than in GEPR-3s. Fewer studies have been undertaken with serotonergic than with noradrenergic neuroanatomy of seizure regulation. As a result, this serotonergic area of inquiry is relatively rudimentary.

GAER neuroanatomy

The generation and/or propagation of electroencephalographic abnormalities in the GAER may involve the same brain structures identified for the feline penicillin model of generalized absence seizures (McLachlan *et al.*, 1984a,b; Gloor & Fariello, 1988) and for human absence epilepsy (Williams, 1953). In each of these models and in the human, the spike-and-wave discharges appear to result from an oscillatory pattern of abnormal impulses that propagate in a thalamo-cortical loop.

Other experiments show that specific populations of GABAergic neurons in the brain may have varying influences on spike-and-wave discharges (Depaulis *et al.*, 1988; Liu *et al.*, 1991). In an evaluation of some of these divergent effects, Liu *et al.* (1991) found that the initiation of absence seizures in the GAER probably occurs in response to GABAergic activation in the specific relay nuclei of the medio-lateral thalamus. Apparently, GABA-induced hyperpolarization of GABAergic neurons within thalamic relay nuclei transforms their activity to an oscillatory bursting mode. These oscillations drive the spike-and-wave discharges associated with absence seizures in the GAER.

Epileptic mice neuroanatomy

The noradrenergic excess of the *tottering* has been localized within the cortex (Levitt & Noebels, 1981; Noebels, 1986). This noradrenergic hyperinnervation may be responsible for the epileptic condition of these animals.

Epileptic gerbil neuroanatomy

The behavioral and electrographic characteristics of seizures in the Mongolian gerbil suggest that the principal generator of the epileptic activity is the neocortex (Loskota & Lomax, 1975; Majkowski & Donadio, 1984). The first epileptiform discharges appear in the occipital cortex. However, the initiation of the pathological events appears to result from an abnormal communication between the cerebral cortex and the hippo-campus. In fact, the hippocampus of seizure-sensitive gerbils displays several morphological abnormalities (Paul *et al.*, 1981; Ribak & Khan, 1987; Peterson & Ribak, 1989). Also, while epileptiform activity in the Mongolian gerbil apparently emanates from the cortico-hippocampal circuitry, the thalamus seems to be significantly involved in controlling the spread of seizures (Lee *et al.*, 1989). An exact map of all the brain structures and pathways involved in the generation, propagation, and termination of seizures in the Mongolian gerbil, however, has yet to be elucidated.

Baboon neuroanatomy

The fronto-rolandic cortex as the site of initial appearance of ILS-induced paroxysmal activity is supported by several studies (Naquet *et al.*, 1972; Stutzmann *et al.*, 1980; Menini & Naquet, 1980; Menini *et al.*, 1981; Silva-Barrat & Menini, 1984, 1990; Brailowsky *et al.*, 1987, 1989; Fukuda *et al.*, 1988; Silva-Barrat *et al.*, 1988a). Once paroxysmal activity becomes evident in the fronto-rolandic cortex, secondary expressions of epileptic electroencephalographic activity may appear in divergent areas of the brain (Menini *et al.*, 1970, 1981; Wada *et al.*, 1973; Silva-Barrat & Menini, 1984, 1990; Silva-Barrat *et al.*, 1986; Brailowsky *et al.*, 1989). Non-specific visual cortical areas are necessary for ILS-induced seizures, since neurons derived therefrom innervate the fronto-rolandic cortex to initiate parox-ysmal discharges. Seemingly, ILS induces electrographic and biochemical alterations in the occipital cortex that are translated into paroxysmal discharges in the fronto-rolandic cortex (Naquet & Valin, 1990; Silva-Barrat & Menini, 1990). Cortically induced initiation of seizure activity in the reticular formation occurs as the seizure progresses (Fischer-Williams *et al.*, 1968; Catier *et al.*, 1970; Naquet *et al.*, 1972; Pumain *et al.*, 1985; Silva-Barrat *et al.*, 1986, 1988b; Fukuda *et al.*, 1988; Silva-Barrat & Menini, 1990). This secondary activation apparently heightens cerebral excitability as a tertiary effect. These combined events underlie intrinsically maintained seizure activity. The reticular activation probably results from direct cortico-reticular excitatory input and from loss of caudally directed and cortically derived inhibitory influences.

Genetically epileptic animals as models of human epilepsy

A complete understanding of the applicability of genetic models to the human epilepsies awaits additional data. Progress depends partly on further clarification of the nature of human epilepsy. A reciprocal relationship characterizes the generation of more complete and accurate concepts relative to the human epilepsies and the epilepsies of the various animal models. Improved phenomenological and mechanistic hypotheses derived from either investigative arena should prove to be a powerful stimulus for general advancement.

Presently, we know that, as a group, the genetic animal models and human epileptic patients exhibit similarities in seizure predisposition. Both have exaggerated responsiveness to convulsant stimuli such as pentylene-tetrazol. Both experience seizures in response to stimuli that do not cause seizures in neurologically normal subjects. These aspects of seizure predisposition in the genetic models have been described in pertinent sections of this chapter. The analogous traits in human epileptics have also been documented (Kaufman *et al.*, 1947; Gastaut, 1950; Garretson *et al.*, 1966; Wolf & Goosses, 1986; Shorvon, 1990; Tassinari *et al.*, 1990).

Both the genetic models and humans with epilepsy develop resident triggering mechanisms that produce seizures. These epileptic discharges may or may not become secondarily generalized. A small fraction of genetically epileptic animals exhibits spontaneous status epilepticus. Humans also rarely develop status epilepticus. Following a period of postpartum development, the seizure prone characteristics of developing epileptic animals become evident. Similarly, most cases of human epilepsy also become evident during an initial period of development but before maturation is completed. Many of the genetic models retain seizure predisposition throughout their lives. This protracted period of susceptibility is similar to many forms of human epilepsy.

Some of the genetic models are excessively sensitive to limbic kindling. Arguments supporting the concept that kindled seizures can serve as a model of human complex partial seizures have been summarized by McNamara (1984, 1986; see also Chapter 1, this volume). Within this context, relevant genetic models can be used to elucidate the underlying processes that might cause people with epileptic predisposition to develop kindled epilepsy. Appropriately, some of the genetic models may provide a means for determining the mechanistic contributions of seizure predisposition to the stimulus-dependent development of epilepsy.

Clinically useful anti-epileptic drugs produce specific anticonvulsant effects in many of the genetic models (Consroe *et al.*, 1979; Loscher, 1984; Dailey & Jobe, 1985). Moreover, with at least some of the genetic models, drugs useful in non-convulsive epilepsy can be separated from those that are useful for suppression of convulsive seizures in humans.

Epileptic seizures in both humans and the animal models described in the current review have genetic determinants (Newmark & Penry, 1980; Jobe & Laird, 1981). Because these models are characterized by a biologically inherited predisposition to seizures, they appear to be relevant for studies of human predisposition to seizures.

Finally, some humans with seizure predisposition and some of the genetic models may be characterized similarly with regard to neurochemical deficits. Many of the etiologically significant neurobiological defects characteristic of the genetic models described herein have also been reported for human epilepsy. A review of this latter topic is beyond the scope of this chapter.

Summary and conclusions

Seizure-triggering mechanisms

The genetic models of the epilepsies provide the means for examining key questions in epileptology. These models are characterized by a marked degree of seizure predisposition. Stimuli that do not cause seizures in normal subjects do so in the genetic models. Some animal models exhibit seizures in response to specific sensory stimuli or to other non-specific stimuli, whereas normal animals do not. Moreover, many of the genetic models experience spontaneous seizures. Consequently, it is clear that these animals have endogenous neuronal dysfunctions that act as triggering devices for initiation of seizure activity in defined regions of the brain. For example, the electrographic discharges of audiogenic seizures in GEPRs and DBA/2 mice probably appear first within the inferior colliculus. In epileptic gerbils, novelty-induced seizures appear first in the occipital cortex. Photogenic seizures in epileptic *Papio papio* appear to originate in the fronto-rolandic cortex. In normal animals, the interactions between sensory input and other key elements of the nervous system do not result in seizure activity. The genetic models, however, offer a means for examining seizure-triggering devices that express their activity when the topographically corresponding neuronal circuits in normal animals do not. In what ways do the seizure-generating neuronal arrangements and interactions of epileptic animals differ from anatomically correspond-ing neuronal groups in normal brain? Existing evidence indicates that both the 'wiring diagrams' and the neurons within the circuits are different. Accordingly, the density of GABAergic neurons is elevated in the seizure-triggering areas of the GEPR and those of the epileptic gerbil. Moreover, the density of noradrenergic fibers is deficient in GEPRs. Abnormal functioning of neurons within the circuits is supported by the observations (a) that not only do GEPRs have a deficiency in the number of noradrenergic processes but they release too little norepinephrine per existing neuron, and (b) that the compensatory mechanisms of the post-synaptic receptor processes are deficient.

Another type of seizure-triggering device also exists in the genetic models. Not only do they have unique generators, they also have those that exist in normal animals. For example, both types of animal have the triggering mechanisms that respond to the various types of electroshock and convulsant drugs such as pentylenetetrazol. Also, the GAER has the thalamo-cortically localized absence epilepsy-triggering mechanism that is also present in normal animals. However, even these triggers in the genetic models do not operate normally; they are seemingly hyper-responsive. Smaller doses of pentylenetetrazol and smaller electric currents are required to generate seizures in many of the genetic models as compared to non-epileptic controls. The trigger for absence seizures in the GAER is activated innately in response to internal biological vari-ations. It can also be activated by experimentally applied GABAergic agents, as can the more resistant absence epilepsy trigger in normal animals.

In close association with these ideas, seizure predisposition appears to be broadly represented in the brains of genetically epileptic animals. Thus, through the use of genetic models, investigators have an opportunity to discover contributions to seizure generation stemming from interactions between uniquely operative triggering mechanisms and the broader elements of the determinants of seizure predisposition.

These issues have provided an impetus for research with the genetic models of the epilepsies. Many of the principal issues have already been opened experimentally. Some have just recently emerged in preliminary form. Highlights of some of the areas of investigation are summarized below.

Epileptic mechanisms outside the site of initial electrographic appearance

In addition to their use in studies of seizure-triggering mechanisms, the genetic models are useful for elucidating the interactions between the site of initial appearance of electrographic seizure discharges and other etiologically dysfunctional areas of the brain (see Chapter 2, this volume). These key participating areas of seizure predisposition may enable the point of initial appearance to express seizure discharges when, under the influence of the same stimulus, the identical site in a neurologically normal animal does not. It seems increasingly unlikely that the primary etiological dysfunction in the various forms of the epilepsies resides almost exclusively within the point of initial appearance of electrographic discharges. Rather, epilepsy appears to result from a broader array of interacting components. This interactional concept is not in disharmony with the well-documented findings that epileptic discharges can occur under the correct experimental conditions in isolated tissue slices obtained from normal brain. It does, however, emphasize the idea that epilepsy, in contradistinction to seizures in simplified and isolated systems or seizures in normal intact brain, may derive from interactions between various epileptic components of the brain even though these other components do not serve as sites in which epileptic discharges are first detected.

Some evidence in the GEPR suggests that the enabling effects of sites outside the point of origin are important determinants of seizure triggering devices in epileptic brain. Accordingly, noradrenergic deficits within the inferior colliculus do not appear to be a determinant of susceptibility to audiogenic seizures in the GEPR. Nevertheless, noradrenergic deficits in other parts of the brain, possibly the midbrain excluding the inferior colliculus, apparently subserve this function. In absence of such deficits, the audiogenic seizures of the GEPR do not occur. Yet seizure discharges appear first in the inferior colliculus. Within this context, a particular conceptual dichotomy often invoked in epileptology may be partly counterproductive. We sometimes rationalize the site of initial appearance of electrographic seizure activity to be the region of primary scientific interest. Mechanistically, the behavior of the so-called focus may be subject to elucidation only when considered in concert with the etiologically significant 'non-seizing' epileptic neurons.

Additional interdisciplinary studies of the neuronal networks which determine various elements of seizure predisposition in the genetic models is clearly warranted. Impressive progress has been made in the study of neuronal networks with the use of the kindling models (see Chapter 1, this volume). Some of the information rapidly emerging from these investigations should provide guidance for studies with genetic models.

Mechanisms by which seizure predisposition exacerbates seizure-induced neuronal dysfunction

A large number of studies have been undertaken to determine the pathophysiological consequences of seizures or electrographic after-discharges on brain function. Many of these have been with kindling in normal animals. Others have been with status epilepticus in normal animals treated with convulsant agents. However, studies to determine the effects of seizures or kindling on genetically epileptic animals have been relatively few. Existing data in GEPRs and audiogenic-seizure-susceptible mice show that the consequences of seizures or of 'subliminal stimuli' on subsequent neuronal functioning are more pronounced than in normal animals. Perhaps some cases of epilepsy are the result of seemingly inconsequential stimuli impacting a genetically seizure prone nervous system, with the same stimuli in a normal brain failing to result in epilepsy. Genetic models in which spontaneous seizures are rare or non-existent provide a means for determining the mechanisms by which such deleterious events occur. They should also serve as a way to detect novel means of prevention.

Mechanisms of seizure progression

Some genetic models appear to experience absence seizures. Others exhibit convulsive seizures that appear to be sustained by forebrain circuitry. Still others exhibit the tonic–clonic seizures characteristic of brainstem circuitry. Other genetic models experience various combinations of these dysfunctions. In some, seizure predisposition of the brainstem is seemingly more pronounced than that of the forebrain. Other genetic models are a little more similar to non-epileptic controls in that seizure responsiveness of the forebrain is dominant despite its seizure prone condition. These models provide useful biological systems for studies of seizure progression. What abnormal mechanisms in the predisposed nervous system might foster the conversion of absence seizures into convulsive seizures? What are the processes by which forebrain seizures activate the seizure circuitry of the brainstem? Typically, forebrain seizures do not evoke such a conversion, but they appear to be more common in some of the genetic models, particularly at crucial ages.

Shared etiologically significant neural dysfunctions

A few etiologically significant dysfunctions now seem to be shared by several of the genetic models of the epilepsies. A few years ago, the role of GABA in seizure predisposition in the genetic models of the epilepsies was unclear. Pharmacological studies suggested that GABAergic deficits should characterize these models and that these abnormalities might contribute to the seizure prone condition of the animals. However, neurochemical and neuroanatomical assessments suggested the existence of excessive GABAergic influences in some genetic models. Since that time, some resolution has been possible. Although elements of excessive GABAergic function may exist in some of the genetic models, other processes seemingly exert a greater influence so that a net functional GABAergic deficit dominates. Within this context, GABAergic deficits now appear to contribute to epileptogenesis in the GEPR, DBA/2 and *el* mice, epileptic gerbil and the photo-epileptic baboon. The evidence supporting this commonality is stronger for some models than for others. In all cases, it is incomplete, but our overall interpretation is less ambivalent than it was in earlier assessments (Jobe & Laird 1981, 1987).

Perhaps it is premature to identify shared abnormalities in the action of excitatory amino acids in the genetic models of the epilepsies. The weight of evidence supports the existence of excessive glutamatergic and/or aspartatergic influences as partial causes of seizure predisposition in the GEPR. Initial data also point toward a possible etiological contribution of excitatory amino acids in some genetic mouse models and in the epileptic baboon. Data are inadequate to support speculation relative to the GAER.

Existing evidence supports the hypothesis that noradrenergic deficits function as determinants of seizure predisposition in the GEPR, GAER and epileptic baboon. For the GEPR, the supporting evidence is extensive and unequivocal. Noradrenergic studies in the GAER and the epileptic baboon provide positive leads but are insufficient. Assessments of noradrenergic regulation of seizure predisposition in the epileptic gerbil have produced negative results. The experimental approaches employed in the gerbil, however, form an insufficient basis for accepting or rejecting hypotheses of etiological significance. Additional specific pharmacological and neurochemical studies are needed to formulate definitive conclusions about the noradrenergic systems in the particular animals.

Evidence implicates serotonergic deficits as determinants of seizure predisposition in the GEPR, some epileptic mice, and *Papio papio*. These positive findings must be interpreted against an overall insufficient data base.

Neurobiological paradoxes

There are some common etiological factors in the different genetic models. Other factors act as a cause of the seizure prone condition in one model but have no influence in another model. Still others appear to have opposite effects in the process of seizure predisposition. Several of these anomalies exist. GABAergic, noradrenergic, dopaminergic and thyroid abnormalities are examples of these paradoxes.

Present evidence shows that GABAergic influences in the GAER are opposite to those in other genetic models of the epilepsies. Drugs that augment GABAergic activity exacerbate absence epilepsy seizures in the GAER. In contrast, they suppress convulsive seizures in the GEPR, DBA/2 and *el* mice, epileptic gerbil and photo-epileptic baboon. Seemingly, some of these GABAergic deficits involve synaptic interactions with the $GABA_A$ receptor complex. In some cases, deficits in other GABAergic systems may contribute to seizure predisposition.

Arguments that GABAergic influences are excitatory in absence epilepsy seizures but suppressive in convulsive seizures are increasingly persuasive. The seeming paradox between GABAergic influences in the GAER and the other epilepsy models might be rationalized in conformity with this functional dichotomy. Except for the GAER, these other models exhibit convulsive seizures. Perhaps, the 'pure' absence epilepsy seizure of the GAER is derived from excessive GABAergic influences within thalamo-cortical circuitry. Anticonvulsant effects of GABA in other models may derive from seizure-suppressing activity in alternative circuits. For example, pro-GABAergic influences appear to be unequivocally inhibitory in brainstem seizures and in partial convulsive seizures emanating from the limbic components of forebrain circuitry.

The intermingling of biological factors responsible for convulsive and absence epilepsy seizures exhibited by the *tottering* mouse and epileptic gerbil may complicate the interpretation of results from experiments designed to examine GABAergic influences. Perhaps the antiseizure effects of pro-GABAergic effects in these models stems from the suppression of circuits that drive convulsive seizures and that interact with absence epilepsy seizure networks.

The divergence that characterizes noradrenergic influences in the *tottering* mouse versus those in the GEPR, GAER, and possibly the epileptic baboon, deserves clarification. The possibility that noradrenergic influences are opposite in animals with absence epilepsy seizures versus those with convulsive seizures seems remote. Pro-noradrenergic effects appear to suppress spike-and-wave discharges in the GAER and in audiogenic convulsions in the GEPR. The possibility that at least some seizures in *mice* are facilitated or caused by excessive noradrenergic influences deserves scrutiny.

As a companion issue, mice and rats appear to be influenced oppositely by thyroid deficiency. In the mouse, thyroid deficiency seemingly causes an anticonvulsant effect, whereas in rats it is proconvulsant. Are the direct effects of thyroid deficiency on brains of the two species opposite? Alternatively, are the direct effects the same, but the secondary effects opposite? Thyroid deficiency appears to alter noradrenergic function. Perhaps this neuronal alteration has effects of its own that, in mice, are the opposite of those in other species.

Molecular genetics

Through the use of molecular genetics techniques, the genetic models of the epilepsies provide a means for determining aberrations in the sequencing of the contiguous nucleotidyl moieties in DNA that give rise to innate epileptic triggers. As noted by Engel (1989), the use of genetic models in this way allows the issues of epileptology to be approached from a direction different from that which can be obtained from the use of normal animals exposed to a seizure-provoking stimulus. Overall, the science of epileptology should optimize achievements by giving an increased emphasis to the molecular genetics of epilepsy while continuing an energetic pursuit of the neurochemical, neuroanatomical and electrophysiological mechanisms of seizure predisposition. A more advanced understanding of the last three factors will provide invaluble guidance for designating experimentation in the domain of molecular genetics.

Anti-epileptic drugs

The clarification of basic and theoretical issues of epileptology through the use of genetic models has been emphasized throughout this chapter. The emerging concepts suggest that application of these models to the development of new anti-epileptic drugs has the potential to provide practical benefits to mankind. The unique features of the genetically

epileptic animals highlight their potential usefulness in developing novel
drugs that can selectively ameliorate underlying seizure-predisposing
dysfunctions. Presently, only some of these etiologically significant abnormalities are known. Additional mechanistically pertinent experimentation
is needed. Elucidation of the biological causes of seizure predisposition
in the genetic models is in harmony with the increasing recognition that
epilepsy mechanisms should become an important cornerstone in future
drug development strategies (Rogawski & Porter, 1990). The current
anti-epileptic drugs suppress symptoms. New drugs developed through a
thorough understanding of the genetically determined epileptic states and
their interactions with environmental factors should augment the potential for development of preventions and cures.

Acknowledgments

This work was supported in part by NIH grant NS22672. We are grateful
to Mss Hazel Williamson, Kim Dannenberg & Sue Ann Munge for
editorial assistance. We also appreciate Dr Ron Browning's review of our
manuscript and his helpful recommendations.

References

Abood, L. G. and Gerard, R. W. (1955). A phosphorylation defect in the
    brains of mice susceptible to audiogenic seizure. In *Biochemistry of the
    Developing Nervous System*, ed. H. Waelsh, pp. 467–72. New York: Academic
    Press.
Alexander, G. J. & Kopeloff, L. M. (1976). Audiogenic seizures in mice.
    Research Communications in Chemical Pathology and Pharmacology, **14**:
    437–47.
Altshuler, H. L., Killam, E. K. & Killam, K. F. (1976). Biogenic amines and the
    photomyoclonic syndrome in the baboon *Papio papio. Journal of
    Pharmacology and Experimental Therapeutics*, **196**: 156–66.
Anlezark, G. M., Horton, R. W. & Meldrum, B. S. (1978). Dopamine agonists
    and audiogenic seizures: the relationship between protection against
    seizures and changes in monoamine metabolism. *Biochemical
    Pharmacology*, **27**: 2821–8.
Anlezark, G., Marrosu, F. & Meldrum, B. (1981). Dopamine agonists in reflex
    epilepsy. In *Neurotransmitters, Seizures and Epilepsy*, ed. P. L. Morselli,
    K. G. Lloyd, W. Loscher, B. Meldrum & E. H. Reynolds, pp. 251–62. New
    York: Raven Press.
Anlezark, G. M. & Meldrum, B. S. (1975). Effects of apomorphine, ergocornine
    and piribedil on audiogenic seizures in DBA/2 mice. *British Journal of
    Pharmacology*, **53**: 419–26.
Anlezark, G. & Meldrum, B. (1978). Blockade of photically induced epilepsy by
    'dopamine agonist' ergot alkaloids. *Psychopharmacology*, **57**: 57–62.

Anlezark, G., Pycock, C. & Meldrum, B. (1976). Ergot alkaloids as dopamine agonists: comparison in two rodent models. *European Journal of Pharmacology*, **37**: 295–302.

Benavides, J., Guilloux, F., Allam, D. E., Uzan, A., Mizoule, J., Renault, C., Dubroeucq, M. C., Gueremy, C. & Le Fur, G. (1984). Opposite effects of an agonist, R05-4864, and an antagonist PK 11195, of the peripheral type benzodiazepine binding sites on audiogenic seizures in DBA/2J mice. *Life Sciences*, **34**: 2613–20.

Boggan, W. O., Freedman, D. X., Lovell, R. A. & Schlesinger, K. (1971). Studies in audiogenic seizure susceptibility. *Psychopharmacology*, **20**: 48–56.

Boggan, W. O. & Seiden, L. S. (1971). Dopa reversal of reserpine enhancement of audiogenic seizure susceptibility in mice. *Physiology and Behavior*, **6**: 215–17.

Booker, J. G., Dailey, J. W., Jobe, P. C. and Lane, J. D. (1986). Cerebral cortical GABA and benzodiazepine binding sites in genetically seizure prone rats. *Life Sciences*, **39**: 799–806.

Brailowsky, S., Menini, C., Silva-Barrat, C. & Naquet, R. (1987). Epileptogenic gamma-aminobutyric acid-withdrawal syndrome after chronic, intracortical infusion in baboons. *Neuroscience Letters*, **74**: 75–80.

Brailowsky, S. & Naquet, R. (1976). Effects of drugs modifying brain levels of catecholamines on photically induced epilepsy in *Papio papio*. *Epilepsia*, **17**: 271–4.

Brailowsky, S., Silva-Barrat, C., Menini, C., Riche, D. & Naquet, R. (1989). Effects of localized, chronic GABA infusions into different cortical areas of the photosensitive baboon *Papio papio*. *Electroencephalography and Clinical Neurophysiology*, **72**: 147–56.

Brailowsky, S., Silva-Barrat, C., Menini, C., Riche, D. & Naquet, R. (1990). Anticonvulsant effects of intracortical chronic infusion of GABA in generalized epilepsy. In *Generalized Epilepsy: Neurobiological Approaches*, ed. M. Avoli, P. Gloor, G. Kostopoulos & R. Naquet, pp. 126–36. Boston, MA: Birkhäuser.

Browning, R. A. (1987). Effect of lesions on seizures in experimental animals. In *Epilepsy and the Reticular Formation: The Role of the Reticular Core in Convulsive Seizures*, ed. G. H. Fromm, C. L. Faingold, R. A. Browning & W. M. Burnham, pp. 137–62. New York: Alan R. Liss.

Browning, R. A., Lanker, M. L. & Faingold, M. L. (1989*a*). Injections of noradrenergic and GABAergic agonists into the inferior colliculus: effects on audiogenic seizures in genetically epilepsy-prone rats. *Epilepsy Research*, **4**: 119–25.

Browning, R. A., Wade, D. R., Marcinczyk, M., Long, G. L. & Jobe, P. C. (1989*b*). Regional brain abnormalities in norepinephrine uptake and dopamine beta-hydroxylase activity in the genetically epilepsy-prone rat. *Journal of Pharmacology and Experimental Therapeutics*, **249**: 229–35.

Browning, R. A., Wang, C., Lanker, M. L. & Jobe, P. C. (1990). Electroshock and pentylenetetrazol-induced seizures in genetically epilepsy-prone rats: differences in threshold and pattern. *Epilepsy Research*, **6**: 1–11.

Burnham, W. M. (1987). Electrical stimulation studies: generalized convulsions triggered from the brainstem. In *Epilepsy and the Reticular Formation: The Role of the Reticular Core in Convulsive Seizures*, ed. G. H. Fromm, C. L. Faingold, R. A. Browning & W. M. Burnham, pp. 25–38. New York: Alan R. Liss.

Carl, G. F., Critchfield, J. W., Thompson, J. L., Holmes, G. L., Gallagher, B. B. & Keen, C. L. (1990). Genetically epilepsy-prone rats are characterized by altered tissue trace element concentrations. *Epilepsia*, **31**: 247–52.

Catier, J., Choux, M., Cordeau, J. P., Dimov, S., Riche, D., Eberhard, A. & Naquet, R. (1970). Résultats préliminaires des effets électrographiques de la section du corps calleux chez le *Papio papio* photosensible. *Review of Neurology*, **122**: 521–2.

Cepeda, C., Tanaka, T., Besselievre, R., Pottier, P., Naquet, R. & Rossier, J. (1981). Proconvulsant effects in baboons of beta-carboline, a putative endogenous ligand for benzodiazepine receptors. *Neuroscience Letters*, **24**: 53–7.

Cepeda, C., Worms, P., Lloyd, K. G. & Naquet, R. (1982). Action of progabide in the photosensitive baboon *Papio papio*. *Epilepsia*, **23**: 463–70.

Chambon, J. P., Brochard, J., Hallot, A., Heaulme, M., Brodin, R., Roncucci, R. & Biziere, K. (1985). A structural novel anticonvulsant in mice, rats and baboons. *Journal of Pharmacology and Experimental Therapeutics*, **233**: 836–44.

Champney, T. H. (1989). Transection of the pineal stalk produces convulsions in male Mongolian gerbils (*Meriones unguiculatus*). *Epilepsy Research*, **4**: 14–19.

Chapman, A. G., Cheetham, S. C., Hart, G. P., Meldrum, B. S. & Westerberg, E. (1985). The effect of two convulsant beta-carboline derivatives, DMCM and beta-CCM, on regional neurotransmitter amino acid levels and on in vitro D-[^{3}H]-aspartate release in rodents. *Journal of Neurochemistry*, **45**: 370–81.

Chapman, A. G., Faingold, C. L., Hart, G. P., Bowker, H. M. & Meldrum, B. S. (1986). Brain regional amino acid levels in seizure susceptible rats: changes related to sound-induced seizures. *Neurochemistry International*, **8**: 273–9.

Chapman, A. G., Horton, R. W., & Meldrum, B. S. (1978). Anticonvulsant action of 1,5-benzodiazepine, clobazam, in reflex epilepsy. *Epilepsia*, **19**: 293–9.

Chapman, A. G. & Meldrum, B. S. (1987). Epilepsy-prone mice: genetically determined sound-induced seizures. In *Neurotransmitters and Epilepsy*, ed. P. C. Jobe & H. E. Laird II, pp. 9–29. Clifton, NJ: Humana Press.

Chermat, R., Lachapelle, F., Baumann, N. & Simon, P. (1979). Anticonvulsant effect of yohimbine in quaking mice: antagonism by clonidine and prazosine. *Life Sciences*, **25**: 1471–6.

Consroe, P., Picchioni, A. & Chin, L. (1979). Audiogenic seizure susceptible rats. *Federation Proceedings*, **38**: 2411–16.

Croucher, M., De Sarro, G., Jensen, L. & Meldrum, B. S. (1984). Behavioral and convulsant actions of two methyl esters of β-carboline-3-carboxylic acid in photosensitive baboons and in DBA/2 mice. *European Journal of Pharmacology*, **104**: 55–60.

Dailey, J. W. & Jobe, P. C. (1984). Effect of increments in the concentration of dopamine in the central nervous system on audiogenic seizures in DBA/2J mice. *Neuropharmacology*, **23**: 1019–24.

Dailey, J. W. & Jobe, P. C. (1985). Anticonvulsant drugs and the genetically epilepsy-prone rat. *Federation Proceedings*, **44**: 2640–4.

Dailey, J. W. & Jobe, P. C. (1986). Indices of noradrenergic function in the central nervous system of seizure-naive genetically epilepsy-prone rats. *Epilepsia*, **27**: 665–70.

Dailey, J. W., Lasley, S. M., Bettendorf, A. F., Burger, R. L. & Jobe, P. C. (1988). Aspartame does not facilitate pentylenetetrazol-induced seizures in genetically epilepsy-prone rats. *Epilepsia*, **29**: 651.

Dailey, J. W., Mishra, P. K., Penny, J., Reigel, C. E., Ko, K. H. & Jobe, P. C. (1991). Noradrenergic abnormalities in the central nervous system of seizure-naive genetically epilepsy-prone rats. *Epilepsia*, **32**: 168–73.

Dailey, J. W., Reigel, C. E., Mishra, P. K. & Jobe, P. C. (1989). Neurobiology of seizure predisposition in the genetically epilepsy-prone rat. *Epilepsy Research*, **3**: 3–17.

Davis, W. M. & King, W. T. (1966). Pharmacogenetic factor in the convulsive responses of mice to flurothyl. *Experientia*, **23**: 214–15.

Depaulis, A., Vergnes, M., Marescaux, C., Lannes, B. & Warter, J.-M. (1988). Evidence that activation of GABA receptors in the substantia nigra suppresses spontaneous spike-and-wave discharges in the rat. *Brain Research*, **448**: 20–9.

Ducis, I., Norenberg, L.-O. B. & Norenberg, M. D. (1990). The benzodiazepine receptor in cultured astrocytes from genetically epilepsy-prone rats. *Brain Research*, **531**: 318–21.

Duplisse, B. R. (1976). Mechanism of susceptibility of rats to audiogenic seizure. Dissertation, University of Arizona.

Duplisse, B. R., Picchioni, A. L., Chin, L. & Consroe, P. F. (1974). Relationship of the inferior colliculus and gamma-aminobutyric acid (GABA) to audiogenic seizure in the rat. *Federation Proceedings*, **33**: 468.

Engel, J., Jr (1989). Basic mechanisms of epilepsy. In *Seizures and Epilepsy*, Chapter 4, pp. 71–111. Philadelphia: F. A. Davis Company.

Faingold, C. L. & Boersma-Anderson, C. A. (1988). Inferior colliculus (IC) unit activity and audiogenic seizures (AGS) in behaving genetically epilepsy-prone rats (GEPRs). *Society for Neuroscience Abstracts*, **14**: 253.

Faingold, C. L. & Copley, C. A. (1988). Effects of MK-801, a non-competitive excitant amino acid (EAA) antagonist on audiogenic seizures (AGS) in the genetically epilepsy-prone rat (GEPR). *Epilepsia*, **29**: 693.

Faingold, C. L., Copley, C. A. & Boersma, C. A. (1987). Blockade of audiogenic seizures (AGS) in genetically epilepsy-prone rats (GEPR) by the microinjection into inferior colliculus (IC) blockers of inhibitory and excitant amino acid (EAA) metabolism. *Society for Neuroscience Abstracts*, **13**: 1158.

Faingold, C. L., Copley, C. A. & Boersma, C. A. (1988a). Effects of microinjection of a new excitant amino acid (EAA) antagonist, CPP, into inferior colliculus (IC) and amygdala (AMG) on audiogenic seizures (AGS) in the genetically epilepsy-prone rat (GEPR). *FASEB Journal*, **2**: A1067.

Faingold, C. L., Gehlbach, G. & Caspary, D. M. (1985). Effects of GABA on inferior colliculus neuronal responses to acoustic stimuli. *Society for Neuroscience Abstracts*, **11**: 247.

Faingold, C. L., Gehlbach, G. & Caspary, D. M. (1986a). Decreased effectiveness of GABA-mediated inhibition in the inferior colliculus of the genetically epilepsy-prone rat. *Experimental Neurology*, **93**: 145–59.

Faingold, C. L., Gehlbach, G., Travis, M. A. & Caspary, D. M. (1986b). Inferior colliculus neuronal response abnormalities in genetically epilepsy-prone rats: evidence for a deficit of inhibition. *Life Sciences*, **39**: 869–78.

Faingold, C. L., Millan, M. H., Boersma, C. A. & Meldrum, B. S. (1988b). Excitant amino acids and audiogenic seizures in the genetically epilepsy-prone rat. I. Afferent seizure initiation pathway. *Experimental Neurology*, **99**: 678–86.

Faingold, C. L., Millan, M. H., Boersma, C. A. & Meldrum, B. S. (1989). Induction of audiogenic seizures in normal and genetically epilepsy-prone rats by focal microinjection of an excitant amino acid into auditory and reticular formation nuclei. *Epilepsy Research*, **3**: 199–205.

Faingold, C. L. & Naritoku, D. K. (1992). The genetically epilepsy-prone rat: neuronal networks and actions of amino neurotransmitters. In *Drugs for the Control of Epilepsy: Actions on Neuronal Networks Involved in Seizure Disorders*, ed. C. L. Faingold & G. H. Fromm, pp. 277–308. Boca Raton, FL: CFC Press.

Faingold, C. L., Travis, M. A., Gehlbach, G., Hoffmann, W. I., Jobe, P. C., Laird, H. E. II. & Caspary, D. M. (1986c). Neuronal response abnormalities in the inferior colliculus of the genetically epilepsy-prone rat. *Electroencephalography and Clinical Neurophysiology*, **63**: 296–305.

Fischer-Williams, M., Poncet, M., Riche, D. & Naquet, R. (1968). Light induced epilepsy in the baboon *Papio papio*, cortical and depth recordings. *Electroencephalography and Clinical Neurophysiology*, **25**: 557–69.

Franck, J. E., Ginter, K. L. & Schwartzkroin, P. A. (1989). Developing genetically epilepsy-prone rats have an abnormal seizure response to flurothyl. *Epilepsia*, **30**: 1–6.

Frey, H. (1987). Induction of seizures by air blast in gerbils: stimulus duration/effect relationship. *Epilepsy Research*, **1**: 262–4.

Fukuda, H., Valin, A., Bryere, P., Riche, D., Wada, J. A. & Naquet, R. (1988). Role of the forebrain commissure and hemispheric independence in photosensitive response of epileptic baboon *Papio papio*. *Electroencephalography and Clinical Neurophysiology*, **69**: 363–70.

Garretson, H., Gloor, P. & Rasmussen, T. (1966). Intracarotid amobarbital and metrazol test for the study of epileptiform discharges in man: a note on its technique. *Electroencephalography and Clinical Neurophysiology*, **21**: 607–10.

Gastaut, H. (1950). Combined photic and metrazol activation of the brain. *Electroencephalography and Clinical Neurophysiology*, **2**: 249–61.

Geddes, J. W., Cooper, S. M., Cotman, C. W., Patel, S. & Meldrum, B. S. (1989). *N*-Methyl-D-aspartate receptors in the cortex and hippocampus of baboon (*Papio anubis* and *Papio papio*). *Neuroscience*, **32**: 39–47.

Gloor, P. & Fariello, R. G. (1988). Generalized epilepsy: some of its cellular mechanisms differ from those of focal epilepsy. *Trends in Neuroscience*, **11**: 63–8.

Goldblatt, D. (1968). Seizure disorder in gerbils. *American Academy of Neurology Program*, **18**: 303–4.

Green, M. & Sidman, R. L. (1962). Tottering – a neuromuscular mutation in the mouse. *Journal of Heredity*, **53**: 233–7.

Hansen, S., Perry, T. L., Wada, J. A. & Sokol, M. (1973). Brain amino acids in baboons with light-induced epilepsy. *Brain Research*, **50**: 480–3.

Heller, A. H., Dichter, M. A. & Sidman, R. L. (1983). Anticonvulsant sensitivity of absence seizures in the tottering mutant mouse. *Epilepsia*, **25**: 25–34.

Hjeresen, D. L., Franck, J. E. & Amend, D. L. (1987). Ontogeny of seizure incidence, latency, and severity in genetically epilepsy prone rats. *Developmental Psychobiology*, **20**: 355–63.

Holmes, G. L., Thompson, J. L., Marchi, T. A., Gabriel, P. S., Hjogan, M. A., Carl, F. G. & Feldman, D. S. (1990). Effects of seizures on learning, memory, and behavior in the genetically epilepsy-prone rat. *Annals of Neurology*, **27**: 24–32.

Horton, R., Anlezark, G. & Meldrum, B. S. (1980). Noradrenergic influences on sound-induced seizures. *Journal of Pharmacology and Experimental Therapeutics*, **214**: 437–42.

Horton, R. W. & Meldrum, B. S. (1973). Seizures induced by allylglycine, 3-mercaptopropionic acid and 4-deoxy-pyridoxine in mice and photosensitive baboons, and different models of inhibition of cerebral glutamic acid decarboxylase. *British Journal of Pharmacology*, **49**: 52–63.

Horton, R. W., Prestwich, S. A. & Jazrawi, S. P. (1984). Neurotransmitter receptor binding in genetically seizure susceptible mice. In *Neurotransmitters, Seizures and Epilepsy* II, ed. R. G. Fariello, P. L. V. Morselli, K. G. Lloyd, L. F. Quesney & J. Engel Jr, pp. 191–200, New York: Raven Press.

Horton, R. W., Prestwich, S. A. & Meldrum, B. S. (1982). Gamma-aminobutyric acid and benzodiazepine binding sites in audiogenic seizure susceptible mice. *Journal of Neurochemistry*, **39**: 864–70.

Huxtable, R. & Laird, H. (1978). The prolonged anticonvulsant action of taurine on genetically determined seizure-susceptibility. *Journal Canadien Des Sciences Neurologiques*, **5**: 215–21.

Jobe, P. C. (1981). Pharmacology of audiogenic seizures. In *Pharmacology of Hearing: Experimental and Clinical Bases*, ed. R. D. Brown & E. A. Daigneault, pp. 271–304. New York: John Wiley & Sons, Inc.

Jobe, P. C. (1987). Spinal seizures induced by electrical stimulation. In *Epilepsy and the Reticular Formation: The Role of the Reticular Core in Convulsive Seizures*, ed. G. H. Fromm, C. L. Faingold, R. A. Browning & W. M. Burnham, pp. 81–91. New York: Alan R. Liss.

Jobe, P. C., Brown, R. D. & Dailey, J. W. (1981). Effect of Ro 4-1284 on audiogenic seizure susceptibility and intensity in epilepsy-prone rats. *Life Sciences*, **28**: 2031–8.

Jobe, P. C., Brown, R. D., Dailey, J. W., Ray, T. B., Woods, T. W., Mims, M. E. & Bairnsfather, S. (1980). Effects of multiple exposures to intense acoustical stimulation on audiogenic seizures susceptibility and intensity in rats. I. A developmental study in progeny from a genetically susceptible colony. *Society for Neuroscience Abstracts*, **6**: 824.

Jobe, P. C., Dailey, J. W. & Reigel, C. E. (1986). Noradrenergic and serotonergic determinants of seizure susceptibility and severity in genetically epilepsy-prone rat. *Life Sciences*, **39**: 775–82.

Jobe, P. C., Ko, K. H. & Dailey, J. W. (1984). Abnormalities in norepinephrine turnover rate in the central nervous system of the GEPR. *Brain Research*, **290**: 357–60.

Jobe, P. C. & Laird, H. E., II (1981). Neurotransmitter abnormalities as determinants of seizure susceptibility and intensity in the genetic models of epilepsy. *Biochemical Pharmacology*, **30**: 3137–44.

Jobe, P. C. & Laird, H. E., II (1987). Neurotransmitter systems and the epilepsy models: distinguishing features and unifying principles. In *Neurotransmitters and Epilepsy*, ed. P. C. Jobe & H. E. Laird, pp. 339–66. Clifton, NJ: Humana Press.

Jobe, P. C., Laird, H. E., Ko, K. H., Ray, T. B. & Dailey, J. W. (1982). Abnormalities in monoamine levels in the central nervous system of the genetically epilepsy-prone rat. *Epilepsia*, **23**: 359–66.

Jobe, P. C., Lasley, S. M., Bettendorf, A. F., Frasca, J. J. & Dailey, J. W. (1988). Studies of aspartame on supramaximal electroshock seizures in epileptic and non-epileptic rats. *FASEB Journal*, **2**: A1067.

Jobe, P. C., Mishra, P. K. & Dailey, J. W. (1992). Genetically
  epilepsy-prone rat: actions of antiepileptic drugs and monoaminergic
  neurotransmitters. In *Drugs for the Control of Epilepsy: Actions on
  Neuronal Networks Involved in Seizure Disorders*, ed. C. L. Faingold &
  G. H. Fromm, pp. 253–75. Boca Raton, FL: CRC Press.
Jobe, P. C., Picchioni, A. L. & Chin, L. (1973*a*). Role of brain norepinephrine in
  audiogenic seizure in the rat. *Journal of Pharmacology and Experimental
  Therapeutics*, **184**: 1–10.
Jobe, P. C., Picchioni, A. L. & Chin, L. (1973*b*). Role of 5-hydroxytryptamine
  in audiogenic seizure in the rat. *Life Sciences*, **13**: 1–13.
Jobe, P. C., Picchioni, A. L. Chin, L. (1973*c*). Effect of lithium carbonate and
  alpha-methyl-*p*-tyrosine (alpha-MPT) on audiogenic seizure intensity.
  Journal of Pharmacy and Pharmacology, **25**: 830–1.
Kaplan, H. (1975). What triggers seizures in the gerbil, *Meriones unguiculatus?*
  Life Sciences, **17**: 693–8.
Kaplan, B. J., Seyfried, T. N. & Glaser, G. H. (1979). Spontaneous polyspike
  discharges in an epileptic mutant mouse (tottering). *Experimental
  Neurology*, **66**: 577–86.
Kaufman, I. C., Marshall, C. & Walker, A. E. (1947). Activated
  electroencephalography. *Archives of Neurology and Psychiatry*, **58**:
  533–49.
Kellogg, C. (1971). Serotonin metabolism in the brains of mice sensitive or
  resistant to audiogenic seizures. *Journal of Neurobiology*, **2**: 209–19.
Kellogg, C. (1976). Audiogenic seizures: relation to age and mechanisms of
  monoamine neurotransmission. *Brain Research*, **106**: 87–103.
Killam, E. K. (1976). Measurement of anticonvulsant activity in the *Papio papio*
  model of epilepsy. *Federation Proceedings*, **35**: 2264–9.
Killam, E. K. & Killam, K. F., Jr (1984). Evidence for neurotransmitter
  abnormalities related to seizure activity in the epileptic baboon. *Federation
  Proceedings*, **43**: 2510–15.
Killam, K. F., Killam, E. K. & Naquet, R. (1966*a*). Etudes pharmacologiques
  realisées chez des singes présentant une activité EEG paroxystique
  particulière à la stimulation lumineuse intermittente. *Journal de Physiologie
  (Paris)*, **58**: 543–4.
Killam, K. F., Killam, E. K. & Naquet, R. (1966*b*). Mise en evidence chez
  certains singes d'un syndrome photomyoclonique. *Comptes Rendus de
  l'Académie des Sciences*, **262**: 1010–12.
Killam, K. F., Killam, E. K. & Naquet, R. (1967). An animal model of
  light-sensitive epilepsy. *Electroencephalography and Clinical
  Neurophysiology*, **22**: 497–513.
Killam, K. F., Naquet, R. & Bert, J. (1966*c*). Paroxysmal responses to
  intermittent light stimulation in a population of baboons (*Papio papio*).
  Epilepsia, **7**: 215–19.
Ko, K. H., Dailey, J. W. & Jobe, P. C. (1982). Effect of increments in
  norepinephrine concentrations on seizure intensity in the genetically
  epilepsy-prone rat. *Journal of Pharmacology and Experimental Therapy*,
  222: 662–9.
Ko, K. H., Dailey, J. W. & Jobe, P. C. (1984). Evaluaton of monoaminergic
  receptors in the genetically epilepsy-prone rat. *Experientia*, **40**: 70–3.
Laird, H. E., II & Huxtable, R. J. (1976). Effect of taurine on audiogenic seizure
  response in rats. In *Taurine*, ed. R. Huxtable & A. Barbeau, pp. 267–74.
  New York: Raven Press.

Laird, H. E., II & Huxtable, R. J. (1978). Taurine and audiogenic epilepsy. In *Taurine and Neurological Disorders*, ed. A. Barbeau & R. J. Huxtable, pp. 339–57. New York: Raven Press.

Lasley, S. M., Burger, R. L., Dailey, J. W. & Jobe, P. C. (1989). Regional brain content of amino acid transmitters in genetically epilepsy-prone rats (GEPR). *Society for Neuroscience Abstracts*, **15**: 1215.

Lasley, S. M., Yan, Q.-S. & Burger, R. L. (1990). Diminished *in vivo* potassium (K^+)-stimulated GABA release in genetically epilepsy-prone rats (GEPR). *Society for Neuroscience Abstracts*, **16**: 780.

Lauterborn, J. C. & Ribak, C. E. (1989). Differences in dopamine β-hydroxylase immunoreactivity between the brains of genetically epilepsy-prone and Sprague-Dawley rats. *Epilepsy Research*, **4**: 161–76.

Lee, R. J., Bajorek, J. G. & Lomax, P. (1984). Similar anticonvulsant, but unique, behavioural effects of opioid agonists in the seizure-sensitive Mongolian gerbil. *Neuropharmacology*, **23**: 517–24.

Lee, R. J., Depaulis, A., Lomax, P. & Olsen, R. W. (1989). Anticonvulsant effect of muscimol injected into the thalamus of spontaneously epileptic Mongolian gerbils. *Brain Research*, **487**: 363–7.

Lee, R. J., McCabe, R. T., Wamsley, J. K., Olsen, R. W. & Lomax, P. (1986). Opioid receptor alterations in a genetic model of generalized epilepsy. *Brain Research*, **380**: 76–82.

Lehmann, A. (1967). Audiogenic seizure data in mice supporting new theories of biogenic amine mechanisms in the central nervous system. *Life Sciences*, **6**: 1423–31.

Lehmann, A. (1989). Abnormalities in the levels of extracellular and tissue amino acids in the brain of the seizure-susceptible rat. *Epilepsy Research*, **3**: 130–7.

Lehmann, A., Sandberg, M. & Huxtable, R. J. (1986). In vivo release of neuroactive amines and amino acids from the hippocampus of seizure-resistant and seizure-susceptible rats. *Neurochemistry International*, **8**: 513–20.

Levitt, P. & Noebels, J. L. (1981). Mutant mouse tottering: selective increase of locus coeruleus axons in a defined single locus mutation. *Proceedings of the National Academy of Sciences, USA*, **78**: 4630–4.

Lints, C. E., Willott, J. F., Sze, P. Y. & Nenja, L. H. (1980). Inverse relationship between whole brain monoamine levels and audiogenic seizure susceptibility in mice: failure to replicate. *Pharmacology, Biochemistry and Behavior*, **12**: 385–8.

Liu, Z., Vergnes, M., Depaulis, A. & Marescaux, C. (1991). Evidence for a critical role of GABAergic transmission within the thalamus in the genesis and control of absence seizures in the rat. *Brain Research*, **545**: 1–7.

Lloyd, K. G., Scatton, B., Voltz, C., Bryere, P., Valin, A. & Naquet, R. (1986). Cerebrospinal fluid amino acid and monoamine metabolite levels of *Papio papio*: correlation with photosensitivity. *Brain Research*, **363**: 390–4.

Löscher, W. (1984). Genetic animal models of epilepsy as a unique resource for the evaluation of anticonvulsant drugs. A review. *Methods and Findings in Experimental and Clinical Pharmacology*, **6**: 531–47.

Löscher, W. (1985). Influence of pharmacological manipulation of inhibitory and excitatory neurotransmitter systems on seizure behavior in the Mongolian gerbil. *Journal of Pharmacology and Experimental Therapeutics*, **233**: 204–13.

Löscher, W. & Czuczwar, S. J. (1985). Evaluation of the 5-hydroxytryptamine receptor agonist 8-hydroxy-2-(DI-*n*-Propylamino) tetralin in different rodent models of epilepsy. *Neuroscience Letters*, **60**: 201–6.

Löscher, W., Nolting, B. & Honack, D. (1988). Evaluation of CPP, a selective NMDA antagonist, in various rodent models of epilepsy. Comparison with other NMDA antagonists, and with diazepam and phenobarbital. *European Journal of Pharmacology*, **152**: 9–17.

Loskota, W. J. & Lomax, P. (1975). The Mongolian gerbil (*Meriones unguiculatus*) as a model for the study of the epilepsies: EEG records of seizures. *Electroencephalography and Clinical Neurophysiology*, **38**: 597–604.

Loskota, W. J., Lomax, P. & Rich, S. T. (1974). The gerbil as a model for the study of the epilepsies. *Epilepsia*, **15**: 109–19.

Ludvig, N., Farias, P. A. & Ribak, C. E. (1991). An analysis of various environmental and specific sensory stimuli on the seizure of the Mongolian gerbil. *Epilepsy Research*, **8**: 30–5.

Ludvig, N., Gyorgy, L., Folly, G. & Vizi, E. S. (1985*a*). Yohimbine cannot exert its anticonvulsant action in genetically audiogenic seizure-prone mice. *European Journal of Pharmacology*, **115**, 123–4.

Ludvig, N., Harsing, L. G., Hideg, J. & Vizi, E. S. (1985*b*). Reduced cyclic-AMP responsiveness in the colliculus inferior of audiogenic seizure-prone rats. *Biochemical Pharmacology*, **34**: 2042–4.

Ludvig, N. & Moshé, S. L. (1989). Different behavioral and electrographic effects of acoustic stimulation and dibutyryl cyclic AMP injection into the inferior colliculus in normal and in genetically epilepsy-prone rats. *Epilepsy Research*, **3**: 185–90.

Majkowski, J. & Donadio, M. (1984). Electro-clinical studies of epileptic seizures in Mongolian gerbils. *Electroencephalography and Clinical Neurophysiology*, **57**, 369–77.

Marescaux, C., Vergnes, M., Kiesmann, M., Depaulis, A., Micheletti, G. & Warter, J. M. (1987). Kindling of audiogenic seizures in wistar rats: an EEG study. *Experimental Neurology*, **97**: 160–8.

Marley, R. J., Gaffney, D. & Wahner, J. M. (1986). Genetic influences on GABA-related seizures. *Pharmacology, Biochemistry and Behavior*, **24**: 665–72.

Maxson, S. C., Fine, M. D., Ginsburg, B. S. & Koniecki, D. L. (1983). A mutant for spontaneous seizures in C57 BL/10Bg mice. *Epilepsia*, **24**: 15–24.

McGreer, E. G., Ikeda, H., Asakura, T. & Wada, J. A. (1969). Lack of abnormality in brain aromatic amines in rats and mice susceptible to audiogenic seizures. *Journal of Neurochemistry*, **16**, 945–50.

McLachlan, R. S., Avoli, M. & Gloor, P. (1984*a*). Transition from spindles to generalized spike and wave discharges in the cat: simultaneous single-cell recordings in cortex and thalamus. *Experimental Neurology*, **85**: 413–25.

McLachlan, R. S., Gloor, P. & Avoli, M. (1984*b*). Differential participation of some 'specific' and 'non-specific' thalamic nuclei in generalized spike and wave discharges of feline generalized penicillin epilepsy. *Brain Research*, **307**: 277–87.

McNamara, J. O. (1984). Kindling: an animal model of complex partial epilepsy. *Annals of Neurology*, **16**: S72–S76.

McNamara, J. O. (1986). Kindling model of epilepsy. *Advances in Neurology*, **44**, 303–18.

Meldrum, B. S. (1984). GABAergic agents as anticonvulsants in baboons with photosensitive epilepsy. *Neuroscience Letters*, **47**, 345–9.

Meldrum, B. S., Balzano, E., Gadea, M. & Naquet, R. (1970). Photic and drug-induced epilepsy in the baboon (*Papio papio*): the effects of isoniazid, thiosemicarbazide, pyridoxine and aminooxyacetic acid. *Electroencephalography and Clinical Neurophysiology*, **29**: 333–47.

Meldrum, B. S., Balzano, E., Wada, J. A. & Vuillon-Cacciutto, G. (1972). Effects of L-tryptophan, L-3,4-dihydroxyphenylalanine and tranylcypromine on the electroencephalogram and on photically-induced epilepsy in the baboon *Papio papio*. *Physiological Behavior*, **9**: 615–21.

Meldrum, B. S., Brailowsky, S. & Naquet, R. (1977). Approche pharmacologique de l'épilepsie photosensible du *Papio papio*. *Actualités Pharmacologiques* (*Paris*), **30**: 81–99.

Meldrum, B. S., Chir, B., Horton, R. W. & Toseland, P. A. (1975). A primate model for testing anticonvulsant drugs. *Archives of Neurology*, **32**: 289–94.

Meldrum, B. S., Croucher, M. J., Badman, G. & Collins, J. F. (1983*a*). Antiepileptic action of excitatory amino acid antagonists in the photosensitive baboon, *Papio papio*. *Neuroscience Letters*, **39**: 101–4.

Meldrum, B. S., Croucher, M. J., Czuczwar, S. J., Collins, J. F., Curry, K. Joseph, M. & Stone, T. W. (1983*b*). A comparison of the anticonvulsant potency of ($\pm$) 2-amino-5-phosphono-pentanoic acid and ($\pm$) 2-amino-7-phosphonoheptanoic acid. *Neuroscience*, **9**, 925–30.

Meldrum, B. S. & Horton, R. W. (1971). Convulsive effects of 4-deoxypyridoxine and of bicuculline in photosensitive baboons (*Papio papio*) and in rhesus monkeys (*Macaca mulatta*). *Brain Research*, **35**: 419–36.

Meldrum, B. S. & Horton, R. (1978). Blockade of epileptic responses in the photosensitive baboon, *Papio papio*, by two irreversible inhibitors of GABA-transaminase, gamma-acetylenic GABA (4-amino-hex-5-enoic acid) and gamma-vinyl GABA (4-amino-hex-enoic acid). *Psychopharmacology*, **59**: 47–50.

Meldrum, B. S. & Horton, R. W. (1979). Anticonvulsant activity, in photosensitive baboons *Papio papio*, of two new 1,5-benzodiazepines. *Psychopharmacology*, **60**: 277–80.

Meldrum, B. S. & Horton, R. W. (1980). Effects of the bicyclic GABA agonist, THIP, on myoclonic and seizure responses in mice and baboons with reflex epilepsy. *European Journal of Pharmacology*, **61**: 231–7.

Meldrum, B. S., Menini, C., Naquet, R., Laurent, H. & Stutzmann, J. M. (1979). Proconvulsant, convulsant and other actions of D- and L-stereoisomers of allylglycine in the photosensitive baboon, *Papio papio*. *Electroencephalography and Clinical Neurophysiology*, **47**: 389–95.

Meldrum, B. S., Millan, M, Patel, S. & DeSarro, G. (1988). Anti-epileptic effects of focal micro-injection of excitatory amino acid antagonist. *Journal of Neural Transmission*, **72**: 191–200.

Meldrum, B. S. & Naquet, R. (1971). Effects of psilocybin, dimethyltryptamine, mescaline and various lysergic acid derivatives on the EEG and on photically induced epilepsy in the baboon. *Papio papio*. *Electroencephalography and Clinical Neurophysiology*, **31**: 563–72.

Menini, Ch., Dimov, S., Vuillon-Cacciuttolo, G. & Naquet, R. (1970). Réponses corticales evoquées par stimulation lumineuse chez le *Papio papio*. *Electroencephalography and Clinical Neurophysiology*, **29**: 233–45.

Menini, Ch. & Naquet, R. (1980). Generalized photosensitive epilepsy in the Senegalese baboon (*Papio papio*). In *Advances in Epileptology*, ed. R. Canger, F. Angeleri & K. Penry, pp. 265–72. New York: Raven Press.

Menini, Ch., Silva-Comte, C., Stutzmann, J. M. & Dimov, S. (1981). Cortical unit discharges during photic intermittent stimulation in the *Papio papio*. Relationships with paroxysmal fronto-rolandic activity. *Electroencephalography and Clinical Neurophysiology*, **53**: 42–9.

Menini, Ch., Stutzmann, J. M., Laurent, H. & Valin, A. (1977). Les crises induités – ou non – par la stimulation lumineuse intermittente chez le *Papio papio* après l'injection d'allylglycine. *Review of Electroencephalography and Clinical Neurophysiology*, **7**: 232–8.

Micheletti, G., Marescaux, C., Vergnes, M., Rumbach, L. & Warter, J. M. (1985). Effect of GABA mimetics and GABA antagonists on spontaneous nonconvulsive seizures in Wistar rats. In *L.E.R.S. Monograph Series*, *3*, ed. G. Bartholini, L. Bossi, K. G. Lloyd & M. L. Morselli, pp. 129–37. New York: Raven Press.

Micheletti, G., Warter, J. M., Marescaux, C., Depaulis, A., Tranchant, C., Rumbach, L. & Vergnes, M. (1987). Effects of drugs affecting noradrenergic neurotransmission in rats with spontaneous petit mal-like seizures. *European Journal of Pharmacology*, **135**: 397–402.

Millan, M. H., Meldrum, B. S., Boersma, C. A. & Faingold, C. L. (1988). Excitant amino acids and audiogenic seizures in the genetically epilepsy-prone rat. II. Efferent seizure propagating pathway. *Experimental Neurology*, **99**: 687–98.

Millan, M. H., Meldrum, B. S. & Faingold, C. L. (1986). Induction of audiogenic seizure susceptibility by focal infusion of excitant amino acid or bicuculline into the inferior colliculus of normal rats. *Experimental Neurology*, **91**: 634–9.

Mills, S. A., Razani-Boroujerdi, S., Reigel, C. E., Jobe, P. C. & Savage, D. D. (1990). Decrease in hippocampal [^{3}H]vinylidene kainic acid binding in genetically epilepsy-prone rats. *Neuroscience*, **35**: 519–24.

Mills, S. A. & Savage, D. D. (1988). Evidence of hypothyroidism in the genetically epilepsy-prone rat. *Epilepsy Research*, **2**: 102–10.

Mimaki, T., Yabuuchi, H., Laird, H. E., II & Yamamura, H. I. (1984). Effects of seizures and antiepileptic drugs on benzodiazepine receptors in rat brain. *Pediatric Pharmacology*, **4**: 205–11.

Mishra, P. K., Dailey, J. W., Reigel, C. E. & Jobe, P. C. (1988*a*). Brain norepinephrine and convulsions in the genetically epilepsy-prone rat: sex-dependent responses to Ro 4-1284 treatment. *Life Sciences*, **42**: 1131–7.

Mishra, P. K., Dailey, J. W., Reigel, C. E., Tomsic, M. L. & Jobe, P. C. (1988*b*). Sex-specific distinctions in audiogenic convulsions exhibited by severe seizure genetically epilepsy-prone rats (GEPR-9s). *Epilepsy Research*, **2**: 309–16.

Mishra, P. K., Dailey, J. W., Wang, C., Browning, R. A. & Jobe, P. C. (1990). Effects of 6-hydroxydopamine (6-OHDA) injected into the locus ceruleus (LC) on indices of forebrain and brainstem seizures in genetically epilepsy-prone rats (GEPRs). *Epilepsia*, **31**: 633–4.

Mishra, P. K., Dailey, J. W., Reigel, C. E. & Jobe, P. C. (1989). Audiogenic convulsion in moderate seizure genetically epilepsy-prone rats (GEPR-3's). *Epilepsy Research*, **3**: 191–8.

Mori, A. (1988). El mice: neurochemical approach to the seizure mechanism. *Neurosciences*, **14**: 275–85.

Naquet, R. (1973). L'épilepsie photosensible du *Papio papio*. Un modèle de l'épilepsie photosensible de l'homme. *Archives Italiennes de Biologie*, **111**: 516–26.

⁎ Naquet, R. & Meldrum, B. S. (1972). Photogenic seizures in baboon. In *Experimental Models of Epilepsy – A Manual for the Laboratory Worker,* ed. D. P. Purpura, J. K. Penny, D. M. Woodbury, D. B. Tower & R. D. Walter, pp. 373–406. New York: Raven Press.

Naquet, R. & Meldrum, B. S. (1986). Myoclonus induced by intermittent light stimulation in the baboon: neurophysiological and neuropharmacological approaches. In *Advances in Neurology,* vol. 43 *Myoclonus,* ed. S. Fahn, C. D. Marsden & M. von Waert, pp. 611–27. New York: Raven Press.

Naquet, R., Menini, Ch. & Catier, J. (1972). Photically induced epilepsy in *Papio papio.* The initiation of discharges and the role of the frontal cortex and of the corpus callosum. In *Synchronization of the EEG in the Epilepsies,* ed. H. Petsche & M. A. B. Brazier, pp. 347–67. Vienna: Springer-Verlag.

Naquet, R., Menini, Ch., Riche, D., Silva-Barrat, C. & Valin, A. (1988). Photic epilepsy in man and in the baboon, *Papio papio.* In *Anatomy of Epileptogenesis,* ed. B. S. Meldrum, J. A. Ferrendelli & H. G. Wieser, pp. 107–26. London: John Libbey and Company Ltd.

Naquet, R. & Valin, A. (1990). Focal discharges in photosensitive generalized epilepsy. In *Generalized Epilepsy: Neurobiological Approaches,* ed. M. Avoli, P. Gloor, G. Kostopoulos & R. Naquet, pp. 273–85. Boston, MA: Birkhäuser.

Naritoku, D. K., Mecozzi, L. B. & Faingold, C. L. (1988). Effects of repeated audiogenic seizures (AGS) on seizure severity and EEG in two substrains of the genetically epilepsy-prone rats (GEPRs). *Society for Neuroscience Abstracts,* **14**: 252.

Naritoku, D. K., Mecozzi, L. B., Randall, M. E. & Faingold, C. L. (1989*a*). Infusions of GABA agonists or 2-APH into amygdala (AMY) or medial geniculate (MGB) reversibly reduce seizure duration and clonus after repeated audiogenic seizures (AGS) in the genetically epilepsy-prone rat (GEPR-9). *Society for Neuroscience Abstracts,* **15**: 46.

Naritoku, D. K., Randall, M. E. & Faingold, C. L. (1989*b*). Microinfusions of GABA agonists or 2-APH into amygdala reduce seizure duration and clonus in repeated audiogenic seizures (AGS) of the genetically epilepsy-prone rat (GEPR-9s). *Epilepsia,* **30**: 698.

Naruse, H., Kato, M., Kurokawa, M., Haba, R. & Yabe, T. (1960). Metabolic defects in a convulsive strain of mouse. *Journal of Neurochemistry,* **5**: 359–69.

Newmark, M. E. & Penry, J. K. (1980). *Genetics of Epilepsy: A Review,* pp. 3–84. New York: Raven Press.

Nicoletti, F., Barbaccia, M. L., Iadarola, M., Pozzi, O. & Laird, H. E., II (1986). Abnormality of alpha-1-adrenergic receptors in the frontal cortex of epileptic rats. *Journal of Neurochemistry,* **46**: 270–3.

Noebels, J. L. (1979). Analysis of inherited epilepsy using single locus mutations in mice. *Federation Proceedings,* **38**: 2405–10.

Noebels, J. L. (1984). A single gene error of noradrenergic axon growth synchronizes central neurons. *Nature,* **310**: 409–11.

Noebels, J. L. (1986). Mutational analysis of inherited epilepsies. In *Advances in Neurology,* vol. 44, ed. A. V. Delgado-Escueta, A. A. Ward Jr, D. M. Woodbury & R. J. Porter, pp. 97–113. New York: Raven Press.

Noebels, J. L. & Sidman, R. L. (1979). Inherited epilepsy: spike–wave and focal motor seizures in the mutant mouse tottering. *Science,* **204**: 1334–6.

Olsen, R. W., Wamsley, J. K., McCabe, R. T., Lee, R. J. & Lomax, P. (1985). Benzodiazepine/gamma-amino-butyric acid receptor deficit in the midbrain of the seizure-susceptible gerbil. *Proceedings of the National Academy of Sciences, USA*, **82**: 6701–5.

Palayoor, S. T. & Seyfried, T. N. (1984a). Genetic study of cationic ATPase activities and audiogenic seizure susceptibility in recombinant inbred and congenic strains of mice. *Journal of Neurochemistry*, **42**: 529–33.

Palayoor, S. T. & Seyfried, T. N. (1984b). Genetic association between Ca^{2+}-ATPase activity and audiogenic seizures in mice. *Journal of Neurochemistry*, **42**: 1771–4.

Patrick, D. L. & Faingold, C. L. (1989). Auditory brainstem responses (ABRs) and effects of microinjection into inferior colliculus (IC) of an excitant amino acid (EEA) antagonist or GABA agonist on audiogenic seizures (AGS) in thyroid deficient (THX) or genetically epilepsy-prone rats (GEPRs). *Society for Neuroscience Abstracts*, **15**: 46.

Patrick, D. L. & Faingold, C. L. (1990). Sensitivity differences to blockade of audiogenic seizures (AGS) in thyroid deficient (THX) or genetically epilepsy-prone rats (GEPRs): microinjection into brainstem auditory nuclei. *Society for Neuroscience Abstracts*, **16**: 785.

Paul, L. A., Fried, I., Watanabe, K., Forsythe, A. B. & Scheibel, A. B. (1981). Structural correlates of seizure behavior in the Mongolian gerbil. *Science*, **213**: 924–6.

Pedley, T. A., Horton, R. W. & Meldrum, B. S. (1979). Electroencephalographic and behavioral effects of a GABA agonist (muscimol) on photosensitive epilepsy in the baboon, *Papio papio*. *Epilepsia*, **20**: 409–16.

Pellow, S. & File, S. E. (1984). Behavioral actions Ro 5-4864: a peripheral-type benzodiazepine? *Life Sciences*, **35**: 229–40.

Peterson, G. M. & Ribak, C. E. (1989). Relationship of the hippocampal GABAergic system and genetic epilepsy in the seizure-sensitive gerbil. In *The Hippocampus – New Vistas*, pp. 483–97. New York: Alan R. Liss.

Philo, R. (1982). Catecholamines and pinealectomy-induced convulsions in the gerbil (*Meriones unguiculatus*). In *The Pineal and Its Hormones*, pp. 233–41. New York: Alan R. Liss.

Pumain, R., Louvel, J. & Kurcewicz, I. (1986). Long-term alterations in amino acid-induced ionic conductances in chronic epilepsy. In *Excitatory Amino Acids and Epilepsy*, ed. R. Schwarcz & Y. Ben-Ari, pp. 439–77. New York: Plenum Press.

Pumain, R., Menini, Ch., Heinemann, U., Louvel, J., & Silva-Barrat, C. (1985). Chemical synaptic transmission is not necessary for epileptic seizures to persist in the baboon *Papio papio*. *Experimental Neurology*, **89**: 250–8.

Razani Boroujerdi, S. & Savage, D. D. (1990). Evidence of transient neonatal hypothyroidism in the moderate seizure genetically epilepsy-prone (GEPR-3) rat. *Society for Neuroscience Abstracts*, **16**: 781.

Reigel, C. E. & Aldrich, W. M. (1990). Kanamycin-induced audiogenic seizure (AGS) susceptibility requires monoamine depletion in Sprague-Dawley (SD) rats. *Society for Neuroscience Abstracts*, **16**: 781.

Reigel, C. E., Dailey, J. W. & Jobe, P. C. (1986). The genetically epilepsy-prone rat: an overview of seizure-prone characteristics and responsiveness to anticonvulsant drugs. *Life Sciences*, **39**: 763–74.

Reigel, C. E., Jobe, P. C., Dailey, J. W. & Savage, D. D. (1989a). Ontogeny of sound-induced seizures in the genetically epilepsy-prone rat. *Epilepsy Research*, **4**: 63–71.

Reigel, C. E., Jobe, P. C., Dailey, J. W. & Stewart, J. J. (1988). Responsiveness of genetically epilepsy-prone rats to intracerebroventricular morphine-induced convulsions. *Life Sciences*, **42**: 1743–9.

Reigel, C. E., Joliff, J. L., Jobe, P. C. & Mishra, P. K. (1987a). Ontogeny of monoaminergic determinants of seizure susceptibility and severity in the genetically epilepsy-prone rat. *Society for Neuroscience Abstracts*, **13**: 943.

Reigel, C. E., Mishra, P. K., Jobe, P. C. & Joliff, J. L. (1987b). Ontogeny of noradrenergic determinants of seizure susceptibility and severity in the genetically epilepsy-prone rat. *Federation Proceedings*, **46**: 706.

Reigel, C. E., Randall, M. E. & Faingold, C. L. (1989b). Developmental hearing impairment and audiogenic seizure (AGS) susceptibility in the genetically epilepsy-prone rat. *Society for Neuroscience Abstracts*, **15**: 46.

Riaz, A. & Faingold, C. L. (1989). Effects of excitant amino acid (EAA) antagonists on audiogenic seizures (AGS) during ethanol withdrawal (EXT) and in genetically epilepsy-prone rats (GEPRs). *Society for Neuroscience Abstracts*, **15**: 46.

Ribak, C. E., Byun, M. Y., Ruiz, G. T. & Reiffenstein, R. J. (1988a). Increased levels of amino acid neurotransmitters in the inferior colliculus of the genetically epilepsy-prone rat. *Epilepsy Research*, **2**: 9–13.

Ribak, C. E., Ghaderi, L. & Byun, M. Y. (1989). Seizure severity correlates with an increase in the number of GABAergic neurons in the moderate seizure line of genetically epilepsy-prone rat. *Epilepsia*, **30**: 698.

Ribak, C. E. & Khan, S. U. (1987). The effect of knife cuts of hippocampal pathways on epileptic activity in the seizure-sensitive gerbil. *Brain Research*, **418**, 146–51.

Ribak, C. E., Roberts, R. C., Byun, M. Y. & Kim, H. L. (1988b). Anatomical and behavioral analyses of the inheritance of audiogenic seizures in the progeny of genetically epilepsy-prone and Sprague-Dawley rats. *Epilepsy Research*, **2**: 345–55.

Roberts, R. C., Kim, K. H. & Ribak, C. E. (1985a). Increased numbers of neurons occur in the inferior colliculus of the young genetically epilepsy-prone rat. *Developmental Brain Research*, **23**: 277–81.

Roberts, R. C. & Ribak, C. E. (1986). Anatomical changes of the GABAergic system in the inferior colliculus of the genetically epilepsy-prone rat. *Life Sciences*, **39**, 789–98.

Roberts, R. C., Ribak, C. E. & Oertel, W. H. (1985b). Increased numbers of GABAergic neurons occur in the inferior colliculus of an audiogenic model of genetic epilepsy. *Brain Research*, **36**: 324–38.

Robertson, H. A. (1980). Audiogenic seizures: increased benzodiazepine receptor binding in a susceptible strain of mice. *European Journal of Pharmacology*, **66**: 249–52.

Rogawski, M. A. & Porter, R. J. (1990). Antiepileptic drugs: pharmacological mechanisms and clinical efficacy with consideration of promising developmental stage compounds. *Pharmacological Review*. **43**: 223–86.

Rosenblatt, D. E., Lauter, C. J. & Trams, E. G. (1976). Deficiency of a Ca^{2+}-ATPase in brains of seizure prone mice. *Journal of Neurochemistry*, **27**, 1299–304.

Savage, D. D., Mills, S. A., Jobe, P. C. & Reigel, C. E. (1988). Elevation of naloxone-sensitive ^{3}H-dihydromorphine binding in hippocampal formation of genetically epilepsy-prone rats. *Life Sciences*, **43**: 239–46.

Savage, D. D., Reigel, C. E. & Jobe, P. C. (1986). Angular bundle kindling is accelerated in rats with a genetic predispositon to acoustic stimulus-induced seizures. *Brain Research*, **376**: 412–15.

Sax, D. A., Hirano, A. & Shofer, R. J. (1968). Staggerer, a neurological murine mutant: an electron microscopic study of the cerebellar cortex in the adult. *Neurology*, **18**: 1093–100.

Schlesinger, K., Boggan, W. & Freedman, D. X. (1965). Genetics of audiogenic seizures. I. Relation to brain serotonin and norepinephrine in mice. *Life Sciences*, **4**: 2345–51.

Schlesinger, K., Boggan, W. O. & Freedman, D. X. (1970). Genetics of audiogenic seizures. III. Time response relationships between drug administration and seizure susceptibility. *Life Sciences*, **9**:721–9.

Schwartzkroin, P. A. (1986). Hippocampal slices in experimental and human epilepsy. In *Advances in Neurology*, vol. 44, ed. A. V. Delgado-Escueta, A. A. Ward Jr, D. M. Woodbury & R. J. Porter, pp. 991–1010. New York: Raven Press.

Seregi, A., Forstermann, U., Heldt, R. & Hertting, G. (1985). The formation and regional distribution of prostaglandins D_2 and F_2 in the brain of spontaneously convulsing gerbils. *Brain Research*, **337**, 171–4.

Seregi, A., Forstermann, U. & Hertting, G. (1984). Decreased levels of brain cyclo-oxygenase products as a possible cause of increased seizure susceptibility in convulsion-prone gerbils. *Brain Research*, **305**: 393–5.

Seyfried, T. N., Glaser, G. H. & Yu, R. K. (1979). Thyroid hormone influence on the susceptibility of mice to audiogenic seizures. *Science*, **205**: 598–600.

Seyfried, T. N., Glaser, G. H. & Yu, R. K. (1981). Thyroid hormone can restore the audiogenic seizure susceptibility of hypothyroid DBA/2J mice. *Experimental Neurology*, **71**: 220–5.

Seyfried, T. N., Glaser, G. H. & Yu, R. K. (1984). Genetic analysis of serum thyroxine content and audiogenic seizures in recombinant inbred and congenic strains of mice. *Experimental Neurology*, **83**: 423–8.

Shorvon, S. D. (1990). The routine EEG. In *Comprehensive Epileptology*, **25**, ed. M. Dam & L. Gram, pp. 321–38. New York: Raven Press.

Silva-Barrat, C., Brailowsky, S., Levesque, G. & Menini, C. (1988*a*). Epileptic discharges induced by intermittent light stimulation in photosensitive baboons: a current source density study. *Epilepsy Research*, **2**: 1–8.

Silva-Barrat, C., Brailowsky, S., Riche, D. & Menini, C. (1988*b*). Anticonvulsant effects of localized chronic infusions of GABA in cortical and reticular structures of baboons. *Experimental Neurology*, **101**: 418–27.

Silva-Barrat, C. & Menini, Ch. (1984). The influence of light stimulation on potentials evoked by single flashes in photosensitive and non-photosensitive *Papio papio*. *Electroencephalography and Clinical Neurophysiology*, **57**: 448–61.

Silva-Barrat, C. & Menini, Ch. (1990). Photosensitive epilepsy of the baboon: a generalized epilepsy with a motor cortical origin. In *Generalized Epilepsy: Neurobiological Approaches*, ed. M. Avoli, P. Gloor, G. Kostopoulos & R. Naquet, pp. 286–97. Boston, MA: Birkhäuser.

Silva-Barrat, C., Menini, Ch., Bryere, P. & Naquet, R. (1986). Multiunitary activity analysis of cortical and subcortical structures in paroxysmal discharges and grand mal seizures in photosensitive baboons. *Electroencephalography and Clinical Neurophysiology*, **64**: 455–68.

Stark, L. G., Killam, K. F. & Killam, E. K. (1970). The anticonvulsant effect of phenobarbital, diphenylhydantoin and two benzodiazepines in the baboon *Papio papio. Journal of Pharmacology and Experimental Therapy*, **173**: 125–32.

Stutzmann, J. M., Laurent, H., Valin, A. & Menini, Ch. (1980). Paroxysmal visual evoked potentials (PVEP) in *Papio papio*. II. Evidence for a facilitatory effect of photic intermittent stimulation. *Electroencephalography and Clinical Neurophysiology*, **50**: 365–74.

Suzuki, J. & Nakamoto, Y. (1977). Seizure patterns and electroencephalograms of El mouse. *Electroencephalography and Clinical Neurophysiology*, **43**: 229–311.

Tacke, U. & Braestrup, C. (1984). A study of benzodiazepine receptor binding in audiogenic seizure-susceptible rats. *ACTA Pharmacology and Toxicology*, **55**: 252–9.

Tassinari, C. A., Rubboli, G. & Michelucci, R. (1990). Reflex epilepsy. In *Comprehensive Epileptology*, **17**, ed. M. Dam & L. Gram, pp. 233–46. New York: Raven Press.

Thiessen, D. D., Lindzey, G. & Friend, H. C. (1968). Spontaneous seizures in the Mongolian gerbil. *Psychonomatic Science*, **11**: 227–8.

Ticku, M. K. (1979). Differences in γ-aminobutyric acid receptor sensitivity in inbred strains of mice. *Journal of Neurochemistry*, **33**: 1135–8.

Toth, E., Lajtha, A., Sarhan, S. & Seiler, N. (1983). Anticonvulsant effects of some inhibitory neurotransmitter amino acids. *Neurochemical Research*, **8**: 291–302.

Trams, E. G. & Lauter, C. J. (1978). Ecto-ATPase deficiency in glia of seizure-prone mice. *Nature*, **271**, 270–1.

Trimble, M. R. (1977). Effect of nomifensine on brain amines and epilepsy in photosensitive baboons. *British Journal of Clinical Pharmacology*, **4**: 101S–107S.

Valin, A., Dodd, R. A., Liston, D. R., Potier, P. & Rossier, J. (1982). Methyl-β-carboline-induced convulsions are antagonized by Ro-15-1788 and by propyl-β-carboline. *European Journal of Pharmacology*, **85**: 93–7.

Valin, A., Kaijima, M., Bryere, P. B. Naquet, R. (1983). Differential effects of the benzodiazepine antagonist Ro15-1788 on two types of myoclonus in baboon *Papio papio. Neuroscience Letters*, **38**: 79–84.

Vergnes, M., Kiesmann, M., Marescaux, C., Depaulis, A., Micheletti, G. & Warter, J. M. (1987*a*). Kindling of audiogenic seizures in the rat. *International Journal of Neuroscience*, **36**: 167–76.

Vergnes, M., Marescaux, C., Depaulis, A., Micheletti, G. & Warter, J.-M. (1987*b*). Spontaneous spike and wave discharges in thalamus and cortex in a rat model of genetic petit mal-like seizures. *Experimental Neurology*, **96**: 127–36.

Vergnes, M., Marescaux, C., Depaulis, A., Micheletti, G. & Warter, J.-M. (1990). Spontaneous spike-and-wave discharges in Wistar rats: a model of genetic generalized nonconvulsive epilepsy. In *Generalized Epilepsy: Neurobiological Approaches*, ed. M. Avoli, P. Gloor, G. Kostopoulos & R. Naquet, pp. 238–53. Boston, MA: Birkhäuser.

Vergnes, M., Marescaux, C., Micheletti, G., Depaulis, A., Rumbach, L. & Warter, J.-M. (1984). Enhancement of spike and wave discharges by GABAmimetic drugs in rats with spontaneous petit-mal-like epilepsy. *Neuroscience Letters*, **44**: 91–4.

Vergnes, M., Marescaux, C., Micheletti, G., Reis, J., Depaulis, A., Rumbach, L. & Warter, J.-M. (1982). Spontaneous paroxysmal electroclinical patterns in rat: a model of generalized non-convulsive epilepsy. *Neuroscience Letters,* **33**: 97–101.

Vuillon-Cacciuttolo, G. & Balzano, E. (1972). Action de quatre derivés de l'ergot sur la photosensibilité et l'EEG du *Papio papio. Journal of Pharmacology,* **3**: 31–45.

Vuillon-Cacciuttolo, G., Meldrum, B. S. & Balzano, E. (1973). Electroretinogram and afferent visual transmission in the epileptic baboon, *Papio papio*; effects of drugs influencing monoaminergic systems. *Epilepsia,* **14**: 213–21.

Wada, J. A., Balzano, E., Meldrum, B. S. & Naquet, R. (1972). Behavioral and electrographic effects of l-5-hydroxytryptan and d,l-parachlorophenyl-alanine on epileptic Senegalese baboon (*Papio papio*). *Electroencephalography and Clinical Neurophysiology,* **33**: 520–6.

Wada, J. A., Catier, J., Charmasson, G., Menini, Ch. & Naquet, R. (1973). Further examination of neural mechanisms underlying photosensitivity in the epileptic Senegalese baboon *Papio papio. Electroencephalography and Clinical Neurophysiology,* **34**: 786.

Walter, S., Balzano, E., Vuillon-Cacciuttolo, G. & Naquet, R. (1971). Effets comportementaux et électrographiques du diethylamide de l'acide d-lysergique (LSD 25) sur le *Papio papio* photosensible. *Electroencephalography and Clinical Neurophysiology,* **30**: 294–305.

Wang, C., Jobe, P. C. & Browning, R. A. (1990). Effect of 6-OHDA-induced lesions of the medial forebrain bundle (MFB) on audiogenic seizures in genetically epilepsy-prone rats (GEPR-3s). *Society for Neuroscience Abstracts,* **16**: 781.

Warter, J. M., Vergnes, M., Depaulis, A., Tranchant, C., Rumbach, L., Micheletti, G. & Marescaux, C. (1988). Effects of drugs affecting dopaminergic neurotransmission in rats with spontaneous petit mal-like seizures. *Neuropharmacology,* **27**: 269–74.

Waterhouse, B. D. (1986). Electrophysiological assessment of monoamine synaptic function in neuronal circuits of seizure susceptible brains. *Life Sciences,* **39**: 807–18.

Williams, D. (1953). A study of thalamic and cortical rhythms in petit mal. *Brain,* **76**: 50–69.

Wolf, P. & Goosses, R. (1986). Relation of photosensitivity to epileptic syndromes. *Journal of Neurology, Neurosurgery and Psychiatry,* **49**, 1368–91.

Wolf-Dieter, R., Heuschneider, G., Sperk, G. & Riederer, P. (1989). Biochemical events in spontaneous seizures in the Mongolian gerbil. *Metabolic Brain Disease,* **4**: 3–7.

Yan, Q.-S., Berger, R., Jobe, P. C. & Dailey, J. W. (1990*a*). Anticonvulsant doses of fluoxetine increase dialyzable serotonin from the thalamus of genetically epilepsy-prone rats (GEPRs). *FASEB Journal,* **4**: A465.

Yan, Q.-S., Jobe, P. C. & Dailey, J. W. (1990*b*). Parenteral carbamazepine: effect on convulsions and on dialyzable hippocampal serotonin (5-HT) in genetically epilepsy-prone rats (GEPRs). *Society for Neuroscience Abstracts,* **16**: 784.

Yourick, D. L., LaPlaca, M. & Meyerhoff, J. L. (1990). Norepinephrine-stimulated inositol phosphate accumulation in cortex, amygdala/pyriform cortex and hippocampus of genetically epilepsy-prone and kindled rats. *Society for Neuroscience Abstracts,* **16**: 780.

4

Noradrenergic modulation of excitability: transplantation approaches to epilepsy research

OLLE LINDVALL

Introduction

The first attempts to implant central nervous system (CNS) tissue into the adult mammalian brain were performed a century ago (Thompson, 1890), seemingly with very poor graft survival. Although developing CNS tissue had been shown by Dunn (1917) and Le Gros Clark (1940) to survive transplantation, the ability of such grafts to establish extensive afferent and efferent connections with the recipient's brain and to influence the behavior of the host was not demonstrated until the late 1970s (for a historical overview see e.g., Björklund & Stenevi, 1985). Since then, grafting of fetal neural tissue into the mammalian CNS has emerged as a widely used experimental tool with which to study a diversity of neuro-biological problems, for example mechanisms of neural development, plasticity and regeneration. Much basic research has been devoted to the morphological and functional analysis of neural grafts in animal models of human neurological disorders, such as Parkinson's disease, Huntington's disease, and dementia. This has led to the first clinical trials with intrastriatal implantation of fetal dopamine-rich mesencephalic tissue in patients with Parkinson's disease (see e.g., Lindvall et al., 1990).

Considerably less work has been performed with neural grafts in experimental epilepsy. Recent animal data seem to indicate that neural grafts can reduce the hyperexcitability of an epileptic brain region (Barry et al., 1987; Buzsáki et al., 1988), and have thus provided the necessary impetus for further studies using this approach. The objective of this chapter is to discuss the usefulness and limitations of the neural grafting technique both for studies on pathophysiological mechanisms in experimentally induced seizures and as a tool to reduce neuronal hyperexcitability. The main emphasis is on transplantation of fetal norepinephrine-rich tissue from the pontine locus coeruleus region, which

141

seems to provide a highly suitable model system. First, considerable evidence has accumulated which indicates that intrinsic locus coeruleus neurons act to dampen epileptic activity in the CNS (see e.g., Chauvel & Trottier, 1986); second, the anatomy of this system is well known, and the locus coeruleus neurons can easily be demonstrated microscopically and are also susceptible to relatively specific destruction using the neurotoxin 6-hydroxydopamine (6-OHDA) (see e.g., Björklund & Lindvall, 1986); third, there is an extensive knowledge of the biochemical, pharmacological and physiological characteristics of pre- and postsynaptic noradrenergic mechanisms (see e.g., Foote *et al.*, 1983); fourth, grafted locus coeruleus neurons have been shown to grow into the host brain and modify the function and behavior of the host (Björklund *et al.*, 1979, 1986; Buchanan & Nornes, 1986; Barry *et al.*, 1987; Semenova *et al.*, 1987; Buzsáki *et al.*, 1988; Collier *et al.*, 1988; Yakovleff *et al.*, 1989).

Transplantation techniques

Figure 4.1 illustrates one attractive feature of the neural grafting approach in epilepsy research, i.e., that it allows for a detailed analysis of the

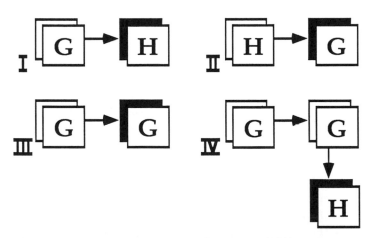

Fig. 4.1. Schematic representation of some possibilities of combining graft (G) and host (H) when neural transplantation is used for epilepsy research. Black shadow denotes hyperexcitability. I, influence of one or more grafts on the epileptic host brain (most suitable transplantation techniques are Solid and Dissociated in Fig. 4.2); II, influence of the normal host brain on an epileptic graft (Solid and Dissociated); III, influence of a graft on an epileptic graft (Intraocular); and IV, influence of one graft, regulated or activated by another graft, on the epileptic host brain (Solid).

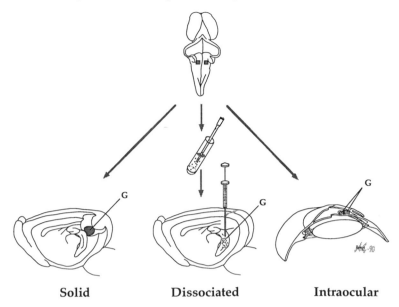

Solid   Dissociated   Intraocular

Fig. 4.2. Schematic illustration of three different transplantation techniques that can be used in epilepsy research, for example to study the influence of noradrenergic locus coeruleus grafts (G) on hyperexcitability in the hippocampus. The tissue is taken from rat fetuses (as illustrated here the developing locus coeruleus region) and implanted as a solid piece into a cortical cavity adjacent to the structure to be innervated (in this case the hippocampus) or prepared as a cell suspension and injected stereotaxically directly into the brain parenchyma. Pieces of fetal tissue can also be transplanted to the anterior chamber of the eye.

interaction between non-epileptic and epileptic graft and host neurons in various combinations. To achieve this it is important that the transplantation technique is carefully selected on the basis of the aim of the study. There are three main grafting procedures in which: (a) tissue pieces are put into a premade cavity (Solid in Fig. 4.2); (b) dissociated tissue is injected stereotaxically directly into the brain (Dissociated in Fig. 4.2); and (c) tissue pieces are placed in the anterior chamber of the eye (Intraocular in Fig. 4.2). As will be described below, each of these techniques have advantages and disadvantages for epilepsy research. Only immature CNS tissue survives transplantation, and for each region there is a time interval during development that is optimal for grafting. One factor of importance for the degree of graft survival is that the dissection of the fetal tissue is carried out before the cell type in question has begun to extend long axonal processes. (For a detailed description of the dissection of fetal neural tissue for transplantation, see Seiger, 1985.)

Intracerebral grafts of solid tissue

Implantation of tissue pieces into the brain (Fig. 4.2; for details, see Stenevi *et al.*, 1985) most often requires the removal of host tissue to form a transplantation cavity. Intraventricular grafts (see e.g., Freed, 1985) are useful only when the objective is to influence areas immediately adjacent to the ventricles. Injected solid CNS tissue survives poorly and gives rise to large necrotic areas around the transplant. Much better conditions for survival and growth are created if the grafts are placed in cavities (produced by suction) in the cortex, exposing the blood vessels in the choroidal fissure. For example, in order to obtain a graft-derived innervation of the hippocampal formation from solid locus coeruleus implants, two locations of cortical cavities have been found to be particularly useful (Björklund *et al.*, 1979). (a) The *caudal site* in the occipital–retrosplenial cortex on the pia overlying the superior colliculus (illustrated schematically in Fig. 4.2). This cavity transects the perforant path input to the dorsal hippocampal formation. (b) The *rostral site* between septum and hippocampus. The cavity transects the fornix, hippocampal fimbria, dorsal routes of cholinergic, noradrenergic and serotonergic afferents to the hippocampus, as well as the major commissural connections running in the hippocampal commissure. This placement has also beeen used in many studies for fetal acetylcholine-rich grafts from the septum-diagonal band region to provide the hippocampal formation with a new cholinergic innervation (Björklund & Stenevi, 1977). In order to get good graft survival in areas outside the choroidal fissure, the cavity is created first and the transplantation of the solid CNS tissue pieces performed several weeks later, when blood vessels have formed on the walls of the cavity.

The *limitations* of this transplantation technique are related primarily to the removal of tissue when a cavity is being created. This makes it more traumatic to the host brain than using stereotaxic injections of dissociated tissue (see below). The main *advantages* are:

(1) The graft is easily accessible from outside, even after long survival times. This allows, for example, for injections of tracers or different pharmacological agents as well as for electrophysiological recordings within selected portions of the graft to be made under direct visual control. Moreover, the graft is in most cases well delineated so that it can be destroyed selectively.

(2) Since the implantation is performed under visual guidance the

placement, orientation and possibilities for interaction between several individual grafts can be well controlled. This allows for studies on the interaction (a) between selected neuronal populations and their target tissue, both of which are placed in a cavity, and (b) between the grafts and the host brain. For example, pieces of fetal locus coeruleus have thus been observed to reinnervate pieces of fetal hippocampus placed in the same cortical cavity (U. Stenevi, unpublished results).

Intracerebral grafts of dissociated tissue

The procedure involves three major steps (Fig. 4.2; for technical details, see Brundin *et al.*, 1985). First, there is dissection and collection of CNS tissue from several fetuses; second, a dissociation step, which may or may not include incubation in trypsin, followed by washing and mechanical dissociation of the tissue by pipetting. In case of fetal locus coeruleus, trypsinization leads to poor graft survival and should therefore be avoided. The third step is the stereotaxic injection of the cell suspension into the host brain. The major *limitation* of this transplantation technique is that suspension grafts become diffusely delineated and less well organized internally than are solid grafts. Tracer injections or electrical recordings in the graft are therefore much more difficult to perform than on solid tissue pieces placed in superficial cavities. One possibility for overcoming this problem is to record in slice preparations that also include the graft (see e.g., Segal *et al.*, 1988).

The *advantages* are:

(1) Transplantation can be performed with a minimum of damage to the recipient's brain and the graft tissue can be implanted at any predetermined site in the CNS. These include structures that are difficult to reach with solid grafts in premade cavities such as the substantia nigra and the amygdala (see below).

(2) Multiple implantation sites are possible, which allow for reinnervation of larger areas of the host brain. This may be necessary in order to effect a significant change of seizure susceptibility in some epilepsy models.

(3) Different cell populations can be mixed before transplantation, which in epilepsy research could be of interest, for example to implant two types of inhibitory neurons such as noradrenergic and GABAergic cells.

Intraocular grafts of solid tissue

In this technique pieces of fetal brain tissue are introduced into the anterior chamber of the adult eye and placed on the iris (Fig. 4.2; for technical details see Olson *et al.*, 1983; Olson & Hoffer, 1985).

The major *limitation* of this technique in epilepsy research is that it cannot be used for studies of graft influences on convulsive behavioral parameters in the host.

The *advantages* can be summarized as follows:

(1) The morphological and functional interaction between multiple grafts can be studied.
(2) The grafts are easily accessible for electrochemical and electrophysiological recordings.
(3) Pharmacological agents and electrical stimuli can be applied directly to the grafts and epileptogenic drugs can be administered locally.

Mechanisms of action of locus coeruleus grafts

Although functional effects after transplantation of fetal neural tissue to the CNS have been demonstrated in many different animal model systems, the exact mechanisms by which the graft influences the host brain often remain more or less unclear. Obviously, control experiments must first be performed to exclude non-specific effects of, for example, the transplantation surgery or the volume increase of the graft. If a specific graft effect can be demonstrated, four mechanisms of action seem possible (Björklund *et al.*, 1987). (a) The fetal graft tissue could have a trophic influence on the host brain and stimulate recovery mechanisms such as sprouting from intrinsic neurons. This does not require long-term survival of the graft and could probably be exerted by any type of fetal CNS tissue. (b) The graft could act as a biological mini-pump, establish no, or very few, synaptic contacts with host neurons, and release transmitter substances into the surrounding parenchyma or cerebrospinal fluid in a diffuse, hormonal manner. (c) The grafted neurons could reinnervate elements in the host brain, form synaptic contacts and provide a tonic, unregulated (or auto-regulated) release of neurotransmitter, sufficient to restore tonic activation, inhibition or disinhibition of host circuitry. (d) The grafted neurons could be more completely integrated, anatomically and functionally, into the host brain by establishing extensive afferent and efferent connections.

Grafts obtained from the locus coeruleus region of rat fetuses have been reported to improve spinal reflexes and locomotor activity in the lesioned spinal cord (Buchanan & Nornes, 1986; Yakovleff *et al.*, 1989), avoidance learning in aged rats (Collier *et al.*, 1988), open field locomotion in 6-OHDA-lesioned rats (Semenova *et al.*, 1987), and development of epileptic phenomena in 6-OHDA lesioned (Barry *et al.*, 1987) or fimbria-fornix lesioned rats (Buzsáki *et al.*, 1988). The most detailed morphological analysis has been performed on locus coeruleus grafts in the hippocampus. Several studies have shown (Björklund *et al.*, 1979, 1986; Barry *et al.*, 1987) that grafted locus coeruleus neurons survive and form a new noradrenergic terminal plexus in the denervated hippocampus with a pattern similar to that of the intrinsic innervation (Fig. 4.3). Also without previous denervation, the grafted neurons are able to grow into the hippocampus and give rise to a low density noradrenergic innervation in addition to the normal one. The graft-derived noradrenergic terminal axons seem to form synaptic contacts with host neurons in both the denervated and non-denervated hippocampus (Murata *et al.*, 1990).

Intrahippocampal locus coeruleus suspension grafts restore total norepinephrine levels in the denervated hippocampus to a mean of 55% of normal levels (Björklund *et al.*, 1986). In animals with good graft-derived reinnervation, the norepinephrine synthesis rate (measured as the rate of 3,4-dihydroxyphenylalanine (dopa) accumulation after synthesis inhibition) was found to be close to normal. Furthermore, intracerebral microdialysis has demonstrated that grafted locus coeruleus neurons are able to restore extracellular norepinephrine in the denervated hippocampus to near-normal levels under baseline conditions (Bengzon *et al.*, 1991).

In summary, available data indicate, first, that grafted noradrenergic locus coeruleus neurons exert their functional effects through a synaptic release of norepinephrine and, second, that they are spontaneously active. Much less is known about which mechanisms are important for regulating the activity of, and norepinephrine release from, the grafted locus coeruleus neurons and which receptors are involved in the postsynaptic effects. It has not yet been clarified whether there is an autoregulation of transmitter release from these neurons similar to what seems to be the case for intrastriatal grafts of mesostriatal dopaminergic neurons (Strecker *et al.*, 1987). Microdialysis studies have, however, provided some evidence that the host brain can influence the release of norepinephrine from grafted locus coeruleus neurons. First, electrical stimulation of the lateral habenula induces an approximately two-fold increase of extracellular

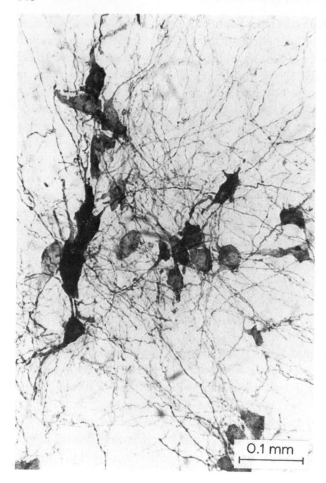

Fig. 4.3. Rat noradrenergic locus coeruleus neurons in an intrahippocampal cell suspension graft as demonstrated by tyrosine hydroxylase immunocytochemistry.

norepinephrine levels in the grafted, previously denervated, hippocampus (Kalén *et al.*, 1991); second, a generalized kindled seizure leads to a three-fold increase of norepinephrine release in both the stimulated and non-stimulated hippocampus (see below and Fig. 4.5; Bengzon *et al.*, 1991). These data suggest that the locus coeruleus grafts to some extent are integrated functionally and probably also anatomically with the host brain. In fact, morphological evidence has been provided for a possible innervation of the grafted locus coeruleus neurons by the host (Murata *et al.*, 1990).

Of major importance is of course what level of integration of the graft with the host neuronal circuitry is necessary for a particular functional effect in the recipient's brain. Experiments with intrastriatal dopamine-rich grafts in Parkinsonian rats have shown that simple motor abnormalities can easily be reversed by the grafts (Björklund & Stenevi, 1979; Perlow *et al.*, 1979), whereas deficits in at least some complex behaviors are not improved (Dunnett *et al.*, 1987). The absence of a functional effect may reflect the lack of appropriate anatomical and functional connections between the host and the ectopically placed graft. It remains to be elucidated how much integration with the host is required for a graft to have effects on neuronal excitability and seizure activity. The temporally well-defined, transient and marked increase of norepinephrine release from grafted locus coeruleus neurons that occurs concomitantly with their seizure-suppressant action (Bengzon *et al.*, 1991) and in a manner similar to that of the intrinsic system, may reflect a necessary integration with the host.

Locus coeruleus grafts in experimental models of epilepsy

Hippocampal kindling in norepinephrine-depleted forebrain

Rats with extensive 6-OHDA-induced lesions of forebrain NA neurons exhibit a marked facilitation of the rate of amygdala and hippocampal kindling due to the powerful inhibitory influence on the development of kindled seizures normally exerted by the locus coeruleus system (McIntyre *et al.*, 1979; Corcoran & Mason, 1980; McIntyre & Edson, 1981, 1982; Araki *et al.*, 1983). A series of grafting experiments has been initiated in such animals with the following main objectives. First, to explore the capacity of locus coeruleus grafts to reverse the functional deficit induced by the 6-OHDA lesion, i.e., to retard the kindling rate in norepinephrine-depleted, hyperexcitable rats; second, to elucidate the mechanisms underlying the functional effect of the grafts in kindled seizures; and, third, to obtain more information on the role and mode of action of the intrinsic locus coeruleus system in kindling. In the first study (Barry *et al.*, 1987), locus coeruleus grafts implanted bilaterally into the hippocampus were found to retard the development of hippocampal kindling in norepinephrine-depleted rats (Fig. 4.4). The noradrenergic neurons in the grafts had reinnervated the dorsal two-thirds of the hippocampal formation, whereas only few graft-derived noradrenergic axons were observed outside the hippocampus. The retardation of seizure development was significantly correlated with the degree of noradrenergic axonal ingrowth

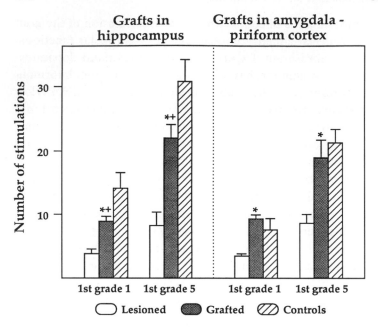

Fig. 4.4. Number of electrical kindling stimulations in the caudal hippocampus to reach the first grade 1 and 5 seizures, respectively, in normal rats and in 6-OHDA-treated rats with either bilateral locus coeruleus grafts in the hippocampus or in the amygdala–piriform cortex or with bilateral sham vehicle grafts. (*) Grafted rats significantly different from lesioned at $P < 0.05$ (amygdala–piriform cortex group) or at $P < 0.01$ (hippocampus group); ($+$) grafted rats significantly different from controls at $P < 0.05$. One-way analysis of variance (ANOVA) with post hoc Newman–Keul's test. Bars indicate S.E.M.s. (Redrawn and modified from Barry et al., 1989.).

into the stimulated hippocampus (primary kindling site), supporting the view that the seizure-suppressant action of the grafts was mediated via noradrenergic mechanisms. In a subsequent study, this effect was only obtained with bilateral grafts and could not be demonstrated after implantation of locus coeruleus tissue unilaterally in the hippocampus ipsilateral to the stimulating electrode (Barry et al., 1989).

The functional capacity of locus coeruleus grafts has also been tested after implantation into a region distant to the stimulating electrode (Barry et al., 1989). The amygdala–piriform cortex was chosen as implantation site, since this region has been proposed to be of central importance for the development and expression of kindled seizures (Racine & Burnham, 1984; McIntyre & Racine, 1986). The locus coeruleus grafts, placed bilaterally into the amygdala–piriform cortex, retarded kindling rate evoked by hippocampal stimulation to the same degree as if they had been implanted into the hippocampus (Fig. 4.4). In this experiment it was not possible to determine the degree of noradrenergic reinnervation by the grafts and their mechanisms of action therefore remain to be elucidated. However, the working hypothesis is that the grafted locus coeruleus neurons have influenced kindling rate through norepinephrine release at denervated postsynaptic sites in the amygdala–piriform cortex. Restoration of noradrenergic neurotransmission in this area, remote from the stimulation site, thus seems to be sufficient to normalize the susceptibility of the norepinephrine-depleted animals to kindled seizures, elicited by stimulation in the hippocampus.

A major objective for subsequent studies has been to provide further evidence that the seizure-suppressant action of the locus coeruleus grafts is mediated through noradrenergic mechanisms. Using intracerebral microdialysis it has been shown that intrahippocampal locus coeruleus grafts respond with a three-fold increase of norepinephrine release to generalized kindled seizures in a way very similar to the intrinsic system (Fig. 4.5; Bengzon *et al.*, 1991). Furthermore, the seizure-suppressant action of intrahippocampal locus coeruleus grafts is blocked by systemic administration of the α-2 adrenergic receptor antagonist, idazoxan, before each kindling stimulation (Bengzon *et al.*, 1990*b*). This may suggest (cf. Gellman *et al.*, 1987) that norepinephrine released from these grafts influences kindling rate via activation of postsynaptic α-2 adrenergic receptors.

Spontaneous and picrotoxin-induced seizures in subcortically denervated hippocampus

Buzsáki *et al.* (1988) have described an epilepsy model that is created by removing major parts of the subcortical inhibitory input to the hippocampus. The lesion, which involves aspiration of the medial portion of the parietal cortex and cingulate cortex, transects the cingulate bundle, the supracallosal stria, the corpus callosum, the dorsal fornix, the fimbria and the ventral hippocampal commissure (similar to the 'rostral site' transplantation cavity, see above). According to Buzsáki *et al.* (1988) this leads to the removal of cholinergic and GABAergic afferents from the septal area, noradrenergic afferents from the locus coeruleus, serotonergic afferents from the mesencephalic raphe, several minor pathways from other subcortical nuclei, the commissural pathways and the subcortical efferent projection of the hippocampal formation. Animals with this lesion

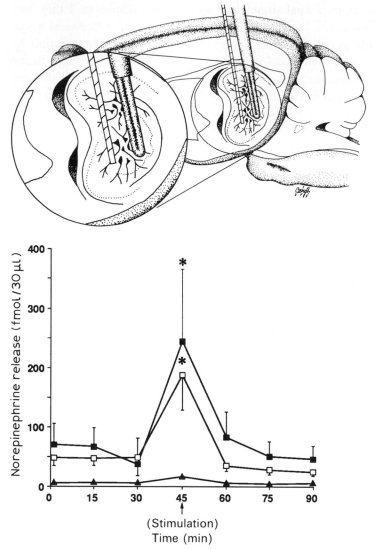

Fig. 4.5. (Top) Schematic illustration of the location of the microdialysis probe and the kindling stimulation electrode in the hippocampus of previously norepi-nephrine-depleted rats with intrahippocampal locus coeruleus cell suspension grafts. (Botton) Extracellular levels of hippocampal norepinephrine in intact rats (□), in 6-OHDA treated animals with bilateral intrahippocampal locus coeruleus grafts (■) and in rats with 6-OHDA lesion alone (▲), respectively. Norepinephrine release is shown during steady-state conditions and during generalized seizures (duration 2–3 min) evoked by electrical kindling stimulation of the hippocampus ipsilateral to the probe. (*) Significantly different from the preceding steady-state level. $P < 0.001$ in the normal group and $P < 0.01$ in the grafted group (Student's two-tailed paired t test). Bars indicate s.e.m.s. (From Bengzon et al., 1991).

Grafts in hippocampus

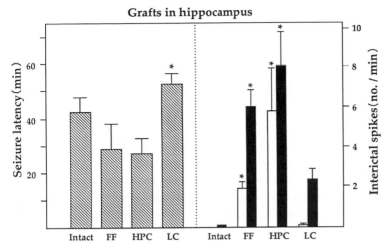

Fig. 4.6. (Left) Latency to convulsive behavioral symptoms following picrotoxin (1 mg/kg, i.p.) in intact animals and in rats either with subcortical denervation of the hippocampus alone (fimbria–fornix lesion, FF) or in combination with bilateral intrahippocampal grafts of dissociated tissue prepared from the fetal hippocampus (HPC) or locus coeruleus (LC). (*) Significantly different from FF and HPC groups ($P < 0.01$). (Right) Frequency of interictal spikes in the different groups one day before (open columns) and one day after (filled columns) six hippocampal seizures (one seizure per day) induced by electrical stimulation of the perforant path. (*) Significantly different from intact and LC groups ($P < 0.02$). Means ± s.e.m. ANOVA with post hoc Fisher test.

show increased susceptibility to picrotoxin-induced behavioral seizures, and a higher frequency of interictal spikes in the hippocampus both before and after repeated hippocampal seizures evoked by electrical stimulation of the perforant path (Fig. 4.6; Buzsáki *et al.*, 1988). Grafts of dissociated fetal locus coeruleus tissue implanted bilaterally into the hippocampus of lesioned animals reduced the incidence of interictal spikes in the host hippocampus and protected against picrotoxin-induced behavioral seizures (Fig. 4.6; Buzsáki *et al.*, 1988). Control grafts consisting of fetal hippocampal tissue had the opposite effects. The locus coeruleus grafts contained noradrenergic neurons from which axonal processes extended into the host hippocampus. Buzsáki *et al.* (1988) proposed that the grafted locus coeruleus neurons may have influenced seizure susceptibility in this model either through a direct action of norepinephrine on hippocampal pyramidal cells (reducing after-hyperpolarizations and preventing population synchrony) or by competing for vacant (after the lesion) postsynaptic sites with sprouting axons of host neurons, thereby limiting excessive collateral excitation.

Penicillin-induced seizures in fetal hippocampus in oculo

Pieces of fetal hippocampus placed on the iris in the anterior chamber of the eye in adult animals grow and develop a laminar neuronal organization. The grafts also form the intrinsic excitatory and inhibitory circuitries typical of the hippocampus in situ (Olson *et al.*, 1977). Seizures can be induced in such grafts by electrical stimulation, penicillin superfusion and cobalt iontophoresis (Hoffer *et al.*, 1977). Using sequential double brain tissue grafts, it is possible to innervate an intraocular hippocampal graft with norepinephrine-containing fibres from a locus coeruleus transplant (Olson *et al.*, 1979). The locus coeruleus neurons give rise to a dense noradrenergic hyperinnervation of the hippocampal graft (Olson *et al.*, 1980).

Seizures induced in single hippocampal grafts by penicillin superfusion were not seen in the precence of co-grafts of fetal locus coeruleus tissue (Fig. 4.7; Taylor *et al.*, 1980). Local application of GABA followed by glutamate on to the grafted locus coeruleus neurons led to generation and suppression, respectively, of penicillin-induced epileptiform activity

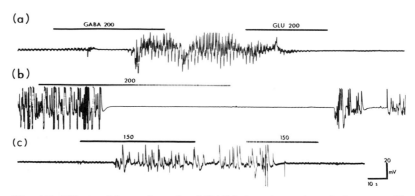

Fig. 4.7. Effects of iontophoresis of GABA (continuous) and glutamate (dotted line) into locus coeruleus grafts on hippocampal EEG in locus coeruleus–hippocampus double grafts. (a), (b) and (c) are from three different grafts. In all cases the graft is superfused with penicillin but no epileptic activity is present until GABA is iontophoresed. Subsequent iontophoresis of glutamate terminates the seizure. In graft (b), only the glutamate response is shown. Numbers after microiontophoretically applied drugs (sodium glutamate (0.5 M, pH 7.5), GABA (1 M, pH 5.0)) refer to injection current in nA.

in the hippocampus (Fig. 4.7). This suggested that a functional inhibitory innervation had developed between the locus coeruleus graft and neurons in the hippocampal graft. The inhibitory influence was blocked by administration of reserpine, supporting the involvement of noradrenergic mechanisms.

Further support for the seizure-suppressant action of norepinephrine in this model has been obtained in experiments where sympathetic adrenergic nerve fibres from the host iris have reinnervated single hippocampal grafts implanted in oculo (Freedman *et al.*, 1979). Electrical stimulation of the cervical sympathetic trunk activating these noradrenergic afferents reduced both the amplitude and frequency of penicillin-induced epileptiform activity. This effect could be blocked by administration of a β-adrenergic receptor antagonist.

Limitations of the neural grafting technique

Graft tissue contains mixture of cells

For the interpretation of results obtained after implantation of fetal neural tissue, it must be remembered that the specific cell population of interest, for example the norepinephrine-producing neurons, represents only a minor fraction of the total number of cells. If we take the example of implants of locus coeruleus tissue, any graft-derived functional effects cannot therefore directly, without proper control experiments, be referred to noradrenergic mechanisms. For this, a significant survival of noradrenergic neurons within the graft must be demonstrated and preferably the extent of axonal growth from the graft should be correlated with the degree of functional effect. Implantation of fetal CNS tissue not containing noradrenergic neurons should not have the same functional consequences. However, even such a control experiment must be interpreted cautiously, since there could of course be a specific effect exerted by certain non-adrenergic neuronal populations also in the control tissue. Further evidence for the involvement of noradrenergic mechanisms, for example, must therefore often be obtained in experiments demonstrating that the graft-induced effects are reduced or prevented by drugs interfering with norepinephrine transmission, e.g., specific receptor antagonists or a norepinephrine-depleting agent.

It seems possible that in the future, cell sorting procedures will allow for the enrichment of noradrenergic or other transmitter-characterized neurons in cell suspension grafts. Although implantation of a 'pure' population of norepinephrine-producing neurons would probably be favorable when functional effects are examined, it cannot be excluded that the survival and axonal outgrowth of such a graft could in fact be impaired because of the lack of other cell elements. Another possible approach that might overcome such a problem would be to use cells that have been genetically engineered to produce norepinephrine (see below).

Axonal outgrowth from graft is region specific

It seems likely that the ability of fetal CNS grafts to change neuronal excitability in the host brain, at least partly, is dependent on the extent and density of the graft-derived innervation. Two characteristics of the target region are of major importance in the determination of the degree of axonal outgrowth from the graft. First, to what extent is this region normally innervated by a given cell population? This is clearly observed when comparing the axonal growth from fetal locus coeruleus neurons implanted into the hippocampus and striatum, respectively (P. Brundin, unpublished results). In the hippocampus, which normally contains a dense noradrenergic innervation, there is extensive outgrowth from the graft. In the striatum, on the other hand, which is poorly innervated by locus coeruleus neurons, the graft survives well but there is very little growth of noradrenergic axons into the surrounding parenchyma of the host. Second, is the target region denervated prior to transplantation? When locus coeruleus neurons are implanted into the intact hippocampus, the density of the graft-derived innervation is 20–30% of that of the normal noradrenergic innervation (O. Lindvall, unpublished results). On the other hand, if the intrinsic innervation has been removed by a previous neurotoxic lesion, the density of the innervation originating from the graft becomes normal or even above normal.

Choice of epilepsy model is critical

The time course of axonal outgrowth from the graft and synapse formation with neuronal elements in the host brain must be taken into account when the experimental model is chosen. For example, reinnervation of the denervated hippocampus by noradrenergic axons from a locus coeruleus graft occurs over a period of two to three months. Obviously, no meaningful information will be obtained if locus coeruleus neurons are implanted into animals with experimental epilepsy that will resolve spontaneously within one or two months. An alternative approach is then to induce the epileptic syndrome in grafted animals after reinnervation has been completed and to compare the results with those obtained in appropriate controls.

Even under optimal conditions in rat-to-rat grafting experiments, there is a variability in the degree of graft survival within a group of recipients. In order to allow for correlation analysis between, for example, cell number or density of reinnervation from the graft and various parameters of the epileptic syndrome (e.g., seizure threshold), it is therefore important that the model used is highly reproducible. Furthermore, the epileptogenic agent must not have any toxic effects on the grafted neurons. This could cause either poor cell survival or inhibited outgrowth, or degeneration if the induction of epilepsy is carried out after the graft has grown into the host brain. The repeated electrical stimulations performed in kindling seem to have no such adverse effects on grafted locus coeruleus neurons (O. Lindvall, unpublished results). In contrast, the application of cobalt leads to few surviving noradrenergic neurons and restricted axonal ramifications from locus coeruleus implants (S. Trottier, unpublished results).

Present and future lines of research

The further application of neural transplantation in experimental epilepsy will probably follow two major and partly interrelated research lines. This approach will be used: (a) to disclose in more detail the normal functional role in seizures exerted by different regions and neuronal systems in the CNS; and (b) to explore the possibility that grafting of inhibitory neurons can be used as a tool to reduce hyperexcitability and suppress seizure activity in the epileptic brain. It seems likely that this research will supply new information on both the pathophysiology of epileptic seizures and the possible anti-epileptogenic and anticonvulsant action of neural grafts, which may eventually lead to clinical trials with transplantation of inhibitory cell systems in human epilepsy. In the following, examples will be given of how the neural grafting approach already has provided important data on these issues. Furthermore, some current problems and possible future developments will be discussed briefly.

Grafting as a tool to study the pathophysiology of epileptic seizures

The capacity of locus coeruleus grafts to influence kindled seizures has been shown in animals with a lesion-induced deficit in the intrinsic noradrenergic system following intraventricular administration of 6-OHDA (Barry *et al.*, 1987, 1989). The results obtained are in close agreement with what could be expected on the basis of previous studies on the role of locus coeruleus neurons during the development of kindling in the intact brain (McIntyre *et al.*, 1979; Corcoran & Mason, 1980; McIntyre & Edson, 1981, 1982; Araki *et al.*, 1983). The hyperexcitability caused by the lesion could thus be reversed by the grafts, giving further support for a seizure-suppressant action of the locus coeruleus system. Interestingly, while the lesion causes an extensive noradrenergic denervation throughout the forebrain, the noradrenergic reinnervation produced by the grafts was confined to the hippocampal formation. This suggests that reinstatement of norepinephrine transmission locally in a stimulated structure, i.e., in the hippocampus, is sufficient to suppress the development of seizures in norepinephrine-depleted animals.

A similar experimental strategy can be used to explore the influence on neuronal excitability also of other transmitter-characterized neuron systems. For example, selective lesions of forebrain 5-hydroxytryptamine (5-HT)-producing neurons can be induced by intraventricular or intracerebral administration of 5,6- or 5,7-dihydroxytryptamine (Jonsson, 1983). Grafting of 5-HT-rich tissue from the fetal mesencephalic raphe region into brains pretreated in this way provides a new model for studies on the role of the 5-HT system in epileptic seizures. It has been demonstrated that raphe implants give rise to a new serotonergic innervation of the denervated hippocampus and restore hippocampal 5-HT levels and release (Daszuta *et al.*, 1988, 1989). The effects of a lesion of forebrain 5-HT neurons and a subsequent graft-derived reinnervation of the hippocampus on seizure susceptibility remain to be clarified. According to Lerner-Natoli *et al.* (1986) local destruction of 5-HT terminals in the rat olfactory bulb, induced by direct injection of 5,6-dihydroxytryptamine, facilitates the development of kindling evoked by electrical stimulation in the same structure. Camu *et al.* (1990) have reported that 5-HT-rich raphe grafts reinnervating the olfactory bulb can reverse the facilitatory effect on olfactory bulb kindling caused by local neurotoxin-induced lesions of 5-HT neurons.

Also, more non-selective lesions and the subsequent implantation of defined cell populations can be useful. As described above, a subcortical denervation leads to hyperexcitability in the hippocampus, which is probably due to the removal of a large number of afferent inputs to this structure including noradrenergic, serotonergic, GABAergic and cholinergic ones. Buzsáki *et al.* (1988) have shown that this hyperexcitability can be reduced by bilateral intrahippocampal locus coeruleus grafts. Similarly, it would be of interest, for example, to implant acetylcholine-rich tissue from the septum-diagonal band and 5-HT-rich tissue from the mesencephalic raphe into the hippocampus in this model and to monitor changes in excitability. This could provide information on the functional action of cholinergic and serotonergic neurons. It is also possible to implant, in the same animal, two or more different neuronal populations (e.g. noradrenergic and GABAergic ones) to study possible interactions and to optimize inhibition. The cells can be transplanted together either as a mixed cell suspension, which is injected stereotaxically into the brain, or as solid pieces in a cortical cavity.

Of major importance would be if implantation of neural grafts into the epileptic brain could disclose some changes in transmitter-characterized neuron systems underlying the development and maintenance of seizure activity. Taking the example from the kindling model of epilepsy, it has been proposed that the development of kindling could be due to a progressive impairment of noradrenergic mechanisms, occurring either at the pre- or postsynaptic level (for references, see Bengzon *et al.*, 1990*a*). Transplantation of locus coeruleus neurons to fully kindled animals could, if it leads to suppression of stimulus-evoked seizure activity, provide evidence for a deficit in the intrinsic noradrenergic system as an important factor in kindling development and maintenance. In fact, this hypothesis is supported by recent data obtained with intracerebral microdialysis, indicating that the interictal, steady-state release of norepinephrine is significantly lower in kindled compared to non-kindled animals (Bengzon *et al.*, 1990*a*).

Another possible approach to obtain more insights into changes underlying hyperexcitability is to study interactions between the epileptic host brain and a non-epileptic graft of a suitable CNS region, placed in a cavity. Embryonic neural tissues from various areas grow and mature in such a cavity, forming a 'microbrain', which can be made to fuse with the adjoining host brain tissue, thereby promoting the formation of afferent and efferent axonal connections (Kromer *et al.*, 1979, 1983). If the graft is implanted into a fully kindled animal, for example, the effects of kindling stimulations in the (non-kindled) graft tissue itself (focal or generalized seizures, i.e., class 1 or class 5 (Racine, 1972) in the host) could reveal some of the pathophysiological mechanisms in kindling epilepsy. Additional information might be obtained if the 'microbrain' is combined with various transmitter-characterized grafts, e.g., epinephrine- and/or 5-HT-rich ones, in the same transplantation cavity.

The neural grafting technique also provides new possibilities for studies on the importance of various brain regions (also outside the epileptic focus) for the spread and generalization of seizures. For this purpose, grafts can be placed uni- or bilaterally and at single or multiple sites in animals subjected to different forms of experimentally induced seizures. As described above, bilateral locus coeruleus grafts in the amygdala–piriform cortex retard the development of seizures evoked by kindling stimulations in the hippocampus to the same degree as bilateral intra-hippocampal implants (Barry *et al.*, 1989). This supports previous findings obtained with other experimental approaches suggesting a central role for this region in the generalization and expression of kindled seizures (Racine & Burnham, 1984; McIntyre & Racine, 1986).

Grafting as a tool to suppress epileptic seizures

Particularly from the clinical perspective, it seems highly warranted to explore to what extent neural grafts can suppress the generation, spread, severity and duration of convulsive activity in the epileptic brain. Available studies suggest that intrahippocampal locus coeruleus grafts can inhibit epileptogenesis, as seen with hippocampal kindling in norepinephrine-depleted rats (Barry *et al.*, 1987), and also reduce the severity of seizures, as observed on spontaneous hippocampal interictal spikes and after administration of picrotoxin in subcortically denervated rats (Buzsáki *et al.*, 1988). A similar inhibition of penicillin-induced seizure activity has been observed with hippocampus–locus coeruleus co-grafts in the anterior chamber of the eye (Freedman *et al.*, 1979).

The principal strategy underlying the transplantation approach seems very simple, i.e., to reduce neuronal hyperexcitability in an epileptic brain region by implanting cells, leading to increased inhibition. The further progress of this research is complicated, however, by two major problems. First, there is a lack of any identified deficit in a particular transmitter system underlying most forms of experimental as well as clinical epilepsy. This is in contrast to the situation for transplantation in Parkinson's disease, in which the implantation of neural tissue aims at restoring dopamine synthesis, storage, and release at synaptic sites through a reinnervation of the striatum by grafted mesencephalic dopaminergic neurons. Second, it is largely unknown whether the addition of 'inhibitory' neurons to an epileptic brain region without a deficit in that particular neuron system leads to increased inhibition. For example, if GABA-producing neurons from the striatum survive implantation into the hippocampus, it remains to be established to what extent they are anatomically and functionally integrated with the host brain. If so, one must consider the possibility not only of a seizure-suppressant action but also that the resultant functional action exerted by a population of these neurons placed at an ectopic site could be an increased excitation. It is interesting in this context that intrahippocampal implants of fetal hippocampus in hyperexcitable rats, despite the fact that the grafts contained GABA-immunoreactive neurons, induced epileptic activity (Buzsáki *et al.*, 1988).

From a theoretical point of view it seems at present most appropriate to focus on transplantation of tissue rich in two types of neurons, norepinephrine- and GABA-producing. These cells seem to be the most suitable candidates for grafting experiments intended to reduce neuronal excitability. In the following, some important scientific issues related to the use of norepinephrine and GABA cells for this purpose will be discussed.

Functional capacity of locus coeruleus grafts

Three main problems should be addressed. (a) Can grafted locus coeruleus neurons inhibit convulsive activity in a larger variety of experimental epilepsy models? (b) Can grafted locus coeruleus neurons reduce neuronal excitability after implantation into a region without prior denervation of the intrinsic noradrenergic input? (c) Can the threshold for generalization of seizures be raised by locus coeruleus neurons grafted to a region distant from the epileptic focus? The intracerebral implantation of locus coeruleus neurons into animals subjected to forms of hyperexcitability other than kindling and subcortical denervation of the hippocampus will be important in order to clarify whether the seizure-suppressant action of these grafts is a general phenomenon. Mainly through the results of lesion experiments, the intrinsic locus coeruleus system has been proposed to have an inhibitory role in several other epilepsy models, including cobalt-, Metrazol-, and electroshock-induced seizures (Chauvel & Trottier, 1986). The primary objective of the first grafting experiments will be to reverse the hyperexcitability in these models evoked by a lesion of the noradrenergic system.

Mechanisms of action of locus coeruleus grafts

Transplantation of locus coeruleus neurons into the norepinephrine-depleted hippocampus of rats subjected to hippocampal kindling provides one useful model to study how grafts exert their seizure-suppressant effects and to what extent their functional action is regulated by the host brain. One major scientific issue relates to whether and by which mechanisms the grafted inhibitory neurons are activated by the seizures, and if this activation is necessary for the seizure-suppressant effect. In the intact brain, generalized kindled seizures have been reported to involve an increased firing rate of locus coeruleus neurons (Jimenez-Rivera & Weiss, 1989), which is accompanied by increased release of norepinephrine (Kokaia *et al.*, 1989). Transection experiments support the suggestion that the activation of the intrinsic locus coeruleus system in kindled seizures occurs mainly through an influence at the cell body level in the pons (Bengzon *et al.*, 1991). Grafted locus coeruleus neurons show similar changes in norepinephrine release in response to a generalized seizure as regards both temporal course and magnitude (Bengzon *et al.*, 1991), but it is not known if there is also a change in their electrical activity. Seizures therefore seem to activate grafted neurons also, although the underlying mechanisms are unclear. Since the locus coeruleus neurons are placed ectopically in the hippocampus, they have lost their normal afferent input and cannot be regulated via the same neuronal pathways as in the intact brain. However, some data indicate that intrahippocampal cell suspension grafts of locus coeruleus tissue are innervated by the host brain (Murata *et al.*, 1990). It is important to identify the origins of these afferents and to clarify their involvement in the graft response to seizures. It should also be tested whether release of norepinephrine from grafted locus coeruleus neurons to a larger extent than from the intrinsic system is influenced by local regulatory mechanisms at the nerve terminals. In fact, Nelson *et al.* (1980) have provided evidence for local control of hippocampal norepinephrine release in kainic acid-induced seizures.

Another major subject for further study concerns how norepinephrine release from locus coeruleus grafts can change the excitability of host neurons. First, are specific postsynaptic receptors involved? As pointed out above, some evidence has been obtained that suggests that the retardation of hippocampal kindling rate exerted by locus coeruleus grafts could be at least partly mediated via α-2 adrenergic receptors. Second, is it necessary for the functional effect that norepinephrine release takes place at synaptic sites? Electronmicroscopical evidence has been obtained for synaptic contacts between grafted noradrenergic locus coeruleus neurons and host hippocampal neurons (Murata *et al.*, 1990). When genetically engineered cells producing norepinephrine become available, they will be very useful in clarifying whether the same seizure-suppressant effect can be demonstrated with non-synaptic transmitter release, and the degree of importance of a regulatory influence on this release exerted by the host brain.

Survival and functional capacity of GABA-producing grafts

So far, no conclusive experimental evidence has been presented indicating that implantation of GABA-rich tissue can influence epileptic activity. Stevens *et al.* (1988*b*) have reported that grafts of fetal cerebellar or cortical tissue placed in the deep prepiriform area of amygdala-kindled rats (intended to provide the host brain with additional GABA neurons at a 'critical' site) transiently raised seizure thresholds but only in a minority of animals. Furthermore, these authors were not able to demonstrate any glutamic acid decarboxylase-immunopositive, i.e., presumed GABAergic, cells in the grafts. This illustrates that a major, initial problem for the strategy of increasing GABA-transmission within a brain region using neural grafts is the difficulty of finding a suitable source of GABA-rich tissue. Although GABA neurons from the striatum can survive both in the normal and in the kainic acid-treated epileptic hippocampus, the grafts are often small and poorly integrated with the host brain (Schwartzkroin & Kunkel, 1988; O. Lindvall, unpublished results). This is in contrast to what happens when the grafts are placed in the lesioned striatum, where they form extensive afferent and efferent connections with the host brain (Wictorin *et al.*, 1988, 1989; Wictorin & Björklund, 1989) and release GABA (Sirinathsinghji *et al.*, 1988). Other possible sources of GABA neurons such as fetal substantia nigra should also be tested but it seems likely that grafts from these regions would be unfavorable when implanted at ectopic sites. Enriched GABAergic neurons, prepared by cell sorting, could represent one future alternative. Another attractive possibility may be the implantation of genetically engineered GABA-producing cells. If such cells are non-neuronal it remains to be established, whether non-synaptic release of GABA is sufficient for a seizure-suppressant action and whether this effect requires the activation of the graft. This either could occur in response to the seizures, as seems to be the case for locus coeruleus grafts, or may require priming of the graft pharmacologically.

Available experimental evidence suggests that GABA-producing cells might influence epileptic phenomena after implantation into at least two, principally different sites. First, in the epileptic focus where some reports have described a deficit of GABAergic transmission, for example after hippocampal kindling (Kamphuis *et al.*, 1986, 1989) and application of cobalt (Emson & Joseph, 1975; Ross & Craig, 1981) or alumina cream (Ribak *et al.*, 1979). However, even with normal intrinsic GABA transmission, grafting of GABA cells to the epileptic focus might possibly counteract hyperexcitability caused by impairment in some other neuronal system. Second, in those regions which have been proposed to be of crucial importance for the spread and generalization of epileptic seizures. One such site is the substantia nigra pars reticulata; bilateral micro-injections of GABA agonists into this region suppress electroconvulsive shock seizures (Iadarola & Gale, 1982), and chemically induced seizures (Iadarola & Gale, 1982; Turski *et al.*, 1986), as well as kindled seizures (Le Gal La Salle *et al.*, 1983; McNamara *et al.*, 1984). A similar functional effect could possibly also be exerted by GABA neurons implanted into the substantia nigra. Another 'critical' region that might be suitable for transplantation of GABA neurons is the 'area tempestas', in the deep prepiriform area (Piredda & Gale, 1985; see also Chapter 2, this volume). Infusion of a GABA agonist or a transaminase inhibitor into this region has been shown to suppress both chemically induced and kindled seizures (Piredda & Gale, 1986; Stevens *et al.*, 1988a). As described above, some, largely negative, attempts of implanting GABA-rich tissue have already been performed in the deep prepiriform region (Stevens *et al.*, 1988b).

Concluding remarks

The use of neural grafting as an investigative tool in epilepsy research is still in its infancy. The potential value of this approach is, however, already indicated by experimental evidence showing that neural grafts can suppress epileptic phenomena in the CNS and that such grafts also may induce seizure activity. At this early stage, it is most important to clarify in further detail whether and to what extent different parts of the epileptic syndrome can be influenced by neural grafts. This involves the implantation of various cell populations in different brain regions of animals subjected to a variety of experimental epilepsy models. The mechanisms of action of neural grafts in epilepsy should also be explored. Do the grafts act via synaptic release of a particular transmitter, which then influences specific receptors? Which level of anatomical and functional integration into the host neuronal circuitry is necessary for grafts to modulate neuronal excitability and convulsive phenomena? The major objective of this chapter has been to illustrate the usefulness of norepinephrine-rich locus coeruleus grafts for some of these studies. Similar experimental strategies could be applied for other transmitter-characterized cell systems such as those producing GABA, acetylcholine or 5-HT. Obviously, more general advances in the field of neural transplantation will also have a direct impact on its application in epilepsy research. These include, for example, the development of cell sorting procedures and the production of genetically engineered cells, making possible implantation of a pure population of transmitter-characterized cells. It is conceivable that this research will give more insights into the pathophysiology of seizures and, it is to be hoped, will also provide the necessary experimental basis for future attempts at reducing neuronal hyperexcitability in human epilepsy using cell transplantation.

Acknowledgments

The research carried out in this laboratory and reviewed here was supported by grants from the Swedish Medical Research Council (14X-8666), The Thorsten and Elsa Segerfalk Foundation and the Bank of Sweden Tricentenary Fund.

References

Araki, H., Aihara, H., Watanabe, S., Ohta, H., Yamamoto, T. & Ueki, S. (1983). The role of noradrenergic and serotonergic systems in the hippocampal kindling effect. *Japan Journal of Pharmacology*, **33**: 57–64.

Barry, D. I., Kikvadze, I., Brundin, P., Bolwig, T. G., Björklund, A. & Lindvall, O. (1987). Grafted noradrenergic neurons suppress seizure development in kindling-induced epilepsy. *Proceedings of the National Academy of Sciences, USA*, **84**: 8712–15.

Barry, D. I., Wanscher, B., Kragh, J., Bolwig, T. G., Kokaia, M., Brundin, P., Björklund, A. & Lindvall, O. (1989). Grafts of fetal locus coeruleus neurons in rat amygdala–piriform cortex suppress seizure development in hippocampal kindling. *Experimental Neurology*, **106**: 125–32.

Bengzon, J., Brundin, P., Kalen, P., Kokaia, M. & Lindvall, O. (1991). Host regulation of noradrenaline release from grafts of seizure-suppressant locus coeruleus neurons. *Experimental Neurology*, **111**: 49–54.

Bengzon, J., Kalen, P. & Lindvall, O. (1990a). Evidence for long-term reduction of noradrenaline release after kindling in the hippocampus. *Brain Research*, 535: 353–7.

Bengzon, J., Kokaia, M., Brundin, P. & Lindvall, O. (1990b). Seizure suppression in kindling epilepsy by intrahippocampal locus coeruleus grafts: evidence for an *alpha*-2-adrenoreceptor mediated mechanism. *Experimental Brain Research*, **81**: 433–7.

Björklund, A. & Lindvall, O. (1986). Catecholaminergic brain stem regulatory systems. In *Handbook of Physiology – The Nervous System IV, Intrinsic Regulatory Systems in the Brain*, ed. F. E. Bloom, pp. 155–235. Bethesda, MD: American Physiological Society.

Björklund, A., Lindvall, O., Isacson, O., Brundin, P., Wictorin, K., Strecker, R. E., Clarke, D. J. & Dunnett, S. B. (1987). Mechanisms of action of intracerebral neural implants: studies of nigral and striatal grafts to the lesioned striatum. *Trends in Neurosciences*, **10**: 509–16.

Björklund, A., Nornes, H. & Gage, F. H. (1986). Cell suspension grafts of noradrenergic locus coeruleus neurons in rat hippocampus and spinal cord: reinnervation and transmitter turnover. *Neuroscience*, **18**: 685–98.

Björklund, A., Segal, M. & Stenevi, U. (1979). Functional reinnervation of rat hippocampus by locus coeruleus implants. *Brain Research*, **170**: 409–26.

Björklund, A. & Stenevi, U. (1977). Reformation of the severed septohippocampal cholinergic pathway in the adult rat by transplanted septal neurons. *Cell and Tissue Research*, **185**: 289–302.

Björklund, A. & Stenevi, U. (1979). Reconstruction of the nigrostriatal dopamine pathway by intracerebral nigral transplants. *Brain Research*, **177**: 555–60.

Björklund, A. & Stenevi, U. (1985). Intracerebral neural grafting: a historical perspective. In *Neural Grafting in the Mammalian CNS*, ed. A. Björklund & U. Stenevi, pp. 3–14. Amsterdam: Elsevier Science Publishers, B.V.

Brundin, P., Isacson, O., Gage, F. H., Stenevi, U. & Björklund, A. (1985). Intracerebral grafts of neuronal cell suspensions. In *Neural Grafting in the Mammalian CNS*, ed. A. Björklund & U. Stenevi, pp. 51–9. Amsterdam: Elsevier Science Publishers, B.V.

Buchanan, J. T. & Nornes, H. O. (1986). Transplants of embryonic brainstem containing the locus coeruleus into spinal cord enhance the hindlimb flexion reflex in adult rats. *Brain Research*, **381**: 225–36.

Buzsáki, G., Ponomareff, G., Bayardo, F., Shaw, T. & Gage, F. H. (1988). Suppression and induction of epileptic activity by neuronal grafts. *Proceedings of the National Academy of Sciences, USA*, **85**: 9327–30.

Camu, W., Marlier, L., Lerner-Natoli, M., Rondouin, G. & Privat, A. (1990). Transplantation of serotonergic neurons into the 5,7-DHT-lesioned rat olfactory bulb restores the parameters of kindling. *Brain Research*, **518**: 23–30.

Chauvel, P. & Trottier, S. (1986). Role of noradrenergic ascending system in extinction of epileptic phenomena. In *Advances in Neurology*, ed. A. V. Delgado-Escueta, A. A. Ward Jr, D. M. Woodbury & R. I. Porter, vol. 44, pp. 475–87. New York: Raven Press.

Collier, T. J., Gash, D. M. & Sladek, J. R. Jr (1988). Transplantation of norepinephrine neurons into aged rats improves performance of a learned task. *Brain Research*, **448**: 77–87.

Corcoran, M. E. & Mason, S. T. (1980). Role of forebrain catecholamines in amygdaloid kindling. *Brain Research*, **190**: 473–84.

Dailey, J. W. & Jobe, P. C. (1986). Indices of noradrenergic function in the central nervous system of seizure-naive genetically epilepsy-prone rats. *Epilepsia*, **27**: 665–70.

Daszuta, A., Strecker, R. E., Brundin, P. & Björklund, A. (1988). Serotonin neurons grafted to the adult rat hippocampus. I. Time course of growth as studied by immunohistochemistry and biochemistry. *Brain Research*, **458**: 1–19.

Daszuta, A., Kalen, P., Strecker, R. E., Brundin, P. & Björklund, A. (1989). Serotonin neurons grafted to the adult rat hippocampus. II. 5-HT release as studied by intracerebral microdialysis. *Brain Research*, **498**: 323–32.

Dunn, E. H. (1917). Primary and secondary findings in a series of attempts to transplant cerebral cortex in the albino rat. *Journal of Comparative Neurology*, **27**: 565–82.

Dunnett, S. B., Whishaw, I. Q., Rogers, D. C. & Jones, G. H. (1987). Dopamine-rich grafts ameliorate whole body motor asymmetry and sensory neglect but not independent limb use in rats with 6-hydroxydopamine lesions. *Brain Research*, **415**: 63–78.

Emson, P. C. & Joseph, M. H. (1975). Neurochemical and morphological changes during the development of cobalt-induced epilepsy in the rat. *Brain Research*, **93**: 91–110.

Foote, S. L., Bloom, F. E. & Aston-Jones, G. (1983). Nucleus locus coeruleus: new evidence of anatomical and physiological specificity. *Physiological Reviews*, **63**: 844–911.

Freed, W. J. (1985). Transplantation of tissues to the cerebral ventricles: methodological details and rate of graft survival. In *Neural Grafting in the Mammalian CNS*, ed. A. Björklund & U. Stenevi, pp. 31–40. Amsterdam: Elsevier Science Publishers, B.V.

Freedman, R., Taylor, D. A., Seiger, Å., Olson, L. & Hoffer, B. J. (1979). Seizures and related epileptiform activity in hippocampus transplanted to the anterior chamber of the eye: modulation by cholinergic and adrenergic input. *Annals of Neurology*, **6**: 281–95.

Gellman, R. L., Kallianos, J. A. & McNamara, J. O. (1987). *Alpha*-2 receptors mediate an endogenous noradrenergic suppression of kindling development. *Journal of Pharmacology and Experimental Therapeutics*, **241**: 891–8.

Hoffer, B. J., Seiger, Å., Taylor, D., Olson, L. & Freedman, R. (1977). Seizures and related epileptiform activity in hippocampus transplanted to the anterior chamber of the eye. I. Characterization of seizures, interictal spikes and synchronous activity. *Experimental Neurology*, **54**: 233–50.

Iadarola, M. J. & Gale, K. (1982). Substantia nigra: site of anticonvulsant activity mediated by γ-aminobutyric acid. *Science*, **218**: 1237–40.

Jimenez-Rivera, C. A. & Weiss, G. K. (1989). The effect of amygdala kindled seizures on locus coeruleus activity. *Brain Research Bulletin*, **22**: 751–8.

Jonsson, G. (1983). Chemical lesioning techniques: monoamine neurotoxins. In *Handbook of Chemical Neuroanatomy*, vol. 1 *Methods in Chemical Neuroanatomy*, ed. A. Björklund & T. Hökfelt, pp. 463–507. Amsterdam: Elsevier Science Publishers, B.V.

Kalén, P., Cenci, M. A., Lindvall, O. & Björklund, A. (1991). Host brain regulation of fetal locus coeruleus neurons grafted to the hippocampus in 6-hydroxydopamine-treated rats. An intracerebral microdialysis study. *European Journal of Neuroscience*, **3**, 905–18.

Kamphuis, W., Huisman, E., Wadman, W. J. & Lopes da Silva, F. H. (1989). Decrease in GABA immunoreactivity and alteration of GABA metabolism after kindling in the rat hippocampus. *Experimental Brain Research*, **74**: 375–86.

Kamphuis, W., Wadman, W. J., Buijs, R. M. & Lopes da Silva, F. H. (1986). Decrease in number of hippocampal gamma-aminobutyric acid (GABA) immunoreactive cells in the rat kindling model of epilepsy. *Experimental Brain Research*, **64**: 491–5.

Kokaia, M., Kalén, P., Bengzon, J. & Lindvall, O. (1989). Noradrenaline and 5-hydroxytryptamine release in the hippocampus during seizures induced by hippocampal kindling stimulation: an in vivo microdialysis study. *Neuroscience*, **32**: 647–56.

Kromer, L. E., Björklund, A. & Stenevi, U. (1979). Intracephalic implants: a technique for studying neuronal interactions. *Science*, **204**: 1117–19.

Kromer, L. E., Björklund, A. & Stenevi, U. (1983). Intracephalic embryonic neural implants in the adult rat brain. I. Growth and mature organization of brain stem, cerebellar, and hippocampal implants. *Journal of Comparative Neurology*, **218**: 433–59.

Le Gal La Salle, G., Kaijima, M. & Feldblum, S. (1983). Abortive amygdaloid kindled seizures following microinjection of γ-vinyl-GABA in the vicinity of substantia nigra in rats. *Neuroscience Letters*, **36**: 69–74.

Le Gros Clark, W. E. (1940). Neuronal differentiation in implanted foetal cortical tissue. *Journal of Neurology and Psychiatry*, **3**: 263–84.

Lerner-Natoli, M., Rondouin, G., Malafosse, A., Sandillon, F., Privat, A. & Baldy-Moulinier, M. (1986). Facilitation of olfactory bulb kindling after specific destruction of serotoninergic terminals in the olfactory bulb of the rat. *Neuroscience Letters*, **66**, 299–304.

Lindvall, O., Brundin, P., Widner, H., Rehncrona, S., Gustavii, B., Frackowiak, R., Leenders, K. L., Sawle, G., Rothwell, J. C., Marsden, C. D. & Björklund, A. (1990). Grafts of fetal dopamine neurons survive and improve motor function in Parkinson's disease. *Science*, **247**: 574–7.

McIntyre, D. C. & Edson, N. (1981). Facilitation of amygdala kindling after norepinephrine depletion with 6-hydroxydopamine in rats. *Experimental Neurology*, **74**: 748–57.

McIntyre, D. C. & Edson, N. (1982). Effect of norepinephrine depletion on dorsal hippocampus kindling in rats. *Experimental Neurology*, **77**: 700–4.

McIntyre, D. C. & Racine, R. J. (1986). Kindling mechanisms: current progress of an experimental epilepsy model. *Progress in Neurobiology*, **27**: 1–12.

McIntyre, D. C., Saari, M. & Pappas, B. A. (1979). Potentiation of amygdala kindling in adult or infant rats by injections of 6-hydroxydopamine. *Experimental Neurology*, **63**: 527–44.

McNamara, J. O., Galloway, M. T., Rigsbee, L. C. & Shin, C. (1984). Evidence implicating substantia nigra in regulation of kindled seizure threshold. *Journal of Neuroscience*, **4**: 2410–17.

Murata, Y., Chiba, T., Brundin, P., Björklund, A. & Lindvall, O. (1990). Formation of synaptic graft-host connections by noradrenergic locus coeruleus neurons transplanted into the adult rat hippocampus. *Experimental Neurology*, **110**: 258–67.

Nelson, M. F., Zaczek, R. & Coyle, J. T. (1980). Effects of sustained seizures produced by intrahippocampal injection of kainic acid on noradrenergic neurons: evidence for local control of norepinephrine release. *Journal of Pharmacology and Experimental Therapeutics*, **214**: 694–702.

Olson, L., Freedman, R., Seiger, Å. & Hoffer, B. (1977). Electrophysiology and cytology of hippocampal formation transplants in the anterior chamber of the eye. 1. Intrinsic organization. *Brain Research*, **119**: 87–106.

Olson, L. & Hoffer, B. (1985). In oculo transplantation technique. In *Neural Grafting in the Mammalian CNS*, ed. A. Björklund & U. Stenevi, pp. 15–21. Amsterdam: Elsevier Science Publishers, B.V.

Olson, L., Seiger, Å., Hoffer, B. J. & Taylor, D. (1979). Isolated catecholaminergic projections from substantia nigra and locus coeruleus to caudate, hippocampus and cerebral cortex formed by intraocular sequential double brain grafts. *Experimental Brain Research*, **35**: 47–67.

Olson, L., Seiger, Å. & Strömberg, I. (1983). Intraocular transplantation in rodents. A detailed account of the procedure and examples of its use in neurobiology with special reference to brain tissue grafting. In *Advances in Cellular Neurobiology*, vol. 4. ed. S. Fedoroff & L. Hertz, pp. 407–42. New York: Academic Press.

Olson, L., Seiger, Å., Taylor, D., Freedman, R. & Hoffer, B. J. (1980). Conditions for adrenergic hyperinnervation in hippocampus. I. Histochemical evidence from intraocular double grafts. *Experimental Brain Research*, **39**: 277–88.

Perlow, M. J., Freed, W. J., Hoffer, B. J., Seiger, Å., Olson, L. & Wyatt, R. J. (1979). Brain grafts reduce motor abnormalities produced by destruction of nigrostriatal dopamine system. *Science*, **204**: 643–7.

Piredda, S. & Gale, K. (1985). A crucial epileptogenic site in deep prepyriform cortex. *Nature*, **317**: 623–5.

Piredda, S. & Gale, K. (1986). Anticonvulsant action of 2-amino, 7-phosphonoheptanoic acid and muscimol in the deep prepiriform cortex. *European Journal of Pharmacology*, **120**: 115–18.

Racine, R. J. (1972). Modification of seizure activity by electrical stimulation. II. Motor seizures. *Electroencephalography and Clinical Neurophysiology*, **32**: 281–94.

Racine, R. J. & Burnham, W. M. (1984). The kindling model. In *Electrophysiology of Epilepsy*, ed. P. A. Schwartzkroin & H. V. Wheal, pp. 153–71. London: Academic Press.

Ribak, C. E., Harris, A. B., Vaughn, J. E. & Roberts, E. (1979). Inhibitory, GABAergic nerve terminals decrease at sites of focal epilepsy. *Science*, **205**: 211–14.

Ross, S. M. & Craig, C. R. (1981). γ-Aminobutyric acid concentration, L-glutamate 1-decarboxylase activity and properties of the γ-aminobutyric acid postsynaptic receptor in cobalt epilepsy in the rat. *Journal of Neuroscience*, **1**: 1388–96.

Schwartzkroin, P. A. & Kunkel, D. D. (1988). Viability of GABAergic striatal neurons grafted into normal hippocampus. *Society for Neuroscience Abstracts*, **233**: 8.

Segal, M., Azmitia, E., Björklund, A., Greenberger, V. & Richter-Levin, G. (1988). Physiology of graft–host interactions in the rat hippocampus. In *Transplantation into the Mammalian CNS*, ed. D. M. Gash & J. R. Sladek Jr, pp. 95–101. Amsterdam: Elsevier Science Publishers, B.V.

Seiger, Å. (1985). Preparation of immature central nervous system regions for transplantation. In *Neural Grafting in the Mammalian CNS*, ed. A. Björklund & U. Stenevi, pp. 71–7. Amsterdam: Elsevier Science Publishers, B.V.

Semenova, T. P., Gromova, E. A., Grischenko, N. I., Nesterova, I. V., Kulikov, A. V., Smirnova, G. N., Tretyak, T. M., Bragin, A. G. & Vinogradova, O. S. (1987). Behavioural, biochemical and histochemical effects of locus coeruleus transplantation in rats with neurotoxic lesions of the catecholaminergic system. *Neuroscience*, **22**: 993–1002.

Sirinathsinghji, D. J. S., Dunnett, S. B., Isacson, O., Clarke, D. J., Kendrick, K. & Björklund, A. (1988). Striatal grafts in rats with unilateral neostriatal lesions. II. *In vivo* monitoring of GABA release in globus pallidus and substantia nigra. *Neuroscience*, **24**: 803–11.

Stenevi, U., Kromer, L. F., Gage, F. H. & Björklund, A. (1985). Solid neural grafts in intracerebral transplantation cavities. In *Neural Grafting in the*

Mammalian CNS, ed. A. Björklund & U. Stenevi, pp. 41–49. Amsterdam: Elsevier Science Publishers, B.V.

Stevens, J. R., Phillips, I. & de Beaurepaire, R. (1988a). γ-Vinyl GABA in endopiriform area suppresses kindled amygdala seizures. *Epilepsia*, **29**: 404–11.

Stevens, J. R., Phillips, I., Freed, W. J. & Poltorak, M. (1988b). Cerebral transplants for seizures: preliminary results. *Epilepsia*, **29**: 731–7.

Strecker, R. E., Sharp, T., Brundin, P., Zetterström, T. & Björklund, A. (1987). Autoregulation of dopamine release and metabolism by intrastriatal nigral grafts as revealed by intracerebral dialysis. *Neuroscience*, **22**, 169–78.

Taylor, D., Freedman, R., Seiger, Å., Olson, L. & Hoffer, B. J. (1980). Conditions for adrenergic hyperinnervation in hippocampus. II. Electrophysiological evidence from intraocular double grafts. *Experimental Brain Research*, **39**: 289–99.

Thompson, W. G. (1890). Successful brain grafting. *New York Medical Journal*, **51**, 701–2.

Turski, L., Cavalheiro, E. A., Schwarz, M., Turski, W. A., De Moraes Mello, L. E. A., Bortolotto, Z. A., Klockgether, T. & Sontag, K. (1986). Susceptibility to seizures produced by pilocarpine in rats after microinjection of isoniazid or γ-vinyl-GABA into the substantia nigra. *Brain Research*, **370**: 294–309.

Wictorin, K. & Björklund, A. (1989). Connectivity of striatal grafts implanted into the ibotenic acid-lesioned striatum. II. Cortical afferents. *Neuroscience*, **30**, 297–311.

Wictorin, K., Isacson, O., Fischer, W., Nothias, F., Peschanski, M. & Björklund, A. (1988). Connectivity of striatal grafts implanted into the ibotenic acid-lesioned striatum. I. Subcortical afferents. *Neuroscience*, **27**, 547–62.

Wictorin, K., Simerly, R. B., Isacson, O., Swanson, L. W. & Björklund, A. (1989). Connectivity of striatal grafts implanted into the ibotenic acid-lesioned striatum. III. Efferent projecting graft neurons and their relation to host afferents within the grafts. *Neuroscience*, **30**, 313–30.

Yakovleff, A., Roby-Brami, A., Guezard, B., Mansour, H., Bussel, B. & Privat, A. (1989). Locomotion in rats transplanted with noradrenergic neurons. *Brain Research Bulletin*, **22**, 115–21.

5

Sensitivity of the immature central nervous system to epileptogenic stimuli

SOLOMON L. MOSHÉ, PATRIC K. STANTON, and ELLEN F. SPERBER

Introduction

During the last ten years, there has been an increased interest in investigating the basic mechanisms of epilepsy in the immature brain. It was already known that the behavioral manifestations of seizures were age dependent but it was widely believed that in the immature central nervous system (CNS) inhibitory events predominated (Purpura & Housepian, 1961; Purpura, 1969, 1972). Therefore, it was assumed that the immature brain was not prone to seizures. However, the preponderance of recently acquired data indicates that the developing CNS is more susceptible to seizures than is the adult CNS. This concept is based on both epidemiological (Gibbs & Gibbs, 1963; Vernadakis & Woodbury, 1969; Hauser & Kurland, 1975; Woodbury, 1977) and experimental (Moshé et al., 1983; Albala et al., 1984; Schwartzkroin, 1984; Swann & Brady , 1984; Cavalheiro et al., 1987; Sperber & Moshé, 1988; Moshé, 1989) studies. Additional data have revealed that epileptogenesis during development may not be a linear event. There appear to be periods of increased seizure susceptibility, followed by relatively more resistant 'developmental windows' (Schwartzkroin, 1984; Moshé 1989; Moshé et al., 1992). Furthermore, since brain areas do not mature at the same time, epileptogenesis may differ from site to site. As a result, the sequelae of recurrent seizures may depend on the cause and site of origin of seizures as well as on the age of the animal (Moshé et al., 1992).

The study of the mechanisms underlying the development and maintenance of the epileptic state requires the use of appropriate animal models that can depict the age-related changes in seizure susceptibility. These models should be reliable and easily reproduced. We have found that a single model may not be adequate; rather, a combination of models and techniques may be more useful in elucidating the factors governing epileptic processes early in life.

The kindling model

Background information

In the kindling model, repetitive, localized, intracranial, low intensity stimulations lead initially to the development of focal afterdischarges (ADs), behavioral automatisms and, in time, to the development of generalized motor convulsions of increasing severity and complexity (Goddard *et al.*, 1969; Moshé, 1981). This gradual alteration in brain function and expression, once induced, is permanent in that the same stimulus will reproduce the seizures even if the animal has remained stimulation-free for a long time (Goddard *et al.*, 1969). Eventually, spontaneous seizures may occur (Wada *et al.*, 1974; Pinel & Rovner, 1978). Kindling can be produced by several chemical means including the systemic or intracranial, periodic administration of drugs (chemical kindling). More often, kindling is produced by the repeated application of electrical stimuli to discrete areas of the brain (for a review, see Moshé & Ludvig, 1988).

To induce kindling, the electrical stimuli must be delivered at regular intervals (Goddard *et al.*, 1969). In adult animals, kindling cannot be induced if the stimulation is continuous or is delivered at intervals of less than 20–30 min (Goddard *et al.*, 1969; Racine *et al.*, 1973; Peterson *et al.*, 1981; Moshé & Albala, 1983; Moshé *et al.*, 1983). Starting with one hour intervals, the effectiveness of the stimulus increases as the interstimulation period is increased (Goddard *et al.*, 1969). The most common form of stimulation consists of sinusoidal or rectangular current at about 60 Hz delivered for 1–2 s; however, all frequencies above 25 Hz are equally effective (Goddard *et al.*, 1969; Racine, 1978; Moshé & Ludvig, 1988). Low frequency stimuli (1.5–3 Hz) will also induce kindling as long as the current is delivered for a longer period of time (10–60 s) and the stimulus intensity is increased (Cain & Corcoran, 1981; Lothman *et al.*, 1985). The occurrence of ADs is required for kindling to happen (Racine, 1972*a,b*). While subthreshold for ADs, stimulations can eventually decrease the AD threshold; the repeated failure to elicit an AD suggests that the site cannot be kindled. Thus, the determination of the AD threshold can be considered as an index of local epileptogenicity, although the AD threshold does not accurately predict the ease with which generalized kindled seizures will emerge (Moshé *et al.*, 1981; Racine *et al.*, 1977; Racine, 1972*a*; Zaide, 1974).

Table 5.1. *Classification of kindling-induced motor behaviors following amygdala stimulations as a function of age in the rat*

| Kindling stage | Motor behavior[a] | |
	Pups	Adults
0	Behavioral arrest	Behavioral arrest
1	Mouth clonus	Chewing
2	Head bobbing	Head bobbing
3	Unilateral forelimb clonus and ±hindlimb clonus; 'wet dog shakes'	Unilateral forelimb clonus
3.5	Alternating forelimb clonus	
4	Bilateral forelimb clonus	Bilateral forelimb clonus
5	Bilateral forelimb clonus with rearing and falling over	Bilateral forelimb clonus with rearing and falling over
6	Wild running and jumping with or without vocalizations	Wild running and jumping with vocalizations
7	Tonus	Tonus
8	Spontaneous seizures	Spontaneous seizures

From Haas *et al.* (1992).
[a] Pups aged 14–16 days; adults aged 90–120 days.

The behavioral manifestations of kindled seizures depend on the stimulated site and on the animal species. In the adult rat, amygdala-kindled seizures progress through predictable and characteristic stages (Table 5.1). Stages 0–3 represent focal (partial) seizures, although by the time stage 3 seizures occur, the seizure activity has propagated throughout the ipsilateral hemisphere. Stages 4 and 5 represent generalized seizures of different severity. Further stimulations will induce progressively more severe seizures, classified as stages 6–8 (Pinel & Rovner, 1978). Most investigators consider the development of stage 4 or 5 generalized seizures as the end point of kindling (Goddard *et al.*, 1969; Burchfiel & Applegate, 1989; Moshé, 1989; Racine *et al.*, 1972). The number of stimulations required for the development of a generalized (stage 4 or 5) convulsion has been termed kindling rate and is a measure of the ability of the focus to propagate to distant sites involved in the behavioral expression of seizures, as well as the ability of surrounding and remote brain regions to limit this spread. Animals with short kindling rates are considered to be more seizure prone than animals with long kindling rates.

Kindling has been induced experimentally in a variety of adult animal species, including frogs, reptiles, rodents, cats, dogs, and primates (for a review, see Moshé & Ludwig, 1988). In contrast, in developing animals, kindling has been induced in rats and cats (Moshé & Ludwig, 1988; Moshé *et al.*, 1988; Shouse *et al.*, 1990). In both these animal species, kindling was produced by the repeated application of electrical stimuli to discrete areas of the brain. Chemical kindling has not been reported in developing animals.

Anesthesia and surgery

Almost all kindling studies in developing animals have been performed in rats older than 14 days. There are several reasons for this. First, rats younger than 12 days are susceptible to the effects of anesthetic agents and thus may not survive the anesthesia even when minuscule doses are used. Cooling has been employed as an anesthetic agent but the possible detrimental effects of cooling have not been adequately studied. To lower the temperature, the rat pup is placed on ice for 3–4 min (W. Paredes, personal communication). Second, the electrodes tend to become displaced because the skull is too thin to allow for the insertion of anchoring screws and the brain and skull grow fast at this age. Because of these limitations, kindling must be carried out as soon as the rat recovers from anesthesia, without any recuperation period. To date, only one study has been reported in very young rats (seven days old) using the 'rapid kindling' technique of Michelson & Lothman (1991). The latter authors found that the kindling response was attenuated on the second day, although the rats had already experienced generalized seizures during the first day. This loss of response may be due to electrode movement. Finally, surgery must be modified because the rats cannot be easily placed in a stereotaxic instrument, since the ear canals are still closed and the pup's snout is too small to help in the positioning of the head. Although methods have been described for stereotaxic implantations in neonatal rats (Cain & Dekergommeaux, 1979; Heller *et al.*, 1979; Lithgow & Barr, 1982), the first two limitations cannot be easily bypassed.

Correlative ontogenetic studies indicate that a seven to ten day old rat may be equivalent in some respects to newborn human infants (Gottlieb *et al.*, 1977; Moshé, 1987; Moshé *et al.*, 1992). The ear canals of rat pups are open by 12 days and therefore these pups can be easily placed in the stereotaxic apparatus. Surgery is conducted under anesthesia with a mixture of ketamine (70 mg/kg) and xylazine (6 mg/kg) i.p., using a ten-fold dilution of the solution used in adults. The depth of surgical anesthesia can be maintained by supplemental administration of

Table 5.2. *Coordinates for electrode placements in amygdala or hippocampus in 13–17 day old rats*

Site	Angle	Anterior–posterior	Lateral	Depth
Amygdala	—	−1.8	±3.5	7.2–7.4
Amygdala	15° forward	+0.5	±3.5	7.5–7.7
Hippocampus	—	−3.2	±3.0	2.8

Coordinates are in millimeters and referenced from bregma, except for the depth coordinate that is measured from skull surface. Stereotaxic implantations are conducted with the incisor bar set at −3.5 mm.

methoxyflurane whenever necessary. Rats are allowed two days of recuperation to permit both physical recovery and clearance of the anesthetic compound. During this period the rats are kept with their dams and are hydrated with subcutaneously administered fluids as necessary.

In our laboratory, stereotaxic implantation of the electrodes is conducted with the incisor bar set at −3.5 mm, and the electrodes are fixed to the skull with two or three screws and dental acrylic. The coordinates depend on the site that is to be stimulated, and the number of the electrodes that are implanted. Because in rat pups the surface of the skull is small, electrodes are often inserted at an angle. Table 5.2 depicts coordinates for amygdala and hippocampus.

Recently, kindling was induced in weaned kittens (Shouse *et al.*, 1990). The mortality rate in the postoperative period was 30.5%. Deaths occurred within a week of surgery and, in 73%, were due to thermoregulatory instability associated with anesthesia. The remaining 27% died from upper respiratory disease. The anesthesia employed was sodium pentobarbital 35 mg/kg, i.p. The coordinates were modified from adult coordinates. Because the maturational process is slower in kittens than in rats, the kittens were allowed to recuperate for one to two weeks.

Stimulation paradigms

In our laboratory, kindling stimulations consist of a 1 s train of 60 Hz sinusoidal current, 400 µA, peak to peak. In pups, the usual pattern of stimulation used in adults (one to three stimulations/day) cannot be used because by the time kindling is finished, the pups are grown rats. In addition, the electrodes may fall off as the skull grows. Kindling can be induced with stimuli delivered every hour (Moshé, 1981). However, we have found this stimulation paradigm taxing because of the time constraints. For the past several years, we have been inducing kindling by stimulating rat pups at 15 min intervals (Moshé *et al.*, 1983; Wurpel *et al.*, 1990; Haas *et al.*, 1992; Sperber *et al.*, 1990). Electroencephalographic (EEG) recordings are taken prior to each kindling stimulation to establish a stable baseline, and immediately following stimulation to record the complete seizure AD. Through relays, the same electrodes can be used for stimulation and EEG recordings. In rat pups, once kindling is induced, it produces a permanent change in seizure susceptibility, irrespective of whether the rat pups are kindled with stimulations delivered quarter-hourly or hourly (Moshé & Albala, 1982, 1983). To test the permanence of kindling, the electrodes must be first surgically removed, the pups allowed to grow and then new electrodes must be inserted. To date, kittens have been stimulated with daily stimulations (Shouse *et al.*, 1990). It will be interesting to determine the characteristics of kindling in kittens using shorter interstimulus intervals. The permanence of the kindling phenomenon in kittens has not been studied.

The AD threshold (ADT) is defined as the lowest current intensity capable of inducing an AD and is frequently used as an index of local excitability. The ADT is often determined as follows: each pup receives an initial 50 µA stimulus and is stimulated once per minute, with the stimulus intensity increasing by 50 µA increments until an AD occurs. The stimulus intensity is then reduced by 25 µA and the pup stimulated once more (Moshé *et al.*, 1981; Moshé & Albala, 1982).

Adult animals can be kindled with 10 s trains of low frequency (10 Hz) stimulation presented every 5 min (Lothman *et al.*, 1985). The current intensity is higher than that used for conventional kindling. This regimen results in kindling in two to three hours. 'Rapid kindling' can be triggered in developed animals (Holmes & Thompson, 1987; Michelson & Lothman, 1991). Holmes & Thompson (1987) have reported that in prepubescent, 26–29 day old rats, 'rapid kindling' can occur when either the amygdala or the hippocampus is stimulated with 10 s trains. High frequency (60 Hz) stimulation may be more effective than low frequency frequency (10 Hz) stimulation of equal duration. While 'rapid kindling' provides a convenient way of establishing generalized seizures in a matter of minutes, the overall kindling rate is no different from that observed with conventional stimuli. Holmes & Thompson (1987) observed also that in 'rapid kindling', the progression of seizures is not smooth with frequent digressions or jumps. These characteristics are not age specific.

The classic kindling procedure can be modified in order to study specific aspects of epileptogenesis. Instead of stimulating one site at a time, Burchfiel and his colleagues stimulated two sites on an alternating basis in adult rats (Duchowny & Burchfiel, 1981; Applegate *et al.*, 1986, 1987; Burchfiel *et al.*, 1986; Burchfiel & Applegate, 1989). This procedure allows for the examination of inhibitory interactions between the stimulated foci and has been named kindling antagonism. The same paradigm can be used in immature animals to determine the ease with which multiple seizure foci develop as a function of age (Haas *et al.*, 1992; Sperber *et al.*, 1990).

Another variant of the kindling protocol allows for the determination of the intensity of postictal refractoriness that follows a generalized seizure (Engel & Ackermann, 1980; Engel *et al.*, 1981; Moshé & Albala, 1983). In this paradigm, rats are kindled, using conventional techniques, until they consistently develop generalized seizures. Subsequently, they are exposed to eight consecutive stimulations each delivered at 2 min intervals. The paradigm is useful only if the first stimulus of the series elicits a generalized seizure. The severity and duration of elicited convulsions during the 16 min period is recorded and two indices of the intensity of postictal refractoriness are obtained. These are the seizure and the AD index. The seizure index is obtained by adding the numerical value depicting the seizure severity according to an age-appropriate kindling scale (Table 5.1) and dividing the sum by the total number of stimulations. The AD index is similarly obtained by adding the AD duration of each seizure and dividing by the total number of stimulations. In general, the smaller the two indices, the greater the intensity of postictal refractoriness, but a dissociation may also occur. Using this method, Moshé & Albala (1983) were able to demonstrate that the intensity of postictal refractoriness increases with age and they suggested that the lack of effective postictal refractoriness may be responsible for the propensity of immature rats to develop status epilepticus.

In adults, status epilepticus has been obtained by exposing kindled rats to continuous stimulations for one hour (McIntyre *et al.*, 1982). Status can also be obtained by continuously stimulating naive animals (Ackermann *et al.*, 1986). Neither paradigm has yet been applied in developing animals.

Classification of seizures

The behavioral expression of seizures depends on the maturational stage of the CNS, including the extent of myelination of intrinsic connections and motor pathways. Table 5.1 compares the kindling stages of adult rats and 15–18 day old rats stimulated from the amygdala. Hippocampal kindling follows similar characteristics but 'wet dog shakes' occur immediately after the stimulation (Haas *et al.*, 1992; Sperber *et al.*, 1990). As the other ictal events emerge, the incidence of 'wet dog shakes' diminishes. In amygdala-kindled rats, 'wet dog shakes' appear after the pups have experienced at least unilateral forelimb clonus (Moshé, 1989).

Shouse *et al.* (1992) have reported that the behavioral manifestations of amygdala kindling in kittens are similar to those observed in adult cats. However, after the completion of kindling, a large percentage of kittens, aged less than 5.5 months, experienced spontaneous generalized seizures. Most of the spontaneous seizures were similar to stimulation-induced seizures but a new type, labeled 'catnip seizure', was also seen. These seizures consist of long periods of staring, associated with purring and periods of retropulsion of the head and jackknife-like jerks. 'Catnip seizures' may be the sequel of bilateral amygdala stimulation during kindling.

Advantages

Kindling offers several unique opportunities to study several aspects of epileptogenesis in animals, and perhaps by extrapolation allow for better understanding of the pathophysiology of some human epileptic syndromes (Wada, 1986). In the kindling model, the investigator has precise control of the site of seizure initiation, as well as of seizure development and maintenance. The introduced convulsive patterns are easily recognizable, reproducible, and age specific. The seizures can be quantified by severity (see Kindling stages, Table 5.1) and duration (electrographic ADs). Finally, spontaneous seizures may eventually occur (Pinel & Rovner, 1978; Wada *et al.*, 1974; Wada & Osawa, 1976). Thus, kindling satisfies most of the prerequisite characteristics of an 'ideal' model of epilepsy (Wada, 1986) and it may allow for the determination, in vivo, of the site of action of drugs against seizures of varying intensity (for a review, see Moshé & Ludwig, 1988).

Before the introduction of kindling as a model of epilepsy in developing animals (Moshé, 1981), the few available studies performed in immature animals did not depict the changes in seizure susceptibility observed in humans as a function of age (Moshé, 1989). Although studies using chemoconvulsants suggested that immature animals require smaller doses to develop seizures than do adults, the chemical approach may be complicated by several factors such as drug absorption, distribution, metabolism, and the maturational state of the blood–brain barrier (Moshé, 1989). These limitations do not appear to play a major role in electrical kindling.

Kindling is a particularly useful model for evaluating the excitability of different brain sites in developing animals. Characteristics of kindling that are age specific (Moshé *et al.*, 1992) include:

(1) Kindling is inducible in immature animals with short interstimulus intervals that fail to induce kindling in adults.
(2) Bilateral seizure manifestations occur faster in immature animals than in adults.
(3) Kindling antagonism does not occur in immature rats.
(4) In immature rats, kindling progresses at a similar rate irrespective of whether the animal is stimulated from the amygdala or hippocampus.
(5) Immature rats develop severe kindled seizures, stages 6 and 7, faster than adults do.
(6) Immature rats have very short periods of postictal refractoriness.

Kindling is best suited to studying propagation patterns including the progressive recruitment of various structures that may modify seizure susceptibility. Thus, kindling in combination with the deoxyglucose technique (Engel *et al.*, 1978; Ackermann *et al.*, 1986) was instrumental in developing the nigral hypothesis, namely that the substantia nigra pars reticulata is an important site capable of modifying seizure severity as a function of age (Moshé, 1989; Moshé *et al.*, 1986; Ackermann *et al.*, 1989; Moshé & Sperber, 1990).

Disadvantages

Kindling studies are time consuming and require a degree of technical expertise for the insertion of several electrodes or cannulae into very small and fragile animals. The breech of the blood–brain barrier induced by the insertion of the electrodes may, by itself, enhance seizure susceptibility (Remler & Marcussen, 1984). The precise mechanism by which kindling operates is unknown. Yet, the discrete developmental stages allow for the possible combination of kindling with other techniques such as electro-graphic monitoring in vivo and in vitro or metabolic mapping using the deoxyglucose technique.

Systemic convulsants

In our laboratory we use two drugs capable of inducing seizures of varying intensity when administered systemically: flurothyl and kainic acid.

Flurothyl-induced seizures

Flurothyl (bis-2,2,2-triflurothyl ether) is a volatile convulsant agent established as an effective technique for measuring the brain's threshold to generalized seizures (Truitt *et al.*, 1960; Prichard *et al.*, 1969). The convulsions produced by the inhalation of flurothyl are considered to represent a model of generalized seizures, since flurothyl produces seizures by diffusely opening neuronal sodium channels (Woodbury, 1980).

The procedure used for flurothyl eliminates the stress of the injection associated with other systemic convulsants. The rats are placed in an airtight 9.2 liter chamber and liquid flurothyl is delivered via a Harvard pump at the constant rate of 20 μl/min to a filter pad from which it vaporizes (Okada *et al.*, 1986; Sperber *et al.*, 1987; Wong & Moshé, 1987). When a generalized seizure occurs, the flurothyl infusion can be stopped. Between trials, the chamber is flushed with room air and the filter changed. The following variables can be analyzed: latency to onset of forelimb clonus, latency to onset of tonic–clonic seizures with loss of posture as well as seizure duration. These indices are consistent both within and between animals (Truitt *et al.*, 1960; Prichard *et al.*, 1969).

To determine whether the susceptibility to flurothyl-induced seizures varies with age, Sperber & Moshé (1988) tested adult rats and 16 day old pups in different size chambers. The sizes of the chamber were chosen so that the rats of both groups were near the filter pad from which flurothyl vaporized and to account for the differences in body size. Flurothyl was administered at the constant rate of 20 μl/min in both groups. The latencies to the onset of three different stages – forelimb clonus, loss of posture, and development of tonic seizures – were the measurements of the convulsive thresholds. Rat pups developed age-specific patterns. Overall, their seizure latency was shorter than that of adult rats and the sequence of convulsive events occurred rapidly; indeed the three stages were often indistinguishable. This was not the case with adult rats. For both age groups, seizure thresholds varied as a function of chamber size: the smaller the chamber, the faster seizures occurred.

Continuous administration of flurothyl can produce status epilepticus. In adults rats, flurothyl-induced status epilepticus produces neuronal damage in several discrete brain regions, even when the animals are kept well oxygenated (Nevander *et al.*, 1985). If the rats are not well oxygenated, they die. In contrast, rat pups can undergo an hour of continuous tonic–clonic seizures with low mortality rates (S. L. Moshé, unpublished results). Furthermore, these rats are not prone to develop brain lesions similar to those observed in surviving adults (S. L. Moshé, unpublished results; Wasterlain & Dwyer, 1983).

Advantages

An advantage of the flurothyl model is that it avoids the stress of the injection associated with systemic convulsions. In addition, many animals can be tested simultaneously. Another advantage is that seizures will always occur. Since flurothyl is constantly infused, changes in latency depict the amount of flurothyl administered. Thus, animals with short flurothyl latencies require smaller amounts of flurothyl to have a convulsion than animals with long latencies. Changes in the latencies and seizure severity can readily distinguish whether pharmacological manipulations produce a facilitation or a partial suppression of convulsions. If the infusion is not stopped then the animals may experience status epilepticus that lasts as long as flurothyl is administered. This is particularly the case with immature rats, since adult rats may die quickly (S. L. Moshé, unpublished results). The ease and reliability of flurothyl-induced seizures permit its use together with other more invasive techniques such as intracranial lesions or cannulae implantation. This is especially pertinent for studies of the epileptic process in immature animals. Since the flurothyl model, in contrast to kindling, does not require any surgery, the animals will be exposed to only one anesthetic and surgical procedure related to the variable the investigator plans to study.

Disadvantages

Flurothyl, when inhaled, can induce seizures in humans (Chatrian & Petersen, 1960). Thus, a special chamber must be used and the investigator must take all necessary precautions to avoid massive or chronic subacute exposure to this agent. The mechanism by which flurothyl induces seizures is unknown. It has been suggested that it may produce seizures by opening sodium channels diffusely (Woodbury, 1980). The site of action of flurothyl also is not not known.

Flurothyl levels in serum and brain are not routinely measured. Since flurothyl is absorbed by the lungs, physiological parameters that influence the respiratory rate may alter the rate of absorption of flurothyl. For example, administration of GABAergic agents in the substantia nigra often induces intense stereotypes (Sperber et al., 1987) and the increased motor activity may affect the respiratory rate (Anlezark et al., 1977; Hedner et al., 1981). Therefore, this variable must be controlled for, when comparative studies are performed.

Kainic acid seizures

Kainic acid is an excitatory amino acid, capable of producing electrographic and behavioral seizures when injected systematically or intracerebrally (Ben-Ari et al., 1981; Lothman & Collins, 1981). Kainic acid has an affinity for limbic structures and consequently the behavioral seizures include manifestations that can be elicited by direct stimulation of limbic sites (Ben-Ari et al., 1981; Lothman & Collins, 1981). However, the seizure manifestations are age specific (Albala et al., 1984; Okada et al., 1984). For example, seizures in adult animals are characterized by chewing, 'wet dog shakes', rearing, forelimb clonus, and eventually generalized clonic–tonic seizures. 'Wet dog shakes' are rare in 15–18 days old rat pups, while scratching is often the first manifestation, especially when relatively low doses of kainic acid are used. Rat pups younger than 15 days exhibit 'swimming movements' before the expression of tonic seizures. In general, the younger the rat, the higher the probability that status epilepticus will occur. Status epilepticus is often lethal in rats of all ages, although younger animals have a higher mortality rate than adults (Albala et al., 1984). Rats exposed to kainic acid-induced seizures may develop, later on, spontaneous seizures (Cavalheiro et al., 1982). The occurrence of spontaneous seizures is age dependent. Rats younger than 30 days rarely develop spontaneous seizures (Thompson et al., 1990).

Adult animals that experience severe kainic acid-induced seizures are found to have lesions of specific neuronal groups within the limbic structures. The neuropathological damage is considered to be the result of a process that is secondary to seizures (Nadler et al., 1978;

Schwob *et al.*, 1980; Nadler, 1981) and not the result of toxic kainic acid accumulation (Scherer-Singler & McGeer, 1979). The lesions induced by kainic acid seizures have a topography similar to that of the lesions found in the temporal lobes of human epileptics suffering from intractable seizures (mesial temporal sclerosis) (Falconer *et al.*, 1964; Scheibel *et al.*, 1974). It has been suggested that mesial temporal sclerosis may be the result of seizures occurring early in life, although the available evidence is controversial (Moshé, 1987). The results of ontogenetic studies of kainic acid seizures suggest that the neuropathological damage is age dependent; the older the animal the higher the probability that seizures will be associated with hippocampal gliotic lesions (Albala *et al.*, 1984; Nitecka *et al.*, 1984; Okada *et al.*, 1984; Holmes & Thompson, 1988; Sperber *et al.*, 1991). The route of administration of kainic acid as well as the species of animal used in the study of kainic acid seizures may have an important role. Thus, in immature rabbits, systemic, but not intra-cerebral, injections of kainic acid may produce lesions (Franck & Schwartzkroin, 1984).

Kainic acid can be administered systemically or intracerebrally dissolved in a buffered solution. The doses depend on the route of administration as well as the age of the animal. In rats, the dose of systemically administered kainic acid is in the range 2.5–20 mg/kg. Rat pups require doses between 2.5–10 mg/kg (Albala *et al.*, 1984). The dose of intracerebrally injected kainic acid is in the range of 0.005–1 µg in adult rats and 1–7.5 µg in developing rats (Cook & Crutcher, 1985, 1986).

Advantages

Kainic-acid-induced seizures are prolonged. Thus, this model is useful for studying several types of status epilepticus and the sequelae that may result from the long seizures. The occurrence of characteristic lesions is a particularly important advantage because it allows for the study of how 'epileptic' damage may occur. The existence of spontaneous seizures that persist long after the acute administration of kainic acid indicates that this model may create a type of 'epileptic dysfunction' similar to the human epileptic condition (Sutula *et al.*, 1988; Sutula *et al.*, 1989; Haas *et al.*, 1990; Sperber *et al.*, 1991; Babb, 1992). Combined with other techniques, such as in-vitro brain slices, this method may provide powerful insights of the pathophysiological substrates of seizures.

Disadvantages

The limitations pertaining to all systemically administered chemoconvulsants, relating to drug absorption and metabolism, are pertinent in this model too. Furthermore, this model does not easily allow the study of the effects of short seizures, since the acutely induced seizures worsen with time and may lead to the animal's death. The seizures are sometimes difficult to treat with standard anticonvulsants and thus difficult to stop. The behavioral manifestations of the seizures do not depict accurately what is going on electrically in the brain. Kainic acid seizures often produce subclinical status epilepticus, and brief behavioral seizures may be associated with continuous generalized electrographic discharges (Moshé, 1987). This observation suggests that EEG monitoring is important in this model. Furthermore, since the seizures are prolonged, drugs that are effective against them may not be optimal to treat brief seizures because they may produce unacceptable side effects. Finally, kainic acid seizures may be a model of epilepsy specifically related to activation of excitatory amino acid receptors. Correlation with findings obtained from other models is important in order to confirm that the data are not model specific.

Tissue slices

Background information

The study of basic physiological mechanisms of neuronal communication has been advanced by the development of the brain slice preparation. Slices contain a network of neurons and glia that is capable of supporting both normal synaptic transmission and epileptiform activity. Thus, this preparation allows the separate investigation of intrinsic membrane properties and synaptic connectivity contributing to epileptiform firing. There are two broad classes of experiments typically performed on brain slices. In the first, a convulsant compound, such as the GABAergic antagonist bicuculline, is applied acutely to the slice to induce epileptiform burst firing similar to activity recorded in vivo. The second involves prior induction of seizures using some in-vivo model system such as kindling; brain slices from animals with seizures are compared to slices from normal control animals for persistent differences in cellular and/or synaptic properties.

The majority of studies to date have focused on epileptogenesis in slices from adult animals. However, there is a growing use of slices to study sensitivity in vitro of the immature brain to epileptogenic stimuli (Schwartzkroin, 1982; Mueller *et al.*, 1984; Swann & Brady, 1984; Stanton *et al.*, 1987*a,b*; Hamon & Heinemann, 1988; Ben-Ari *et al.*, 1989; Hablitz *et al.*, 1989; Haglund & Schwartzkroin, 1990). Again, experimental approaches can involve either investigation of the sensitivity of slices from young animals to acutely applied convulsants, or comparisons of the effects of prior induction of seizures in vivo on electrophysiological responses in slices. The first approach yields information on factors controlling the generation and propagation of epileptiform bursts in normal neuronal tissue, and the second yields data about long-term cellular changes associated with maintenance of seizure activity.

Methodology

Techniques of preparation of thin slices for in-vitro electrophysiological recordings are currently in wide use. While a number of slicing procedures have been employed, the highest viability slices are cut with vibrating tissue slicers known as vibratomes. Histological comparisons of 400 μm thick slices prepared with a vibratome with those prepared with a McIlwain chopper have shown that chopped slices have 50 μm thick layers of severe tissue damage, while vibratomed slices contain healthy neurons within 10 μm of the cut surfaces. This difference is especially important in the preparation of slices from immature brain, where the fragility of the tissue is greater.

There are two types of chamber typically used to maintain slices: interface and submerged recording chambers. In the first, the slice sits at the interface between artificial cerebrospinal fluid (ACSF) below, and humidified 95% O_2/5% CO_2 gas mixture above, the tissue. As the name suggests, the submerged slice is completely immersed in ACSF saturated with O_2. In general, the interface preparation can maintain tissue at temperatures closer to physiological (34–36 °C), probably due to better oxygenation, while the submerged preparation has been favored for minimizing fluid movement for stability of intracellular recording. A typical ACSF composition is (mM): NaCl 126, KCl 5, NaH_2PO_4 1.25, $MgSO_4$ 2, $CaCl_2$ 2, $NaHCO_3$ 26, glucose 10. Glass micropipettes for extracellular recording are filled with NaCl, while intracellular electrodes can be filled with a variety of ionic mixtures depending upon experimental needs. The tip size for intracellular electrodes is in the range 0.2–0.5 μm, although optimal size and shape can vary widely depending upon the cell types to be impaled. Stimulating electrodes that supply the best focal stimulation are bipolar twisted wire, where the tip size is of the order of 25 μm diameter for insertion into the slice, and tip separation is minimal (see also, Mody et al., 1988).

Another important issue concerns the design of experiments comparing slices from animals in which seizures have been induced with controls. Although these experiments are not always so structured, the use of age-matched sham-operated controls that are examined in parallel on the same day is far preferable in controlling for confounding variables unrelated to epileptogenesis.

It is relatively recently that the slice technique has begun to be exploited in the study of developmental changes in neuronal response to epilepto-genic stimuli, as well as other developmental changes in electrophysio-logical and biochemical properties. An essential feature of such studies is the comparison, by the same investigators, of responses in slices obtained from immature rats at varying stages of postnatal development with identically recorded responses in slices from adult animals. With this approach, variations in methodology between laboratories which may obscure reliable differences between immature and mature brain tissue can be controlled for.

Preparation of slices from different areas

The hippocampus is not the only site that has been examined with slice techniques. A number of other areas including visual (Scharfman & Sarvey, 1987), pyriform (McIntyre & Wong, 1986) and entorhinal (Stanton et al., 1987b) cortex have been examined, as well as subcortical preparations such as locus coeruleus (Williams et al., 1984) and substantia nigra (Llinas et al., 1984; Nakanishi et al., 1987). These preparations, of immense potential, have yet to be exploited for the study of neuronal development. This may be due partly to the greater technical difficulties they present. Potential problems include greater sensitivity to ischemic damage during dissection, tissue fragility and architectural diffuseness. Techniques used to minimize ischemic damage during dissection include cooling the bathing media, application of N-methyl-D-aspartate (NMDA) receptor antagonists or voltage-dependent calcium channel antagonists while cutting, and lowering potassium concentration in the bathing media. While cooling and lowering extracellular potassium concentration are probably helpful and rational, the use of pharmacological agents has considerable potential for long-term alterations in slice physiology and should be avoided.

Mechanical fragility of a particular neuronal area can be a difficult problem. Factors that are under the experimenter's control in vibratoming slices include the rate and length of blade vibration, speed of blade advance, and orientation of slicing. In general, the most rapid vibration speed coupled with the slowest rate of advance yields the best results. In cutting, white matter usually poses the greatest problems, and pulling on associated axonal pathways can be extremely damaging. Cutting through the area of interest last is usually the best strategy for minimizing mechanical damage.

Synaptic plasticity in the immature nervous system

High-frequency stimulation of a number of neuronal pathways in the central nervous system elicits an extremely stable increase in synaptic efficacy known as long-term potentiation (LTP) (Bliss & Lømo, 1973), which has been implicated as a possible substrate for learning and memory. The range of high-frequency trains that generate LTP, when applied repeatedly, will lead to kindling in both immature and adult animals. Interestingly, it appears that LTP is not present in the early development of neonatal rats. Several reports suggest that the ability to induce LTP in area CA1 of a hippocampal slice from rat pup appears during the second week after birth (Baudry *et al.*, 1981; Harris & Teyler, 1984). It has been shown that NMDA receptor mechanisms, presynaptic plasticity, calcium regulation, and synaptic inhibitory circuitry all change markedly between postnatal day 7 and day 15 (Muller *et al.*, 1989). These and similar studies make it clear that there are significant developmental phases in the expression of LTP, phases whose contribution to seizure susceptibility of the immature brain is largely unknown. The slice preparation will be useful in answering a number of these questions.

Other studies have uncovered a second form of synaptic plasticity in hippocampal and cortical neurons. Long-term depression (LTD) of synaptic transmission occurs when presynaptic activity occurs while the postsynaptic neuron is hyperpolarized and inactive (Stanton & Sejnowski, 1989). Since LTD seems to involve non-NMDA receptor mechanisms (Chattarji *et al.*, 1989), we have begun examining LTD induced by stimulation while blocking LTP with an NMDA antagonist. LTD induced in slices from 15 day old rats was significantly greater than that observed in adult slices (P. K. Stanton, unpublished results). Like LTP, it seems likely that LTD may make important contributions to the regulation of seizure susceptibility and development in the immature brain.

Transmitter systems in the immature nervous system

Another approach that has been underutilized is the study of development of transmitter systems, many of which are associated with epileptiform activity. Recent studies have shown that GABAergic receptors in the immature hippocampus exhibit different responses from GABA agonists than are typically observed in adult slices (Mueller *et al.*, 1984; Chesnut & Swann, 1989). Muller *et al.* (1989) compared NMDA responses of 7–9 and 12–15 day postnatal rat hippocampus, and found a larger NMDA contribution to evoked responses in the younger animals.

While the slice technique has been employed effectively to study postnatal development of a number of physiological parameters, this technique also lends itself to the study of the effects of prenatal insults upon subsequent neuronal development. One such study addressed the effects of fetal alcohol exposure on postnatal development of multiple transmitter systems linked to phosphoinositide turnover, and on norepinephrine-stimulated ionic fluxes in hippocampal slices (Stanton *et al.*, 1987*a*). These experiments compared slices from fetal alcohol-treated and age-matched control animals at various ages from 6 to 50 days postnatal. Remarkable agreement in the levels of impairment of noradrenergic function was observed in both biochemical and electrophysiological paradigms. There is great potential for this approach provided care is taken to provide for age-matched and cross-fostered controls and comparisons across development which include slices from adult animals.

Kindling and immature brain slices

There is a great deal of untapped potential for studies comparing the responses of immature and adult slices to epileptogenic stimuli such as kindling. While work at the in-vivo level has focused on variations in seizure susceptibility of the immature brain, these efforts would be complemented by comparison of slices from immature kindled animals with age-matched non-kindled controls. Until now, this experimental paradigm has not been employed.

Advantages

The slice preparation offers a number of advantages that complement in-vivo approaches. Chief among these is the control of the extracellular milieu, allowing alteration of extracellular ionic constituents, contents or temperature of bath, or local drug application, and biochemical study of transmitter release. Slices offer superior stability of intracellular impalements, and easy stimulation of multiple afferent and efferent pathways under visual placement. It is also well suited for combining electro-physiological and anatomical techniques, since intracellular electrodes can be filled with a number of substances, such as horseradish peroxidase or Lucifer yellow, for imaging cell location and morphology after recording.

It is important to note that the slice is a synaptically interconnected network of neurons in a relatively normal glial and interstitial environment, capable of exhibiting epileptiform burst activity that propagates through the tissue in ways similar to in vivo (Knowles *et al.*, 1987). Thus, the slice offers simultaneous access to single cell membrane properties and their alterations in the seizure state, and access to a neuronal system, its extracellular milieu and interconnected activity.

Disadvantages

One of the obvious limitations of the slice preparation is the absence of normal afferent and efferent interconnections with other brain areas. This may be a significant problem in the study of generalization of seizure activity, antagonism between kindling foci and secondary focus formation. The level and patterns of spontaneous activity in slice preparations are probably quite different from the whole animal, and many (but not all) fiber tracts that can be stimulated in the slice originate from cell bodies outside the preparation. This latter point should be borne in mind when one is considering possible transmitter depletion associated with pro-longed high frequency firing induced by convulsants or stimulation.

Conclusion

Current research suggests that the immature CNS is highly susceptible to the development of seizures when exposed to epileptogenic stimuli. Similar stimuli may fail to induce seizures in older animals. There are at least two basic questions.

(1) What are the substrates underlying the increased seizure susceptibility of the developing brain?

(2) Do the sequelae of seizures vary as function of age?

The most likely answer to the first question is that the causes of increased seizure susceptibility are multifactorial. For convenience, the process of epileptogenesis can be separated into three probably interrelated series of events. The first includes the mechanism by which an aggregate of neurons initiates the paroxysmal discharge locally. The second involves the mechanisms of seizure propagation and the third is the processes that lead to the suppression of seizures. All three categories may be capable of altering the normal developmental process, leaving some degree of permanent sequelae that also appear to be age dependent (Moshé, 1987).

Within each event, several factors may operate including changes in molecular biology, cell morphology, basic electrical properties, receptor development, local connectivity (microcircuitry) and afferent and efferent connections to and from distal sites (macrocircuitry). There is already evidence that in the developing CNS, excitatory synapses mature before inhibitory synapses, at least in some areas such as the CA1 region of the hippocampus (Schwartzkroin, 1982, 1984; Schwartzkroin *et al.*, 1982). In the same region, there may be an enhanced sensitivity to excitatory amino acids that is expressed by large influxes of calcium in the neurons (Hamon & Heineman, 1988). However, the molecular consequences of this increased influx are poorly understood. In the CA3 region, changes in seizure susceptibility may be due, in part, to differences in the location of synapses in the dendritic tree, abundant local networks of recurrent excitation and perhaps differences in the nature of cations regulating the NMDA receptor (Swann & Brady, 1984; Swann *et al.*, 1988, 1992, Chapter 6, this volume). There appear to be age-related differences in the GABA-mediated inhibition both in the hippocampus and the substantia nigra pars reticulata. The former may enhance local excitatory circuits, the latter alters the proposed inhibitory-to-seizures role of the substantia nigra pars reticulata. This is achieved by changing both local responses as well as the structures that are activated as a result of the altered local response as a function of age (Moshé & Sperber, 1990; Moshé *et al.*, 1992).

To test the various hypotheses, we use combinations of the models we described above. For example, we are investigating local changes in the dentate-CA3 circuitry of the hippocampus before and after the induction of seizures of varying severity and duration, which in turn produce different levels of synaptic reorganization. This requires the use of hippocampal slices. These slices can be obtained from normal animals, or animals exposed to kindling or kainic acid. Kindled animals have permanent changes in seizure susceptibility irrespective of the age at which they are initially kindled (Moshé & Albala, 1982; Moshé *et al.*, 1983). Kainic acid-induced seizures do not induce gliotic lesions early in life, even when status epilepticus has occurred (Haas *et al.*, 1990; Sperber *et al.*, 1991). This suggests that the immature CNS may have inherent compensatory mechanisms to protect itself from its propensity to respond with seizures to stimuli that may be incapable of producing convulsions later on (Albala *et al.*, 1984; Okada *et al.*, 1984; Holmes & Thompson, 1988; Thompson *et al.*, 1990).

Other experiments are designed to test the hypothesis that the age-related different response of substantia nigra pars reticulata neurons to GABA-mimetic drugs is responsible for the failure of the immature CNS to contain seizures and prevent acute seizure recurrences. We have proposed that there are two factors that may play a role: (a) a relative paucity of nigral $GABA_A$ high affinity receptors and (b) an age-dependent nigral anticonvulsant effect mediated by $GABA_B$ receptor (Wurpel *et al.*, 1988; Sperber *et al.*, 1989a,b). We use flurothyl seizures to test the pharmacology of nigral GABAergic infusions and the slice technique to determine the microcircuitry and local responsivity to the administration of the same drugs that have vastly different and often opposite effects on seizures as a function of age.

Acknowledgments

This work was supported by NIH grant NS-20253 (S.L.M.), NRSA training grant NS-07183 from the NINDS and a Klingenstein Foundation fellowship (P.K.S.).

References

Ackermann, R. F., Chugani, H. T., Handforth, A., Moshé, S. L., Caldecott-Hazard, S. & Engel, J. J. (1986). Autoradiographic studies of cerebral metabolism and blood flow in rat amygdala kindling. In *Kindling 3*, ed. J. A. Wada, pp. 78–87. New York: Raven Press.

Ackermann, R. F., Moshé, S. L. & Albala, B. J. (1989). Restriction of enhanced ^{14}C-2-deoxyglucose utilization to rhinencephalic structures in immature amygdala-kindled rats. *Experimental Neurology*, **104**: 73–81.

Albala, B. J., Moshé, S. L. & Okada, R. (1984). Kainic-acid-induced seizures: a developmental study. *Developmental Brain Research*, **13**: 139–48.

Anlezark, G., Collins, J. & Meldrum, B. (1977). GABA agonists and audiogenic seizures. *Neuroscience Letters*, **7**: 337–40.

Applegate, C. D., Burchfiel, J. L. & Konkol, R. J. (1986). Kindling antagonism: effects of norepinephrine depletion on kindled seizure suppression after concurrent alternating stimulation in rats. *Experimental Neurology*, **94**: 379–90.

Applegate, C. D., Konkol, R. J. & Burchfiel, J. L. (1987). Kindling antagonism: a role for hindbrain norepinephrine in the development of site suppression following concurrent, alternate stimulation. *Brain Research*, **407**: 212–22.

Babb, T. L. (1992). Research on the anatomy and pathology of epileptic tissue. In *Epilepsy Surgery*, ed. H. Lüders, pp. 719–28. New York: Raven Press.

Baudry, M., Arst, D., Oliver, M. & Lynch, G. (1981). Development of glutamate binding sites and their regulation by calcium in the rat hippocampus. *Development Brain Research*, **1**, 37–48.

Ben-Ari, Y., Cherubini, E., Corradetti, R. & Gaiarsa, J. (1989). Giant synaptic potentials in immature rat CA3 hippocampal neurons. *Journal of Physiology*, **416**, 303–25.

Ben-Ari, Y., Riche, D., Ghilini, G. & Naquet, R. (1981). Electrographic, clinical and pathological alterations following systemic administration of kainic acid, bicuculline or pentetrazol: metabolic mapping using the deoxyglucose method with special reference to the pathology of epilepsy. *Neuroscience*, **6**: 1361–91.

Bliss, T. V. P. & Lømo, T. (1973). Long-lasting potentiation of synaptic transmission in the dentate area of the anaesthetized rabbit following stimulation of the perforant path. *Journal of Physiology*, **232**: 331–56.

Burchfiel, J. L. & Applegate, C. D. (1989). Stepwise progression of kindling: perspectives from the kindling antagonism model. In *Neuroscience and Biobehavioral Reviews*, ed. D. P. Cain & D. Teskey, pp. 289–308. New York: Pergamon.

Burchfiel, J. L., Applegate, C. D. & Konkol, R. J. (1986). Kindling antagonism: a role for norepinephrine in seizure suppression. In *Kindling 3*, ed. J. A. Wada, pp. 213–29. New York: Raven Press.

Cain, D. P. & Corcoran, M. E. (1981). Kindling with low frequency stimulation: generality, transfer, and recruiting effects. *Experimental Neurology*, **73**: 219–32.

Cain, D. P. & Dekergommeaux, S. E. (1979). Electrode implantation in small rodents for kindling and long term brain recording. *Physiology and Behavior*, **22**: 799–801.

Cavalheiro, E. A., Riche, D. A. & Le Gal La Salle, G. (1982). Long-term effects of intrahippocampal kainic acid injection in rats: a method for inducing spontaneous recurrent seizures. *Clinical Neurophysiology*, **53**: 581–9.

Cavalheiro, E. A., Silva, D. F., Turski, W. A., Calderazzo-Filho, L. S., Bartolotto, Z. & Turski, L. (1987). The susceptibility of rats to pilocarpine-induced seizures is age dependent. *Developmental Brain Research*, **37**: 43–58.

Chatrian, G. E. & Petersen, M. C. (1960). The convulsive patterns provoked by Indoklon, Metrazol and electroshock: some depth electrographic observations in human patients. *Electroencephalography and Clinical Neurophysiology*, **12**: 715–25.

Chattarji, S., Stanton, P. K. & Sejnowski, T. J. (1989). Induction of associative long-term depression (LTD) in hippocampal field CA3 is not mediated by NMDA receptors. *Society for Neuroscience Abstracts*, **16**: 165.

Chesnut, T. J. & Swann, J. W. (1989). Disinhibitory actions of the GABA$_A$ agonist muscimol in immature hippocampus. *Brain Research*, **502**: 365–74.

Cook, T. M. & Crutcher, A. (1985). Extensive target cell loss during development results in mossy fibers in the regio superior (CA1) of the rat hippocampal formation. *Developmental Brain Research*, **21**: 19–30.

Cook, T. M. & Crutcher, K. A. (1986). Intrahippocampal injection of kainic acid produces significant pyramidal cell loss in neonatal rats. *Neoroscience*, **18**, 79–92.

Duchowny, M. S. & Burchfiel, J. F. (1981). Facilitation and antagonism of kindled seizures development in the limbic system of the rat. *Electroencephalography and Clinical Neurophysiology*, **51**: 403–16.

Engel, J. Jr & Ackermann, R. F. (1980). Interictal EEG spikes correlate with decreased, rather than increased, epileptogenicity in amygdaloid kindled rats. *Brain Research*, **190**: 543–8.

Engel, J. Jr, Ackermann, R. F., Caldecott-Hazard, S. & Kuhl, D. E. (1981). Epileptic activation of antagonistic systems may explain paradoxical features of experimental and human epilepsy: a review and hypothesis. In *Kindling 2*, ed. J. A. Wada, pp. 193–217. New York: Raven Press.

Engel, J. Jr, Brown, L. L. & Wolfson, L. (1978). Anatomical correlates of electrical and behavioral events related to amygdaloid kindling. *Annals of Neurology*, **3**: 538–44.

Falconer, M. A., Serafetinides, E. A. & Corsellis, J. A. N. (1964). Etiology and pathogenesis of temporal lobe epilepsy. *Archives of Neurology*, **10**: 233–48.

Franck, J. E. & Schwartzkroin, P. A. (1984). Immature rabbit hippocampus is damaged by systemic but not intraventricular kainic acid. *Developmental Brain Research*, **13**: 219–27.

Gibbs, F. A. & Gibbs, E. L. (1963). Age factor in epilepsy. *New England Journal of Medicine*, **269**: 1230–6.

Goddard, G. V., McIntyre, D. C. & Leech, C. K. (1969). A permanent change in brain function resulting from daily electrical stimulation. *Experimental Neurology*, **25**: 295–330.

Gottlieb, A., Keydor, I. & Epstein, H. T. (1977). Rodent brain growth stages. An analytical review. *Biology of Neonate*, **32**: 166–76.

Haas, K., Sperber, E. F. & Moshé, S. L. (1992). Kindling in developing animals: expression of severe seizures and enhanced development of bilateral foci. *Developmental Brain Research*, **68**: 140–3.

Haas, K., Sperber, E. F., Moshé, S. L. & Stanton, P. K. (1990). Persistent alterations of dentate gyrus inhibition following kainic acid-induced status epilepticus in mature, but not immature, rats. *Society of Neuroscience Abstracts*, **16**: 281.

Hablitz, J. J., Tehrani, M. H. & Barnes, E. M. J. (1989). Chronic exposure of developing cortical neurons to GABA down-regulates GABA/benzodiazepine receptors and GABA-gated chloride currents. *Brain Research*, **501**: 332–8.

Haglund, M. M. & Schwartzkroin, P. A. (1990). Role of Na–K pump potassium regulation and IPSPs in seizures and spreading depression in immature rabbit hippocampal slices. *Journal of Neurophysiology*, **63**: 225–39.

Hamon, B. & Heinemann, U. (1988). Developmental changes in neuronal sensitivity to excitatory amino acids in area CA1 of the rat hippocampus. *Brain Research*, **466**: 286–90.

Harris, K. H. & Teyler, T. J. (1984). Developmental onset of long-term potentiation in area CA1 of the rat hippocampus. *Journal of Physiology*, **346**: 27–48.

Hauser, W. A. & Kurland, L. T. (1975). The epidemiology of epilepsy in Rochester, Minnesota, 1935–1967. *Epilepsia*, **16**: 1–66.

Hedner, J., Hedner, T., Jonason, J. & Lundberg, D. (1981). GABAergic mechanisms in central respiratory control in anesthesized rat. *Naunyn-Schmiedeberg's Archives of Pharmacology*, **317**: 315–20.

Heller, A., Hutchens, J. O., Kirby, M. L., Karapas, F. & Fernandez, C. (1979). Stereotaxic electrode placement in the neonatal rat. *Journal of Neuroscience Methods*, **1**: 41–76.

Holmes, G. L. & Thompson, J. L. (1987). Rapid kindling in the prepubescent rat. *Brain Research*, **433**: 281–4.

Holmes, G. L. & Thompson, J. L. (1988). Effects of kainic acid on seizure susceptibility in the developing brain. *Developmental Brain Research*, **39**: 51–9.

Knowles, W. D., Traub, R. D. & Strowbridge, B. W. (1987). The initiation and spread of epileptiform bursts in the in vitro hippocampal slice. *Neuroscience*, **21**: 441–55.

Lithgow, T. & Barr, G. A. (1982). A method for stereotaxic implantation in neonatal rats. *Developmental Brain Research*, **2**: 315–20.

Llinas, R., Greenfield, S. A. & Jahnsen, H. (1984). Electrophysiology of pars compacta cells in the in vitro substantia nigra – a possible mechanism for dendritic release. *Brain Research*, **294**: 127–32.

Lothman, E. W. & Collins, R. C. (1981). Kainic acid induced limbic seizures: metabolic, behavioral, electroencephalographic and neuropathological correlates. *Brain Research*, **218**: 299–318.

Lothman, E. W., Zorumski, C. F., Hatlelid, J. M., Conry, J. A., Moon, P. F. & Perlin, J. B. (1985). Kindling with rapidly recurring hippocampal seizures. *Brain Research*, **360**: 83–91.

McIntyre, D. C., Nathanson, D. & Edson, N. (1982). A new model of partial status epilepticus based on kindling. *Brain Research*, **250**: 53–63.

McIntyre, D. C. & Wong, R. K. S. (1986). Cellular and synaptic properties of amygdala-kindled pyriform cortex in vitro. *Journal of Neurophysiology*: **55**: 1295–1307.

Michelson, H. B. & Lothman, E. W. (1991). An ontogenetic study of kindling using rapidly recurring hippocampal seizures. *Developmental Brain Research*, **61**: 79–85.

Mody, I., Stanton, P. K. & Heinemann, U. (1988). Activation of N-methyl-D-aspartate (NMDA) receptors parallels changes in cellular and synaptic properties of dentate gyrus granule cells after kindling. *Journal of Neurophysiology*, **59**: 1033–54.

Moshé, S. L. (1981). The effects of age on the kindling phenomenon. *Developmental Psychobiology*, **14**: 75–81.

Moshé, S. L. (1987). Epileptogenesis and the immature brain. *Epilepsia*, **28** (Suppl), S3–S15.

Moshé, S. L. (1989). *Ontogeny of Seizures and Substantia Nigra Modulation*, pp. 247–62. Baltimore, MD: Johns Hopkins Press.

Moshé, S. L., Ackermann, R. F., Albala, B. J. & Okada, R. (1986). The role of substantia nigra in seizures of developing animals. In *Kindling 3*, ed. J. A. Wada, pp. 91–106. New York: Raven Press.

Moshé, S. L. & Albala, B. J. (1982). Kindling in developing rats: persistence of seizures into adulthood. *Developmental Brain Research*, **4**: 67–71.

Moshé, S. L. & Albala, B. J. (1983). Maturational changes in postictal refractoriness and seizure susceptibility in developing rats. *Annals of Neurology*, **13**: 552–7.

Moshé, S. L., Albala, B. J., Ackermann, R. F. & Engel, J. Jr (1983). Increased seizure susceptibility of the immature brain. *Developmental Brain Research*, **7**: 81–5.

Moshé, S. L. & Ludvig, N. (1988). Kindling. In *Recent Advances in Epilepsy 4* ed. T. A. Pedley & B. S. Meldrum, pp. 21–44. Edinburgh: Churchill Livingstone.

Moshé, S. L., Sharpless, N. S. & Kaplan, J. (1981). Kindling in developing rats: afterdischarge thresholds. *Brain Research*, **211**: 190–5.

Moshé, S. L. & Sperber, E. F. (1990). Substantia nigra-mediated control of generalized seizures. In *Generalized Epilepsy: Neurobiological Approaches*, ed. M. Avoli, P. Gloor, G. Kostopoulos & R. Naquet, pp. 355–67. Boston, MA: Birkhäuser.

Moshé, S. L., Sperber, E. F., Brown, L. L., Tempel, A. & Wurpel, J. N. D. (1988). Experimental epilepsy: developmental aspects. *Cleveland Clinic Journal of Medicine*, **56** (Suppl. 1), S92–S99.

Moshé, S. L., Sperber, E. F., Haas, K., Xu, S. & Shinnar, S. (1992). Effects of the maturational process on epileptogenesis. In *Epilepsy Surgery*, ed. H. Lüders, pp. 741–8. New York: Raven Press.

Mueller, A. L., Taube, J. S. & Schwartzkroin, P. A. (1984). Development of hyperpolarizing inhibitory postsynaptic potentials and hyperpolarizing response to gamma-aminobutyric acid in rabbit hippocampus studied in vitro. *Journal of Neuroscience*, **4**: 860–7.

Muller, D., Oliver, M. & Lynch, G. (1989). Developmental changes in synaptic properties in hippocampus of neonatal rats. *Developmental Brain Research*, **49**: 105–14.

Nadler, J. V. (1981). Minireview: kainic acid as a tool for the study of temporal lobe epilepsy. *Life Sciences*, **29**: 2031–42.

Nadler, J. V., Perry, B. W. & Cotman, C. W. (1978). Intraventricular kainic acid preferentially destroys hippocampal pyramidal cells. *Nature*, **271**: 676–7.

Nakanishi, H., Kita, H. & Kitai, S. T. (1987). Intracellular study of rat substantia nigra pars reticulata neurons in an in vitro slice preparation: electrical membrane properties and response characteristics to subthalamic stimulation. *Brain Research*, **437**: 45–55.

Nevander, G., Ingvar, M., Auer, R. & Siesjø, B. K. (1985). Status epilepticus in well-oxygenated rats causes neuronal necrosis. *Annals of Neurology*, **19**: 281–90.

Nitecka, L., Tremblay, E., Charton, G., Bouillot, J. P., Berger, M. L. & Ben-Ari, Y. (1984). Maturation of kainic acid seizure–brain damage syndrome in the rat. II. Histopathological sequelae. *Neuroscience*, **13**: 1073–94.

Okada, R., Moshé, S. L. & Albala, B. J. (1984). Infantile status epilepticus and future seizure susceptibility in the rat. *Developmental Brain Research*, **15**: 177–83.

Okada, R., Moshé, S. L., Wong, B. Y., Sperber, E. & Zhao, D. (1986). Age-related substantia nigra-mediated seizure facilitation. *Experimental Neurology*, **93**, 180–7.

Peterson, S. L., Albertson, T. E. & Stark, L. G. (1981). Intertrial intervals and kindled seizures. *Experimental Neurology*, **71**: 144–53.

Pinel, J. P. J. & Rovner, L. I. (1978). Experimental epileptogenesis: kindling induced epilepsy in rats. *Experimental Neurology*, **58**: 190–202.

Prichard, J. W., Gallagher, B. B. & Glaser, G. H. (1969). Experimental seizure threshold testing with flurothyl. *Journal of Pharmacology and Experimental Therapeutics*, **166**: 170–8.

Purpura, D. P. (1969). Stability and seizure susceptibility of immature brain. In *Basic Mechanisms of the Epilepsies*, ed. H. H. Jasper, A. A. Ward & A. J. Pope, pp. 481–505. Boston, MA: Little, Brown.

Purpura, D. P. (1972). Ontogenetic models in studies of cortical seizure activitics. In *Experimental Models of Epilepsy*, ed. D. P. Purpura, J. K. Penry, D. Tower, D. M. Woodbury & R. Walter, pp. 531–6. New York: Raven Press.

Purpura, D. P. & Housepian, E. M. (1961). Morphological and physiological properties of chronically isolated immature neocortex. *Experimental Neurology*, **4**, 377–401.

Racine, R. J. (1978). Kindling: the first decade. *Neurosurgery*, **3**: 234–52.

Racine, R. J., Okujava, V. & Senera, C. (1972). Modification of seizure activity by electrical stimulation. III. Mechanisms. *Electroencephalography and Clinical Neurophysiology*, **32**: 295–9.

Racine, R. J., Rose, P. A. & Burnham, W. M. (1977). Afterdischarge thresholds and kindling rates in dorsal and ventral hippocampus and dentate gyrus. *Canadian Journal of Neurological Sciences*, **4**: 273–8.

Racine, R. J. (1972a). Modification of seizure activity by electrical stimulation. II. Motor seizures. *Electroencephalography and Clinical Neurophysiology*, **32**: 281–94.

Racine, R. J. (1972b). Modification of seizure activity by electrical stimulation. I. After-discharge threshold. *Electroencephalography and Clinical Neurophysiology*, **32**: 269–79.

Racine, R. J., Burnham, W. M., Gartner, J. G. & Levitan, D. (1973). Rates of motor seizure development of rats subjected to electrical brain stimulation: strain and interstimulation interval effects. *Electroencephalography and Clinical Neurophysiology*, **35**: 553–6.

Remler, M. P. & Marcussen, W. H. (1984). The blood–brain barrier lesion and the systemic convulsant model of epilepsy. *Epilepsia*, **25**: 574–7.

Scharfman, H. E. & Sarvey, J. M. (1987). Responses to GABA recorded from identified rat visual cortical neurons. *Neuroscience*, **23**: 407–22.

Scheibel, M. E., Crandall, P. H. & Scheibel, A. B. (1974). The hippocampal–dentate complex in temporal lobe epilepsy. *Epilepsia*, **15**: 55–80.

Scherer-Singler, U. & McGeer, E. G. (1979). Distribution and persistence of kainic acid in brain. *Life Sciences*, **24**: 1015–22.

Schwartzkroin, P. A. (1982). Development of rabbit hippocampus: physiology. *Developmental Brain Research*, **2**: 469–86.

Schwartzkroin, P. A. (1984). Epileptogenesis in the immature CNS. In *Electrophysiology of Epilepsy*, ed. P. A. Schwartzkroin & H. V. Wheal, pp. 389–412. New York: Academic Press.

Schwartzkroin, P. A., Kunkel, D. D. & Mathers, L. H. (1982). Development of rabbit hippocampus: anatomy. *Developmental Brain Research*, **2**: 453–68.

Schwob, J. E., Fuller, T., Price, J. L. & Olney, J. W. (1980). Widespread patterns of neuronal damage following systemic or intracerebral injections of kainic acid: a histological study. *Neuroscience*, **5**: 991–1014.

Shouse, M. N., King, A., Langer, J., Vreeken, T., King, K. & Richkind, M. (1990). The ontogeny of feline temporal lobe epilepsy: kindling a spontaneous seizure disorder in kittens. *Brain Research*, **525**: 215–24.

Sperber, E. F., Haas, K., & Moshé, S. L. (1990). Mechanisms of kindling in developing animals. In *Kindling 4*, ed. J. A. Wada, pp. 157–68. New York: Plenum Press.

Sperber, E. F., Haas, K., Stanton, P. K. & Moshé, S. L. (1991). Resistance of the immature hippocampus to seizure-induced synaptic reorganization. *Developmental Brain Research*, **60**: 88–93.

Sperber, E. F. & Moshé, S. L. (1988). Age-related differences in seizure susceptibility to flurothyl. *Developmental Brain Research*, **39**: 295–7.

Sperber, E. F., Wong, B. Y., Wurpel, J. N. D. & Moshé, S. L. (1987). Nigral infusions of muscimol or bicuculline facilitate seizures in developing rats. *Developmental Brain Research*, **37**: 243–50.

Sperber, E. F., Wurpel, J. N. D. & Moshé, S. L. (1989a). Evidence for the involvement of nigral $GABA_B$ receptors in seizures in rat pups. *Developmental Brain Research*, **47**: 143–6.

Sperber, E. F., Wurpel, J. N. D., Zhao, D. Y. & Moshé, S. L. (1989b). Evidence for the involvement of nigral $GABA_A$ receptors in seizures of adult rats. *Brain Research*, **480**: 378–82.

Stanton, P. K., Bommer, M., Heinemann, U. & Noble, E. P. (1987a). In utero alcohol exposure impairs postnatal development of hippocampal noradrenergic sensitivity. *Neuroscience Research Communications*, **1**: 145–52.

Stanton, P. K., Jones, R. S. G., Mody, I. & Heinemann, U. (1987b). Epileptiform activity induced by lowering extracellular $[Mg^{2+}]$ in combined hippocampal–entorhinal cortex slices: modulation by receptors for norepinephrine and *N*-methyl-D-aspartate. *Epilepsy Research*, **1**: 53–62.

Stanton, P. K. & Sejnowski, T. J. (1989). Associative long-term depression in the hippocampus induced by hebbian covariance. *Nature*, **339**: 215–18.

Sutula, T., Cascino, G., Cavazos, J. & Parada, I. (1989). Mossy fiber synaptic reorganization in the epileptic human temporal lobe. *Annals of Neurology*, **26**: 321–30.

Sutula, T., Xiao-Xian, H., Cavazos, J. & Scott, G. (1988). Synaptic reorganization in the hippocampus induced by abnormal functional activity. *Science*, **239**: 1147–50.

Swann, J. W. & Brady, R. J. (1984). Penicillin-induced epileptogenesis in immature rats CA3 hippocampal cells. *Developmental Brain Research*, **12**: 243–54.

Swann, J. W., Brady, R. J., Smith, K. L. & Pierson, M. G. (1988). Synaptic mechanisms of focal epileptogenesis in the immature nervous system. In *Disorders of the Developing Nervous System: Changing View on their Origins, Diagnoses, and Treatment*, ed. J. W. Swann & A. Messer, pp. 19–49. New York: Alan R. Liss.

Swann, J. W., Smith, K. L. & Brady, R. (1990). Neural networks and synaptic transmissions in immature hippocampus. In *Excitatory Amino Acids and Neuronal Plasticity. Advances in Experimental Medicine and Biology*, ed. Y. Ben-Ari, pp. 161–71. New York: Plenum Press.

Thompson, J. L., Stafstrom, C. E., Chronopoulos, A., Thurber, S. & Holmes, G. L. (1990). Effect of age on seizure susceptibility following kainic acid induced status epilepticus. *Epilepsia*, **32**: 634.

Truitt, E. B., Ebesberg, E. M. & Ling, A. S. G. (1960). Measurement of brain excitability by use of hexaflurodiethyl ether (Indoclon). *Journal of Pharmacology and Experimental Therapeutics*, **129**: 445–53.

Vernadakis, A. & Woodbury, D. M. (1969). The developing animal as a model. *Epilepsia*, **10**: 163–78.

Wada, J. A. (1986). Preface. *Kindling 3*, ed. J. A. Wada, pp. v–vi. New York: Raven Press.

Wada, J. A. & Osawa, T. (1976). Spontaneous recurrent seizure state induced by daily electric amygdaloid stimulation in Senegalese baboons. *Neurology*, **26**: 273–86.

Wada, J. A., Sato, M. & Corcoran, M. E. (1974). Persistent seizure susceptibility and recurrent spontaneous seizures in kindled cats. *Epilepsia*, **15**: 465–78.

Wasterlain, C. G. & Dwyer, B. E. (1983). Brain metabolism during prolonged seizures in neonates. In *Status Epilepticus*, ed. A. V. Delgado-Escueta, C. G. Waterlain, D. M. Treiman & R. J. Porter, pp. 241–60. New York: Raven Press.

Williams, J. T., North, R. A., Shefner, A., Nishi, S. & Egan, T. M. (1984). Membrane properties of rat locus coeruleus neurons. *Neuroscience*, **13**: 137–56.

Wong, B. Y. & Moshé, S. L. (1987). Mutual interactions between repeated flurothyl convulsions and electrical kindling. *Epilepsy Research*, **1**: 159–64.

Woodbury, D. M. (1980). Convulsant drugs; mechanism of drug action. *Advances of Neurology*, **27**: 249–303.

Woodbury, L. A. (1977). Incidence and prevalence of seizure disorders including the epilepsies in the USA. A review and analysis of the literature. In *Plan for the Nationwide Action on Epilepsy*, Vol. 4, pp. 24–77. DHEW Publication no. (NIH) 78–276.

Wurpel, J. N. D., Sperber, E. F. & Moshé, S. L. (1990). Baclofen inhibits amygdala kindling in immature rats. *Epilepsy Research*, **5**: 1–7.

Wurpel, J. N. D., Tempel, A., Sperber, E. F. & Moshé, S. L. (1988). Age-related changes of muscimol binding in the substantia nigra. *Developmental Brain Research*, **43**: 305–7.

Zaide, J. (1974). Differences between Tryon Bright and Dull rats in seizure activity evoked by amygdala stimulation. *Physiology and Behavior*, **12**: 527–34.

Section 2
Features of the epileptogenic brain

Introduction

The chapters in the previous section focused on questions that could be addressed with intact-animal models of the epilepsies. In Section 2, there is an attempt to deal more directly with mechanisms that may underlie epileptiform properties that give rise to, for example, the models discussed in Section 1. Two broad issues are addressed by the chapters in this section. (a) What are the features of epileptic brain, i.e. what are the mechanisms that might underlie the production of abnormal epileptiform activities? (b) What do we know about the processes of epileptogenesis itself, i.e., how does the epileptic brain become epileptic? Most of our understanding of underlying mechanisms is derived from studies on brain (or brain tissue) that is already epileptic; we have a still minimal insight into the process of epileptogenesis. Studies have begun to establish which brain attributes are correlated with epileptiform (i.e., abnormal) activities and are providing clues about the consequences of seizure activity; however, initial 'cause' is, in most cases (and models) still to be determined. It has been tricky to separate the underlying features of epileptogenesis from characteristics of the already epileptic tissue.

Many of these studies on the mechanisms of epileptiform activities have been carried out in neocortical and hippocampal preparations – perhaps not surprisingly, since a majority of the epilepsies (at least in mature brain) appear to be associated with cortical sites of abnormality (i.e., cortical foci). Given this association of 'cortex' and epilepsy, it is tempting to speculate about unique properties of cortical tissue that preferentially support the abnormal hyperexcitability and synchrony associated with epileptiform discharge. For example, do cortical neurons have intrinsic properties that are likely to result in hyperexcitable discharge if unchecked? Is the laminar structure of cortical tissue advantageous for the development of hyperexcitability and/or synchrony? Are the local circuitries of cortical tissues, especially the inhibitory circuitries, particularly vulnerable to damage? Are the modulatory influences to cortical regions – e.g., as exerted by the brainstem projection systems – so delicately balanced that small perturbations will lead to abnormal electrical activity? Is it simply coincidence that cortical regions – brain areas clearly involved in normal learning and experience-dependent behaviors, and thus presumably 'plastic' – are the most common sites of epileptic abnormalities? One could argue that mechanisms that are responsible for the plasticities underlying normal behaviors are just those features that support epileptiform activities. Is there really something special about these cortical structures that has encouraged the development of so many models – or is it simply convenient to carry out experiments on a focus in the neocortex and/or hippocampus?

Despite the emphasis on the cortex and hippocampus, other regions of the brain have been implicated in various forms of seizure activity. For example, thalamo-cortical circuitry has long been implicated in spike-and-wave discharge (Gloor & Fariello, 1988), and modern studies have supported the critical role played by thalamic neurons in such activity (McCormick & Pape, 1990). The thalamic relay cells display a marked 'transient' low threshold calcium conductance (Coulter *et al.*, 1989) that, when interposed in a circuit with cells of the reticular nucleus of the thalamus (which also show pronounced, albeit somewhat different transient calcium currents; Coulter *et al.*, 1989), provides a unique system for generating rhythmic excitatory bursts and intervening hyperpolarizing waves (Steriade & Deschenes, 1984). Recent studies have implicated also such unlikely structures as the inferior colliculus and deep regions of the superior colliculus as important in the generation of some types of seizure activity (Snyder-Keller & Pierson, 1992). This region of the brainstem appears to be involved in mediating audiogenic seizures, quite common in a number of genetically seizure prone animal models. Finally, it is now clear that brainstem structures, alone and/or in combination with the spinal cord, may be critical in generating some behavioral seizure types that have been largely ignored because of the apparent absence of correlated electroencephalographic (EEG) activity (Mizrahi & Kellaway, 1987). With recent emphasis on seizure activities in the immature brain (see Swann *et al.*, Chapter 6, this volume), the various forms of 'epilepsy' characteristic of the immature nervous system have come under greater scrutiny. Some immature forms of 'seizure' do not show typical EEG activation patterns (Chugani *et al.*, 1992); they may be modeled by such experimental 'brainstem preparations'.

Given the great diversity of seizure types and models, there should be no problem in determining what factors are characteristic of epileptic brain, what changes must occur to produce the abnormal epileptiform phenomena. But it is just this variety and wealth of information that make the task so difficult. We have still to solve apparently elementary issues in our approach to these issues. Simplistically stated, we must still answer the question 'What are we looking for?' One strategy is to start with phenomenological characteristics of human epileptic brain, and attempt to mimic those features in an animal model in which the underlying mechanisms could be investigated in a controlled experimental manner. As is reviewed here by Avoli (Chapter 7), a number of laboratories have now looked at tissue from human epileptic neocortex and hippocampus. The in-vitro technique used for such studies gives the investigator significant technical power – particularly to look at (or for) unique properties of the epileptic neuron. However, the in-vitro preparation complicates, as well as simplifies, some aspects of the investigation. Particularly when examining human tissue, investigators have had considerable difficulty in defining what they are studying in excised pieces of brain (Schwartzkroin & Knowles, 1984). In a sense, the human brain slice itself becomes an in-vitro model system. How do we determine, in these preparations, the site of the epileptic focus? Can we be sure whether the piece of tissue under investigation is really epileptic, only partially epileptic, or normal; that is, what defines the epileptogenicity? Also problematic in studying human epileptic tissue, in vivo or in vitro, is whether the tissue features under investigation are critical to the generation of seizure activity, or simply the result of a long history of seizures in the patient. Since seizures may result in positive feedback by which seizure activity is maintained, the effects of seizures may also be causal.

A striking feature of epileptic tissue in many experimental models is how 'ordinary' it may appear (Schwartzkroin & Prince, 1978). As seen electrophysiologically, cellular activities in tissue slices of neocortex and hippocampus from human epileptic patients are generally quite normal. In some sense, this observation parallels the older data obtained from acute animal models, in which the electrophysiological properties (intrinsic and synaptic) of cells in an epileptic focus were found to be indistinguishable from control cells except during the period of burst discharge or seizures (Schwartzkroin & Wyler, 1980). Given the relatively normal appearance of cells in slices from epileptic brain, we might conclude that we have somehow missed the critical site, the epileptic focus. Alternatively, it may be that the epileptic activity generated in vivo is a function of larger pieces of tissue (a critical mass), or requires more extensive circuitry than is provided by the in-vitro preparation. Perhaps the epileptiform features of this tissue may be so subtle as to be 'invisible' in qualitative evaluations. That a quantitative, cell-by-cell analysis of these tissues might be necessary is suggested by a number of the recent studies of animal models (see Connors and Amitai, Chapter 12, this volume). The basis for such careful, quantitative studies in epileptic tissue must be a clear definition of the normal characteristics of the various elements in the brain region in question – the intrinsic properties of neurons and the nature of synaptic connections (including the various transmitters and receptor subtypes). It is critical to learn as much as possible about the *normal* brain in order to understand what is different about the epileptic tissue. In such detailed investigations, the techniques of molecular neurobiology will undoubtedly prove to be of crucial significance. These techniques should allow us to quantify receptors and their subunits, identify cells of various types on the basis of neurochemical markers, determine changes in protein as a function of activity, etc. Indeed, much of the impetus for studying immediate early genes (Morgan *et al.*, 1987) comes from this need to *quantify* the features of the normal tissue, so as to evaluate better the abnormalities in epileptic brain.

At present, it is still not clear what tissue features are likely to be altered in epileptic tissue. Given that structural damage is a generally consistent marker of epileptic brain (Babb *et al.*, 1984; Meldrum & Corsellis, 1984; de Lanerolle *et al.*, 1989), one strategy for gaining insights into functional epileptic abnormalities has been to correlate electrophysiological (Schwartzkroin & Knowles, 1984), pharmacological (Hosford *et al.*, 1991), and biochemical (Robbins *et al.*, 1991; Sherwin *et al.*, 1991) changes with the morphological abnormalities. In doing so, however, investigators must face the issue of whether damage is itself a cause of seizure activity, or simply another variable associated with seizures. That question has become a major controversy in the field. Since epilepsy has been historically defined as an electrical (i.e., EEG) disorder, another strategy for defining the epileptogenic region has been to focus on electrophysiological criteria. Other approaches, based on other measures (e.g. positron emission tomography identification of metabolic abnormality; Engel *et al.*, 1982), have been basically correlative. Since it is so difficult to identify a given feature of tissue that defines it as epileptic, investigators have begun to put together constellations of abnormalities which constitute various epileptic syndromes.

In recent years, the structure of choice for much of the in-vitro work on defining underlying mechanisms of the epilepsies has been the hippocampus. The selection of the hippocampus is due partly to its widespread implication in clinical seizure activity; mesial temporal abnormalities are perhaps the most common and difficult to treat of the epilepsies. The hippocampus also gives the investigator a relatively tractable preparation on which to work; it has a relatively simple organization (Andersen *et al.*, 1971) (compared to neocortex, for example), there is an extensive background of normative data, and the structure has a low threshold for inducing abnormal activities (Dichter & Spencer, 1969). While much of the work has focused on the CA1 and CA3 pyramidal cell regions of hippocampus (Wong & Traub, 1983; see also Chapter 6, this volume) there is accumulating evidence that other cortical regions associated with the hippocampus (the pyriform and entorhinal cortices and associated cell regions) may be even more 'sensitive' than is the hippocampus to epileptogenic insult (Piredda & Gale, 1985; McIntyre & Wong, 1986). A number of studies have also implicated the dentate gyrus (and associated dentate hilus) as a critical gateway to hippocampal epileptogenicity (Stringer & Lothman, 1989). As discussed by Lothman and colleagues (see Chapter 10, this volume), the dentate gyrus (DG) appears to be an essential element in the development of full limbic seizure activity. This emphasis on granule cells is somewhat surprising, given that past studies of the hippocampus have shown the granule cells to be relatively unexcitable (Schwartzkroin & Prince, 1978). Even under conditions in which the pyramidal cells produce epileptiform bursting, the DG is often quiet (the granule cells have very negative resting potentials and high thresholds for discharge). However, Lothman *et al.* suggest that in order for hyperexcitability to spread from the entorhinal cortex through the hippocampus (and presumably through the rest of the brain), there is a requirement that the DG shows a high degree of activation ('maximal dentate activation'). The implication of this finding is that the dentate region normally acts as a brake, to retard recruitment of the rather excitable pyramidal regions of the hippocampus and parahippocampal structures.

Because of their intrinsic cell properties (Brown *et al.*, 1981), and the strong inhibitory circuitry of the dentate region (Sloviter, 1991*a*), the granule cells tend to be relatively inactive under normal conditions. Indeed, when we consider the massive effect that granule cell discharge has on its target neurons in the hilus and CA3 pyramidal region (each granule cell action potential produces a large unitary excitatory postsynaptic potential that is often of sufficient magnitude to trigger an action potential in the postsynaptic neuron) it makes sense that granule cells are difficult to activate. The combination of high activation threshold and large postsynaptic effect leads to a high signal-to-noise for the specific region of the DG that receives a suprathreshold level of excitation. Under conditions of epileptiform activity, however, that selectivity of activation appears to be lost. Large areas of the DG become activated, with subsequent excitation of the rest of the hippocampus.

A number of models have now focused on this role of the DG in the control of excitability. The studies of Lothman and colleagues have shown that with sufficient activation of the DG, it is possible to produce hyperexcitability that is reflected in behavioral seizures in the intact animal. Sloviter (1987) has found that repetitive activation of the DG leads to selective damage, not among the granule cells, but in the dentate hilus. The onset of this lesion effect is correlated with the emergence of granule cell hyperexcitability, and is associated with reduction in functional inhibition of the DG (Sloviter, 1991b). A number of specific cell types in the dentate hilus have been identified that are particularly vulnerable to electrical stimulation (Scharfman & Schwartzkroin, 1990) (and to other types of 'trauma'), and that are lost routinely from the epileptic brain. It has been hypothesized that loss of these vulnerable cells results in the loss of inhibitory controls on the granule cells, with resulting dentate region hyperexcitability (Sloviter, 1987). However, we could argue the other way as well – that hyperexcitability in the granule cells leads to damage of the hilar neurons. If such were the case, this cell loss might not be causally related to the induction of hyperexcitability, but to its result. What is somewhat puzzling in the dentate hilar models, and is reflected also in the intraventricular kainic acid model of hippocampal hyperexcitability (see Franck, Chapter 8, this volume), is that the inhibitory machinery is not obviously disrupted by protocols that give rise to cell loss and development of hyperexcitability (Franck *et al.*, 1988; Sloviter, 1991b). In the kainic acid model (where CA1 inhibition is reduced when CA3 neurons are injured by kainic acid application), GABAergic neurons are present and active, and the CA1 pyramidal cells remain sensitive to GABA (γ-aminobutyric acid) application. One explanation for this apparently paradoxical observation is that the dentate hilar neurons – or the CA3 pyramidal cells – normally provide a tonic excitation to inhibitory elements. Loss of this tonic inhibition releases the granule cells (or CA1 pyramidal cells) from that inhibition, so that they become more excitable in response to stimulation.

Another possible explanation for this increased dentate region excitability is that, with the loss of hilar cells, there is an induction of sprouting. That is, collaterals of granule cell axons – the mossy fibers – turn back to synapse on to themselves, creating a positive feedback loop. Evidence for such sprouting, derived from models involving hilar neuron loss as well as from human epileptic hippocampus, has been presented by a number of laboratories (e.g., Sutula *et al.*, 1989; Babb *et al.*, 1991; see also Sutula, Chapter 9, this volume). In studying this phenomenon, it is critical to determine which effects are primary and which are secondary – which are causally related to the hyperexcitability, and which are a result of it. Using a variety of epileptogenic procedures (including kindling and kainic acid administration), Sutala *et al.* and Babb *et al.* have shown that there is an increase in Timm staining in the inner molecular layer of the granule cell dendrites, reflecting the development of mossy fiber collaterals into that region of the DG. This recurrent excitatory pathway *could* support hyperexcitability. However, the time course of the sprouting phenomenon appears to be very much longer than that for the development of hyperexcitability in the surviving cells (Sloviter, 1992). In initial phases of epileptiform activity, it would appear that there is no abnormal recurrent circuitry to explain the epileptiform bursting activity. Indeed, it could be argued that the degree of hyperexcitability that is monitored following the epileptogenic treatment actually decreases during the time that sprouting occurs into the inner molecular layer of the DG. These data are consistent with the idea that the recurrent mossy fiber collaterals make preferential connections with inhibitory interneurons (Schwartzkroin *et al.*, 1990). It is interesting to note, too, that in tissue from these animal models, and even in tissue from human epileptic hippocampus, hyperexcitability can be induced with minimal blockade of inhibition (Cronin *et al.*, 1992; Chagnac-Amitai & Connors, 1989; see also Chapter 8, this volume). When inhibition is reduced, however, epileptiform discharge does occur – perhaps supported by mossy fiber recurrent excitatory collateralization.

References

Andersen, P., Bliss, T. V. P. & Skrede, K. K. (1971). Lamellar organization of hippocampal excitatory pathways. *Experimental Brain Research*, **13**: 222–38.

Babb, T. L., Brown, W. J., Pretorius, J., Davenport, C. J., Lieb, J. P. & Crandall, P. H. (1984). Temporal lobe volumetric cell densities in temporal lobe epilepsy. *Epilepsia*, **25**: 729–40.

Babb, T. L., Kupfer, W. R., Pretorius, J. K., Crandall, P. H. & Levesque, M. F. (1991). Synaptic reorganization by mossy fibers in human epileptic fascia dentata. *Neuroscience*, **42**: 351–63.

Brown, T. H., Fricke, R. A. & Perkel, D. H. (1981). Passive electrical constants in three classes of hippocampal neurons. *Journal of Neurophysiology*, **46**: 812–27.

Chagnac-Amitai, Y. & Connors, B. W. (1989). Horizontal spread of synchronized activity in neocortex and its control by GABA-mediated inhibition. *Journal of Neurophysiology*, **61**: 747–58.

Chugani, H. T., Shewmon, D. A., Sankar, R., Chen, B. C. & Phelps, M. E. (1992). Infantile spasms. II. Lenticular nuclei and brain stem activation on positron emission tomography. *Annals of Neurology*, **31**: 212–19.

Coulter, D. A., Huguenard, J. R. & Prince, D. A. (1989). Calcium currents in rat thalamocortical relay neurones: kinetic properties of the transient, low-threshold current. *Journal of Physiology*, **414**: 587–604.

Cronin, J., Obenaus, A., Houser, C. & Dudek, F. E. (1992). Electrophysiology of dentate granule cells after kainate-induced synaptic reorganization of the mossy fibers. *Brain Research*, **573**: 305–10.

de Lanerolle, N. C., Kim, J. H., Robbins, R. J. & Spencer, D. D. (1989). Hippocampal interneuron loss and plasticity in human temporal lobe epilepsy. *Brain Research*, **495**: 387–95.

Dichter, M. A. & Spencer, W. A. (1969). Penicillin induced interictal discharges from cat hippocampus. I. Characteristics and topographical features. *Journal of Neurophysiology*, **32**: 649–62.

Engel, J., Jr, Kuhl, D. E., Phelps, M. E. & Mazziotta, J. C. (1982). Interictal cerebral glucose metabolism in partial epilepsy and its relation to EEG changes. *Annals of Neurology*, **12**: 510–17.

Franck, J. E., Kunkel, D. D., Baskin, D. G. & Schwartzkroin, P. A. (1988). Inhibition of kainate-lesioned hyperexcitable hippocampi: physiologic, autoradiographic, and immunocytochemical observations. *Journal of Neuroscience*, **8**: 1991–2002.

Gloor, P. & Fariello, R. G. (1988). Generalized epilepsy: some of its cellular mechanisms differ from those of focal epilepsy. *Trends in Neuroscience*, **11**: 63–8.

Hosford, D. A., Crain, B. J., Cao, Z., Bonhaus, D. W., Friedman, A. H., Okazaki, M. M., Nadler, J. V. & McNamara, J. O. (1991). Increased AMPA-sensitive quisqualate receptor binding and reduced NMDA receptor binding in epileptic human hippocampus. *Journal of Neuroscience*, **11**: 428–34.

McCormick, D. A. & Pape, H.-C. (1990). Properties of a hyperpolarization-activated cation current and its role in rhythmic oscillation in thalamic relay neurons. *Journal of Physiology*, **431**: 291–318.

McIntyre, D. C. & Wong, R. K. S. (1986). Cellular and synaptic properties of amygdala-kindled pyriform cortex in vitro. *Journal of Neurophysiology*, **55**: 1295–307.

Meldrum, B. S. & Corsellis, J. A. N. (1984). Epilepsy. In *Greenfield's Neuropathology*, ed. J. A. N. Corsellis & L. W. Duchen, pp. 921–50. New York: John Wiley.

Mizrahi, E. M. & Kellaway, P. (1987). Characterization and classification of neonatal seizures. *Neurology*, **31**: 1837–44.

Morgan, J. I., Cohen, D. R., Hempstead, J. L. & Curran, T. (1987). Mapping patterns of c-*fos* expression in the CNS after seizure. *Science*, **238**: 797–9.

Piredda, S. & Gale, K. (1985). A crucial epileptogenic site in the deep prepiriform cortex. *Nature*, **317**: 623–5.

Robbins, R. J., Brines, M. L., Kim, J. H., Adrian, T., de Lanerolle, N., Welsh, S. & Spencer, D. D. (1991). A selective loss of somatostatin in the hippocampus of patients with temporal lobe epilepsy. *Annals of Neurology*, **29**: 325–32.

Scharfman, H. E. & Schwartzkroin, P. A. (1990). Responses of cells of the rat fascia dentata to prolonged stimulation of the perforant path: sensitivity of hilar cells and changes in granule cell excitability. *Neuroscience*, **35**: 491–504.

Schwartzkroin, P. A. & Knowles, W. D. (1984). Intracellular study of human epileptic cortex: in vitro maintenance of epileptiform activity? *Science*, **223**: 709–12.

Schwartzkroin, P. A. & Prince, D. A. (1978). Cellular and field potential properties of epileptogenic hippocampal slices. *Brain Research*, **147**: 117–30.

Schwartzkroin, P. A., Scharfman, H. E. & Sloviter, R. S. (1990). Similarities in circuitry between Ammon's horn and dentate gyrus: local interactions and parallel processing. In *Understanding the Brain through the Hippocampus*, ed. J. Storm-Mathisen, J. Zimmer & O. P. Ottersen, pp. 269–86. Amsterdam: Elsevier.

Schwartzkroin, P. A. & Wyler, A. R. (1980). Mechanisms underlying epileptiform burst discharge. *Annals of Neurology*, **7**: 95–107.

Sherwin, A. L., Vernet, O., Dubeau, F. & Olivier, A. (1991). Biochemical markers of excitability in human neocortex. *Canadian Journal of Neurological Science*, **18**: 640–4.

Sloviter, R. S. (1987). Decreased hippocampal inhibition and a selective loss of interneurons in experimental epilepsy. *Science*, **235**: 73–6.

Sloviter, R. S. (1991*a*). Feedforward and feedback inhibition of hippocampal principal cell activity evoked by perforant path stimulation: GABA-mediated mechanisms that regulate excitability *in vivo*. *Hippocampus*, **1**: 31–40.

Sloviter, R. S. (1991*b*). Permanently altered hippocampal structure, excitability, and inhibition after experimental status epilepticus in the rat: the 'dormant basket cell' hypothesis and its possible relevance to temporal lobe epilepsy. *Hippocampus*, **1**: 41–66.

Sloviter, R. S. (1992). Possible functional consequences of synaptic reorganization in the dentate gyrus of kainate-treated rats. *Neuroscience Letters*, **137**: 91–6.

Snyder-Keller, A. M. & Pierson, M. G. (1992). Audiogenic seizures induce c-*fos* in a model of developmental epilepsy. *Neuroscience Letters*, **135**: 108–12.

Steriade, M. & Deschenes, M. (1984). The thalamus as a neuronal oscillator. *Brain Research Review*, **8**: 1–63.

Stringer, J. L. & Lothman, E. W. (1989). Maximal dentate gyrus activation. Characteristics and alterations after repeated seizures. *Journal of Neurophysiology*, **62**: 136–43.

Sutula, T., Cascino, G., Cavazos, J., Parada, I. & Ramirez, L. (1989). Mossy fiber synaptic reorganization in the epileptic human temporal lobe. *Annals of Neurology*, **26**: 321–30.

Wong, R. K. S. & Traub, R. D. (1983). Synchronized burst discharge in disinhibited hippocampal slice. I. Initiation in CA2–CA3 regions. *Journal of Neurophysiology*, **49**: 442–58.

6

Neurophysiological studies of alterations in seizure susceptibility during brain development

JOHN W. SWANN, KAREN L. SMITH,
ROBERT J. BRADY and MARTHA G. PIERSON

Introduction

The basic processes responsible for seizures in an infant's brain are likely to be quite different from those in the central nervous system of an adult. The nervous system of a neonate is so unlike its mature counterpart in basic anatomical, physiological, and metabolic properties that it is obvious even to the most casual observer that many critical issues of pediatric epileptology are different from those addressed by epileptologists concerned with controlling seizures in adults.

Many epileptic syndromes in children occur during restricted phases of nervous system development (O'Donohoue, 1985; Aicardi, 1986; Tharp, 1987); the phrase 'age-specific epilepsies', therefore, has been used to describe these disorders. For example, infantile spasms are observed usually between three months and three years of age (Lacy & Penry, 1976). Thereafter this seizure disorder may evolve into a different form of epilepsy only later to emerge as another syndrome in adulthood. At each stage the seizures are likely to differ not only in their clinical and electrographic features but also in their response to medication (Freeman, 1987).

On the other hand some seizure disorders of childhood have clear counterparts in adulthood. Simple and complex partial seizures are examples (Holmes, 1986, 1987; Wyllie et al., 1989). Characteristically, these seizures arise from localized regions of the brain and are often referred to in experimental epilepsy research as focal seizures. In both infants and adults, the complex partial epilepsies commonly originate from the temporal lobe. However, the clinical manifestations of the seizure episodes in infants are so different from those seen in older children and adults that they are often difficult to classify as the same disorder (Duchowny, 1987). Early-onset complex partial seizures can be very severe. Seizure durations have been reported to be significantly longer, and convulsive movements more extensive, than in older children (Yamamoto *et al.*, 1987). Moreover, complex partial seizures in young children are reported to be particularly difficult to control with anticonvulsant therapy. The likelihood for remission from these seizures has been reported to be low (Kotagal *et al.*, 1987). In recent years, therefore, increasing numbers of children with early-onset complex partial epilepsy have become candidates for epilepsy surgery (Wyllie & Lüders, 1989).

Clinical observations suggest also that even under normal conditions the immature nervous system has an unusually high susceptibility for seizures. For instance, it is well known that children have a marked propensity for seizures induced by high fever (Aicardi, 1986). Before the age of three years, febrile seizures can be quite prolonged. Thus, developmental alterations in the epileptogenicity of brain are likely to be important substrates in determining the types and severity of seizure manifested as a child matures.

Numerous experimental studies in animal models also support the view that during critical stages in development the brain is unusually prone to seizures. In large part these studies have relied on the use of in-vivo models (e.g., responses to convulsant drugs (Vernadakis & Woodbury, 1969), kindling (Moshé, 1987)). However, the advent of in-vitro neurophysiological techniques has offered an unprecedented opportunity to study age-dependent alterations in the physiological mechanisms of epileptogenesis during brain maturation (Swann *et al.*, 1988, 1990). In the following, we review progress made so far in unraveling the cellular mechanisms that contribute to age-specific epileptogenesis. Promising avenues for future study are discussed.

Critical developmental periods of enhanced seizure susceptibility – expression in vitro

When slices of hippocampus, neocortex or entorhinal cortex are taken from rats during the second or third postnatal weeks and subjected to various in-vitro conditions that increase neuronal excitability, the tissue shows a marked capacity to generate electrographic seizures (Schwartzkroin, 1982; Swann & Brady, 1984; Hablitz, 1987). Usually under these conditions slices from mature rats generate only brief interictal events. Extracellular field recordings from the CA3 pyramidal cell body layer, shown in Fig. 6.1, illustrate the observed differences in epileptiform events. In this instance, slices taken from a postnatal day 11 and from a

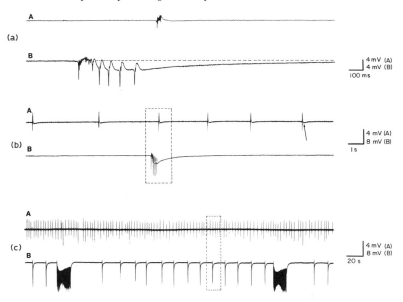

Fig. 6.1. Comparison of spontaneous epileptiform discharges recorded extracellularly from the CA3 cell body layer of a slice taken from a mature rat (traces A) and an 11 day old rat pup (traces B). Slices were bathed in 1.7 mM penicillin. Recordings at three different time bases are shown. Events in (a) are shown framed by dashed line in (b). Likewise, traces in (b) are those framed in (c). (Reproduced, with permission, from Swann & Brady, 1984.)

mature rat (seven to eight weeks) were exposed to the $GABA_A$ receptor antagonist penicillin. Such differences in discharging can also be produced by bath application of other $GABA_A$ receptor antagonists (Brady & Swann, 1984) as well as 4-aminopyridine, tetraethylammonium (Chesnut & Swann, 1988), or by elevating extracellular K^+ to 8–10 mM (Swann *et al.*, 1988). The electrographic seizures recorded at these ages are often 30 s in duration.

On the other hand, during the first postnatal week slices from hippocampus and neocortex are much less likely to undergo electrographic seizures and, when they do occur, neural discharges are far less synchronized than those recorded from tissue taken from rats one week later in life (Swann & Brady, 1984; Kriegstein *et al.*, 1987). Similar observations were made by Purpura and colleagues more than 20 years ago during in-vivo neurophysiological studies of the ontogeny of seizures in kittens (Purpura, 1964, 1969). At that time the immature cortex was considered to be electrophysiologically 'stable'; that is, the kitten neocortex was thought to be less susceptible to seizures than is the cortex of mature animals (see also Prince & Gutnick, 1972). Such findings were thought to be a good reflection of a number of clinical observations in newborn infants. For instance, electroencephalographic correlates of neonatal seizures are frequently dissociated from clinical events. Furthermore, seizures are often restricted to a focus and do not generalize (Mizrahi, 1987). The apparent stability of the neonatal cortex was thought to be the product of several neurophysiological factors, the first of which was the relative inexcitability of immature neurons. It was found that, early in life, action potentials were broader and repetitive discharging was less frequent than in neurons from older animals. Another important contributing factor was thought to be a precocious development of synaptic inhibition relative to that of the emergence of synaptic excitation. Inhibitory postsynaptic potentials (IPSPs) were reported to be large and unusually prolonged early in life.

More recent in-vitro intracellular recordings from brain slices have been consistent with many of these earlier findings. In slices taken from animals during the first postnatal week, intracellular recordings have shown that action potentials routinely have slower rising and falling phases (Schwartzkroin, 1982; Kriegstein *et al.*, 1987). Recent whole-cell patch-clamp and single channel recordings from acutely dissociated neocortical neurons suggest that the age-dependent differences in action potential rate of rise is related to an increase with age in density of Na^+ action potential channels in the neuronal membrane (Huguenard *et al.*, 1988).

In-vitro studies have also supported the earlier in-vivo observations that postsynaptic potentials can be extremely prolonged during the neonatal period. Slow excitatory postsynaptic potentials (EPSPs) as well as IPSPs have been reported in recordings from both the neocortex and the hippocampus. For instance, from studies of neocortical slices, Kriegstein *et al.* (1987) reported the average duration of EPSPs elicited by stimulation of subcortical white matter to be three times longer on days 3–7 than on days 7–14. Similarly, Schwartzkroin (1982) reported ESPSs in CA1 pyramidal cells to be 150–200 ms in duration on days 1–6. While we might speculate on the possible mechanisms underlying EPSP prolongation in early postnatal life, the physiological processes responsible for these slow synaptic events remain unknown.

One possible reason for the prolonged EPSPs recorded in slices taken from neonatal animals is that at these ages IPSPs are not generated in response to electrical stimulation (Schwartzkroin & Altschuler, 1977; Schwartzkroin, 1982; Dunwiddie, 1981; Harris & Teyler, 1983; Kriegstein *et al.*, 1987; Swann *et al.*, 1989). Indeed, this appears to be the clearest distinction that can be made between the early in-vivo reports and in-vitro studies of the immature neocortex and hippocampus.

A late onset of GABAergic inhibition in some cells of the immature nervous system could play a potentially important role in its enhanced susceptibility for seizures. Mature CA1 hippocampal pyramidal cells respond to orthodromic stimulation by producing a brief EPSP followed by a prolonged IPSP. The latter potential has been shown to consist of two separate IPSPs (Alger & Nicoll, 1982*b*). The first component is produced by a $GABA_A$ postsynaptic receptor that is coupled to a Cl^- iontophore. Typically it is 50–100 ms in duration. Blockade of this receptor leads to epileptiform discharging. The second component is more prolonged and can be greater than 1 s in duration. It is thought that this potential is produced by a $GABA_B$ postsynaptic receptor (Newberry & Nicoll, 1984). Activation of this receptor results in an increase in membrane conductance to K^+.

In contrast to recordings from mature animals are responses of both hippocampal CA1 pyramidal cells and neocortical neurons to orthodromic stimulation during the first week of life. Figure 6.2 illustrates recordings from the hippocampus. On postnatal days 4–6, neurons undergo a prolonged depolarization instead of a brief depolarization, followed by a prolonged afterhyperpolarization. During the second postnatal week, intermediate hyperpolarizing events are recorded. By day 30, responses similar to those recorded in mature animals occur in all cells. Clearly in these two brain regions the GABAergic inhibitory system is not fully functional at very early ages. Because the prolonged depolarizing responses result in action potentials, these events must be considered to be excitatory in nature. Many other studies also suggest that neural systems that use GABA as a neurotransmitter are not fully developed at birth. For instance, biochemical markers for GABAergic synaptic transmission are present in only low amounts early in postnatal brain development (see e.g. Swann *et al.*, 1989). Anatomical studies have shown that during the first postnatal week the number of synapses that are immunoreactive for GABA, or the GABA synthetic enzyme glutamic acid decarboxylase (GAD), is fewer than in adults (Kunkel *et al.*, 1986; Seress & Ribak, 1988). Nonetheless, some GABA-containing neurons and synapses are present at these early ages. Thus, several attempts have been made to understand why GABAergic IPSPs are not recorded. Indeed, ultrastructural studies have shown that GAD- and GABA-containing presynaptic nerve terminals present early in life are quite different from their mature counterparts. Nerve terminals have been reported to be small

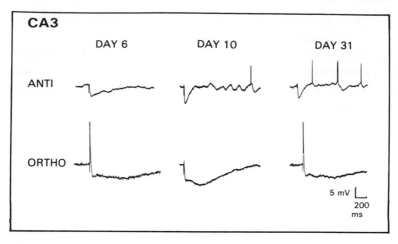

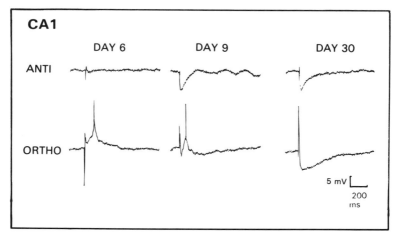

Fig. 6.2. Comparison of responses of rat CA3 and CA1 hippocampal neurons to orthodromic (ORTHO) and antidromic (ANTI) stimulation at three difference postnatal ages. Responses were elicited in each cell by two independently manipulated stimulating electrodes. Responses are averages of three events. Spontaneous action potentials were thus reduced in amplitude. (Reproduced, with permission, from Swann *et al.*, 1989.)

and to contain few synaptic vesicles (Seress *et al.*, 1989). Other synaptic specializations have also been reported not to be fully formed or to be absent (Schwartzkroin & Kunkel, 1982; Kunkel *et al.*, 1986).

In hippocampal area CA1 this immaturity of synaptic specializations coincides with the presence of depolarizing instead of hyperpolarizing responses to exogenously applied GABA (Mueller *et al.*, 1983, 1984). When GABA is applied to the cell bodies of mature pyramidal cells, a hyperpolarization of the membrane potential is observed when cells are near the resting membrane potential. Application of GABA to dendrites, however, produces a depolarization. Alger & Nicoll (1982*a*) were the first to suggest that the receptors mediating GABA depolarizations of mature dendrites were actually extrasynaptic in distribution. Accordingly, Mueller *et al.* (1984) suggested that depolarizing responses produced by application of GABA to the soma in the developing hippocampus may also be mediated by extrasynaptic receptors. This notion is in keeping with the ultrastructural observations mentioned above that showed that GABA synapses are not fully developed on the soma of immature CA1 pyramidal neurons (Kunkel *et al.*, 1986).

More recently, Ben-Ari *et al.* (1989) suggested that, prior to day 5, rat CA3 hippocampal neurons also depolarize in response to bath-applied GABA. However, studies of local application of GABA to the soma of these cells were not reported. Thus, the contribution made by dendritic depolarizing receptors to these responses is unclear. However, at the same time Ben-Ari *et al.* reported that synchronized 'giant' depolarizing synaptic potentials occur both spontaneously and in response to electrical stimulation. Surprisingly these synaptic events were blocked by the GABA antagonist bicuculline. These authors suggest also that the GABA system is therefore not fully developed during the first week of life and that it is predominantly excitatory in its influence.

In sharp contrast to the foregoing observations are results of intracellular recordings made on days 5 and 6 in rat CA3 hippocampal neurons (Swann *et al.*, 1989; see also Schwartzkroin, 1982). As discussed above, in-vivo recordings from kittens suggest that synaptic inhibition is well developed early in life (Purpura, 1969). In contrast to recordings in CA1, by day 5, large GABA-mediated IPSPs can be recorded in the CA3 of rat. Figure 6.2 shows an example of such recordings. Analysis of such IPSPs elicited by antidromic stimulation, revealed that on days 5 and 6 they are quite large and unusually prolonged. IPSP conductances (G_{IPSP}) are, on average, no different from those recorded at 30 days of age. Indeed, during the second week of life G_{IPSP} was three- to four-fold larger than that recorded during week 1 or in one month old animals. The reason for this difference is unexplained at this time. However, it is clear that such IPSPs can, in fact, play a major role in preventing hippocampal seizures. Indeed, as discussed earlier, if $GABA_A$ receptor antagonists are applied to slices during the second and third postnatal week, electrographic seizures are recorded (Brady & Swann, 1984; Swann & Brady, 1984; Fig. 6.1).

Electrographic seizures in immature nervous tissue in vitro

Electrographic seizures recorded in vitro are highly reminiscent of events observed in in-vivo models of epilepsy. The intracellular events that accompany these discharges were first described in penicillin foci in cat neocortex (Matsumoto & Ajmone-Marsan, 1964). As shown in Fig. 6.3, the events consist of an initial paroxysmal depolarization shift followed by rhythmic repetitive intense depolarizations. Dual intracellular recordings suggest that all of these intracellular events occur simultaneously in virtually every neuron of the CA3 subfield. This synchronized discharging of the entire CA3 neuronal population is reflected in large coincident field potentials (Fig. 6.3, trace C).

During the course of an electrographic seizure, individual neurons also undergo a sustained depolarization. The rhythmic and more intense depolarizations of an ictal episode ride the envelope of the slow depolarization. Coincident with the sustained depolarization is a prolonged negative field potential, which is largest in records taken from the basilar dendritic layer. In extracellular recordings from the apical dendritic layer, the slow event has the opposite polarity.

Support for the contention that the electrographic events recorded in slices are very similar to those occurring during seizures in vivo comes

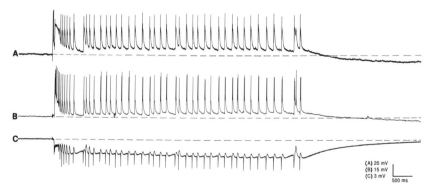

Fig. 6.3. An electrographic seizure recorded in a hippocampal slice taken from a one week old rat pup and exposed to 1.7 mM penicillin. Simultaneous intracellular recordings from two neurons are shown in traces A and B. Trace C is an extracellular field from the proximal portion of the basilar dendritic layer. Notice the remarkable degree of synchronization of neuronal discharging during the course of this ictal episode.

from studies using the anticonvulsant carbamazepine (Smith & Swann, 1987). Carbamazepine is often the drug of first choice in treating children suffering from complex partial epilepsy (Holmes, 1987). However, when treated with carbamazepine, patients with this disorder may become seizure-free while the frequency of interictal discharging actually remains unchanged or may even increase. Carbamazepine, when bath-applied to slices of rat immature hippocampus, has remarkably similar effects. Electrographic seizures are eliminated while interictal discharging continues unabated. The effects of this anticonvulsant in these in-vitro studies are highly dose-dependent and are observed at therapeutic concentrations (Smith & Swann, 1987).

It is also important to note that the electrographic seizures have been shown to arise from the CA3 subfield itself and do not depend on activity in dentate granule cells or CA1 pyramidal cells for their occurrence (Chesnut & Swann, 1988). This has been most clearly demonstrated when segments of rat CA3 subfield are microdissected from slices and placed in an experimental chamber (Swann *et al.*, 1987). Exposure of such minislices to convulsant drugs produced discharges that are structurally very similar to, if not identical with, those recorded in intact slices (see e.g., Fig. 6.7). Studies of these minislices have shown that there is a minimum number of cells required for the elaboration of electrographic seizures. More than 90% of slices that measure 500 μm along the pyramidal cell body layer can generate afterdischarges. Slices larger than this routinely produce electrographic seizures. By comparison, slices measuring approximately 300 μm along the cell body layer generate only burst discharges.

Electrographic seizure discharges are recognized to be an extremely complex physiological phenomenon. One obstacle in the analysis of after discharges is that, while these events are in many ways structurally stereotyped, close examination reveals that from event to event the synchronized events of the afterdischarge have quite different latencies. As an example, in Fig. 6.4(a) the latency of the fifth discharge of the afterdischarge (see arrow) varied from 312 to 420 ms ($\bar{x} = 371 \pm 19$ ms). Thus, one of the simplest signal-processing tools, signal averaging, cannot be applied to these events. Indeed, when conventional averaging is employed, signals such as those shown in Fig. 6.4(a), traces B are obtained in which the afterdischarges are virtually eliminated. However, when procedures referred to as continuous latency corrected averaging (CLCA) are used, a relatively noise-free signal can be obtained (Fig. 6.4(a) traces C). Such procedures have been used routinely in the analysis of evoked potentials in clinical neurophysiology (McGillem & Aunon, 1987), but

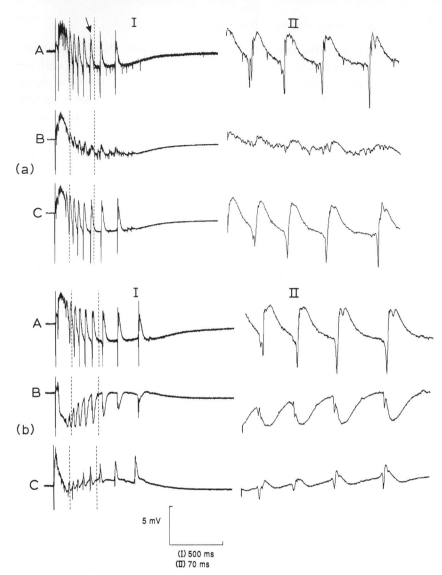

5 mV

(I) 500 ms
(II) 70 ms

Fig. 6.4. Continuous latency corrected averaging (CLCA) of brief synchronized afterdischarges recorded in an immature rat hippocampal slice exposed to penicillin. Events were triggered by orthodromic stimuli. (a) Trace A shows a single response to orthodromic stimulation. Arrow denotes the fifth discharge in the afterdischarge. Trace B is an average of 13 events using conventional averaging techniques. Trace C shows an average of the same event using CLCA techniques. The portion of traces in panel I framed by dashed lines are expanded in panel II. (b) Alterations in the structure of afterdischarges at three different locations in the CA3 hippocampal laminae. Traces A are CLCA averages of five signals from the cell body layer, while B and C are signals recorded at two locations in the apical dendritic layer. As in (a), dashed lines in panel I denote segments of the signal expanded in time in panel II.

they have yet to be applied to studies of complex population discharges recorded in vitro. However, with the availability of powerful desktop computers and workstations, high performance computing is now a reality for neurophysiology laboratories. Computationally intense analyses such as that shown in Fig. 6.4 can now be performed on-line and exploited to permit a better understanding of how seizures are produced. For example, the use of CLCA of laminar field potential and current source density analysis (see Swann *et al.*, 1986*a*) might be used to establish where in a given brain region a certain component of an afterdischarge originates. Figure 6.4(b) shows CLCA traces that indicate how dramatically field potential recordings of an afterdischarge can vary within the CA3 hippocampal laminae. Recordings in trace A were taken from the cell body layer, while B and C were obtained from two different sites in the apical dendritic layer. Being able to pinpoint the sites of generation of the various components of the synchronized discharges of electrographic seizures as well as other more persistent currents (see the Sustained depolarization of electrographic seizures, below) will further understanding of the mechanisms that underlie these events. Ultimately, such procedures are likely to assist significantly in understanding the pronounced susceptibility of the immature nervous system for seizures.

The ionic microenvironment and electrographic seizures in developing brain

The role that extracellular K^+ plays in the generation of seizures in the mature nervous system has long been the subject of much discussion (Dichter *et al.*, 1972; Prince, 1978; Somjen, 1979). Ion-sensitive microelectrode studies have shown that following an interictal spike in the neocortex or hippocampus, extracellular K^+ increases substantially. Recovery to baseline levels can take many seconds. Thus, it has been shown that repeated interictal spiking within short time intervals can lead to temporal summation of extracellular K^+ accumulation. This increase in $[K^+]_o$ is thought to lead to membrane depolarization and thereby to increased neuronal excitability. Thus changes in $[K^+]_o$ have been proposed to play a role in the transition from an interictal state to ictal episodes. Indeed, recent studies in the CA1 subfield in in-vitro slices from adult rats have provided data that most clearly support such a mechanism for the initiation of electrographic seizures (Traynelis & Dingledine, 1988).

Ion-sensitive microelectrode recordings made in vivo (Mutani *et al.*, 1974) and more recent studies in in-vitro preparations suggest that

J. W. Swann et al.

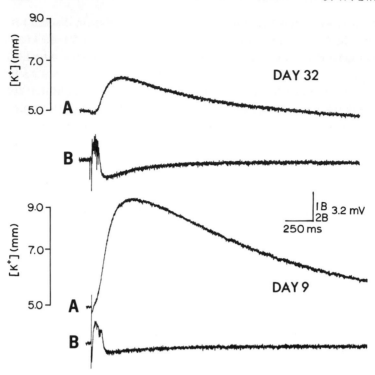

Fig. 6.5. Comparison of changes in extracellular $[K^+]$ (traces A) associated with interictal spike discharging recorded in the rat hippocampal CA3 subfield on postnatal days 32 and 9. Recordings were made in the stratum oriens at the edge of the cell body layer. Extracellular fields recorded simultaneously are shown in traces B. (Reproduced, with permission, from Swann *et al.*, 1986*b*.)

activity-dependent alterations in $[K^+]_o$ change as the brain matures. In the optic nerve, hippocampus and neocortex, unusually large increases in $[K^+]_o$ occur during critical periods in development (Connors *et al.*, 1982; Swann *et al.*, 1986*b*; Hablitz & Heinemann, 1987). Figure 6.5, for instance, compares extracellular $[K^+]$ changes accompanying interictal spikes in the hippocampal CA3 subfield on postnatal days 9 and 32. The changes in K^+ are dramatically larger in immature hippocampus, being on average four- to five-fold greater during the second postnatal week than in one month old rats. Notably, the ages when changes in $[K^+]_o$ are unusually large coincide with the period during which the immature hippocampus demonstrates its marked propensity for seizures. In addition, in the mature brain $[K^+]_o$ has traditionally been shown to reach a 'ceiling level' during the course of an electrographic seizure: typically 10–12 mм. Only under extremely abnormal conditions, such as hypoxia, are these levels exceeded. By contrast, the K^+ ceiling level of the immature nervous system is much higher than that of mature brain, with values of 14–20 mM being observed routinely.

Activity-dependent increases in extracellular $[K^+]$ likely play a role in the propensity of the immature nervous system for seizures. However, like regional variations in the formation of the inhibitory synapses, the relative importance of extracellular $[K^+]$ in epileptogenesis also appears to vary regionally in the developing CNS. Haglund *et al.* (1985) have shown that Na^+–K^+-ATPase activity, an important process regulating $[K^+]_o$, is low in CA1 compared to its activity in area CA3 in one week old rabbit hippocampus. This difference appears to play an important role in the propensity of the CA1 subfield for bouts of spreading depression (Haglund & Schwartzkroin, 1990). The CA3 subfield is relatively resistant to such episodes. Thus, while the late onset of Na^+–K^+ pump activity in the CA1 subfield appears to support a hyperexcitable state during early stages in development, the presence of this K^+ clearing mechanism in the CA3 subfield may prevent similar degrees of extreme excitability in that location. These findings are in keeping with earlier suggestions that the mechanisms for clearing K^+ from the extracellular space are present in the rat hippocampal CA3 subfield at one week of age (Swann *et al.*, 1986*b*, 1988).

Because changes in extracellular K^+ in the CA3 subfield and neocortex follow, and do not precede, the onset of epileptiform events (Swann *et al.*, 1986*b*; Hablitz & Heineman, 1987), it appears that they are in large measure products of the synchronized discharges. Nonetheless, since K^+ changes are so large, they are likely to make an important contribution to the course of seizure events that occur in these regions during development. This notion is supported by studies in which electrographic seizures were produced by increasing the K^+ content of slice perfusate from 5 to 8–10 mM (Swann *et al.*, 1988). This is also true even in studies of isolated segments of immature hippocampal CA3 subfield. Under these conditions the CA3 subfield of mature hippocampus produces only interictal discharges.

In keeping with the idea that epileptiform discharges are generated at discrete sites within the hippocampal and neocortical laminae are observations that changes in extracellular $[K^+]$ accompanying such discharges can also be localized to discrete sites in these regions. Figure 6.6(a) shows a laminar profile of changes in $[K^+]_o$ that accompany interictal discharges in the CA3 subfield of a slice taken from a one month old rat. Changes in $[K^+]_o$ were largest at sites in the proximal portion of the basilar

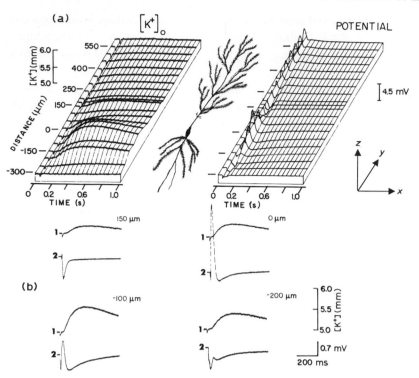

Fig. 6.6. (a) Variations in extracellular $[K^+]$ associated with interictal spike discharging and recorded in the CA3 subfield of a slice taken from a one month old rat. Top left and top right panels are three-dimensional representations of the laminar distribution of changes in extracellular $[K^+]$ and simultaneously recorded extracellular field potentials, respectively. As indicated, x-axis is time. The y-axis is distance from the center of the cell body layer. The center of the stratum pyramidale was assigned a value of 0 μm. Negative values for distances were assigned to positions in the stratum oriens. The z-axis is the amplitude of changes in $[K^+]_o$ and field potentials. Recordings are aligned with a tracing of a CA3 hippocampal pyramidal neuron. (b) Recordings extracted from the three-dimensional plots at the positions indicated and drawn at a faster time base.

dendritic layer. K^+ signals were also recorded in the central portions of both dendritic fields. Field potentials recorded simultaneously are shown on the right. The latter recordings show that negative field potentials are produced in association with K^+ signals.

Changes in $[K^+]_o$ occur at discrete sites in both immature neocortical and hippocampal laminae. There is no measurable difference between the sites in the immature and mature CA3 hippocampal subfields where changes in K^+ are recorded. However, at each of these sites the accumulation of K^+ extracellularly is larger in the immature hippocampus than in the mature hippocampus (Swann *et al.*, 1986*b*). As in mature hippocampus, the site where change of extracellular K^+ is the largest is in the proximal portion of the basilar dendritic layer. The reason why K^+ changes are unusually large at this site could be that a mechanism responsible for K^+ release from neurons is unusually well developed early in life and that this process is non-uniformly distributed in dendrites. Thus, attention has turned to the mechanisms of K^+ release present early in postnatal life.

The sustained depolarization of electrographic seizures

As illustrated in Fig. 6.3, during the course of an electrographic seizure individual neurons are tonically depolarized. In the light of the above discussion, it is noteworthy that a slow negative field potential (Fig. 6.3 trace C) is simultaneously generated in the proximal portion of the basilar dendritic layer, where changes in $[K^+]_o$ are so large.

It is generally agreed that, when an excitatory current like that underlying an EPSP occurs in a neuron, it generates a negativity in the extracellular space while producing a depolarization intracellularly. Thus, it is possible that the basilar dendritic slow potential (of extracellular recordings) and sustained depolarization (of intracellular recordings) are products of the same excitatory process. Other studies have shown that excitatory amino acid antagonists are quite effective in selectively blocking electrographic seizures (Brady & Swann, 1986, 1988). Only at higher concentrations are these same compounds capable of suppressing the paroxysmal depolarization shift. These two observations led us to wonder if the excitatory amino acid antagonists might be blocking synaptically mediated events in the basilar dendrites that were responsible for the genesis of the sustained depolarization and, ultimately, electrographic seizures. In fact, results from experiments in which excitatory amino acid antagonists were applied locally to the basilar dendrites support this contention (Swann *et al.*, 1987). These experiments were performed in small minislices of the CA3 subfield (measuring 500–600 µm along the cell body layer). Figure 6.7 shows recordings of spontaneous epileptiform events that cycle between brief and prolonged seizure discharges. A single droplet of CNQX (6-cyano-7-nitroquinoxaline-2,3-dione) in the basilar dendritic layer abolished the afterdischarges. By contrast, an identical application to the apical dendrites was ineffective in suppressing afterdischarges. These results suggest that an excitatory amino acid synaptic

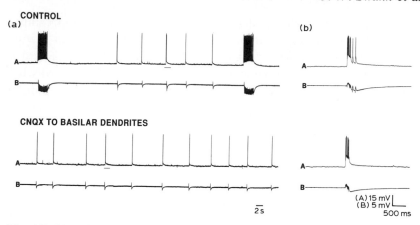

Fig. 6.7. (a) and (b) The effects of local application of a droplet of CNQX (100 µM) to the basilar dendritic layer on epileptiform discharges recorded in a minislice of the hippocampal CA3 subfield taken from a one week old rat pup. The minislices measured 500–600 µm along the cell body layer. Simultaneous intracellular (traces A) and extracellular (traces B) field recordings of spontaneous activity produced by bath-applied penicillin are shown. Recordings underlined in (a) are shown at a faster time base in (b).

event occurring in the basilar dendritic layer plays a key role in afterdischarge generation.

When experiments in larger minislices (700–1000 µm along the cell body layer) were performed, however, somewhat different results were obtained. Local application of kynurenic acid or CNQX to the basilar dendrites near the recording electrode did not block the electrographic seizure but did eliminate the sustained depolarization (Fig. 6.8). This observation indicates that the sustained depolarization is a process separate from that of the repetitive rhythmic depolarizations characterizing ictal episodes. These results also led to the question 'Does the sustained depolarization play a role in afterdischarge generation?' More specifically, we wondered whether the sustained depolarization could be the basilar dendritic synaptic event implicated in seizure generation by the results shown in Fig. 6.7. Further studies have suggested that it is. The following scheme reconciles the contrasting results obtained in different-sized minislices in Figs. 6.7 and 6.8 and supports this conclusion. When CNQX is applied locally to the basilar dendrites in large minislices, the sustained depolarization is suppressed (Fig. 6.8). In these larger minislices, however, there are cells remote from the application site that are not affected by the drug. These cells would be expected to continue

CONTROL   CNQX

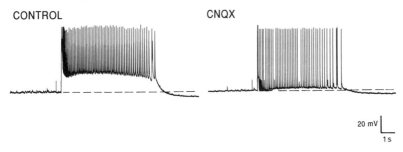

20 mV
1 s

Fig. 6.8. Local application of CNQX (100 μM) to the basilar dendrites in a minislice measuring approximately 900 μm along the cell body layer results in the blockade of the sustained depolarization. Intracellular recordings of an electrographic seizure produced by bath application of penicillin are shown. CNQX was applied by pressure injection from a micropipette. The volume of solution injected was between 5 and 10 nl.

to undergo a sustained depolarization. This population of 'remote' cells might be considered to be seizure 'generator' cells (see Sawa *et al.*, 1968). The generator cells, via recurrent excitatory synapses, would be able to generate epileptiform discharges independently (see Miles & Wong, 1987; Swann *et al.*, 1987). Thus when such a seizure event occurs, the participating cells, through axon collaterals (see Fig. 6.9), would activate the apical dendrites of cells whose basilar dendrites have been treated with CNQX. The latter neurons could under these circumstances be considered to be follower cells. By this scheme every synchronized discharge of the generator cells could result in a discharge in the follower population. The discharge seen in the right-hand panel of Fig. 6.8 would be generated in such a manner.

Results of numerous experiments support this scheme and imply therefore that the occurrence of a sustained depolarization is required in a critical minimum number of cells for seizure generation to occur. The implications of these studies are likely to be far reaching. These data suggest that the sustained depolarization is a single process that plays a pivotal role in seizure generation in the developing hippocampus. This process is mediated by excitatory amino acid synaptic transmission and is restricted to discrete sites on the basilar dendrites of hippocampal pyramidal cells. Moreover, since the ion channel associated with each class of excitatory amino acid receptor is permeable to K^+, it is possible that the unusually large $[K^+]_o$ changes recorded in the CA3 hippocampal basilar dendritic field are, at least in part, a product of excitatory amino acid synaptic transmission. Indeed, glutamate, when applied

CELL I   CELL II

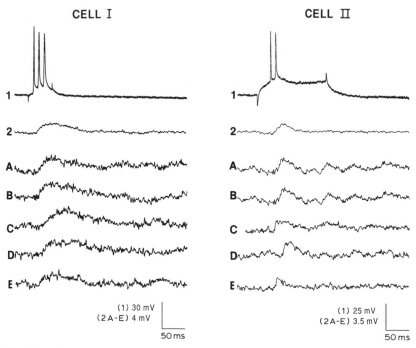

Fig. 6.9. Dual intracellular recordings of polysynaptic EPSPs recorded in a mutually excitatory pair of hippocampal neurons in a minislice taken from a one week old rat pup. IPSPs were blocked with penicillin. Traces 1 show action potentials produced by a brief depolarizing pulse of current injected intracellularly. Traces 2 are averaged ($n = 12$, cross-correlation variable latency averaging techniques were employed) EPSPs recorded in the other cell of the pair. Individual representative responses are shown in traces A–E. Action potentials in cell I produced a prolonged polysynaptically mediated EPSP in cell II. The EPSP produced in cell I by discharging in cell II was shorter in duration.

iontophoretically to the proximal portions of the basilar dendrites, produces large increases in $[K^+]_o$ in the immature hippocampus (Swann *et al.*, 1988).

The supernumerary synapse hypothesis of seizure susceptibility

Results from studies in the CA3 hippocampal subfield suggest that excitatory amino acid synaptic transmission plays a critical role in the propensity of the immature hippocampus for seizures. Could it be that recurrent excitatory synaptic connectivity is unusually well developed in immature hippocampus and responsible not only for the large changes in

$[K^+]_o$ (see discussion above) but also for the propensity to generate the sustained depolarization, and thus seizures? This appears to be the most parsimonious explanation for all our observations. Indeed, taken together, the results are fully consistent with a single unifying hypothesis that during early postnatal life there is a transient overproduction of recurrent excitatory synaptic contacts among CA3 hippocampal neurons (see also Swann *et al.*, 1988, 1990). Moreover, it seems likely that excitatory synaptic interactions in the basilar dendritic layer are particularly well represented during the second postnatal week of life in the rat.

It is well known that the ontogeny of neuronal networks in brain extends well into postnatal life (Purves, 1988). Studies of the developing peripheral and central nervous system have demonstrated that after birth there is often an early 'exuberant' projection of axons to their targets (Purves & Lichtman, 1980; Crepel, 1982; Cowan *et al.*, 1984; Easter *et al.*, 1985). In brain, the use of retrograde anatomical markers has shown that early 'aberrant' projections commonly take place. Adult patterns of innervation are achieved only in part by the death of parent neurons. In fact, the pruning of axonal collaterals is now thought to be a major mechanism of neural circuit rearrangement. These notions are supported by quantitative ultrastructural studies that have shown that far more axons are present in fiber tracts (e.g., the corpus callosum) at birth than exist in adulthood (Koppel & Innocenti, 1983). Whether these exuberant projections make synaptic contacts with target cells is generally unknown. However, electron microscopic studies have demonstrated that at early developmental stages there is an overshoot in the density of synapses in cerebral cortex compared to that of mature brain (Huttenlocher *et al.*, 1982; Huttenlocher, 1984; Rakic *et al.*, 1986). In short, it seems likely that these axons contribute to an increased population of synapses in the central nervous system (CNS) early in postnatal life.

Recent neurochemical studies of excitatory amino acid synaptic trans-mission also support the notion that early in postnatal life dramatic rearrangements take place in CNS neuronal circuits. Biochemical markers for synapses that use an excitatory amino acid as their transmitter undergo a transient overproduction early in postnatal life (for a review, see McDonald & Johnston, 1990). Perhaps the most dramatic example of this is the transient expression of quisqualate receptors in the globus pallidus coincident with an increase in high affinity uptake of glutamate into synaptosomes (Greenmyer *et al.*, 1987). In hippocampal studies, several groups have reported transient overshoots in binding sites for excitatory amino acids. In rat, glutamate binding and *N*-methyl-D-aspartate

(NMDA)-sensitive glutamate binding both exceed adult values during the second postnatal week (Baudry *et al.*, 1981; Tremblay *et al.*, 1988; McDonald & Johnston, 1990). For example, NMDA-sensitive ^{3}H-glutamate binding overshoots levels found in mature animals by 50–130% between days 10 and 28. In the CA3 subfield, NMDA receptor binding reaches maximum values by day 10. Similar overshoots in excitatory amino acid receptor binding have been reported in the neocortex. Thus, studies of the neurochemistry of excitatory amino acid receptors in the hippocampus and neocortex support the notion that an increase in network excitability may be mediated at least in part by a transient overproduction of excitatory synapses. Furthermore, results from numerous anatomical studies reviewed above are likewise consistent with the view that developmental alterations of seizure susceptibility may be mediated by age-dependent rearrangements in neuronal circuitry.

In order to test the hypothesis that alterations in recurrent excitatory synaptic transmission play a key role in the propensity of immature hippocampus for seizures, several lines of study have been undertaken. First, a detailed study of the frequency and features of recurrent EPSPs employing dual intracellular recordings have been undertaken in immature hippocampus. Miles & Wong (1987) have shown that, when synaptic inhibition is suppressed in mature hippocampus, pairs of CA3 hippocampal pyramidal cells that were previously not coupled to each other via recurrent excitatory paths become linked via polysynaptic pathways. Their results suggest that inhibitory interneurons prevent the spread of excitation through the local excitatory networks. Thus, to assay the degree of recurrent excitation in immature hippocampus, recordings were performed in the presence of GABA$_A$ antagonists such as penicillin.

The results obtained are consistent with the hypothesis that recurrent excitatory synapses between hippocampal CA3 neurons are unusually well developed early in postnatal life. In nearly 150 paired recordings from one week old rat hippocampus, action potentials in one cell produced EPSPs in the second in 50% of the pairs (Swann & Smith, 1990). Thirty-five per cent of pairs were found to be polysynaptically coupled; 7% were disynaptically coupled; and 4% were monosynaptically coupled to the follower cell. Six per cent of pairs were mutually excitatory via polysynaptic paths. Figure 6.9 shows examples of polysynaptic EPSPs recorded in a pair of CA3 pyramidal cells that were mutually excitatory. Additionally, the EPSPs recorded could be quite large. On average, unitary monosynaptic EPSPs were nearly 3 mV in amplitude. Disynaptic EPSPs demonstrated similar amplitudes. In some instances unitary EPSPs were unusually prolonged (Swann & Smith, 1990).

Preliminary morphological analyses also appear to support these neurophysiological findings. CA3 hippocampal neurons have been filled with the intracellular markers, biocytin (Horikawa & Armstrong, 1988) or horseradish peroxidase via intracellular recording electrodes. During the second postnatal week an extensive arborization of pyramidal cell axons has been observed in both apical and basilar dendritic layers of the CA3 subfield (Deitch *et al.*, 1990; Gomez *et al.*, 1990). Figure 6.10 is a camera lucida drawing of axon collaterals from a single CA3 pyramidal

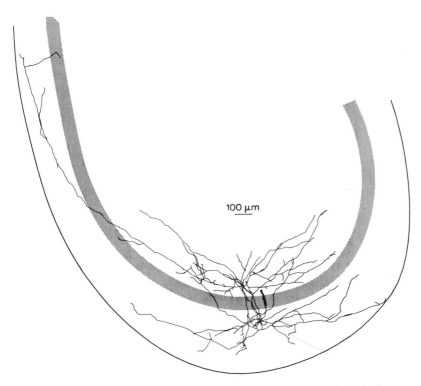

Fig. 6.10. Camera lucida drawing of local axonal arbors of a single rat CA3 hippocampal pyramidal cell injected with biocytin on day 12. The stippled area denotes the pyramidal cell body layer. The cell body of the injected pyramidal cell is included in the drawing but dendrites are not shown. The line that runs parallel to the cell body layer represents the edge of the slice. An extensive axonal arborization occurs in both dendritic layers. A presumed Schaffer collateral projects to the CA1 subfield. In this cell axons were studded with more than 800 varicosities.

cell injected with biocytin on postnatal day 12. These axons are studded
with hundreds of varicosities. Ultrastructural studies have shown the
varicosities to be sites of synaptic contact (Deitch *et al.*, 1991). However,
during the first postnatal week far fewer axons were found to arise from
CA3 pyramidal cells. In mature rats, while axonal arbors still project to
both apical and basilar dendritic layers, the density of axons nonetheless
appears to be less than that observed during the second postnatal week,
especially in the basilar dendritic layer (Gomez *et al.*, 1990). In short, both
physiological and anatomical results obtained so far support the notion
that the enhanced capacity of immature hippocampus for seizures may
be mediated by a transient overproduction of local circuit recurrent
excitatory collaterals.

NMDA receptors and experience-dependent rearrangement of neural circuitry during development

Perhaps the most extensively studied system of synaptic rearrangement
in the developing brain is the postnatal segregation of neural connections
in the visual system (for a review, see Constantine-Paton *et al.*, 1990). In
adult cats and monkeys, projections from the lateral geniculate nucleus
to primary visual cortex (layer IV) are segregated into right- and left-eye
stripes that are referred to as ocular dominance columns. In neonatal
kittens, the terminal fields of lateral geniculate nucleus neurons overlap
widely in visual cortex. However, with maturation a gradual segregation
of terminal fields takes place. This process appears to depend on
competition between converging afferents from each eye. If one eye is
closed during early life the pattern of innervation shifts to one dominated
only by the non-deprived eye. After periods of weeks or months of
monocular deprivation, physiological studies have shown that the deprived
eye loses its ability to drive cortical units, whereas most cortical neurons
respond to the open eye. This phenomenon is referred to as an ocular
dominance shift.

Generally, these observations are explained by the 'correlated activity
rule'. It is thought that coincident activity in afferents leads to the
preferential stabilization of their synaptic connections. By contrast non-
coincidently activated synapses appear to be eliminated. NMDA receptors
have been proposed recently to be the postsynaptic 'detectors' of temporally correlated synaptic events (Cline *et al.*, 1987; Kleinschmidt *et al.*,
1987; Debski *et al.*, 1990). The voltage dependency of its associated ion
channel is thought to provide the NMDA receptor with an ability to detect

the coincident presynaptic activity. According to the prevailing view (Constantine-Paton *et al.*, 1990), one EPSP would depolarize the post-synaptic cell, thereby reducing channel blockade by Mg^{2+}. Upon arrival of a coincident EPSP, a greater depolarization and an increased influx of Ca^{2+} would occur. A cascade of metabolic events initiated by Ca^{2+} is thought to lead to the consolidation of these synapses.

Several laboratories have shown that chronic application of NMDA receptor antagonists, aminophosphonovalerate (APV) or ketamine prevents ocular dominance shifts in monocularly deprived kittens (see e.g., Kleinschmidt *et al.*, 1987; Rauschecher & Hahn, 1987). Similarly, segregation of inputs from normal and supernumerary eyes in tadpoles are blocked by APV and enhanced by NMDA itself (Cline *et al.*, 1987). NMDA receptors appear also to play a key role in the formation of binocular maps in the tectum of *Xenopus* (Scherer & Uden, 1988). In kittens, the critical perod of visual development corresponds to the time at which overshoots in markers for excitatory amino acid synapses take place in the visual cortex (McDonald & Johnston, 1990). At these same times responses by individual cortical neurons to visual inputs as well as local circuit neurons have been reported to be mediated to an unusual extent by NMDA receptors (Tsumoto *et al.*, 1987; Luhmann & Prince, 1990).

Whether NMDA receptors have a role in sculpting the morphology and connectivity of single hippocampal pyramidal cell terminal arbors is unknown. However, it is interesting to consider whether prolonged or abnormal utilization of such excitatory amino acid synapses could lead to their maintenance, thereby resulting in chronically hyperexcitable neural networks, possibly being the cause of epilepsy later in life. Seizures during early childhood may have neurological consequences that are manifested only later in life. For example, numerous epidemiological studies have shown that a number of conditions in childhood are associated with the onset of complex partial seizures many years later (Annegers *et al.*, 1987; Harbord & Manson, 1987; Rocca *et al.*, 1987). One of the most clearly prognostic conditions is severe and complex febrile seizures.

One animal model that may relate NDMA-mediated experience-dependent plasticity to these clinical issues is audiogenic seizure susceptibility. It is well known that NMDA-receptor-mediated synaptic transmission in the inferior colliculus plays a central role in the genesis of these sound-triggered seizures. For instance, the direct infusion of NMDA into normal inferior colliculi can elicit either outright or sound-triggered wild running seizures with subsequent convulsions (Millan *et al.*, 1986). Moreover, infusion of low concentrations of the NMDA antagonists 2-amino-7-phosphonoheptanoic acid (APH) (Jones *et al.*, 1984; McCowen *et al.*, 1987; Faingold *et al.*, 1988) or APV (Faingold *et al.*, 1989) into the colliculi of genetically susceptible rats blocks such seizures. Correspondingly, brain slice studies of inferior colliculus demonstrate that epileptiform activity in bicuculline-disinhibited slices of normal inferior colliculi is blocked by bath application of APV (Pierson *et al.*, 1989). NMDA channel blockers ketamine (Bourne *et al.*, 1983) and MK-801 (Pierson *et al.*, 1990), when systemically administered, also have been found to block audiogenic seizures in susceptible rodents.

However, apart from the direct role played by NMDA receptors in audiogenic seizure initiation, it appears that this receptor may play a role in the induction of seizure susceptibility, possibly by establishing hyperexcitable circuitry in the inferior colliculus. Since 1967, it has been known that auditory deprivation during a critical period of development can induce audiogenic susceptibility in seizure-resistant mouse strains. This deprivation can arise as ear-plugging (Chen *et al.*, 1973; McGinn *et al.*, 1973), the administration of low doses of cochleotoxic drugs (kanamycin) (Norris *et al.*, 1977; Tepper & Schlesinger, 1980; Chen & Aberdeen, 1981; Pierson & Swann, 1988) or may involve simply a single exposure to intense high frequency sound (Henry, 1967; Iturrian & Fink, 1969; Pierson & Swann, 1991). A second common feature of all of the above studies of effective susceptibility-inducing paradigms was that, in order to be effective, the auditory deprivation had to occur during a critical development period. For example, in the Wistar rat it was found that intense noise exposure might induce chronic audiogenic seizure susceptibility if administered between postnatal days 14 and 32, although days 14–16 were found to be the most sensitive developmental period (Pierson & Swann, 1991). Figure 6.11 demonstrates two features of induced audiogenic seizure susceptibility: (a) shows there is a critical developmental period for the induction of such susceptibility; (b) shows that the age when seizures are actually expressed may be quite a bit later than the age (day 14) of the initiation of susceptibility. In short, numerous studies indicate that auditory deprivation during a critical period, a time when the projection from the cochlea to the central auditory pathway is occurring, appears to be the basis of experience-induced audiogenic seizure susceptibility. Age-dependent relationships such as these are reminiscent of the timing of events surrounding the ocular dominance shifts occurring in visual cortex following monocular deprivation in kittens. However, it is

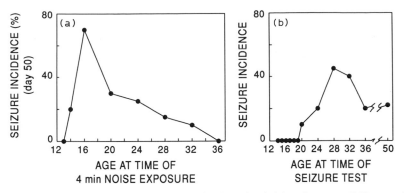

Fig. 6.11. Developmental features of (a) noise-initiated susceptibility and (b) eventual noise-triggered expression of audiogenic seizures. In (a), groups of ten rats at various ages were exposed to a fire alarm bell (128 dBA); susceptibility was tested only on day 50 (adulthood). In (b), all groups of ten rats were exposed to noise on day 14, but each group was tested for susceptibility at only one later age. This strain of rats has never ($n > 4000$) expressed seizure susceptibility without some prior experimental treatment.

only recently that NMDA receptors also were implicated in establishing auditory deprivation-induced audiogenic seizure susceptibility. It was found that acute single administrations of MK-801 or phencyclidine prior to relatively weak noise exposure on day 14 in the rat greatly promotes the development of adult seizure susceptibility (from an expected 20% to an observed 90–100% on day 50) (Pierson *et al.*, 1990). While the mechanism by which short-term NMDA receptor blockade promotes the induction of audiogenic seizure susceptibility remains to be elucidated, these initial findings suggest that the induction process is in some way dependent on a form of use-dependent plasticity mediated by NMDA receptors.

Heterogeneity of neurotransmitter receptors: implications for studies of epileptogenesis throughout development

Application of molecular biological techniques to the study of neuro-transmitter receptors has revolutionized our understanding of both the types and the function of neurotransmitter receptors in the central nervous system. For example, numerous subunits of the GABA$_A$ receptor (Sieghart, 1989) and the nicotinic acetylcholine receptor (Boulter *et al.*, 1987), among others, have been identified. The diversity of the receptors formed in the CNS due to the different possible combinations of the subunits was unsuspected only four or five years ago. Moreover, their differential expression in various brain regions (Wisden, 1989), classes of neurons (Shivers *et al.*, 1989), and at various stages of development are only now becoming appreciated. Such findings will doubtless transform our understanding of seizure generation as a function of brain maturation and how childhood seizure disorders may be controlled or prevented.

Results from several electrophysiological and neurochemical studies predict that a different form of the NMDA receptor exists in the immature hippocampus than has been described previously. For instance, Ben-Ari *et al.* (1988) reported that during the first postnatal week, responses of some CA3 hippocampal neurons to NMDA lack voltage dependency. Nadler *et al.* (1990) have reported that NMDA receptors in CA1 neurons are less sensitive to changes in Mg^{2+} than are the same cells in mature animals. McDonald & Johnston (1990) have shown that, while NMDA receptor binding overshoots during the second and third postnatal weeks of life in rat hippocampus, strychnine-insensitive glycine binding does not overshoot and N-(1-[thienyl]cyclohexypiperidine (TCP) binding does not parallel the ontogeny of either of these two components of the NMDA receptor channel complex. The authors suggested that a differential expression of these receptor components probably occurs during development, the implications being that isoforms of the NMDA receptor exist (see pp. 503–4).

In the CA3 subfield of one week old rat hippocampus, the NMDA receptor demonstrates a voltage dependency similar to that of receptors in mature rats. However, recent studies suggest that this voltage dependency arises in a unique manner in early development. Extracellular Ca^{2+} appears to contribute significantly to the voltage dependency of the NMDA ion channel in these cells (Brady *et al.*, 1990).

In the light of this finding it is interesting that lowering extracellular Ca^{2+} from 2 mM to 1 mM enhances electrographic seizure generation in immature CA3 neurons. This is also an age-dependent phenomenon, since similar changes in Ca^{2+} have no effect on epileptiform discharges in mature CA3 neurons. Importantly, the effect of Ca^{2+} on epileptiform discharging is prevented by bath application of NMDA antagonists. Thus the presence of Ca^{2+}-mediated NMDA voltage dependency may serve to promote seizure susceptibility in the developing hippocampus.

During repetitive discharging in the CNS the concentration of Ca^{2+} in the extracellular space decreases (see e.g., Heinemann *et al.*, 1981). Thus at early ages a positive feedback system could exist at the NMDA receptor in immature CA3 hippocampal neurons. With synaptic activity, extracellular $[Ca^{2+}]$ should decrease and lead to a reduction of $[Ca^{2+}]$ at the mouth of the channel. This, in turn, could lead to enlarged synaptic potentials due to a reduction in voltage dependency, and to further Ca^{2+} entry.

The existence of such a unique postsynaptic mechanism may be particularly important during development when synapse stabilization is activity dependent. In keeping with the temporally correlated activity rule, the presence of Ca^{2+}-mediated NMDA voltage-dependency could cause those processes responsible for synapse stabilization to be more easily induced. In this instance, consolidation of a synapse might not be mediated by the NMDA receptor solely by the temporal summation of EPSPs.

Like alterations in $[K^+]_o$ (see Fig. 6.7) changes in extracellular Ca^{2+} occur at discrete sites in the cortical lamina. However, the ionic changes occur over tens, if not hundreds, of micrometers in a given lamina. Since terminal arbors of individual CA3 pyramidal cells overlap in space, it seems entirely possible that decreases in extracellular $[Ca^{2+}]$ may act as a signal allowing NMDA receptors to detect activity in neighboring pyramidal cells in the local circuit. This could lead to the preferential stabilization of synapses within a region, even if the synapses are on other cells. If indeed such a process were to be at work early in postnatal life, then, during abnormal activity such as that associated with prolonged seizures, any supernumerary excitatory amino acid synapses existing would be more likely to become consolidated. This could lead to a permanent network of hyperexcitable neurons and enhanced seizure susceptibility later in life. Clearly, this discussion is quite speculative. However, the availability of in-vitro neurophysiological techniques should permit the experimental exploration of the role NMDA receptors play not only in seizures early in life but also in conditions that lead to chronic seizure susceptibility and epilepsy upon maturation.

Conclusion

As a first step in understanding the biological origin of childhood seizure disorders, numerous laboratories have explored the basic physiological processes that underlie the enhanced susceptibility of the immature nervous system for seizures. The use of in-vitro neurophysiological techniques has greatly expanded our understanding of how the physiological properties of individual neurons change as the brain matures. As a consequence, the age-specific processes underlying epileptogenesis are now being described. Results suggest that the mechanisms which underlie seizures not only vary with age but differ between given brain regions at the same stage in nervous system development. Perhaps the most dramatic example of this is in hippocampal formation. In the CA1 subfield, a late onset of GABAergic synaptic inhibition and an inability of this tissue to regulate $[K^+]_o$ appear to contribute significantly to the propensity of this area for seizures and for episodes of spreading depression. On the other hand, at the same age area CA3 has well-developed GABA IPSPs and Na^+–K^+ pump activity. However, since this subfield also has a marked propensity for electrographic seizures, some other mechanism must account for it. The most parsimonious explanation for the results obtained thus far in area CA3 is that seizures may in large part be the product of a transient overproduction of local circuit excitatory synapses during this critical stage in development. It is suggested that these local circuit synapses make an important contribution to the genesis of the sustained depolarization of electrographic seizures, which plays a pivotal role in electrographic seizure generation. The sustained depolarization appears to be generated by an excitatory amino acid neurotransmitter.

In recent years the NMDA receptor has been implicated as an important participant in the rearrangement of neural microcircuits that occurs during normal brain development. The voltage dependency of the NMDA channel is thought to provide this receptor channel complex with the ability to detect temporally correlated presynaptic activity. Under conditions of correlated activity, Ca^{2+} entry into post-synaptic cells through this channel is thought to act as a second messenger that initiates synapse consolidation. One important avenue of future study will be in determining whether abnormal neuronal activity, such as that occurring during early-onset seizures, has an effect on synaptic rearrangements that occur during development. Audiogenic seizure susceptibility induced by auditory deprivation early in life may serve as a useful model in this regard.

Several laboratories have recently suggested the NMDA receptor of the immature hippocampus has unique physiological properties that may contribute to the enhanced susceptibility of the immature nervous system for seizures. The reported Ca^{2+}-mediated voltage dependency of the NMDA receptor-linked ionophore in immature CA3 hippocampal pyramidal cells could have important implications for synapse consolidation during normal and abnormal brain development.

Acknowledgments

This work was supported by grants NS18309, NS23071 and the Epilepsy Foundation of America.

References

Aicardi, J. (1986). *Epilepsy in Children*. New York: Raven Press.

Alger, B. E. & Nicoll, R. A. (1982*a*). Pharmacological evidence for two kinds of GABA receptors on rat hippocampal pyramidal cells in vitro. *Journal of Physiology*, **328**: 125–41.

Alger, B. E. & Nicoll, R. A. (1982*b*). Feed forward dendritic inhibition in rat hippocampal pyramidal cells in vitro. *Journal of Neurophysiology*, **328**: 105–23.

Annegers, J. F., Hauser, W. A., Shirts, S. B. & Kurland, L. T. (1987). Factors prognostic of unprovoked seizures after febrile convulsions. *New England Journal of Medicine*, **316**: 493–8.

Baudry, M., Arst, D., Oliver, M. & Lynch, G. (1981). Development of glutamate binding sites and their regulation by calcium in rat hippocampus. *Developmental Brain Research*, **1**: 37–48.

Ben-Ari, Y., Cherubini, E., Corradetti, R. & Galarska, J.-L. (1989). Giant synaptic potentials in immature rat CA3 hippocampal neurones. *Journal of Physiology*, **416**: 303–25.

Ben-Ari, Y., Cherubini, E. & Krnjevic, K. (1988). Changes in voltage dependence of NMDA currents during development. *Neuroscience Letters*, **94**: 88–92.

Boulter, J., Connolly, J., Deneris, E., Goldman, D., Heinemann, S. & Patrick, J. (1987). Functional expression of the two neuronal nicotinic acetylcholine receptors from cDNA clones identified as a gene family. *Proceedings of the National Academy of Sciences, USA*, **84**, 7763–7.

Bourne, W. M., Yang, D. J. & Davisson, J. N. (1983). Effect of ketamine enantiomers on sound-induced convulsions in epilepsy prone rats. *Pharmacological Research Communications*, **15**: 815–24.

Brady, R. J., Smith, K. L. & Swann, J. W. (1990). Calcium modulation of the *N*-methyl-D-aspartate (NMDA) response and electrographic seizures in immature hippocampus. *Neuroscience Letters*, **124**: 92–6.

Brady, R. J. & Swann, J. W. (1984). Postsynaptic actions of baclofen associated with its antagonism of bicuculline-induced epileptogenesis in hippocampus. *Cellular and Molecular Neurobiology*, **4**: 403–8.

Brady, R. J. & Swann, J. W. (1986). Ketamine selectively suppresses synchronized afterdischarges in immature hippocampus. *Neuroscience Letters*, **69**: 143–9.

Brady, R. J. & Swann, J. W. (1988). Suppression of ictal-like activity by kynurenic acid does not correlate with its efficacy as an NMDA receptor antagonist. *Epilepsy Research*, **2**: 232–8.

Chen, C. S. & Aberdeen, G. C. (1981). The sensitive period for induction of susceptibility to audiogenic seizures by kanamycin in mice. *Archives of Otorhinolaryngology*, **232**: 215–20.

Chen, C. S., Gates, G. R. & Bock, G. R. (1973). Effect of priming and tympanic membrane destruction on development of AGS susceptibility in BALB/c mice. *Experimental Neurology*, **39**: 277–84.

Chesnut, T. J. & Swann, J. W. (1988). Epileptiform activity induced by 4-aminopyridine in immature hippocampus. *Epilepsy Research*, **2**: 187–95.

Cline, H. T., Debski, E. A. & Constantine-Paton, M. (1987). N-methyl-D-aspartate receptor antagonists desegregate eye-specific stripes. *Proceedings of the National Academy of Sciences, USA*, **84**: 4342–5.

Connors, B. E., Ransom, B. R., Kunis, D. M. & Gutnick, M. J. (1982). Activity-dependent K$^+$ accumulation in the developing rat optic nerve. *Science*, **216**: 1341–3.

Constantine-Paton, M., Cline, H. T. & Debski, E. (1990). Patterned activity, synaptic convergence, and the NMDA receptor in developing visual pathways. *Annual Review of Neuroscience*, **13**: 129–54.

Cowan, W. M., Fawcett, J. W., O'Leary, D. D. M. & Stanfield, B. B. (1984). Regressive events in neurogenesis. *Science*, **225**: 1258–65.

Crepel, F. (1982). Regression of functional synapses in the immature mammalian cerebellum. *Trends in Neurosciences*, **5**: 266–9.

Debski, E. A., Cline, H. T. & Constantine-Paton, M. (1990). Activity-dependent tuning and the NMDA receptor. *Journal of Neurobiology*, **21**: 18–32.

Deitch, J. S., Smith, K. L., Lee, C. L., Swann, J. W. & Turner, J. N. (1990). Confocal scanning laser microscope images of hippocampal neurons intracellularly labeled with biocytin. *Journal of Neuroscience Methods*, **33**: 61–76.

Deitch, J. S., Smith, K. C., Swann, J. W. & Turner, J. N. (1991). Ultrastructural investigation of neurons identified and localized using the confocal scanning laser microscope. *Journal of Electron Microscopy Technique*, **18**: 82–90.

Dichter, M. A., Herman, C. J., Hofmeier, G. & Seltzer, M. (1972). Silent cells during interictal discharges and seizures in hippocampal penicillin foci: evidence for the role of extracellular K$^+$ in the transition from the interictal state to seizures. *Brain Research*, **48**: 173–83.

Duchowny, M. S. (1987). Complex partial seizures in infancy. *Archives of Neurology*, **44**: 911–14.

Dunwiddie, T. V. (1981). Age-related differences in the in vitro rat hippocampus. Development of inhibition and the effects of hypoxia. *Developmental Neuroscience*, **4**: 165–75.

Easter, S. S., Jr, Purves, D., Rakic, P. & Spitzer, N. C. (1985). The changing view of neural specificity. *Science*, **230**: 507–11.

Faingold, C. L., Hoffmann, W. E. & Caspary, D. M. (1989). Effects of excitant amino acids on acoustic responses of inferior colliculus. *Hearing Research*, **40**: 127–36.

Faingold, C. L., Millan, M. H., Boersma, C. A. & Meldrum, B. S. (1988). Excitant amino acids and audiogenic seizures in the genetically epilepsy prone rat. I. Afferent seizure initiation pathway. *Experimental Neurology*, **99**: 678–86.

Freeman, J. M. (1987). A clinical approach to the child with seizures and epilepsy. *Epilepsia*, **28** (Suppl.): S103–S109.

Gomez, C. M., Rice, F. L., Smith, K. L. & Swann, J. W. (1990). Morphologic studies of CA3 hippocampal neurons in the developing rat. *Society for Neuroscience Abstracts*, **16**: 1290.

Greenmyre, J. T., Penny, J. B., Young, A. B., Hudson, C., Silverstein, F. S. & Johnston, M. V. (1987). Evidence for transient perinatal glutamatergic innervation of globus pallidus. *Journal of Neuroscience*, 7: 1022–30.

Hablitz, J. J. (1987). Spontaneous ictal-like discharges and sustained potential shifts in the developing rat neocortex. *Journal of Neurophysiology*, **58**: 1052–65.

Hablitz, J. J. & Heinemann, U. (1987). Extracellular K^+ and Ca^{2+} changes during epileptiform discharges in the immature rat neocortex. *Developmental Brain Research*, **36**: 299–303.

Haglund, M. M. & Schwartzkroin, P. A. (1990). Role of Na–K pump potassium regulation and ipsps in seizures and spreading depression in immature rabbit hippocampal slices. *Journal of Neurophysiology*, **63**: 225–39.

Haglund, M. M., Stahl, W. L., Kunkel, D. D. & Schwartzkroin, P. A. (1985). Developmental and regional differences in the localization of Na, K-ATPase activity in the rabbit hippocampus. *Brain Research*, **343**: 198–203.

Harbord, M. G. & Manson, J. I. (1987). Temporal lobe epilepsy in childhood: reappraisal of etiology and outcome. *Pediatric Neurology*, **3**: 263–8.

Harris, K. & Teyler, T. J. (1983). Evidence for late development of inhibition in area CA1 of the rat hippocampus. *Brain Research*, **268**: 339–43.

Heinemann, U., Konnerth, A. & Lux, H. D. (1981). Stimulation induced changes in extracellular free calcium in normal cortex and chronic alumina cream foci of cats. *Brain Research*, **213**: 246–50.

Henry, K. R. (1967). Audiogenic seizure susceptibility induced in C57B1/6J mice by prior auditory exposure. *Science*, **158**: 938–40.

Holmes, G. L. (1986). Partial seizures in children. *Pediatrics*, **77**: 725–31.

Holmes, G. L. (1987). Partial seizures. In *Diagnosis and Management of Seizures in Children*, vol. 30 *Major Problems in Clinical Pediatrics*, pp. 125–61. Philadelphia: W. B. Saunders Co.

Horikawa, K. & Armstrong, W. E. (1988). A versatile means of intracellular labeling: injection of biocytin and its detection with avidin conjugates. *Journal of Neuroscience Methods*, **25**: 1–11.

Huguenard, J. R., Hamill, O. P. & Prince, D. A. (1988). Developmental changes in Na^+ conductances in rat neocortical neurons: appearance of a slowly inactivating component. *Journal of Neurophysiology*, **59**: 778–95.

Huttenlocher, P. R. (1984). Synapse elimination and plasticity in developing human cerebral cortex. *American Journal of Mental Deficiency*, **88**: 488–96.

Huttenlocher, P. R., deCourten, C., Garey, L. J. & Van Der Loos, H. (1982). Synaptogenesis in human visual cortex – evidence for synapse elimination during normal development. *Neuroscience Letters*, **33**: 247–52.

Iturrian, W. B. & Fink, G. B. (1969). Influence of age and brief auditory conditioning upon experimental seizures in mice. *Developmental Psychobiology*, **2**: 10–18.

Jones, A. W., Croucher, M. J., Meldrum, B. S. & Watkins, J. C. (1984). Suppression of audiogenic seizures in DBA/2 mice by two new dipeptide NMDA receptor antagonists. *Neuroscience Letters*, **45**: 157–61.

Kleinschmidt, A., Bears, M. F. & Singer, W. (1987). Blockade of NMDA receptors disrupt experience-dependent plasticity in kitten striate cortex. *Science*, **238**: 355–8.

Koppel, H. & Innocenti, G. M. (1983). Is there a genuine exuberancy of callosal projections in development? A quantitative electron microscopic study of the cat. *Neuroscience Letters*, **41**: 33–40.

240   *J. W. Swann* et al.

Kotagal, P., Rothner, A. D., Erenberg, G., Cruse, R. P. & Wyllie, E. (1987). Complex partial seizures of childhood onset. A five year follow-up study. *Archives of Neurology*, **44**: 1177–80.

Kriegstein, A. R., Suppes, T. & Prince, D. A. (1987). Cellular and synaptic physiology and epileptogenesis of developing rat neocortical neurons in vitro. *Developmental Brain Research*, **34**: 161–71.

Kunkel, D. D., Hendrickson, A. E., Wu, J.-Y. & Schwartzkroin, P. A. (1986). Glutamic acid decarboxylase (GAD) immunocytochemistry of developing rabbit hippocampus. *Journal of Neuroscience*, **6**: 541–52.

Lacy, J. R. & Penry, J. K. (1976). *Infantile Spasms*. New York: Raven Press.

Luhmann, H. J. & Prince, D. A. (1990). Transient expression of polysynaptic NMDA receptor-mediated activity during neocortical development. *Neuroscience Letters*, **111**: 109–15.

Matsumoto, H. & Ajmone-Marsan, C. A. (1964). Cortical cellular phenomena in experimental epilepsy: ictal manifestation. *Experimental Neurology*, **9**: 305–26.

McCowen, T. J., Givens, B. S. & Breese, G. R. (1987). Amino acid influences on seizures elicited within the inferior colliculus. *Journal of Pharmacology and Experimental Therapeutics*, **243**: 603–8.

McDonald, J. W. & Johnston, M. V. (1990). Physiological and pathophysiological roles of excitatory amino acids during central nervous system development. *Brain Research Reviews*, **15**: 14–70.

McGillem, C. D. & Aunon, J. I. (1987). Analysis of event-related potentials. In *Methods of Analysis of Brain Electrical and Magnetic Signals. EEG Handbook* (revised series, vol. 1), ed. A. S. Gevins & A. Remond, pp. 131–69. North-Holland: Elsevier Science Publishers B.V. (Biomedical Division).

McGinn, M. D., Willott, J. F. & Henry, K. R. (1973). Effects of conductive hearing loss on auditory evoked potentials and audiogenic seizures in mice. *Nature*, **244**: 255–6.

Miles, R. & Wong, R. K. S. (1987). Inhibitory control of local excitatory circuits in the guinea pig hippocampus. *Journal of Physiology*, **388**: 611–29.

Millan, M. H., Meldrum, B. S. & Faingold, C. L. (1986). Induction of audiogenic seizure susceptibility by focal infusion of excitant amino acid or bicuculline into the inferior colliculus of normal rats. *Experimental Neurology*, **91**: 634–9.

Mizrahi, E. M. (1987). Neonatal seizures: problems in diagnosis and classification. *Epilepsia*, **28** (Suppl. 1): S46–S55.

Moshé, S. L. (1987). Epileptogenesis and the immature brain. *Epilepsia*, **28**: 81–5.

Mueller, A. L., Chesnut, R. M. & Schwartzkroin, P. A. (1983). Actions of GABA in developing rabbit hippocampus: an in vitro study. *Neuroscience Letters*, **39**: 193–8.

Mueller, A. L., Taube, J. S. & Schwartzkroin, P. A. (1984). Development of hyperpolarizing inhibitory postsynaptic potentials and hyperpolarizing response to gamma-aminobutyric acid in rabbit hippocampus studied in vitro. *Journal of Neuroscience*, **4**: 860–7.

Mutani, R., Futamachi, K. J. & Prince, D. (1974). Potassium activity in immature cortex. *Brain Research*, **75**: 27–39.

Nadler, J. V., Martin, D., Bowe, M. A., Morrisett, R. A. & McNamara, J. O. (1990). Kindling, prenatal exposure to ethanol and postnatal development selectively alter responses of hippocampal pyramidal cells to NMDA. In *Excitatory Amino Acids in Neuronal Plasticity*, ed. Y. Ben-Ari, pp. 407–17. New York: Plenum Press.

Newberry, N. R. & Nicoll, R. A. (1984). A bicuculline-resistant postsynaptic potential in rat hippocampal pyramidal cells in vitro. *Journal of Physiology*, **348**: 239–54.

Norris, C. H., Cawthorn, T. H. & Carroll, R. C. (1977). Kanamycin priming for audiogenic seizures in mice. *Neuropharmacology*, **16**: 375–80.

O'Donohoue, N. V. (1985). *Epilepsies in Childhood*. London: Butterworth.

Pierson, M., Egid, K. & Swann, J. (1990). Phencyclinoids promote experimental induction of audiogenic seizure susceptibility. *Epilepsia*, **31**: 649.

Pierson, M., Smith, K. L. & Swann, J. W. (1989). A slow NMDA-mediated synaptic potential underlies seizures originating from midbrain. *Brain Research*, **486**: 381–6.

Pierson, M. & Swann, J. W. (1988). The sensitive period and optimum dosage for induction of AGS susceptibility by kanamycin in the Wistar rat. *Hearing Research*, **32**: 1–10.

Pierson, M. & Swann, J. (1991). Ontogenic features of AGS susceptibility induced in immature rats by noise. *Epilepsia*, **32**: 1–9.

Prince, D. A. (1978). Neurophysiology of epilepsy. *Annual Review of Neuroscience*, **1**, 395–415.

Prince, D. A. & Gutnick, M. J. (1972). Neuronal activities in epileptogenic foci of immature cortex. *Brain Research*, **45**: 455–68.

Purpura, D. P. (1964). Relationship of seizure susceptibility to morphological and physiologic properties of normal and abnormal immature cortex. In *Neurologic and Electroencephalographic Correlative Studies in Infancy*, ed. P. Kellaway & I. Petersén, pp. 117–54. New York: Grune and Stratton.

Purpura, D. P. (1969). Stability and seizure susceptibility of immature brain. In *Basic Mechanisms of the Epilepsies*, ed. H. H. Jaspar, A. A. Ward & A. Pope, pp. 481–505. Boston, MA: Little, Brown.

Purves, D. (1988). Regulation of developing neural connections. In *Body and Brain. A Trophic Theory of Neural Connections*, ed. D. Purves, pp. 75–96. Cambridge, MA: Harvard University Press.

Purves, D. & Lichtman, J. W. (1980). Elimination of synapses in the developing nervous system. *Science*, **210**: 153–7.

Rakic, P., Bourgeois, J. P., Eikenhoff, M. F., Zecevic, N. & Goldman-Rakic, P. S. (1986). Concurrent overproduction of synapses in diverse regions of rat prenatal cerebral cortex. *Science*, **232**: 232–8.

Rauschecher, J. P. & Hahn, S. (1987). Ketamine-xylazine anaesthesia blocks consolidation of ocular dominance changes in kitten visual cortex. *Nature*, **326**: 183–5.

Rocca, W. A., Sharbrough, F. W., Hauser, W. A., Annegers, J. F. & Schoenberg, B. S. (1987). Risk factors for complex partial seizures: a population-based case-control study. *Annals of Neurology*, **21**: 22–31.

Sawa, M., Nakamura, K. & Naito, H. (1968). Intracellular phenomena and spread of epileptic seizure discharges. *Electroencephalography and Clinical Neurophysiology*, **24**: 146–54.

Scherer, W. S. & Uden, S. B. (1988). The role of NMDA receptors in the development of binocular maps in *Xenopus tertus*. *Society for Neuroscience Abstracts*, **14**: 675.

Schwartzkroin, P. A. (1982). Development of rabbit hippocampus: physiology. *Developmental Brain Research*, **2**: 469–86.

Schwartzkroin, P. A. & Altschuler, R. J. (1977). Development of kitten hippocampal neurons. *Brain Research*, **134**: 429–44.

Schwartzkroin, P. A. & Kunkel, D. D. (1982). Electrophysiology and morphology of the developing hippocampus of fetal rabbits. *Journal of Neuroscience*, **2**: 448–62.

Seress, L., Frotscher, M. & Ribak, C. E. (1989). Local circuit neurons in both the dentate gyrus and Ammon's horn establish synaptic connections with principal neurons in five day old rats: a morphological basis for inhibition in early development. *Experimental Brain Research*, **78**: 1–9.

Seress, L. & Ribak, C. E. (1988). The development of GABAergic neurons in the rat hippocampal formation: an immunocytochemical study. *Developmental Brain Research*, **44**: 197–209.

Shivers, B. D., Killisch, I., Sprengel, R., Sontheimer, H., Kohler, M., Schofield, P. R. & Seeburg, P. H. (1989). Two novel GABA$_A$ receptor subunits exist in distinct neuronal subpopulations. *Neuron*, **3**: 327–37.

Sieghart, W. (1989). Multiplicity of GABA$_A$-benzodiazepine receptors. *Trends in Pharmacological Sciences*, **10**, 407–11.

Smith, K. L. & Swann, J. W. (1987). Carbamazepine suppresses synchronized afterdischarging in disinhibited immature rat hippocampus in vitro. *Brain Research*, **400**: 371–6.

Somjen, G. G. (1979). Extracellular potassium in the mammalian central nervous system. *Annual Review of Physiology*, **41**: 159–77.

Swann, J. W. & Brady, R. J. (1984). Penicillin-induced epileptogenesis in immature rat CA3 hippocampal pyramidal cells. *Developmental Brain Research*, **12**: 243–54.

Swann, J. W., Brady, R. J., Friedman, R. J. & Smith, K. L. (1986a). The dendritic origins of penicillin-induced epileptogenesis in CA3 hippocampal pyramidal cells. *Journal of Neurophysiology*, **56**: 1718–38.

Swann, J. W., Brady, R. J. & Martin, D. L. (1989). Postnatal development of GABA-mediated synaptic inhibition in rat hippocampus. *Neuroscience*, **28**: 551–61.

Swann, J. W., Brady, R. J. & Smith, K. L. (1986b). Extracellular K$^+$ accumulation during penicillin-induced epileptogenesis in the CA3 region of immature rat hippocampus. *Developmental Brain Research*, **30**: 243–55.

Swann, J. W., Brady, R. J., Smith, K. L. & Pierson, M. G. (1988). Synaptic mechanisms of focal epileptogenesis in the immature nervous system. In *Disorders of the Developing Nervous System: Changing Views on Their Origins, Diagnoses, and Treatments*, ed. J. W. Swann & A. Messer, pp. 19–49. New York: Alan R. Liss.

Swann, J. W. & Smith, K. L. (1990). An analysis of recurrent EPSPs recorded in immature CA3 hippocampal neurons. *Society for Neuroscience Abstracts*, **16**: 1290.

Swann, J. W., Smith, K. L. & Brady, R. J. (1987). Localized synaptic interactions mediate the sustained depolarization of seizure-like discharges in immature hippocampus. *Society for Neuroscience Abstracts*, **13**: 1156.

Swann, J. W., Smith, K. L. & Brady, R. J. (1990). Neural networks and synaptic transmission in immature hippocampus. In *Excitatory Amino Acids and Neuronal Plasticity. Advances in Experimental Medicine and Biology*, ed. Y. Ben-Ari, vol. 268, pp. 161–71. New York: Plenum Press.

Tepper, J. M. & Schlesinger, J. (1980). Acoustic priming and kanamycin-induced cochlear damage. *Brain Research*, **187**: 81–95.

Tharp, B. R. (1987). An overview of pediatric seizure disorders and epileptic syndromes. *Epilepsia*, **28**: S36–S45.

Traynelis, S. F. & Dingledine, R. (1988). Potassium-induced spontaneous electrographic seizures in the rat hippocampal slice. *Journal of Neurophysiology*, **59**: 259–76.

Tremblay, E., Raisin, M. P., Represa, A., Charriant-Marlangue, C. & Ben-Ari, Y. (1988). Transient increased density of NMDA binding sites in developing rat hippocampus. *Brain Research*, **461**: 393–6.

Tsumoto, T., Hagihara, K., Sata, H. & Hata, Y. (1987). NMDA receptors in the cortex of young kittens are more effective than those of adult cats. *Nature*, **327**: 513–14.

Vernadakis, A. & Woodbury, D. M. (1969). The developing animal as a model. *Epilepsia*, **10**: 163–78.

Wisden, W., Morris, B. J., Darlison, M. G., Hunt, S. P. & Barnard, E. A. (1989). Localization of GABA_A receptor alpha-subunit mRNAs in relation to receptor subtypes. *Molecular Brain Research*, **5**: 305–10.

Wyllie, E. & Lüders, H. (1989). Complex partial seizures in children. Clinical manifestations and identification of surgical candidates. *Cleveland Clinic Journal of Medicine*, **56** (Suppl.), Part 1: S43–S52.

Wyllie, E., Rothner, A. D. & Lüders, H. (1989). Partial seizures in children. Clinical features, medical treatment, and surgical considerations. *Pediatric Clinics of North America*, **36**: 343–64.

Yamamoto, N., Watanabe, K., Negoro, T., Takaesu, E., Aso, K., Furune, S. & Takahashi, I. (1987). Complex partial seizures in children: ictal manifestations and their relation to clinical course. *Neurology*, **37**: 1379–82.

7

Electrophysiology and pharmacology of human neocortex and hippocampus in vitro

MASSIMO AVOLI

Introduction

Electrophysiological techniques together with pharmacological procedures have been used extensively to explore the basic mechanisms that underlie the generation of synchronous neuronal activity characteristic of epilepsy (for reviews, see Jasper et al., 1969; Schwartzkroin & Wheal, 1984; Delgado-Escueta et al., 1986; Avoli et al., 1990). In the course of these studies different procedures have been employed to elicit epileptiform activity and, as a result, several models have been developed. These include experimental paradigms in which the processes associated with acute or chronic epileptogenesis can be analyzed by using in-vivo as well as in-vitro preparations. In addition, electrophysiological studies have been performed in genetic models where seizure activity is related to the predisposition of a given animal strain to epileptic attacks, either spontaneously or following physiological stimuli (Kostopoulos & Psarropoulou, 1990; see also Chapter 3, this volume).

The relevance of any mechanism discovered in these studies for understanding the physiopathogenesis of human epileptic syndromes depends on the demonstration that such mechanisms also characterize the human condition. For instance, while it is undisputed that the impairment of γ-aminobutyric acid (GABA) synthesis leads to seizures (Molony & Paramelee, 1954), a decreased efficacy of GABAergic potentials in focal, chronic epilepsy is still a matter of debate (cf. Avoli, 1988; see also p. 266, below). Undoubtedly the most direct approach to the understanding of the human syndromes consists of recording the cellular activity directly in human epileptic tissue. Extracellular single unit recordings from cells located in the human epileptic focus have been performed in situ during surgery for seizures in a number of studies (Ward & Thomas, 1955; Calvin et al., 1973; Wyler et al., 1982; Wyler & Ward,

1986; Isokawa-Akesson *et al.*, 1987). However, these studies have been primarily descriptive. Although they disclosed some important features of the pattern of unitary discharge, limitations imposed by ethical considerations as well as by the impossibility of properly controlling the experimental situation did not allow these investigators to obtain information on the processes taking place at the level of the neuronal membrane.

Many of these constraints have been overcome by the introduction of the in-vitro brain slice technique (for a review, see Dingledine 1984). Thus, following some preliminary reports in which the viability of the human slice preparation was established (Kato *et al.*, 1973; Schwartzkroin & Prince, 1976), more detailed studies on the electrophysiological characteristics of human cortical cells have been undertaken (Schwartzkroin *et al.*, 1983; Avoli & Olivier, 1989). Moreover, the booming interest in the surgical treatment of epilepsy makes it likely that many reports on the electrophysiology of human brain tissue maintained in vitro are about to appear.

In this chapter, I review the findings that have been obtained to date in slices of human neocortex and hippocampus analyzed using electrophysiological techniques. While the point of departure is that of discussing some technical and methodological aspects related to the use of human cortical tissue in vitro, the core of this chapter focuses on those questions that have arisen in this type of experiment. While doing so, I report the results obtained and discuss them in relation to the data that have emerged from studies conducted on animal models of experimental epilepsy.

Methodological and technical aspects

Choice of tissue

Neurosurgical procedures

Human brain tissue to be used for in-vitro studies is obtained by a neurosurgeon during operative procedures for the cure of different neurological diseases. It typically consists of samples of neocortex or hippocampus, although other structures can also be used. In all of these experiments, the tissue used for the in-vitro electrophysiological analysis is part of a block of brain tissue that is removed for strictly therapeutic reasons (i.e., tissue removal is dictated entirely by clinical needs). Human brain specimens from epileptic patients can be obtained only during the limited time frame determined by the length of the operative procedure. Therefore it is at times difficult to establish the temporal profile of ictal and postictal changes. In addition to brain tissue obtained from patients who undergo surgery because of seizures resistant to medical treatment, brain samples for electrophysiological studies can also be obtained during the removal of vascular malformations and neoplasms.

Clinical history and diagnostic findings

Since the biopsies come from patients suffering from various neurological diseases, it is imperative for the neurophysiologist to obtain as much information as possible about the clinical history, the results of brain imaging studies and electrophysiological diagnostic procedures (cf. Sherwin, 1988). The latter are performed before surgery (e.g. extracranial electroencephalograph (EEG) and depth-electrode recordings) and/or intraoperatively (e.g., electrocorticograph (ECoG).

These data are not only relevant for distinguishing epileptic from non-epileptic patients. This type of information is also useful in epileptic patients for localizing the site(s) of origin of epileptic activity and/or the structures to which the epileptiform activity spreads. Furthermore these results are of extreme importance to establish, in patients undergoing surgery for non-epileptic pathologies, the possible presence of epileptic abnormalities that were not clinically relevant (i.e., interictal EEG discharges) as well as to assess the extent of any possible local neuronal damage.

Neuropathological findings

Careful analysis of the samples used for electrophysiological studies is advisable. The histopathological findings that can usually be observed in the neocortical tissue (at least at the Montreal Neurological Institute) are those of moderate gliosis and neuronal loss. This result is obviously biased by the fact that the neurosurgeon always tries to obtain samples for slice studies that do not show gross morphological changes. Data pertaining to the biochemical changes such as those related to adrenoreceptors, amino acids, and enzymes can also provide useful additional information (for reviews, see Sherwin & van Gelder, 1986; Sherwin, 1988).

Types of human cortical sample

In the light of the issues discussed above, three main categories of human neocortical tissue can be analyzed in vitro. First, epileptogenic samples obtained from areas removed from epileptic patients and displaying active interictal spiking in the intraoperative ECoG. Second, juxta-epileptogenic samples, i.e. tissue excised from the lobe of epileptic patients but not showing any sign of epileptic spiking in the ECoG. Third, non-epileptogenic samples, i.e. tissue removed from non-epileptic patients undergoing surgical procedures for pathologies other than epilepsy. Slices obtained from the tissue belonging to this last category can be used as controls for purposes of comparison. However, one must maintain some reservations about tissue normality, since epileptiform abnormalities, due to their intermittent occurrence, might not have been detected at the time when diagnostic tests were performed. Unfortunately it is difficult to apply these characterizations (formulated for the neocortex) to hippocampus. In fact it is practically impossible to obtain non-epileptogenic hippocampal tissues from humans.

Preparation and maintenance of slices

The typical biopsy specimen consists of a piece of neocortex or hippocampus that measures approximately 10 mm × 15 mm × 5 mm. Following the removal, the specimen is immersed within 5–10 s in cold, oxygenated (95% O_2, 5% CO_2), artificial cerebrospinal fluid (ACSF). Slices are cut in a laboratory adjacent to the operating room using a McIlwain tissue chopper. The thickness of the slices varies between 500 and 700 μm and, when neocortex is used, the tissue sample is placed with the pia facing downward on the chopper plate (cf. Schwartzkroin *et al.*, 1983). At the end of the slicing procedure slices are transported to the neurophysiological laboratory, where they are placed in an interphase tissue chamber. Here they are perfused at 34.5 °C with oxygenated ACSF at pH 7.4. The time elapsed between removal and placement in the chamber is approximately 10–15 min. The ionic composition of the standard ACSF used for the human in-vitro studies is similar to that of the ACSF employed by a number of investigators for studies in rat or guinea pig cortical structures (cf. Dingledine, 1984).

Electrophysiological techniques

These are similar to those used in several studies performed in rat, cat, and guinea pig cortex. Conventional current-clamp intracellular recordings are performed with microelectrodes that are back-filled with potassium acetate or KCl solutions. In some experiments the intracellular solution can also contain the lidocaine derivative QX-314 (to block voltage-dependent Na^+ conductance; Connors & Prince, 1982) and/or Cs^+ salts (to block K^+ repolarizing potentials). Signals are fed to a high input resistance amplifier with an internal bridge circuit for passing intracellular current. Single electrode, voltage-clamp recordings from human cortical cells have also been reported (Halliwell, 1986; McCormick & Williamson, 1989). Extracellular field potential recordings or measurements of the concentration of ions in the extracellular space can also be obtained from human samples by using standard procedures similar to those in use for other animal species (cf. Avoli *et al.*, 1987). Electrical stimulation of the human cortex maintained in vitro is performed by applying brief (10–90 μs) pulses of constant current through bipolar or monopolar electrodes (tip diameter 100–150 μm). The stimulating electrode is placed under visual control in the underlying white matter, pia or within the cortical layers. Morphological characterization of the cells analyzed with intracellular recordings is always advisable. This can be obtained, for instance, by including the fluorescent dye Lucifer Yellow in the recording electrode.

Functional properties of human cortical cells

Electrophysiological properties

It is generally accepted that the integrative properties of neuronal networks are strongly dependent upon the electrical properties of the somatodendritic membrane of each single neuron. In the last few years several studies have focused on the characterization of these electrophysiological properties in the mammalian cortex. Therefore it appeared relevant to extend this type of analysis to the human cortex maintained in vitro, since human cells might display passive and active responses of the membrane that might be different both quantitatively and qualitatively from those reported in other mammals. Moreover, knowledge of these properties is a prerequisite to understanding how these cells perform their integrative function such as the conversion of synaptic inputs to action potential coded outputs.

Subthreshold responses

Intracellular recordings performed in slices of the human temporal or frontal neocortex have revealed several responses that deviate from the expected passive behavior of the neuronal membrane during intracellular injection of hyperpolarizing and depolarizing pulses. As shown in Fig. 7.1, a consistent feature is the presence of inward rectification that is seen when the membrane is made 5–15 mV more positive than resting potential. This inward rectification in the depolarizing direction persists during prolonged pulses of current and is blocked by extracellular application of tetrodotoxin (TTX) (Fig. 7.1(C)), indicating that human neocortical cells possess a persistent, or slowly inactivating, Na$^+$ current (Avoli & Olivier, 1989). This current is seen within a range of resting potentials that is subthreshold for the initiation of action potentials. Therefore it might play an important role in the generation of repetitive firing. Furthermore, the ability of the persistent Na$^+$ current readily to follow fast voltage changes such as those changed by a synaptic excitatory input indicates that it contributes to the depolarizing envelope of the EPSP induced by extracellular focal stimuli. A similar type of conductance has been reported to occur in neocortical neurons of cat and guinea pig (Connors *et al.*, 1982; Stafstrom *et al.*, 1984, 1985).

A second subthreshold response seen in human cortex is the inward rectification observed during injection of pulses of hyperpolarizing current (Fig. 7.2(A) and (B)). This response, the so-called anomalous rectifier, is characterized in current-clamp intracellular recordings by a sag of the membrane signal toward a less negative potential than is seen within 15–40 ms after the onset of the hyperpolarizing step. Since this type of rectification is reduced and eventually blocked by the extracellular application of Cs$^+$ (Fig. 7.2(B)) it appears to share pharmacological similarities with the one reported to occur in the sino-atrial node (Brown & DiFrancesco, 1980) and in a number of central neurons in other mammalian species (Halliwell & Adams, 1982; Kubota *et al.*, 1985; Spain *et al.*, 1987; Schwindt *et al.*, 1988a).

Two other types of non-linear response can be recorded in human neocortical cells. The first is characterized by the finding that at the end of a hyperpolarizing pulse the time necessary for the membrane potential to return to resting potential value is longer than the time required to reach the peak in response to the hyperpolarizing command pulse (Fig. 7.2(C) and (D)). Such behavior might suggest the activation of a transient outward current (so-called I_A) similar to that reported in CA3 hippocampal pyramidal cells (Gustafsson *et al.*, 1982). Interestingly, the excitability of the neuron as tested with extracellular focal stimulation (Fig. 7.2(E)) appears to be depressed when a test response is preceded by a hyperpolarizing pulse. The second type of active response is seen during a depolarizing intracellular pulse. It consists of the gradual decline of the

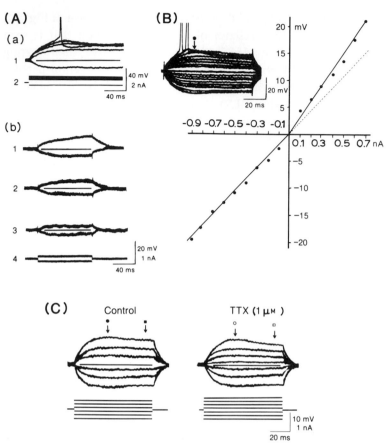

Fig. 7.1. Voltage and time dependence of subthreshold responses to injected current pulses. In (A) the presence of inward rectification in the depolarizing direction is seen both when symmetrical, hyper- and depolarizing pulses are applied over a steady membrane potential (a) and when pulses are injected while changing the membrane potential with steady application of current (b). In (Aa), 1 is the intracellular signal, 2 is the current monitor. In (Ab), 1 is the intracellular response at a membrane potential 8 mV positive to rest, 2 at rest and 3 10 mV negative to rest; 4 is the current monitor. Note in (Aa), the appearance of a 'depolarizing sag' upon injection of larger amounts of depolarizing current. (B) Plot of voltage responses of another neuron to intracellular current pulses; values were computed at the time indicated by the filled circle in the raw data shown in the top left part of the panel. Note, in these intracellularly recorded responses the appearance of both depolarizing and hyperpolarizing sags during the injection of larger amounts of current. (C) Blockade of inward rectification in the depolarizing direction by 1 μM tetrodotoxin (TTX). Note that a depolarizing sag is still evoked in the presence of TTX by the largest depolarizing pulse (+0.7 nA). Cells were recorded in the second temporal gyrus and were characterized by a resting potential of approximately −60 mV. ((A) to (C) from Avoli & Olivier, 1989.).

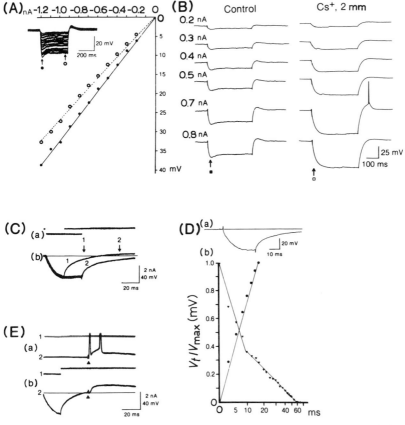

Fig. 7.2. Time and voltage dependence of the membrane responses to injection of hyperpolarizing current pulses. In (A) the I–V plot shows that this type of inward rectification (so-called anomalous rectification) increases when the membrane potential is brought to more hyperpolarized levels; the plotted values were computed at two different times during the hyperpolarizing pulses as indicated by the open and filled dots in the raw data inset. In (B) the anomalous rectification is blocked by the extracellular application of Cs^+. Neurons in (A) and (B) were from the frontal cortex and the second temporal gyrus, respectively. (C) The time required for the V_m to return to resting level at the end of a hyperpolarizing pulse is longer than the time needed to reach the hyperpolarizing level at pulse onset. Arrows 1 and 2 point to the time expected for pulse 1 (duration 20 ms) and 2 (duration 40 ms), respectively, to return to resting V_m. Trace (a) is the current monitor; trace (b) is the intracellular signal. (D) shows a plot (b) of the time required by the V_m to reach the hyperpolarized level (filled circles) and then return to resting V_m (filled triangles) at the end of an intracellular hyperpolarizing pulse of 0.8 nA; raw data are shown in (a). Note that the computed values during repolarization fit two exponential curves. (E) The excitability of the neuron as tested by extracellular focal stimulation (a) is decreased when the stimulus is preceded by a hyperpolarizing pulse (b). In this panel, 1 is the current monitor, 2 is the intracellular signal. ((A) and (B) from Avoli & Olivier, 1989.)

voltage to a steady level following an early peak, so-called depolarizing sag (Fig. 7.1(A) and (C); cf. Stafstrom *et al.*, 1984).

The presence of rectification, i.e. of voltage- and time-dependent responses in the subthreshold range of the membrane potential suggests that human neocortical cells have a very limited, if any, truly passive voltage range. The existence of these subthreshold responses is particularly important in the light of evidence indicating that neuromodulators and exogenous compounds such as anti-epileptic drugs might be capable of modifying voltage-dependent currents.

Generation of action potentials and repetitive firing

Studies performed on the large pyramidal cells of the human neocortex and hippocampus have revealed that most of the cells that are injected with depolarizing current pulses generate rhythmic and regular discharges of fast action potentials (Schwartzkroin *et al.*, 1983; Lacaille *et al.*, 1988; Avoli & Olivier, 1989; McCormick & Williamson, 1989). These action potentials are blocked by extracellular application of TTX or disappear when QX-314 is used in the solution used to fill the intracellular microelectrode, indicating that they are due to voltage-dependent Na^+ currents (Avoli & Olivier, 1989; Hwa *et al.*, 1992). When the repetitive firing of these cells is studied by using depolarizing pulses of increasing intensity, two distinct linear segments of firing are usually seen (so-called primary and secondary ranges of firing; Fig. 7.3(B)). A second characteristic that emerges from these experiments is that the firing rate during the depolarizing pulse declines with time, i.e. the frequency of the repetitive discharge adapts (Fig. 7.3(A); see below).

These data suggest that pyramidal cells in the human neocortex display firing properties that are analogous to those of regularly firing neocortical cells of the guinea pig and rat neocortex maintained in vitro or to hippocampal pyramidal cells (Madison & Nicoll, 1984; McCormick *et al.*, 1985). These results are also remarkably similar to the firing properties of neocortical, long-axoned cells studied in situ (Calvin & Sypert, 1976).

Long-lasting afterhyperpolarizations

As shown in Figs. 7.3(A(b)) and 4(A), the repetitive firing of action potentials induced in neocortical cells by pulses of depolarizing current is often followed by a long-lasting afterhyperpolarization (AHP). This potential displays an equilibrium value that is 15–40 mV more negative

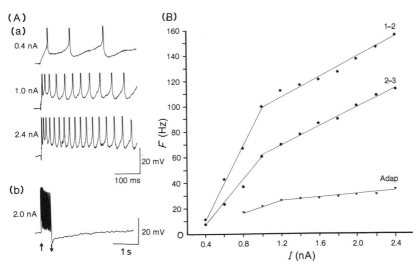

Fig. 7.3. (A) Repetitive firing evoked by depolarizing square pulses of intracellular current in a second temporal gyrus neuron. The firing of the same neuron as in (a) is shown in (b) at low speed. Note in (a) the rhythmic, regular firing of fast action potentials that increases in rate when progressively larger amounts of current are injected and then displays adaptation. (B) Plot of firing frequency versus injected current (F–I curve); same cell as in (A). The three F–I curves were computed for the first (1–2) and second (2–3) intervals as well as for the intervals during the adapted, steady-state firing. Note the primary and secondary ranges of firing detected in all three curves. (From Avoli & Olivier, 1989.)

than rest. This value, as well as the fact that the AHP can be recorded with KCl-filled microelectrodes, suggests that it is mediated by K^+. Furthermore, this AHP is decreased and eventually blocked by extracellular application of Cd^{2+} or Mn^{2+} indicating that it is presumably caused by a Ca^{2+}-dependent K^+ conductance (Fig. 7.4(A)).

This potential appears to play a role in firing adaptation. First, during a depolarizing pulse, neurons with marked adaptation display a hyperpolarizing clamping effect that is pivotal in reducing the rate of firing and is eventually capable of stopping it (e.g., neuron shown in Fig. 7.4(B)), lower panel). Second, during application of Cd^{2+} or Mn^{2+} the ability to adapt decreases in parallel to the diminution of the long-lasting AHP (Fig. 7.4(A)). Like the electrophysiological properties described above, the results pertaining to the ionic mechanisms underlying the long-lasting AHP generated by human neocortical cells are similar to those observed in the cortical cells of other mammals (Madison & Nicoll, 1984; Lancaster & Adams, 1986; Schwindt *et al.*, 1988*b,c*).

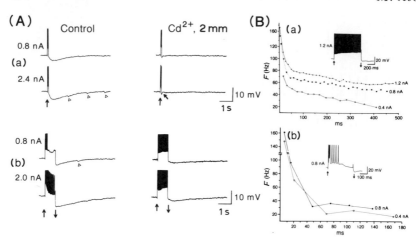

Fig. 7.4. (A) Effects evoked by extracellular application of Cd^{2+} on the AHP evoked by depolarizing pulses of different intensities (leftward numbers) and duration. Note in (a) that Cd^{2+} blocks the AHP and unmasks an early component hyperpolarizing component (curved arrow). Note also in (b) that the reduction of the AHP is accompanied by a loss of adaptation. Open triangles point to spontaneously occurring, synaptic potentials that are blocked by Cd^{2+}. (B) Firing-rate adaptation during steps of injected current. (a) and (b) Plots of instantaneous firing rate (F) versus time in first temporal gyrus (a) and frontal cortex (b) neurons. Zero time indicates the beginning of the depolarizing pulse. Numbers on the right show the amplitude of the injected current. In both panels the inserts are raw data samples of the repetitive firing. Note that the decline in firing rate over time (i.e., adaptation) is more pronounced in the neuron shown in (b). (From Avoli & Olivier, 1989.)

Are the electrophysiological features in epileptogenic and non-epileptogenic tissue samples different?

The large majority of the data reviewed in the preceding sections has been obtained from recordings performed in slices of epileptogenic or juxta-epileptogenic brain tissues. However, preliminary results gathered in my laboratory suggest that similar features can be observed in slices of non-epileptogenic tissue. Moreover, a detailed study of the electrophysiological properties of cells located in the deep layers of neocortex removed from epileptic patients has shown that no difference exists when the values of resting membrane potential, apparent input resistance, and action potential amplitude are compared by segregating the samples into epileptogenic and juxta-epileptogenic types (Avoli & Olivier, 1989). Similar findings have been reported in two preliminary communications by Knowles *et al.* (1988, 1989), although these investigators have observed that neurons recorded from epileptogenic samples have a lower action potential threshold than those studied in tissue displaying little or no epileptogenesis.

Synaptic potentials

Excitatory potentials

As in the case of cells studied in the rodent neocortical slice (Connors *et al.*, 1982; Sutor & Hablitz, 1989), human neurons recorded intracellularly respond to focal extracellular stimuli by generating a short-lasting depolarizing event (Schwartzkroin *et al.*, 1983; Avoli & Olivier, 1987, 1989; McCormick, 1989). Furthermore, when increasingly higher-strength focal stimuli are used, these cells generate in most of the cases a progressively larger-amplitude depolarizing potential that is associated with a single action potential (Fig. 7.5(A)). This response represents a synaptic potential, as its amplitude increases or decreases, respectively, upon injection of hyperpolarizing or depolarizing current. As shown in Fig. 7.5(B(a)) and (C), this procedure often discloses the existence of a hyperpolarizing, inhibitory postsnaptic potential (IPSP, see below). The intracellular event elicited by extracellular focal stimuli is associated with an extracellularly recorded field potential that lasts 15–35 ms (Fig. 7.6(C)). This event attains maximal negative amplitude in the middle layers of the slice.

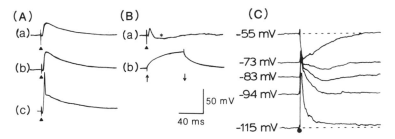

Fig. 7.5. (A) Single shock stimuli delivered in the white matter at progressively higher strength evoke an EPSP that becomes larger in amplitude ((a) and (b)) and is capable of eliciting a single action potential (c). (B(a)) the same stimulus intensity as that used in (A(a)) was delivered while the resting V_m was depolarized by 12 mV; note the presence of a hyperpolarizing IPSP (asterisk) that appears to curtail the initial EPSP. (B(b)) Response of this neocortical cell to a depolarizing intracellular pulse of intensity sufficient to give a response of the same amplitude at the peak of the EPSP shown in (A(b)). ((A) and (B) from Avoli & Olivier, 1989.) (C) Changes in amplitude and polarity of the stimulus-induced EPSP–IPSP sequence during variations of the resting V_m with injection of steady DC current (From McCormick, 1989.)

An interesting finding pertaining to the synaptic responses recorded in human neocortex is the ability of some neurons (approximately one-third of the cells recorded in the deep layers), to generate bursts of action potentials in response to high strength extracellular focal stimuli (Avoli & Olivier, 1987, 1989). The relation between stimulus strength and the appearances of this burst is illustrated in Fig. 7.6(A) and (B). The number of action potentials and the duration of the underlying depolarizing envelope are closely related to the current delivered through the stimulating electrode, i.e., they represent a graded phenomenon rather than an all-or-none event as is the case for the paroxysmal depolarization shift (PDS). As is discussed in more detail below (p. 261), the ability of human neocortical cells to respond to electrical stimuli with a burst of action potentials has been reported in previous studies conducted in different laboratories (Kato *et al.*, 1973; Schwartzkroin & Prince, 1976; Prince & Wong, 1981; Schwartzkroin *et al.*, 1983).

Pharmacological analysis of the stimulus-induced, depolarizing potential generated by neocortical cells suggests that conductances activated through one or more than one receptor subtype for the excitatory amino acid transmitters glutamic and aspartic acids are responsible for this response. Thus this extracellular field potential can be readily blocked by kynurenic acid (Fig. 7.7(A)), a non-specific antagonist of the excitatory amino acid receptors (Ganong *et al.*, 1983). Furthermore, application of the specific antagonist for the NMDA receptor subtype aminophosphonovalerate (APV) does not modify the excitatory postsynaptic potential (EPSP)-type response (Fig. 7.7(B)), while it reduces and eventually blocks the burst in those cells that are capable of generating such response (Fig. 7.7(C)). Therefore in the human neocortex the EPSP is presumably caused by the activation of the non-NMDA receptor subtypes (i.e., those for quisqualate and kainic acid), while the burst is due to conductances that are activated through the NMDA receptor subtype.

Inhibitory mechanisms

As mentioned above, extracellular focal stimuli elicit, under appropriate conditions, an EPSP-hyperpolarizing IPSP sequence. The early component of this IPSP displays a reversal potential that is close to the resting membrane potential (i.e., -65 to -75 mV), is sensitive to intracellular injection of Cl$^-$ (Fig. 7.8(A)) and is reduced by the GABA$_A$ receptor antagonist bicuculline methiodide (Fig. 7.8(B)). Therefore this portion of the stimulus-induced IPSP is presumably caused by an increased

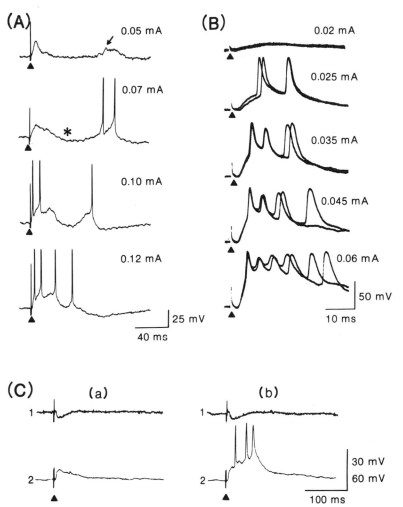

Fig. 7.6. Intracellular responses, to focal stimuli, of two 'bursting' neurons ((A) and (B)) in the deep layers of second temporal gyrus. The neuron in (A) was from the same slice as the neuron shown in Fig. 7.5(A) and (B). (A) The response to low strength stimulation (0.05 mA) consists of a short-latency EPSP followed by a low-amplitude (2 mV) hyperpolarizing IPSP that is interrupted by a late (onset at 180 ms) depolarizing event (arrow). When the stimulus intensity is brought to 0.07 mA, both the EPSP and the IPSP (asterisk) increase in amplitude. When the stimulus strength is further increased, full-blown bursts appear (0.10 and 0.12 mA). (B) Progressive appearance of bursting in response to focal stimuli of increasingly larger intensity. (C) Simultaneous extracellular (1) and intracellular (2) recordings in a slice of the second temporal gyrus. The stimulus duration was 10 μs in (a) and 90 μs in (b). The distance between the intracellular and the extracellular microelectrodes (both at the same depth in the deep layers of the cortical slice) was approximately 0.5 mm. ((A) to (C) from Avoli & Olivier, 1989.).

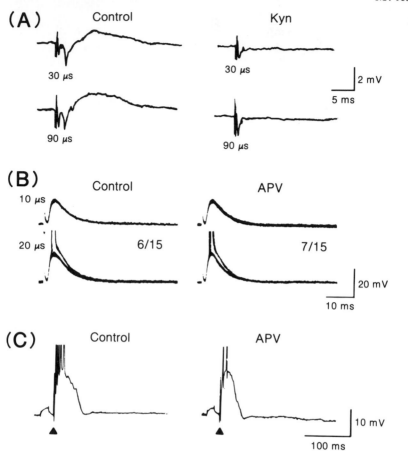

Fig. 7.7. (A) Effects evoked by kynurenic acid (Kyn) on the stimulus-induced response recorded extracellularly following moderate and high strength stimuli. (B) Effects induced by APV on the stimulus-induced EPSP and the EPSP–single action potential. (C) Effects induced by APV on the stimulus-induced bursting response. ((B) and (C) from Avoli & Olivier, 1989.)

conductance of Cl^- due to the activation of the $GABA_A$ receptor (Schwartzkroin *et al.*, 1983; Avoli & Olivier, 1989; McCormick, 1989).

Potentials mediated through the $GABA_B$ receptor subtype also play a role in the human neocortex. As has been reported to occur in the rat neocortex (Avoli, 1986; Connors *et al.*, 1988), the stimulus-induced hyperpolarization becomes biphasic when high strength stimuli are used. Furthermore, the late phase of this hyperpolarization is reduced by the $GABA_B$ antagonist phaclofen (Fig. 7.8(C)). Interestingly, the amplitude

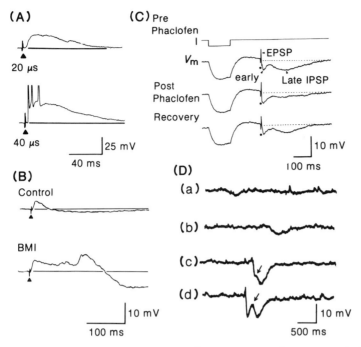

Fig. 7.8. (A) Single shock stimuli delivered at two different strengths induce a pure depolarizing potential that becomes progressively larger in amplitude and more prolonged. The intracellular microelectrode was filled with KCl. Note that the 40 μs stimulus is also capable of eliciting action potentials on top of the depolarizing response. (B) The GABA$_A$ receptor antagonist bicuculline methiodide (BMI) reduces the early hyperpolarizing IPSP and disclosed a late depolarizing potential. (C) Blockade of the late IPSP by phaclofen suggests that this potential is mediated by GABA$_B$ receptors. (D) Progressive development of spontaneously occurring potentials following application of 4-aminopyridine. These potentials are mediated mainly by GABA$_A$ receptors and include the depolarizing GABAergic component. ((A) from Avoli & Olivier, 1989; (B) from Hwa *et al.*, 1992; (C) from McCormick, 1989; (D) from Avoli *et al.*, 1988.)

and duration of the bicuculline-induced burst are potentiated by phaclofen in the human neocortex (McCormick, 1989).

Some evidence also exists for the presence in the human neocortex of conductances that are mediated through GABA$_A$ receptors located in the dendrites. First, the shape of the EPSP–IPSP sequence elicited by extracellular focal stimuli is at times characterized by a transient depolarizing component that occurs between the early and late components of the hyperpolarization (e.g., the synaptic sequence shown in Fig. 7.8(C)). At least in the rat hippocampus this depolarizing component has been shown to be blocked by dendritic application of bicuculline methiodide (Perreault & Avoli, 1988). Second, as illustrated in Fig. 7.8(D), application of 4-aminopyridine induces the appearance of spontaneously occurring, depolarizing potentials that are sensitive to $GABA_A$ receptor antagonists (Avoli et al., 1988). These results are remarkably similar to those obtained in the rat hippocampus and neocortex, where these depolarizations have been shown to be dependent upon the activation of $GABA_A$ receptors located on the apical dendrites of pyramidal cells (Perreault & Avoli, 1989).

In conclusion, these data indicate that GABA is a major inhibitory neurotransmitter in the human cortex and that GABAergic mechanisms are present and important for controlling neuronal excitability in the human brain (see also pp. 266–8). These electrophysiological findings are in keeping with morphological studies in which GABAergic cells have been detected in the human epileptogenic neocortex using immunocyto-chemical and/or histochemical techniques (Schiffmann et al., 1988; Babb et al., 1989). Furthermore biochemical experiments have shown that in the human cortex a GABA receptor of the B subtype plays a role in regulating the release of both newly taken up and endogenous GABA (Bonanno et al., 1989).

Action of other putative transmitters

At least two electrophysiological studies have analyzed the action exerted in the human cortex by transmitters other than glutamate or GABA. By using single electrode voltage-clamp recordings, Halliwell (1986) has shown that neocortical cells generate a muscarine-sensitive, non-inactivat-ing K^+ current that persists when Ca^{2+} flux into neurons is blocked with Cd^{2+}. More recently McCormick & Williamson (1989) have reported that K^+ currents are modulated in the human neocortex by a number of neurotransmitters. Some of these effects are illustrated in Fig. 7.9, which shows that histamine, the muscarine agonist β-methylcholine, nor-epinephrine and serotonin reduce both firing adaptation and the K^+ current associated with the AHP. In addition, McCormick & Williamson (1989) have observed that adenosine, baclofen and in some cases serotonin inhibit neuronal firing by increasing the same K^+ current. These data indicate, therefore, that neurotransmitters/neuromodulators exert their action in the human neocortex and that individual currents are under the control of several putative neurotransmitters.

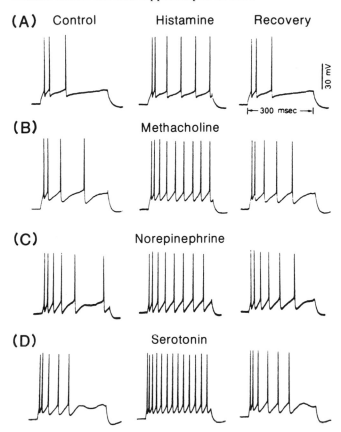

Fig. 7.9. (A) to (D) Histamine, methacholine (β-methylcholine), norepinephrine, and serotonin reversibly reduce spike frequency adaptation in human neocortical neurons. All data were obtained from two different cells in the anterior temporal lobe. (From McCormick & Williamson, 1989.)

Findings relevant to the pathogenesis of human epilepsy

Do human cells generate activity that can be considered abnormal?

This question probably represents the rationale that has been most widely used to analyze the electrophysiological features of human cells in vitro. It has been inspired by the hope that structures removed from the epileptogenic cortex might retain their ability to generate abnormal epileptiform discharges in the slice preparation. If this were true, it would provide a unique opportunity to analyze at the membrane level the mechanisms that underlie the generation of naturally occurring human epileptiform activity. This search is guided by the demonstration that under appropriate conditions, cortical slices obtained from laboratory animals are capable of generating epileptiform discharges that are indistinguishable from those observed in situ following similar pharmacological manipulations (e.g., the interictal PDS induced by penicillin; Prince & Connors, 1986). However, as will be discussed in the following sections, the ability of human epileptogenic tissue maintained in vitro to retain the epileptogenic features encountered in situ is as yet not clearly established.

Stimulus-induced abnormal activity

In the human neocortex maintained in vitro the existence of stimulus-induced responses displaying features that are different from those usually seen in other animal species was originally reported by Kato et al. (1973). In their study, human tissue was obtained during neurosurgical procedures for non-epileptic pathologies, although no electrodiagnostic investigations were performed and therefore the presence or absence of abnormal electrical activity in situ was not established. Kato et al., by employing extracellular single unit recordings, observed that in addition to normal antidromic and orthodromic potentials, some neurons could generate bursts of action potentials in response to extracellular focal stimuli (Fig. 7.10(A)). The occurrence of these bursts was dependent upon stimulus strength. As illustrated in Fig. 7.10(B) and (C) (see also Fig. 7.6), stimulus-induced bursting responses were later observed by a number of investigators to occur in both neocortical and hippocampal (mesial temporal) structures (Schwartzkroin & Prince, 1976; Prince & Wong, 1981; Schwartzkroin et al., 1983; Schwartzkroin & Haglund, 1986; Avoli & Olivier, 1987, 1989).

These results share some interesting features. First, the bursting response does not appear to be elicited by intracellular depolarizing pulses (Fig. 7.10)B)) as it is the case for some subclasses of neocortical cells (Connors et al., 1982; McCormick et al., 1985). Second, with the exception of rare cases (cf. Prince & Wong, 1981; Schwartzkroin & Haglund, 1986), the bursting response is usually graded (i.e., with the number of action potentials and the size of the associated depolarization proportional to the stimulus strength), and not an all-or-none event such as the PDS recorded in the experimentally induced focus (for a review, see Prince & Connors, 1986). Third, at least in those cases in which simultaneous extracellular recordings were performed (Avoli & Olivier, 1989), the stimulus-induced burst is not synchronously generated within a population of neurons (Fig. 7.6(C)). Hence the human bursting response is

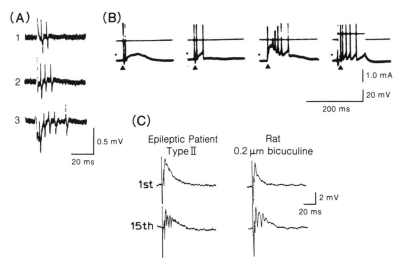

Fig. 7.10. (A) Burst discharge of extracellularly recorded action potential in response to focal stimulation. (B) Cortical neuron producing bursts of action potentials in response to extracellular focal stimuli delivered at progressively (first three panels from left to right) higher strength. Note in the fourth panel (far right) that superimposition of the synaptic response on a depolarized baseline revealed no hyperpolarizing IPSP. (C) Similar field potential responses to low frequency orthodromic stimuli are seen in a hippocampal slice obtained from an epileptic patient and perfused with normal medium and in a rat hippocampal slice perfused with low concentrations of bicuculline. ((A) from Kato *et al.*, 1973; (B) from Schwartzkroin *et al.*, 1983; (C) from Masukawa *et al.*, 1989.)

characterized by a number of features that are different from those of the PDS, the latter being considered the hallmark of interictal epileptogenesis (Prince & Connors, 1986).

The absence of PDS-like potentials in the human epileptogenic neocortical slice might be due to the disruption of the connections with remote cortical and subcortical areas as well as to the artificial microenvironment in which brain slices are maintained. However, this explanation should be limited to the absence of spontaneously occurring bursting events, since human neurons in vitro are indeed capable of generating PDSs and even prolonged synchronous epileptiform activity under appropriate pharmacological manipulation (Schwartzkroin & Haglund, 1986; Avoli *et al.*, 1987; Avoli & Olivier, 1989; Hwa *et al.*, 1992). An alternative explanation for the absence of synchronous epileptiform activity in the studies reviewed here might be related to the fact that only a weak correlation exists between cellular burst firing and interictal ECoG spiking in extracellular single-unit recordings performed on human epileptic foci in situ (Wyler *et al.*, 1982). Also, the occurrence of clear PDSs during interictal spiking is quite uncommon in experimental chronic epileptic foci induced by alumina gel (Prince & Futamachi, 1970; Wyler *et al.*, 1973, 1975). Furthermore, spontaneous or stimulus-induced PDSs are observed only in a small population of neurons recorded in cortical slices obtained from the periphery of freezing lesions which represent another model of chronic epileptogenesis (Lighthall & Prince, 1983). Hence the PDS may not be a key feature of the interictal activity generated by neurons in chronic foci.

However, in spite of the differences existing between the PDS and the stimulus-induced burst response, should one still consider the latter as a pathological event? Schwartzkroin *et al.* (1983) have interpreted the burst as a 'relatively common feature of normal cortex that received synchronous projected activity'. This conclusion was based on two sets of data. First, the observation that in cortex obtained from human epileptic patients, stimulus-induced bursts could occur in both relatively normal (i.e., areas with questionable ECoG relation to the epileptic focus) and epileptic tissue. This finding has later been confirmed in our own studies (Avoli & Olivier, 1989). Second, data obtained in monkeys have indicated that stimulus-induced bursts occur in slices from epileptogenic neocortex treated with alumina gel as well as from normal cortex (Schwartzkroin *et al.*, 1983).

These arguments, however, do not appear to be sufficient to interpret unequivocally the stimulus-induced bursts seen in the human epileptogenic neocortex as a normal physiological event. Indeed, long-term changes in excitability might indeed occur in tissue that is synaptically connected to areas of epileptogenesis. It is therefore difficult to accept even remote (from the focus) areas of the epileptogenic brain as control tissue. Furthermore, cortical areas that did not display any abnormal activity during electro-corticography could possibly have done so at some other time. Therefore it might be hazardous to assume that cortical areas in epileptic brain lying outside the site of onset of the patient's seizure are normal and devoid of epileptogenic potentiality. Interestingly Prince & Wong (1981) reported that burst behavior occurs in nearly 50% of the neurons recorded intracellularly in neocortical areas thought to be involved in epilepto-genesis, while no bursting response was observed in slices obtained from patients who never had clinically documented epileptic discharge. Therefore, until an extensive comparison with findings obtained from cortical areas not involved in any epileptogenic process is accomplished, the question of whether the stimulus-induced burst observed in epilepto-genic samples is a normal or a pathological response must remain open.

As reported above, the stimulus-induced burst, at least in our studies, appears to be mediated by conductances induced by the activation of the NMDA receptor (Avoli & Olivier, 1987, 1989). Furthermore, this type of conductance was not detected in the stimulus-induced EPSP-like response, indicating that NMDA-activated potentials are peculiar to the burst response rather than a common feature of excitatory synaptic transmis-sion in the human neocortex. However, to what extent NMDA-activated conductances found in some human cells are related to the chronic epileptogenicity of the tissue used in our experiments remains speculative. Interestingly, a similar finding has been reported in the kindling model of epilepsy. Thus, although NMDA receptors in the rat dentate gyrus do not normally participate in synaptic transmission, they become actively involved in this mechanism after repetitive stimulation of the amygdala or hippocampal commissures (Mody & Heinemann, 1987; Mody *et al.*, 1988).

A finding that is in line with the presence of abnormal activity in the human epileptogenic tissue has recently been obtained in the dentate gyrus of hippocampus removed from epileptic patients (Masukawa *et al.*, 1989). In this study, multiple population spikes could be elicited by low frequency (1 Hz) stimulation of the perforant pathway (Fig. 7.10(C)). Since a similar epileptiform response was recorded in rat hippocampal slices during perfusion with ACSF containing low concentrations of bicuculline, Masu-kawa *et al.* have proposed that a small reduction of GABA function might occur in the human epileptic hippocampus (see pp. 266–8).

Spontaneous activity

While there appears to be general consensus on the occurrence of stimulus-induced burst responses in some of the cells studied in the human neocortex obtained from epileptic patients, the presence of spontaneous epileptiform events is as yet not clearly established. Spontaneous ab-normal activity has not been observed in any of the studies mentioned above (Schwartzkroin & Prince, 1976; Prince & Wong, 1981; Schwartz-kroin *et al.*, 1983; Avoli & Olivier, 1987, 1989). On the other hand, a short report (Reid & Palovcik, 1989) has appeared that indicates that neocortical slices taken from the epileptogenic region (as identified by ECoG prior to surgical removal) exhibit large-amplitude, spontaneous field potential discharges. Furthermore, this type of in-vitro epileptiform activity was present only in slices taken from the epileptic focus: it was not recorded in slices obtained from adjacent areas that were not considered epileptogenic but were removed in the course of the surgical procedure (so-called juxta-epileptogenic areas in accordance with the tissue characterization described on pp. 246–47) or in non-epileptogenic tissue removed in the course of surgical access to deep lesions (Reid & Palovcik, 1989). The significance of these spontaneous in-vitro discharges awaits further analysis with intracellular recording as well as pharmacological characterization.

Spontaneous potentials can be observed in neocortical and more often hippocampal cells obtained from epileptic patients (Schwartzkroin & Knowles, 1984). This type of activity can be detected extracellularly, suggesting that it represents a synchronous phenomenon. However, as discussed in the following section, these potentials are blocked by bicuculline and thus represent spontaneously occurring inhibitory potentials (Schwartzkroin & Haglund, 1986).

Inhibition in human neocortex and hippocampus

As reported above, human neocortical cells in slices obtained from epileptogenic and juxta-epileptogenic areas generate a GABAergic hyperpolarizing potential in response to extracellular focal stimuli. Both $GABA_A$ and $GABA_B$ receptor subtypes are involved in this response. These findings therefore suggest that the human neocortex retains inhibitory mechanisms that are qualitatively similar to those reported to occur in a number of forebrain structures in other mammals (Krnjević, 1974; Avoli, 1988).

However, there is as yet no conclusive electrophysiological evidence that inhibitory mechanisms are quantitatively different in the human epileptogenic cortex as compared to non-epileptogenic cortex. This type of information would be of paramount importance for the understanding of the physiopathogenesis of human epilepsy, since it has been shown that inhibition appears to be decreased in many experimental models of epilepsy (cf. Avoli, 1988). Schwartzkroin et al. (1983) have reported that cells clearly related to the focus appeared to have less effective inhibitory potentials as compared with cells in slices taken from juxta-epileptogenic tissue. However, a subsequent study performed in my laboratory has indicated that in the deep layers of the human neocortex such a difference is difficult to detect (Avoli & Olivier, 1989). This appears also to be the case for neocortical cells recorded in the superficial layers of slices that belong to the three different sample groups (i.e., epileptogenic, juxta-

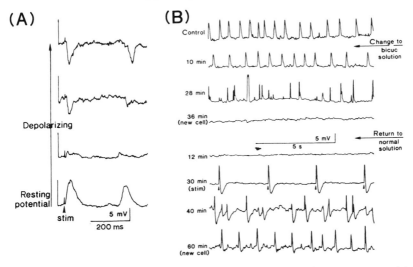

Fig. 7.11. Synchronous rhythmic events recorded in the human temporal lobe. (A) Effects induced by manipulation of the V_m on the stimulus-induced and the spontaneous potentials. (B) Reversible, pharmacological blockage of the spontaneously occurring events by bicuculline (bicuc). (From Schwartzkroin & Haglund, 1986.)

epileptogenic, and non-epileptogenic) (Lacaille *et al.*, 1988; Avoli *et al.*, unpublished results).

The question of whether inhibitory mechanisms are present in human epileptogenic cortex as compared to the non-epileptogenic type has been re-addressed by Schwartzkroin's laboratory (Schwartzkroin & Haglund, 1986). In this study it was shown that cells of the human temporal cortex generate spontaneous rhythmic events that appear to be caused mainly by GABAergic conductances (Fig. 7.11). This type of activity was recorded more often in slices obtained from mesial structures as compared with slices of lateral temporal lobe, suggesting that it reflected the epileptogenicity of the tissue under study (Schwartzkroin & Knowles, 1984; Schwartzkroin & Haglund, 1986). However, these spontaneous potentials have since been observed in normal monkey hippocampus and thus they probably do not reflect the presence of epileptogenicity in the human brain (Schwartzkroin & Haglund, 1986). In the light of these data it has been proposed that these spontaneous events might reflect the propensity of mesial temporal (i.e., hippocampal) tissue to discharge in a rhythmic fashion, which in turn might play a role in the well-known susceptibility of these structures to generate epileptiform activity.

In conclusion, the available electrophysiological data do not indicate that a decrease of inhibitory GABAergic function is a feature of human epileptic cortex. The evidence, though indirect, gathered in the experiments of Masukawa *et al.* (1989) still awaits comparison with data to be obtained in the monkey hippocampus. Given the practical impossibility of gathering human non-epileptogenic hippocampal tissue, the use of this primate for purposes of comparison is the only feasible approach to this problem (cf. Schwartzkroin & Haglund, 1986).

In line with the electrophysiological evidence suggesting no impairment of GABAergic inhibition in the human epileptogenic cortex, a number of biochemical studies have shown no significant differences in GABA, GAD, or GABA transaminase between epileptogenic (spiking) and juxta-epileptogenic (non-spiking) neocortical areas (Schmidt *et al.*, 1984; Sherwin & van Gelder, 1986). Similar negative findings have been reported by Burnham *et al.* (1987) and by Sherwin *et al.* (1986), studying low-affinity GABA-type benzodiazepine binding. More recently Babb *et al.* (1989) have demonstrated that the loss of principal cells in epileptic hippocampi is associated with no decrease of GABAergic neurons and terminals, thus suggesting a GABA hyperinnervation of the remaining pyramidal cells. Babb *et al.* have also suggested that sprouting of GABA terminals or hyperinnervation of the few remnant principal neurons may serve 'to synchronize their membrane potentials so that subsequent excitatory inputs will trigger a large population of neurons for seizure onset' (Babb *et al.*, 1989).

Are epileptiform discharges induced by pharmacological manipulations different in the human neocortex?

A different method of assessing any possible mechanism underlying epileptogenicity in the human tissue obtained from epileptic patients might consist of analyzing the patterns of activity generated following pharmacological manipulations that have been shown to be effective in eliciting synchronous epileptiform activity in animal models. It can be reasoned that such experiments might serve to reveal differences that might exist between epileptogenic and non-epileptogenic tissue under extreme experimental conditions such as for instance, following blockade of the GABA$_A$ receptor subtype. Furthermore this type of study might disclose some characteristics of such activity in the human cortex. The following sections report some of the findings obtained in the course of such studies.

The bicuculline model

As mentioned above, the stimulus-induced, early IPSP is readily blocked by perfusion with the $GABA_A$ antagonist bicuculline methiodide (Avoli & Olivier, 1989; McCormick, 1989; Hwa *et al.*, 1992). As has been reported in lower animal species, this type of change is accompanied by the appearance of an intracellular burst of action potentials in response to electrical, focal stimuli (Fig. 7.12(A) and (B)). Furthermore, this burst is often characterized by the presence of repetitive afterdischarges (Fig. 7.12(B)). As illustrated in Fig. 7.12(C) and (D), the intracellularly recorded epileptiform event is associated with a synchronous, long-lasting field potential that displays different shape and polarity depending on the cortical layer from which it is recorded. Therefore these data indicate that in the human cortex pharmacological blockade of $GABA_A$-mediated conductances induces the appearance of synchronous, epileptiform discharges in response to focal extracellular stimuli.

The epileptiform activity induced by bicuculline in the human cortex shares a number of features with the PDS that is reported to occur in both in-vivo and in-vitro models of focal epilepsy (Prince & Connors, 1986). As already mentioned, these electrophysiological features are different from those of the stimulus-induced bursting response seen in some human cells in control medium. First, the epileptiform response disclosed by bicuculline is an all-or-none event. Second, it has a refractory period. Third, as also suggested by the depth profile analysis, it is a highly synchronized cellular event that can be observed in any given cell studied in any given slice. As shown in Fig. 7.12(E), the stimulus-induced epileptiform discharge recorded in the human cortex in the presence of bicuculline methiodide is a synaptically driven network event, since its amplitude shows a linear relationship with changes in the resting membrane potential (cf. Johnson & Brown, 1984).

The component of the bicuculline-induced epileptiform response that is more sensitive to NMDA-receptor antagonists is the late afterdischarge. This is illustrated in Fig. 7.12(F), which shows that APV does not block the early component while it reversibly abolishes the rhythmic afterdischarge. Therefore we can conclude that NMDA-activated conductances do contribute to this type of epileptiform response mainly by prolonging the depolarizing potential, while other receptor subtypes for excitatory amino acids are involved in the generation of the early part. In conclusion, these results indicate that bicuculline induces synchronous epileptiform discharges. A possible difference between epileptic human and rat or

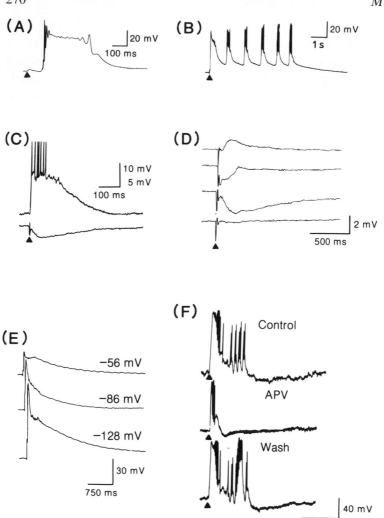

Fig. 7.12. Stimulus-induced epileptiform activity in the presence of bicuculline methiodide. (A) Typical long-latency paroxysmal depolarizing shift (PDS) that is preceded by an EPSP. (B) PDS that is followed by a long-lasting afterdischarge. (C) Simultaneously recorded intracellular (upper) and extracellular (lower) potential following an extracellular stimulus. (D) Changes in shape and polarity of field potentials recorded at different depths in the human neocortical slice bathed in bicuculline methiodide. Upper (first) trace was recorded in the pia; second, third and fourth traces were recorded at 400 μm, 1200 μm and 2400 μm, respectively. (E) Changes in amplitude of the stimulus-induced paroxysmal depolarizing shift during changes in V_m. The microelectrode was filled with potassium acetate and QX-314 to block the occurrence of fast action potentials. (F) Effects induced by the antagonist of the NMDA receptor APV upon the intracellularly recorded epileptiform discharge. (From Hwa et al., 1992.)

guinea pig neocortex is suggested by the occurrence of the prolonged epileptiform activity that is dependent on the involvement of NMDA-activated conductances. Whether there exist differences between the epileptiform discharges recorded in the presence of bicuculline in epileptogenic as compared to non-epileptogenic human neocortex still awaits investigation.

The magnesium-free model

Among the several in-vitro models of epilepsy discovered in the last decade, that induced by Mg^{2+}-free medium shows a number of interesting features. First, since the main cause for the hyperexcitability induced by the Mg^{2+}-free ACSF resides in the relief of the NMDA ionophore from the gating effect of Mg^{2+} (Nowak et al., 1984), this model represents an experimental paradigm for analyzing the role played by the NMDA receptor in the genesis of acute epileptiform discharges (Mody et al., 1987; Tancredi et al., 1990). Second, at least in the rat hippocampus the occurrence of Mg^{2+}-free spontaneous epileptiform discharges is accompanied by the preservation and even the enhancement of inhibitory, GABAergic mechanisms (Mody et al., 1987; Tancredi et al., 1990). Therefore this type of epileptiform activity might constitute an interesting model in which the relation between inhibition and epileptiform activity might be analyzed.

As illustrated in Fig. 7.13, perfusion with Mg^{2+}-free ACSF induces in neocortical slices spontaneous, synchronous discharges. In contrast to the activity induced by bicuculline methiodide, Mg^{2+}-free discharges occur spontaneously and consist of very prolonged events. The experiment illustrated in Fig. 7.13(A) shows also that during each epileptiform event the extracellular concentration of K^+ increases. These findings indicate that NMDA-activated conductances might play a role in triggering spontaneously occurring synchronous activity. Furthermore, the fact that these epileptiform discharges display features reminiscent of ictal discharges might further indicate that NMDA receptors are important for the self-sustaining mechanisms underlying prolonged paroxysmal discharges. The involvement of NMDA-activated conductances in this model is supported by the high sensitivity of the Mg^{2+}-free discharges to antagonists of the NMDA receptors such as APV, CPP, or MK-801 (Fig. 7.13).

Experiments performed on human cortical samples displaying different degrees of epileptogenicity indicate no difference in duration of the epileptiform discharges in the Mg^{2+}-free medium. However, when the

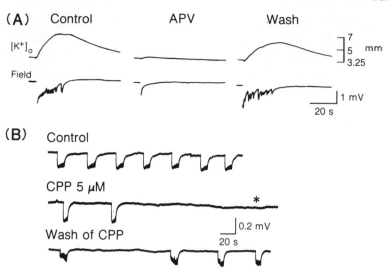

Fig. 7.13. Effects induced by (A) APV and (B) CPP on the epileptiform discharges recorded in two neocortical slices perfused with Mg^{2+}-free medium. (A) The extracellular potassium signal and the field potential were simultaneously recorded. ((A) from Avoli et al., 1987.)

distribution of the changes in the extracellular concentration of potassium associated with each of these discharges is measured through the neocortex there appear to be differences between slices obtained from epileptogenic neocortex as compared with thin non-epileptogenic slices (Avoli et al., unpublished results). These findings might reflect a different localization of NMDA receptors in the epileptogenic as compared to the non-epileptogenic neocortex. This conclusion, however, still awaits further experimental evidence. For instance it would be of pivotal importance to determine whether the different types of human neocortex have different laminar profiles of Ca^{2+} and K^+ signals in response to local applications of excitatory amino acid agonists (cf. Pumain et al. 1986).

Recent studies conducted in my laboratory have also disclosed that the generation of epileptiform bursts in Mg^{2+}-free medium can be controlled by adenosine (Kostopoulos et al., 1989). Thus, as shown in Fig. 7.14(A), the adenosine agonist 2-Cl-adenosine at concentrations of 0.3–3.0 μM is capable of inhibiting the prolonged stimulus-induced bursts recorded in human neocortical slices perfused with Mg^{2+}-free ACSF. Furthermore similar effects could be also observed on both stimulus-induced and spontaneously occurring bursts in an Mg^{2+}-free medium during bath-application of the adenosine-uptake inhibitor nitrobenzylthioinosine

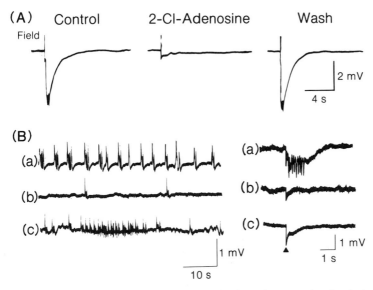

Fig. 7.14. (A) Depressant action of 2-Cl-adenosine on stimulus-induced Mg^{2+}-free epileptiform discharges. (B) Effects induced by nitrobenzylthioinosine upon spontaneously occurring (left traces) and stimulus-induced (right traces) Mg^{2+}-free epileptiform discharges. (a), (b), and (c) show the field potential activity in control, in nitrobenzylthioinosine and after a wash with control Mg^{2+}-free medium, respectively. (From Kostopoulos *et al.*, 1989.)

(Fig. 7.14(B)). Therefore endogenous adenosine in human epileptogenic neocortex can by itself act on adenosine receptors and thus control neuronal excitability.

Conclusions

The results reviewed in this chapter indicate that the electrophysiological analysis of the human cortical tissue maintained in vitro can reveal several aspects of neuronal function, including synaptic and non-synaptic cellular processes. Many of the phenomena so far identified appear remarkably similar to those analyzed in the rodent or feline cortex, yet these studies add relevant information on the membrane mechanisms that regulate excitability in the human brain. Furthermore, in spite of the many similarities to the results obtained in animal species, whether or not human cortical cells have unique pharmacological properties at the subreceptor level still awaits further analysis. For instance, although adenosine exerts clear actions on human neocortical cells, we still do not know what the subreceptor pharmacology of these effects is. The same conclusion applies to a number of biogenic amines and peptides. These findings might be relevant with regard to therapeutic strategies that have been developed recently for the treatment of different neurological diseases, using animal model systems.

Undoubtedly one has to recognize that the human electrophysiological studies have so far been unsuccessful in isolating any definite cellular mechanism that could account for the expression of epileptiform activity in situ. This failure is apparent both when the findings obtained in the epileptogenic human tissue are compared with data gathered in non-epileptogenic samples as well as when comparisons are made with results obtained in other mammalian species. The patterns of activity generated by neurons in human epileptogenic cortex appear in most instances to be remarkably 'normal'. To date some exceptions to this 'normal' behavior of human neurons in epileptogenic cortex include: (a) the ability of part of the cortical cells recorded in slices obtained from epileptic patients to generate bursts of action potentials in response to extracellular focal stimuli (Prince & Wong, 1981; Schwartzkroin *et al.*, 1983; Avoli & Olivier, 1989); (b) the appearance of a synchronous burst response during low frequency stimulation of dentate cells in the epileptogenic hippo-campus (Masukawa *et al.*, 1989); and (c) the occurrence of spontaneous, synchronous epileptiform activity in slices obtained from 'spiking' cortical samples (Reid & Palovcik, 1989). However, these findings are still far from being unequivocally accepted as the hallmark of human epiloptogenicity in vitro. On the one hand they appear to lack a consistent relationship with the degree of epileptogenicity of the analyzed tissue (this criticism does apply mainly to the occurrence of the stimulus-induced burst). On the other hand they have not often been replicated by other investigators.

A well-recognized problem inherent in the electrophysiological study of the human epileptogenic cortex maintained in vitro is that of establish-ing proper control samples: namely, which tissue should be used to obtain a normative baseline? This aspect has been addressed in many of the studies published to date and a pair of alternative solutions has been proposed. First, the use of neocortex and hippocampus obtained from the brain of non-human primates (Schwartzkroin *et al.*, 1983; Schwartzkroin & Haglund, 1986), and, second, the utilization of human samples removed from non-epileptic patients undergoing surgery for pathologies other than epilepsy. This second alternative has been criticized in the light of the possible existence of undetectable abnormalities in any type of human tissue that is surgically removed (Schwartzkroin, 1983). However, we should not overlook the results obtained in biochemical studies that demonstrate differences between epileptogenic and non-epileptogenic cortical areas (Brière *et al.*, 1986; Sherwin & van Gelder, 1986; Sherwin *et al.*, 1984).

A little understood, but not less important, problem that hinders the search for mechanisms that might account for the genesis of human epileptic seizures is that the etiological factors responsible for the occurrence of seizures are heterogeneous. It is not known whether by pooling data from different patients whose seizure disorders are etiologically diverse, it may be difficult to recognize the significance of certain data. A further problem that should be taken into account derives from the fact that so far we have made only a few efforts to study some 'hot' brain structures such as the amygdala. As in studies on the 'epileptic' human hippocampus, however, the only control tissue that we could realistically hope to obtain are samples from the non-human amygdala. Obviously the use of such control is open to criticism.

In the search for future avenues of research to be performed in human brain tissue maintained in vitro one must not underestimate the importance of using models of epileptiform activity that have been developed in animals. When performed in human epileptogenic tissue these studies might disclose patterns of activity that differ from those obtained in other species. Furthermore, these experiments might offer the opportunity to analyze the mechanisms of action of drugs that are used in medical practice or the effects induced by drugs that are being studied for their possible therapeutic anticonvulsant properties.

Acknowledgments

The original work reported in this chapter was supported by the Medical Research Council of Canada (MA-8109), the Fonds en Recherche en Santé du Québec, the Killam Foundation and the Savoy Foundation. I am grateful to C. Drapeau, G. Hwa, G. Kostopoulos, J. Louvel, A. Olivier, R. Pumain, P. Perreault, V. Tancredi and J.-G. Villemure for contributing to many of the experiments described here. I thank Dr P. Gloor for constructive and critical reading of an early draft of the manuscript, and Mr V. Epp for secretarial assistance.

References

Avoli, M. (1986). Inhibitory potentials in neurons of the deep layers of the "in vitro" neocortical slice. *Brain Research*, **370**: 165–70.

Avoli, M. (1988). GABAergic mechanisms and epileptic discharges. In *Neurotransmitter and Cortical Function: From Molecules to Mind*, ed. M. Avoli, T. A. Reader, R. W. Dykes & P. Gloor, pp. 187–205. New York: Plenum Press.

Avoli, M., Gloor, P., Kostopoulos, G. & Naquet, R. (eds.) (1990). *Generalized Epilepsy: Neurobiological Approaches*. Boston: Birkhäuser.

Avoli, M., Louvel, J., Pumain, R. & Olivier, A. (1987). Seizure like discharges induced by lowering $[Mg^{2+}]_o$ in the human epileptogenic neocortex maintained "in vitro". *Brain Research*, **417**: 199–203.

Avoli, M. & Olivier, A. (1987). Bursting in human epileptogenic neocortex is depressed by an *N*-methyl-D-aspartate antagonist. *Neuroscience Letters*, **76**: 249–54.

Avoli, M. & Olivier, A. (1989). Electrophysiological properties and synaptic responses in the deep layers of the human epileptogenic neocortex maintained "in vitro". *Journal of Neurophysiology*, **61**: 589–606.

Avoli, M., Perreault, P., Olivier, A. & Villemure, J.-G. (1988). 4-Aminopyridine induces a long-lasting depolarizing GABA-ergic potential in human neocortical and hippocampal neurons maintained in vitro. *Neuroscience Letters*, **94**: 327–32.

Babb, T. L., Pretorius, J. K., Kupfer, W. R. & Crandall, P. H. (1989). Glutamate decarboxylase-immunoreactive neurons are preserved in human epileptic hippocampus. *Journal of Neuroscience*, **9**: 2562–74.

Bonanno, G., Cavazzani, P., Andrioli, G. C., Asaro, D., Pellegrini, G. & Raiteri, M. (1989). Release-regulating autoreceptors of the $GABA_B$-type in human cerebral cortex. *British Journal of Pharmacology*, **96**: 341–6.

Brière, R., Sherwin, A. L., Robitaille, Y., Olivier, A., Quesney, L. F. & Reader, T. A. (1986). Alpha-1 adrenoceptors are decreased in human epileptic foci. *Annals of Neurology*, **19**: 26–30.

Brown, H. & DiFrancesco, D. (1980). Voltage-clamp investigations of membrane currents underlying pace-maker activity in rabbit sino-atrial node. *Journal of Physiology*, **308**: 331–51.

Burnham, W. M., Hwang, P. A., Hoffman, H.J., Becker, L. E., Murphy, E. G. & Kish, S. J. (1987). Benzodiazepine receptor binding in human epileptogenic cortical tissue. In *Fundamental Mechanisms of Human Brain*, ed. J. Engel, G. A. Ojemann, H. O. Lüders & P. D. Williamson, pp. 227–35. New York: Raven Press.

Calvin, W., Ojemann, G. A. & Ward, A. A. (1973). Human cortical neurons in epileptogenic foci: comparison of inter-ictal firing patterns to those of epileptic neurons in animals. *Electroencephalography and Clinical Neurophysiology*, **34**: 337–51.

Calvin, W. H. & Sypert, G. W. (1976). Fast and slow pyramidal tract neurons: an intracellular analysis of their contrasting repetitive firing properties in the cat. *Journal of Neurophysiology*, **39**: 420–34.

Connors, B. W., Gutnick, M. J. & Prince, D. A. (1982). Electrophysiological properties of neocortical neurons in vitro. *Journal of Neurophysiology*, **48**: 1302–20.

Connors, B. W., Malenka, R. C. & Silva, L. R. (1988). Two inhibitory post-synaptic potentials, and $GABA_A$ and $GABA_B$ receptor-mediated responses in neocortex of rat and cat. *Journal of Physiology*, **406**: 443–68.

Connors, B. W. & Prince, D. A. (1982). Effects of local anaesthetic QX-314 on the membrane properties of hippocampal pyramidal neurons. *Journal of Pharmacology and Experimental Therapeutics*, **220**: 476–81.

Delgado-Escueta, A. V., Ward, A. A., Jr, Woodbury, D. M. & Porter, R. J. (eds.) (1986). *Advances in Neurology*, vol. 44. New York: Raven Press.

Dingledine, R. (ed.) (1984). *Brain Slices.* New York: Plenum Press.

Ganong, A. H., Lanthorn, R. H. & Cotman, C. W. (1983). Kynurenic acid inhibits synaptic and acidic amino acid induced responses in the rat hippocampus and spinal cord. *Brain Research*, **273**: 170–4.

Gustafsson, B., Galvan, M., Grafe, P. & Wigström, H. (1982). A transient outward current in a mammalian central neurone blocked by 4-aminopyridine. *Nature*, **299**: 252–4.

Halliwell, J. V. (1986). M-current in human neocortical neurones. *Neuroscience Letters*, **67**: 1–6.

Halliwell, J. V. & Adams, P. R. (1982). Voltage-clamp analysis of muscarine excitation in hippocampal neurons. *Brain Research*, **250**: 71–92.

Hwa, G. G. C., Avoli, M., Olivier, A. & Villemure, J.-G. (1992). Bicuculline-induced epileptogenesis in the human neocortex maintained in vitro. *Experimental Brain Research*, **83**: 329–39.

Isokawa-Akesson, M., Wilson, C. L. & Babb, T. L. (1987). Structurally stable burst and synchronized firing in human amygdala neurons: auto- and cross-correlation analyses in temporal lobe epilepsy. *Epilepsy Research*, **1**: 17–34.

Jasper, H. H., Ward, A. A., Jr & Pope, A. (eds.) (1969) *Basic Mechanisms of the Epilepsies.* Boston, MA: Little, Brown.

Johnston, D. & Brown, T. H. (1984). Mechanisms of neuronal burst generation. In *Electrophysiology of Epilepsy*, ed. P. A. Schwartzkroin & H. V. Wheal, pp. 277–301. New York: Academic Press.

Kato, H., Ito, Z., Matsuoko, S. & Sakurai, Y. (1973). Electrical activities of neurons in the sliced human cortex *in vitro. Electroencephalography and Clinical Neurophysiology*, **35**: 457–62.

Knowles, W. D., Lüders, H., Hahn, J. F. & Awad, I. A. (1988). In vitro intracellular recordings from epileptic human neocortex and hippocampus. *Epilepsia*, **29**: 711.

Knowles, W. D., Lüders, H., Hahn, J. F. & Awad, I. A. (1989). Intracellular analysis of human epileptic neocortex: a progress report. Paper presented at the Annual meeting, American Association of Neurological Surgeons.

Kostopoulos, G., Drapeau, C., Avoli, M., Olivier, A. & Villemure, J.-G. (1989). Endogenous adenosine can reduce epileptiform activity in the human epileptogenic cortex maintained in vitro. *Neuroscience Letters*, **106**: 119–24.

Kostopoulos, G. & Psarropoulou, C. (1990). In vitro electrophysiology of a genetic model of generalized epilepsy. In *Generalized Epilepsy: Neurobiological Approaches*, ed. M. Avoli, P. Gloor, G. Kostopoulos & R. Naquet, pp. 137–57. Boston: Birkhäuser.

Krnjević, K. (1974). Chemical nature of synaptic transmission in vertebrates. *Physiological Reviews*, **54**: 419–50.

Kubota, M., Nakamura, M. & Tsukahara, N. (1985). Ionic conductance associated with electrical activity of guinea-pig red nucleus neurons in vitro. *Journal of Physiology*, **362**: 161–71.

Lacaille, J. C., Hwa, G. G. C. & Avoli, M. (1988). Electrophysiological properties of neurons in the superficial layers of human temporal cortex. *Society for Neuroscience Abstracts*, **14**: 882.

Lancaster, B. & Adams, P. R. (1986). Calcium-dependent current generating the afterhyperpolarization of hippocampal neurons. *Journal of Neurophysiology*, **55**: 1268–82.

Lighthall, J. W. & Prince, D. A. (1983). Neuronal activity in areas of chronic cortical injury, *Society for Neuroscience Abstracts*, **9**: 907.

Madison, D. V. & Nicoll, R. A (1984). Control of the repetitive discharge of rat CA1 pyramidal neurones in vitro. *Journal of Physiology*, **354**: 310–31.

Masukawa, L. M., Higashima, M., Kim, J. K. & Spencer, D. D. (1989). Epileptiform discharges evoked in hippocampal brain slices from epileptic patients. *Brain Research*, **493**: 168–74.

McCormick, D. A. (1989). GABA as an inhibitory neurotransmitter in human cerebral cortex. *Journal of Neurophysiology*, **62**: 1018–27.

McCormick, D. A., Connors, B. W., Lighthall, J. W. & Prince, D. A. (1985). Comparative electrophysiology of pyramidal and sparsely spiny stellate neurons of the neocortex. *Journal of Neurophysiology*, **54**: 782–806.

McCormick, D. A. & Williamson, A. (1989). Convergence and divergence of neurotransmitter action in human cerebral cortex. *Proceedings of the National Academy of Sciences, USA*, **86**: 8098–102.

Mody, I. & Heinemann, U. (1987). NMDA receptors of dentate gyrus granule cells participate in synaptic transmission following kindling. *Nature*, **326**: 701–4.

Mody, I., Lambert, J. D. C. & Heinemann, U. (1987). Low extracellular magnesium induced epileptiform activity and spreading depression in rat hippocampal slices. *Journal of Neurophysiology*, **57**: 869–88.

Mody, I., Stanton, P. K. & Heinemann, U. (1988). Activation of N-methyl-D-aspartate receptors parallels changes in cellular and synaptic properties of dentate gyrus granule cells after kindling. *Journal of Neurophysiology*, **59**: 1033–54.

Molony, C. J. & Paramelee, A. H. (1954). Convulsions in young infants as a result of pyridoxine (vitamin B6) deficiency. *Journal of the American Medical Association*, **154**: 405.

Nowak, L., Bregestovski, P., Ascher, P., Herbert, A. & Prochiantz, A. (1984). Magnesium gates glutamic activated channels in mouse central neurons. *Nature*, 307: 462–5.

Perreault, P. & Avoli, M. (1988). A depolarizing IPSP activated by synaptically-released GABA under physiological conditions in rat hippocampal pyramidal cells. *Canadian Journal of Physiology and Pharmacology*, **66**: 1100–2.

Perreault, P. & Avoli, M. (1989). Effect of low concentrations of 4-aminopyridine on CA1 pyramidal cells of the hippocampus. *Journal of Neurophysiology*, **61**: 953–70.

Prince, D. A. & Connors, B. W. (1986). Mechanisms of interictal epileptogenesis. In *Advances in Neurology*, vol. 44, ed. A. Delgado-Escueta, A. A. Ward Jr, D. M. Woodbury & R. J. Porter, pp. 275–99. New York: Raven Press.

Prince, D. A. & Futamachi, K. J. (1970). Intracellular recordings from chronic epileptogenic foci in the monkey. *Electroencephalography and Clinical Neurophysiology*, **29**: 496–510.

Prince, D. A. & Wong, R. K. S. (1981). Human epileptic neurons studied in vitro. *Brain Research*, **210**: 323–33.

Pumain, R., Louvel, J. & Kurcewicz, I. (1986). Long-term alterations in amino acid-induced ionic conductances in chronic epilepsy. In *Excitatory Amino Acids and Epilepsy*, ed. R. Schwarcz & Y. Ben-Ari, pp. 439–47. New York: Plenum Press.

Reid, S. A. & Palovcik, R. A. (1989). Spontaneous epileptiform discharges in isolated human cortical slices from epileptic patients. *Neuroscience Letters*, **98**: 200–4.

Schiffmann, S., Campistron, G., Tugendhaft, P., Brotchi, J., Flament-Durand, J., Geffard, M. & Verhaeghen, J.-J. (1988). Immunocytochemical detection of GABAergic nerve cells in the human temporal cortex using a direct γ-aminobutyric acid antiserum. *Brain Research*, **442**: 270–8.

Schmidt, D., Cornaggia, C. & Löscher, W. (1984). Comparative studies of the GABA system in neurosurgical brain specimens of epileptic and non-epileptic patients. In *Neurotransmitters, Seizures, and Epilepsy II*, ed. R. G. Fariello, P. L. Morsellis, K. G. Lloyd, L. F. Quesney & J. Engel Jr, pp. 275–83. New York: Raven Press.

Schwartzkroin, P. A. (1983). Reply to "Chronic epileptogenesis studied in vitro". *Annals of Neurology*, **14**: 596.

Schwartzkroin, P. A. & Haglund, M. M. (1986). Spontaneous rhythmic synchronous activity in epileptic human and normal monkey temporal lobe. *Epilepsia*, **27**: 523–33.

Schwartzkroin, P. A. & Knowles, W. D. (1984). Intracellular study of human epileptic cortex: in vitro maintenance of epileptiform activity? *Science*, **223**: 709–12.

Schwartzkroin, P. A. & Prince, D. A. (1976). Microphysiology of human cerebral cortex studied in vitro. *Brain Research*, **115**: 497–500.

Schwartzkroin, P. A., Turner, D. A., Knowles, W. D. & Wyler, A. R. (1983). Studies of human and monkey "epileptic" neocortex in the in vitro slice preparation. *Annals of Neurology*, **13**: 249–57.

Schwartzkroin. P. A. & Wheal, H. (1984). *Electrophysiology of Epilepsy*. London: Academic Press.

Schwindt, P. C., Spain, W. J. & Crill, W. E. (1988*a*). Influence of anomalous rectifier activation on afterhyperpolarization of neurons from cat sensorimotor cortex in vitro. *Journal of Neurophysiology*, **59**: 468–81.

Schwindt, P. C., Spain, W. J., Foehring, R. C., Chubb, M. C. & Crill, W. E. (1988*b*). Slow conductances in neurons from cat sensorimotor cortex in vitro and their role in slow excitability changes. *Journal of Neurophysiology*, **59**: 450–67.

Schwindt, P. C., Spain, W. J., Foehring, R. C., Stafstrom, C. E., Chubb, M. C. & Crill, W. E. (1988*c*). Multiple potassium conductances and their functions in neurons from cat sensorimotor cortex in vitro. *Journal of Neurophysiology*, **59**: 424–49.

Sherwin, A. L. (1988). Guide to neurochemical analysis of surgical specimens of human brain. *Epilepsy Research*, **2**: 281–8.

Sherwin, A., Matthew, E., Blain, M. & Guevremont, D. (1986). Benzodiazepine receptor binding is not altered in human epileptogenic cortical foci. *Neurology*, **36**: 1380–2.

Sherwin, A. L., Quesney, F., Gauthier, S., Olivier, A., Robitaille, Y., McQuaid, P., Harvey, C. & van Gelder, N. (1984). Enzyme changes in actively spiking areas of human epileptic cerebral cortex. *Neurology*, **36**: 1380–2.

Sherwin, A. L. & van Gelder, N. M. (1986). Amino acid and catecholamine markers of metabolic abnormalities in human focal epilepsy. In *Basic Mechanisms of the Epilepsies*, ed. A. V. Delgado-Escueta, A. A. Ward Jr, D. M. Woodbury & R. J. Porter, pp. 1011–32. New York: Raven Press.

Spain, W. J., Schwindt, P. C. & Crill, W. E. (1987). Anomalous rectification in neurons from cat sensorimotor cortex in vitro. *Journal of Neurophysiology*, **57**: 1555–75.

Stafstrom, C. E., Schwindt, M. C., Chubb, M. C. & Crill, W. E. (1985).
    Properties of persistent sodium conductance and calcium conductance of
    layer V neurons from cat sensorimotor cortex in vitro. *Journal of
    Neurophysiology*, **53**: 153–70.
Stafstrom, C. E., Schwindt, M. C., Flatman, J. A. & Crill, W. E. (1984).
    Properties of subthreshold response and action potential in layer V
    neurons from cat sensorimotor cortex in vitro. *Journal of Neurophysiology*,
    52: 244–63.
Sutor, B., & Hablitz, J. J. (1989). EPSPs in rat neocortical neurons in vitro. I.
    Electrophysiological evidence for two distinct EPSPs. *Journal of
    Neurophysiology*, **61**: 607–20.
Tancredi, V., Hwa, G. G. C., Zona, C., Brancati, A. & Avoli, M. (1990). Low
    magnesium epileptogenesis in the rat hippocampal slice:
    electrophysiological and pharmacological features. *Brain Research*, **511**:
    280–90.
Ward, A. A., Jr & Thomas, L. B. (1955). The electrical activity of single units in
    the cerebral cortex of man. *Electroencephalography and Clinical
    Neurophysiology*, **7**: 135–6.
Wyler, A. R., Fetz, E. E. & Ward, A. A., Jr (1973). Spontaneous firing patterns
    of epileptic neurons in the monkey motor cortex. *Experimental Neurology*,
    40: 567–85.
Wyler, A. R., Fetz, E. E. & Ward, A. A., Jr (1975). Firing patterns of epileptic
    and normal neurons in the chronic alumina focus in undrugged monkeys
    during different behavioral states. *Brain Research*, **98**: 1–20.
Wyler, A. R., Ojemann, G. A. & Ward, A. A. Jr (1982). Neurons in human
    epileptic cortex: correlation between unit and EEG activity. *Annals of
    Neurology*, **11**: 301–8.
Wyler, A. R. & Ward, A. A., Jr (1986). Neuronal firing patterns from
    epileptogenic foci of monkey and human. In *Advances in Neurology*,
    vol. 44, ed. A. V. Delgado-Escueta, A. A. Ward, Jr, D. M. Woodbury &
    R. J. Porter, pp. 967–89. New York: Raven Press.

8

Cell death, plasticity, and epilepsy: insights provided by experimental models of hippocampal sclerosis

JOANN E. FRANCK

Introduction

Many models of epilepsy, or of epileptic foci, take advantage of a genetic predisposition or induce a process(es) either in vivo or in vitro, often in conjunction with the use of convulsant drugs, which results in the most commonly accepted cornerstones of epileptogenicity – neuronal hyper-excitability and synchrony. The mechanisms of this aberrant functioning are then examined for insights they can provide into the genesis of seizures. In one sense seizures are the independent, rather than dependent, variable. The models discussed here, involving selective lesions of hippocampal subfields, are considered relevant for an entirely different reason. Selective cell death in the hippocampus – mesial temporal, or hippocampal, sclerosis (HS) – is observed in the majority of individuals with temporal lobe complex partial seizures and these individuals, as a group, represent the majority of the population with idiopathic, pharmacologically intractable epilepsy. By creating similar patterns of cell loss experimentally and examining the consequences to the functioning of the hippocampal remnants, hyperexcitability and/or synchrony become the dependent variables and the contribution of features of HS to their development can be studied.

Three theoretical positions can be taken. One extreme argues that HS is the benign consequence of seizures and is mechanistically unrelated to their cause except perhaps to provide sufficient neuropil for their propagation or expression. Another extreme argues that the lesion pre-dates and causes the development of temporal lobe epilepsy. This extreme does not preclude the lesion being induced by a seizure event (such as a febrile seizure or post-traumatic seizure); it requires only that the significant features of the lesion are in place before the development and diagnosis of epilepsy as a syndrome (rather than a seizure event). A third, and more tempered, hypothesis is that HS is progressive and develops concurrently with temporal lobe epilepsy as increasing numbers of selectively vulnerable neurons are damaged by repeated seizures. In this scheme aberrant function pre-dates cell loss. However, once produced, the features of the sclerotic lesion, through loss of neural modulation or neuroplastic rearrangement, may become mechanistically incorporated into, and a necessary component of, the seizure focus.

Decades of debate have not resolved which of these three positions is tenable in explaining the significance of HS in the progression of temporal lobe epilepsy. Each choice would predict that seizure activity might be observed in sclerotic hippocampal tissue, as has been demonstrated by presurgical depth recordings and intraoperative recordings from the hippocampal surface. Each would also predict that removing the hippo-campus – by taking out the offending tissue or interrupting a neces-sary pathway of propagation – would 'cure' or improve the epileptic syndrome.

Some of the questions generated by these hypotheses can be approached by creating similar patterns of cell damage in animal models and determining whether these patterns of damage, once produced, lead to chronic excitability changes and, if so, what feature(s) of the lesion is(are) relevant. Two experimental manipulations that selectively destroy vulner-able hippocampal neurons in patterns quite similar to (if not identical with) those seen in HS are the administration of kainic acid (KA) and the production of transient forebrain ischemia (IS).

In what follows, the effects of a loss of specific hippocampal subfields, or neuronal populations, produced by KA injection or IS on the functioning of remaining neurons and the potential relevance that the observed functional changes may have to temporal lobe epilepsy are discussed. Three variables are considered to be significant. Two of these variables – the cell loss per se, and plasticity amongst remaining circuits that may result from such cell loss – are independent variables and their consequences are amenable to experimental evaluation. The third variable – seizures, specifically whether they are a feature of the lesion process, and whether they develop as a consequence of the lesion – is more problematic. The seizure is being measured as a lesion consequence; yet, related lesion consequences (e.g., activity-dependent induction of onco-genes or growth factors) may be quite different if developed on a seizure background versus a normal background. In a sense seizures become both dependent and independent variables.

Hippocampal sclerosis in humans

Cell loss

When the hippocampus of individuals with temporal lobe epilepsy is examined, either at autopsy or following its resection for treatment of intractable seizures, a pattern of damage is observed that is sufficiently consistent to conclude that certain hippocampal subfields and neuronal populations are selectively vulnerable, and others relatively resistant, to degeneration. When a comparison is made with a normal human hippocampus, there is a very striking, and near complete, loss of pyramidal cells seen in both CA1 and CA3; CA3, however, is often variably affected and in many instances some neurons remain in this subfield. There is a relatively abrupt transition between the glial scar, which was once the CA1 pyramidal cell layer, and the subiculum, which often remains quite heavily populated with neurons. Curiously, the dentate gyrus granule cells and an intermediate patch of pyramidal cells, often called the 'resistant sector' and most likely corresponding at least in part to the ill-characterized CA2 region, also survive (Babb & Brown, 1986).

More subtle but equally striking is an apparent pattern of selective vulnerablity and survival of discrete populations of hippocampal local circuit cells. Most neurons in the dentate hilar region appear to be lost (de Lanerolle *et al.*, 1989; Robbins *et al.*, 1991). This includes those containing somatostatin, which project to the outer molecular layer of the dentate gyrus (Bakst *et al.*, 1986) and, most likely, those cells (the mossy cells) forming the commissural/association projection to the inner molecular layer (Ribak *et al.*, 1985; Amaral & Witter, 1989). It has also been demonstrated that local circit neurons containing glutamic acid decarboxylase (GAD), which are presumably inhibitory/GABAergic, survive in all regions of the sclerotic hippocampus (Babb *et al.*, 1989; Sloviter *et al.*, 1991). They are present even in those areas in which principal cells have been lost – a finding that seems paradoxical given our 'expectations' of hyperexcitable tissue and the fact that many experimental models of seizures involve reduced function at inhibitory synapses, or a structural loss of inhibitory neurons.

Plasticity

In addition to this stereotyped pattern of neuron loss, several types of neuroplastic rearrangements amongst remaining cells have been identified. An aberrant pathway that is perhaps most characteristic of sclerotic epileptic hippocampus is formed by mossy fibres of dentate granule cells projecting back through the granule cell layer to form a recurrent terminal field in the region of the granule cell proximal dendrites (Sutula *et al.*, 1989; Babb *et al.*, 1991). While it is unclear whether this is an abnormal pathway, the granule cells have been shown also to project to the pyramidal neurons remaining in the 'resistant sector' (Houser *et al.* 1990).

The picture of hippocampal circuitry with severe sclerosis that is maintained by these surviving neurons has only begun to be determined. If one examines each stage of neuronal processing in the context of the simple trisynaptic circuit of intrinsic hippocampal connectivity, several salient features emerge from this picture. First, the dentate granule cells persist and presumably are still a primary terminal field of limbic cortical inputs, although necrosis is also often observed in these regions as well. GABAergic local circuit cells immediately deep to the granule cell layer also survive and continue to innervate granule cells and, to the extent that the dendrites of these inhibitory neurons extend to the molecular layer, they too presumably receive direct excitation, often at low threshold, from afferent fibres. Thus, the morphological substrates for simple recurrent and feedforward inhibition persist in the dentate gyrus. In addition, the aberrant recurrent mossy fiber projection to the inner molecular layer is positioned ideally to excite both granule cells and inhibitory pyramidal basket cells.

Thus, the altered circuitry of the sclerotic dentate gyrus still has both excitatory and inhibitory components, which appear to interconnect in such a way as to allow rudimentary modulation of neuronal activity. However, the primary terminal field of dentate granule cells, CA3, is either missing or is severely depopulated of pyramidal cells. The mossy fibers from the granule cells do, however, project to the region of the 'resistant sector': this pathway connecting the remnants of the hippocampus may be critical in propagating seizure activity through sclerotic tissue.

Finally, a major source of hippocampal efferents and the last neuron in the trisynaptic circuit, CA1 pyramidal cells, is missing. This is perhaps the most constant feature of human HS and the loss of this subfield raises the interesting question of how locally generated aberrant activity may propagate further through this tissue.

Experimental 'sclerosis' in rat

Each feature of the sclerotic hippocampus may more or less mechanistically contribute to the generation of seizure activity. In the rat animal model, certain characteristics of HS can be duplicated by selective lesioning of hippocampal neurons with KA and IS. One can then ask a relatively simple question: when produced experimentally, do these patterns of cell damage and plasticity promote the development of seizures in vivo or hyperexcitability and synchrony in remaining neurons in vitro?

Systemic kainic acid: lesion

Kainic acid, injected systemically (sys), or into the ventricles (icv), has been used to destroy hippocampal neurons selectively. Each route of administration produces a differing pattern of cell damage and plasticity that can be used as tools in attempts to understand the consequences of such hardwired alterations to epileptogenesis.

Kainic acid injected systemically often produces a variable, but bilateral, pattern of major subfield damage. As seen in Fig. 8.1(a), CA3 is typically lost but CA1 is also often lesioned (Ben-Ari, 1985). Such a pattern of cell loss suggests that several mechanisms of selective vulnerability may be at work; sys KA may kill neurons both by direct receptor interaction in CA3 and by inducing acute recurrent seizures throughout limbic circuits, resulting in seizure-induced damage in CA1.

In addition to the damage observed in major subfields, sys KA also differentially damages local circuit neurons. As in human HS, GAD-containing cells in rats survive sys KA. Unlike human HS, a significant number of dentate hilar somatostatin-containing neurons – particularly in the dorsal and ventral 'blades' of the hilus – also survive sys KA (Fig. 8.1(b)). This route of KA administration does, however, produce a dense band of terminal degeneration in the dentate inner molecular layer, indicating that mossy cells are also damaged (Fig. 8.1(c)).

In addition to this pattern of cell loss, specific patterns of plasticity occur, amongst remaining neurons, that mimic features seen in temporal lobe epilepsy. Most dramatic is the growth of a recurrent mossy fiber pathway, like that shown in Fig. 8.1(d), from the dentate granule cells to the same inner molecular layer region as that observed in humans (Nadler *et al.*, 1980*a*). Evidence suggests that this aberrant pathway most likely does not form in response to the loss of a significant portion of the efferent targets of mossy fibers, CA3 and dentate hilar cells (Laurberg & Zimmer, 1981), but rather grows to reoccupy that portion of the granule cell dendrites deafferented by loss of dentate hilar commissural and association projections.

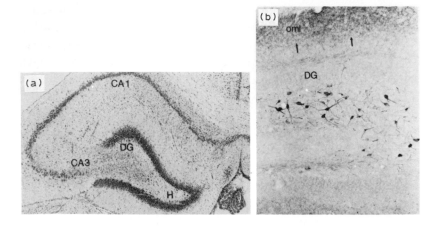

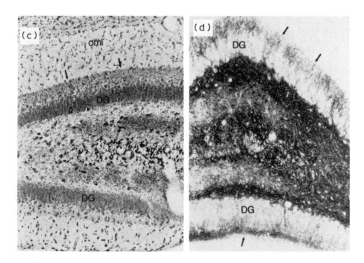

Fig. 8.1. The lesion produced by systemic kainic acid (sys KA) in rat. (a) A Nissl-stained view of a pattern of cell loss produced by sys KA; in this micrograph, CA3 is damaged but CA1 and the dentate gyrus appear relatively spared. (b) Neurons containing somatostatin-like immunoreactivity in the dentate hilus appear to survive sys KA and their terminal field in the outer molecular layer (arrows) is quite apparent (c) In tissue stained for degenerating neurons and terminals, sys KA is seen to destroy some hilar neurons (dying CA3c cells are also apparent): the band of terminal debris in the inner dentate molecular layer (arrows) suggests the presence of dying mossy cells. (d) In Timm-stained material the development of a recurrent mossy fiber pathway following sys KA is shown (arrows). CA1, CA1 subfield of hippocampus; CA3, CA3 subfield of hippocampus; DG, dentate gyrus; H, dentate hilus; oml, outer molecular layer.

Systemic kainic acid: consequences

Spontaneous recurrent behavioral seizures in rats, phenotypically like those seen in human complex partial epilepsy, develop in the days and weeks following sys KA injections (Ben-Ari, 1985; Cronin & Dudek, 1988). These are accompanied by electrographic seizures in limbic cortical regions and throughout the hippocampus. Despite the appearance of this epileptic syndrome and the obvious relevance that the pattern of cell loss and plasticity produced by sys KA has to morphological features of epilepsy there have been surprisingly few studies of the intrahippocampal mechanisms of seizure genesis. Studies examining the postlesion physiology of individual cell types in hippocampus, in attempts to identify substrates of epileptogenesis in this model, have concentrated on dentate granule cells. When these neurons are studied in vitro following sys KA, antidromic stimulation of the mossy fibres has been reported to elicit synaptically mediated multiple population spikes from the granule cell layer (Tauck & Nadler, 1985). Cronin *et al.* (1992) studied similar tissue in vitro but found that granule cells responded normally to antidromic stimulation; multiple population spikes were not observed and chloride-dependent inhibitory postsynaptic potentials (IPSPs) were present. Indeed, Sloviter (1992) has presented data obtained in vivo indicating that inhibition may be enhanced in granule cells following sys KA.

Cronin *et al.* (1992) have shown, however, that if sys KA-lesioned hippocampal slices are perfused with doses of bicuculline that are without effect in normal tissue, single granule cells will respond to stimulation with prolonged aberrant bursts. These data suggest that the morphological features of sys KA-lesioned dentate gyrus are capable of sustaining epileptogenic activity amongst granule cells. The data also required, however, that additional mechanisms exist that perturb apparently enhanced inhibitory function to allow bursting to occur.

Intraventricular kainic acid: lesion

Intraventricularly, in low to moderate doses, KA kills cells associated with high densities of high affinity KA receptors – primarily CA3 pyramidal cells in rat (Nadler *et al.*, 1980*b*). Cells in CA1 remain undamaged, unless significantly higher doses with unacceptable mortality are given (Nadler *et al.*, 1978) and presumably maintain their efferent target relationships with sites outside the hippocampus; these cells have, however, lost roughly 85% of their afferents from the CA3 Schaffer

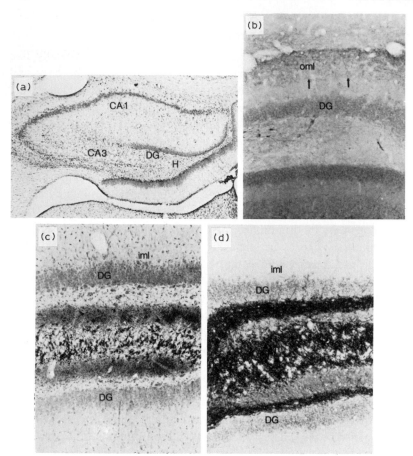

Fig. 8.2. The lesion produced by intraventricular kainic acid (icv KA) in rat. (a) Nissl-stained view of a pattern of cell loss produced by icv KA; CA3 neurons are selectively damaged. (b) Somatostatin-containing cells in the dentate hilus are largely lost; some immunoreactivity does persist in their terminal field in the outer molecular layer (arrows). (c) In silver-stained material, extensive degeneration is seen in CA3 following icv KA; however, from the absence of terminal debris in the inner molecular layer (iml), this does not appear to include significant loss of commissural/association neurons. (d) Intraventricular KA also does not promote the formation of a recurrent mossy fiber pathway in the inner molecular layer. Abbreviations as in Fig. 8.1.

collaterals (Nadler *et al.*, 1980*c*). Dentate granule cells also remain intact (Fig. 8.2(a)).

Intraventricular KA in rats also produces a selective pattern of local circuit cell damage. As in human HS, somatostatin-containing neurons deep in the dentate hilus are lost (Fig. 8.2(b)). On the basis of degeneration stains showing only minimal debris in the inner molecular layer of the dentate gyrus, it appears the icv KA does not significantly damage commissural–association mossy cells (Fig. 8.2(c)) (J. E. Franck, unpublished results). Local circuit cells containing GAD in rat are relatively impervious to icv KA (Franck *et al.*, 1988) and, as is the case in human HS, they survive and maintain their terminal fields in both CA1 and the dentate granule cell layer and they persist, in apparent isolation, in the neuropil of CA3.

Plasticity occurs also amongst remaining circuits following icv KA. Reoccupation of vacated synapses in CA1 is observed; however, the source of these sprouted fibers is unclear (Nadler *et al.*, 1980a). Because simultaneously recorded pairs of CA1 pyramidal neurons fail to show increased synaptic coupling following icv KA lesions, the reinnervating synapses do not appear to represent recurrent collateralization amongst neighboring CA1 cells (Nakajima *et al.*, 1991). They may, however, originate from more temporal CA3 pyramidal cells that survive the lesion.

Unlike sys KA, icv KA does not induce the formation of an appreciable recurrent mossy fiber pathway into the dentate molecular layer (Fig. 8.2(d)). This lack of sprouting with icv KA may be due, in part, to the pattern of hilar cell damage observed. While icv KA kills neurons, such as those containing somatostatin, that project to the outer molecular layer, there is minimal terminal debris in the inner molecular layer following this treatment. Thus, damage to a critical population of neurons with denervation of the inner molecular layer may be required for mossy fiber growth but may not be a feature of icv KA lesions.

Intraventricular kainic acid: consequences

Most studies examining the consequences of icv KA in animal models have concentrated on CA1 pyramidal cells. Although this subfield is typically absent in human HS, studying the mechanisms of hyperexcitability in these cells may provide insight into general mechanisms of epileptogenesis in single neurons from damaged hippocampus. Both bilateral (Franck *et al.*, 1988) and unilateral (Ashwood *et al.*, 1986) injections have been used. When KA is injected bilaterally in rat, CA1 dendrites are deprived of both association and commissural connections from CA3; when unilateral injections are used, the commissural input from contralateral CA3 neurons survives. Despite these morphological differences the physiological properties of CA1 neurons surviving either bilateral or unilateral icv KA are quite similar. When CA1 pyramidal cells are studied in vitro several weeks following icv KA, synchronous, uninhibited burst discharges, which appear to have both an NMDA-dependent and non-NMDA-dependent component, are observed spontaneously and following synaptic stimulation (Lancaster & Wheal, 1984; Ashwood & Wheal, 1987; Franck *et al.*, 1988; Cornish & Wheal, 1989; Simpson *et al.*, 1991; Turner & Wheal, 1991). This aberrant activity is associated with a loss of both early and late IPSPs, in spite of the fact that interneurons remain physiologically viable and pyramidal cells still respond to exogenous GABA (Lancaster & Wheal, 1984; Ashwood *et al.*, 1986; Franck *et al.* 1988; Nakajima *et al.*, 1991). At more prolonged latencies after icv KA, spontaneous ictal events and dramatic afterdischarge activity are no longer prominent in CA1 (Franck & Schwartzkroin, 1985; Franck *et al.*, 1988). However, even at relatively long intervals after KA lesions, multiple action potential discharge, while not as dramatic as that observed several weeks postlesion, can still be evoked from CA1 neurons, and both the early and late IPSPs have been reported to remain depressed, resulting in a relatively chronic deficit in inhibitory function in CA1 (Franck *et al.*, 1988; Cornish & Wheal, 1989).

The finding that functional inhibition is severely compromised in this tissue is notable, since much of the machinery for inhibition remains apparently viable, as in human HS. Neurons containing GAD survive in CA1 and, at the light microscopic level, they maintain a healthy terminal field amongst CA1 pyrimidal cells. Receptors for GABA, at least those associated with the Cl^--dependent $GABA_A$ conductance, are not decreased at times of hyperexcitability (Franck *et al.*, 1988). It is likely that the circuitry necessary to activate GABAergic neurons is either missing, or altered, postlesion. In the hippocampus, feedforward excitation of inhibitory neurons, with subsequent inhibition of pyramidal cells, occurs at lower thresholds than are required for direct pyramidal cell activation; this feed forward pathway appears to be a much more prominent mechanism of inhibiting pyramidal cells than does recurrent inhibition. Loss of CA3 projections may compromise this mode of interneuron activation. While this may account for spontaneously observed burst firing, it is difficult to reconcile a loss of IPSPs with stimulation experiments that demonstrate that local circuit cells are activated concurrently with uninhibited burst discharge in CA1 pyramidal cells (Nakajima *et al.*, 1991). It seems necessary also to postulate that there is a dysfunction at synapses mediating recurrent inhibition – either pyramidal cell onto interneuron or vice versa. The results of Nakajima *et al.* (1991), studying simultaneously recorded pairs of pyramidal cells and interneurons, lend some support to this hypothesis. We found fewer instances of direct synaptic coupling between these two cell populations in KA-lesioned than in normal hippocampus. There is also more recent evidence that suggests that the failure of inhibition in KA-lesioned tissue is due, at least in part, to a decrease in GABA release (Arias *et al.*, 1990).

The lesions, and resulting plasticity, induced by icv and sys KA are distinctly different in some respects (primarily in the fascia dentata) and similar in others (denervation of surviving CA1 pyramidal cells), yet both produce long-term behavioral and electrographic epileptogenesis. In each model hippocampal cell populations have been identified that may mediate aberrant activity. Unfortunately, however, there are significant gaps in experimental information. In order to determine the extent of the differences in the mechanisms of epileptogenesis in these two models it is necessary to examine the fascia dentata following icv KA lesions and the remaining pyramidal cells following sys KA. A priori, there is no reason to hypothesize that loss of a single critical population of neurons, or development of a single critical aberrant pathway, mediates seizures in both these models. Just as in human hippocampal epilepsy with HS, where certain morphological features are frequent but certainly not universal, entirely different *patterns* of morphological change may interact to produce, or permit epileptogenesis.

Ischemia: lesion

Ischemia also selectively damages vulnerable neurons in the hippocampus in patterns that are similar to human HS: in a sense IS 'completes' the stereotyped HS lesion. The pattern of cell loss produced by IS in rat is shown in Fig. 8.3(a). When IS is induced (Pulsinelli & Buchan, 1988), two well-identified populations of neurons in the dentate hilus are destroyed quite rapidly. These include a population of somatostatin containing neurons in the taper of the hilus that normally project to the outer regions of the dentate molecular layer (Johansen *et al.*, 1987; Fig. 8.3(b)) and a population of neurons that is associated with dense terminal debris in the dentate inner molecular layer (Fig. 8.3(c)) and most likely correspond to mossy cells (Crain *et al.*, 1988) as has been shown in other models of selective hilar cell vulnerability (Sloviter, 1987; Scharfman & Schwartz-kroin, 1990*a*). More striking is the complete and consistent loss of pyramidal cells in CA1, which occurs several days following IS (Pulsinelli *et al.*, 1982) and, like HS, disrupts hippocampal–limbic cortical projections; in contrast to KA injection, CA3 pyramidal cells (and local circuit

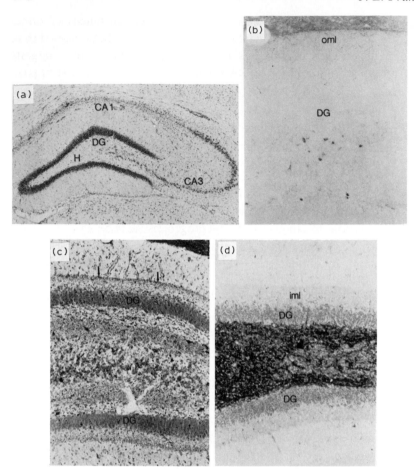

Fig. 8.3. The lesion produced by transient forebrain ischemia (IS) in rat.
(a) Nissl-stained micrograph of the pattern of cell loss produced by IS; most
obvious is a complete loss of subfield CA1. (b) Somatostatin-containing neurons
in the dentate hilus are selectively destroyed by IS. (c) Terminal debris in the inner
dentate molecular layer (arrows) suggest that mossy cells are also lesioned by IS.
(d) Despite significant loss of dentate hilar cells, Timm-stained material suggests
that an aberrant mossy fibre pathway does not develop following IS. Abbreviations as in Figs. 8.1 and 8.2.

neurons) remain undamaged. Again, as in human HS and the KA-
lesioned hippocampus, local circuit neurons containing GABA survive
in regions of primary cell loss (CA1) and in the dentate hilus immediately
beneath the granule cell layer (Johansen *et al.*, 1983).

Plasticity in the hippocampus that occurs following IS has been poorly
characterized. The primary target of CA3 pyrimidal cells, CA1, is gone

and it is unclear whether new (recurrent?) or enhanced terminal fields form in CA2 in response to this damage. There is some suggestion that major redirection of CA3 axons does not occur. First, in rat, in spite of CA1 loss, Shaffer collaterals have been shown to 'die back' very slowly and are perhaps sustained to some extent by connectivity to surviving local circuit cells in CA1. Secondly, at long survival times post-IS, when these axons do begin to disappear in the stratum radiatum of CA1, there appears to be a gradual cell loss in CA3, suggesting that significant and sustaining new synapses have not been formed (Onodera *et al.*, 1990). Most interestingly, in spite of the significant loss of dentate hilar neurons – which appears to be more severe than that seen with sys KA – there is minimal growth of recurrent mossy fibres into the dentate molecular layer (Fig. 8.3(d)). Even in the extreme case shown in Fig. 8.3(d), where the hilus appears shrunken, only occasional patches of staining suggestive of mossy fibres are apparent in the inner molecular layer.

Ischemia: consequences

Fewer data are available on the behavioral and physiological consequences of lesions induced by IS. Results suggest that the functioning of remaining hippocampal tissue in this model stands in marked contrast to that observed following KA lesions. Intrahippocampal multiunit recording in vivo suggests that IS lesions are not associated, either at the time of the lesion (Armstrong *et al.*, 1989; Imon *et al.*, 1991) or several weeks following cell damage (Buzsáki *et al.*, 1989), with seizures or increased excitability – indeed, acute increases in paired-pulse inhibition have been reported (Chang *et al.*, 1989). Single unit and population recordings from remaining hippocampal granule cells and CA3 pyramidal cells in vitro up to six months post-IS also do not support the hypothesis that this pattern of cell loss leads to epileptiform activity or to a loss of early or late IPSPs in surviving neurons (Jensen *et al.*, 1991; Franck, unpublished results).

Significance of morphological changes to epileptogenesis

The lesions produced by IS and KA have certain features in common and others that are characteristic of only one manipulation and each is associated with different physiological consequences at both the single-cell and systems level. This can be used to test hypotheses about the significance of both the cell loss per se and the consequences of the plasticity that occurs in HS.

Dentate hilus damage

The significance of the loss of discrete populations of local circuit cells in the dentate hilus has gained considerable attention because this region appears to be so selectively vulnerable both in human HS and in a variety of animal models (Sloviter, 1987; de Lanerolle *et al.*, 1989; Scharfman & Schwartzkroin, 1990*b*). While numerous populations of neurons can be defined in the hilus based on both morphology (Amaral, 1978) and neurochemistry (Sloviter & Nilaver, 1987), two types that appear highly vulnerable to epileptic damage have commanded particular attention. These are the somatostatin-containing neurons and the source of the commissural–association system, the mossy cells. There is a significant loss of somatostatin immunoreactivity, and of neurons in general, in the epileptic human hilus. Population recordings from granule cells in experimental animals with this pattern of cell loss, induced by intense afferent stimulation, show a reduction of paired-pulse inhibition in the presence of normal numbers of GABAergic neurons (Sloviter, 1987). These findings have fostered the hypothesis that this pattern of cell loss promotes epileptogenesis in granule cells by removing a source of direct inhibitory modulation (somatostatin-containing neurons) and by eliminating a neuronal population (mossy cells) that may be a necessary intermediary in activating GABAergic neurons.

The lesions produced by KA and IS cause similar patterns of hilar cell death in different combinations and the consequences of this damage in these models may shed light on the significance of the cell loss. Intraventricular KA produces a loss of somatostatin cells without extensive damage to commissural–association neurons (based on degeneration stains) and without the growth of recurrent mossy fibres. This would seem an ideal preparation to examine a relatively selective loss of somatostatin-containing hilar cells; it is unfortunate that these granule cells have not been extensively studied.

Systemic KA, on the other hand, spares a significant population of hilar somatostatin-containing neurons but does induce degeneration of commissural–association pathways. As seen, granule cells in this model can sustain epileptogenic activity if challenged appropriately (Cronin *et al.*, 1992). While this model also has other significant morphological alterations, these data lead to the conclusion that loss of somatostatin-containing neurons is not *necessary* for epileptogenesis in the fascia dentata.

The significance of mossy cell loss in this model is difficult to determine. If one examines granule cells in this tissue after cell death has occurred, but before significant neuroplasticity is allowed to compensate for (or contribute to) epileptogenesis, then population hyperexcitability is observed. This suggests that loss of commissural–association neurons may compromise inhibitory function in the tissue (Sloviter, 1992). Alternatively, there may be a transient dysfunction of inhibitory neurons that relies on intrinsic rather than synaptic properties, as has been observed in rat pyramidal cells following KA lesion (Franck & Schwartzkroin, 1985).

Ischemia produces a yet different pattern of morphological change in a manner that does not involve acute seizure induction: both somatostatin neurons and the commissural–association system are damaged, but there is little evidence of plasticity in remaining dentate circuits. Our recordings in this model indicate that this pattern of damage per se does not result in a reduction of inhibition or in consistent excitability changes leading to interictal bursts or to spontaneous or evoked ictal events in dentate granule cells or their synaptic targets, CA3 pyramidal cells, nor does a behavioral epileptic syndrome develop in such animals. These data suggest that the loss of somatostatin-containing neurons and mossy cells are not a *sufficient* condition for epileptogenesis.

CA3 and CA1

In addition to the loss of local circuit neurons, KA and ischemic lesions also allow some hypotheses regarding the significance of major subfield loss to the development of epileptogenesis. In human HS the most consistent loss is subfield CA1. Yet physiological data from animals with IS lesions suggest that loss of this subfield alone – at least without the complete constellation of damage observed in HS – does not lead to temporal lobe seizures.

Rat hippocampi with KA lesions also have lost CA3 and this loss may be critical to the development of granule cell hyperexcitability. CA3 neurons do project axon collaterals back to the dentate hilus, where they may contact neurons that then modulate granule cell activity (Ishizuka *et al.*, 1990; Pokorný & Schwartzkroin, 1991). Increased excitability in CA3 pyramidal cells is associated with dramatic inhibition of granule cells in vitro (Scharfman & Schwartzkroin, 1990b). Thus, by removing both the primary granule cell terminal field and a strong, presumably disynaptic, inhibitory effect, loss of CA3 may be critical to dentate epileptogenicity and to the development of an epileptic syndrome in these animals.

GABAergic circuits

Several aberrant pathways have been identified in HS that also occur to varying degrees in experimental sclerosis, allowing the events critical for their growth and their subsequent effect on surviving neurons to be studied.

One such example is the persistence of GABAergic neurons in experimental and in clinical HS. The evidence that the function of these neurons, and the way they interact with principal cells, may be altered in a dynamic fashion underscores their potential significance, not simply in whether they inhibit other neurons but in whether they may contribute actively to mechanisms of synchronization. Recent data suggest that the axons of GABAergic neurons may sprout and expand their terminal field in the dentate gyrus of KA-lesioned rat tissue (Davenport *et al.*, 1990). Thus, in this tissue, the relative morphological contributions of these neurons to the intrinsic circuitry of the hippocampus may be greater than that seen in normal tissue. While such a phenomenon has not been examined in HS tissue it has been demonstrated that GABAergic cells persist in regions such as the dentate gyrus where granule cells are moderately, but definitely, decreased in number; more notably, GABAergic cells in regions of complete pyramidal cell atrophy, such as CA1, survive and appear to form a 'subfield' of relatively pure inhibitory cells. Whether these neurons functionally interact with each other or with other remaining neurons in the sclerotic hippocampus or even with extrahippocampal regions has not been examined. Spontaneous inhibitory potentials have been observed in human epileptic tissue in vitro (Schwartzkroin & Haglund, 1986) and imaging studies have shown in vivo that the temporal lobes may actually be hypometabolic in all but periods of ictal activity. It is intriguing to speculate that the surviving populations of inhibitory neurons may play a role in these phenomena. Populations of isolated inhibitory neurons are present in both KA- and IS-lesioned tissue and these preparations provide an opportunity for studying the functioning of, and interactions formed by, these cells.

Recurrent mossy fibers

Recurrent mossy fibers in the dentate inner molecular layer are a prominent feature of both human HS and the sys KA lesion. The fascia dentata damaged by sys KA is characterized by the presence of this aberrant pathway and by the loss of commissural–association neurons.

Physiological studies in IS-lesioned tissue suggest that loss of this latter population of cells does not in itself promote epileptogenesis in the dentate gyrus.

Cronin *et al.* (1992) have shed light on this issue by presenting findings that suggest that rat fascia dentata with recurrent mossy fibers may respond normally, or perhaps with increased inhibition (Sloviter, 1992), unless the tissue is perturbed or challenged. They demonstrated that granule cells in tissue lesioned with sys KA responded normally, but they showed also that superfusing the same tissue with doses of bicuculline that had no effect on normal granule cells resulted in burst discharges to antidromic stimulation that correlated with the extent of recurrent mossy fiber innervation. It is noteworthy that human epileptic dentate gyrus studied in vitro responds in a similar fashion. The synaptic and intrinsic properties of single granule cells in this tissue often appear quite normal (but see Masukawa *et al.*, 1989, 1991). If this tissue is exposed to bicuculline, however, a subset of hippocampal biopsies burst to stimulation; this subset has a recurrent mossy fiber plexus in the inner molecular layer of the fascia dentata although non-bursting tissue does not (Pokorný *et al.*, 1991). Here too, however, the finding that such bursting activity requires reduced inhibition indicates that formation of this pathway is not a sufficient condition for epileptogenesis – mechanisms that can episodically perturb such circuitry must also be present. The fact that such activity may not be a constant feature of these granule cells but may be episodic depending on the state of other components of the surviving circuitry has particular relevance to the episodic nature of epileptic seizures. This model may be particularly useful for examining the types and mechanisms of perturbations that may lead to epileptogenic activity resulting from the hardwired mossy fiber substrate.

Seizures

This chapter has reviewed the clinically relevant lesions produced by three different manipulations and, on the basis of the physiological consequences of these lesions, conclusions have been drawn about the significance of morphological changes. Another factor that needs to be considered is whether the damage itself was produced by seizures or by a manipulation that induces seizures. Human HS is, of course, observed in a neural system that has experienced repeated, poorly controlled, seizures, often for decades. Whether or not HS causes seizures, compelling evidence suggests that the reverse is true – seizures in animals induced through appropriate pathways can cause exactly the pattern of damage observed in human HS (Ben-Ari *et al.*, 1979, 1980; Nadler & Cuthbertson, 1980; Nadler *et al.*, 1981; Sater & Nadler, 1987; Sloviter, 1987). Many models of hippocampal epilepsy with cell damage, including the two epileptogenic KA lesions discussed here, also are produced by manipulations that themselves induce acute recurrent seizures. In contrast, the only manipulation discussed here that induces morphological changes like those seen in HS but which does not result in the development of chronic epilepsy, ischemia, does not involve acute seizures. The hypothesis that acute seizures may be a significant variable in determining the outcome of morphological insults to the hippocampus is supported by recent data showing that seizures alone lead to events that not only may underlie cell damage but may lead to long-term phenotypic changes in cells that survive.

Brief seizures have been shown to induce the expressions of proto-oncogenes such as c-*fos* in dentate granule cells (Morgan *et al.*, 1987). Limbic seizures have also been shown to induce a dramatic increase in the expression of nerve growth factor and brain-derived neurotropic factor within the involved tissue – again particularly in dentate granule cells (Gall & Isackson, 1989; Gall *et al.*, 1991; Isackson *et al.*, 1991). Both of these changes in gene expression subside as seizures resolve and, in the case of c-*fos*, cannot be immediately reinduced even with additional seizures. Recent data using the KA model suggest, however, that if an epileptic syndrome develops, as it does in KA-lesioned tissue, c-*fos* activity remains elevated as long as the syndrome persists (J. E. Franck, unpublished results). To the extent that proto-oncogenes are involved in growth factor regulation of neuronal phenotypes, such a persistent change in gene expression could have profound consequences on the aberrant or compensatory responses of the cell.

Activity-dependent modeling of neuronal circuits is a well-established phenomenon in other regions of the brain. In the damaged hippocampus, seizures alone may promote plasticity, or intrinsic alterations in surviving neurons, that, when occurring in relatively 'vacant' neuropil, may be quite different from that produced by either seizures or cell death. Data obtained from the KA and IS models suggest that the issues to be considered are much more complex than simple cell loss, or plasticity in remaining circuits.

Conclusions

Different lesions of hippocampus have been discussed, each having features of cell loss and plasticity like those observed in temporal lobe epilepsy. By comparing each of these lesions on the basis of epileptogenic outcome in each model, some conclusions regarding the significance of discrete cell loss and plasticity to epileptogenesis may be drawn. Almost invariably it has been concluded that loss of a single cell population, or aberrant plasticity of a single pathway in so far as these features are known, does not per se produce an epileptic state. (Perhaps the exception to this is the hyperexcitability that develops in CA1 following CA3 cell loss. However, here too this hyperexcitability may be transient and the relevance of CA1 epileptogenicity is unclear, since this subfield is invariably gone in human epilepsy.)

In a sense this is an artificial analysis – these morphological features do not occur singly in human epileptic tissue and the consequences of them all occurring together may certainly be far different from those discussed here. As an example, sys KA certainly produces an epileptic state in animals, yet the morphological features of this model that are amenable to analysis, such as mossy cell loss (by comparison to a non-epileptic model with similar cell loss (IS)), would not appear to be significant in isolation from other anatomical changes. Similarly, somatostatin-containing neurons are missing in human epileptic hippocampus, yet comparison again with the sclerosis produced by IS would suggest that this is not a sufficient, or even a necessary, condition for the development of epilepsy. A conclusion that remains is that epilepsy depends on all, or a critical combination, of these morphological changes. Preliminary data suggest, however, that even if complete HS is produced experimentally by combined KA and IS (Franck & Roberts, 1991), an epileptic syndrome does not develop.

These data imply that seizures and HS are both symptoms of an underlying pathology: they develop concurrently. While HS may be produced by seizures, the development of epilepsy as a syndrome does not depend on cell loss or plasticity in the hippocampus – seizures clearly occur first. This does not preclude the fact that the anatomical features of HS may become incorporated into, and able to sustain, an epileptic focus; it merely suggests that, at the outset, HS is not able to explain the development of an epileptic syndrome. As such a syndrome develops, the peculiar pattern of morphological changes that occur in the hippocampus may initially be simply permissive to the further progression of seizure activity in temporal lobe epilepsy. It must be remembered, however, that a lesion never tells us what the function of the absent structure is: it simply tells us what the remaining brain is able to accomplish without it. Cell loss and plasticity in the sclerotic hippocampus should not be considered without attention being given to phenotypic changes in neurons that remain, both within and outside the hippocampus. It is these cells that are sustaining seizures.

References

Amaral, D. (1978). A Golgi study of cell types in the hilar region of the hippocampus in the rat. *Journal of Comparative Neurology*, **182**: 851–914.

Amaral, D. & Witter, M. P. (1989). The three dimensional organization of the hippocampal formation: a review of anatomical data. *Neuroscience*, **31**: 571–91.

Arias, C., Montiel, T. & Tapia, R. (1990). Transmitter release in hippocampal slices from rats with limbic seizures produced by systemic administration of kainic acid. *Neurochemical Research*, **15**: 641–5.

Armstrong, D. R., Neill, K. H., Crain, B. J. & Nadler, J. V. (1989). Absence of electrographic seizures after transient forebrain ischemia in the Mongolian gerbil. *Brain Research*, **476**: 174–8.

Ashwood, T. J., Lancaster, B. & Wheal, H. V. (1986). Intracellular electrophysiology of CA1 neurones in slices of the kainic acid lesioned hippocampus of the rat. *Experimental Brain Research*, **62**: 189–98.

Ashwood, T. J. & Wheal, H. V (1987). The expression of *N*-methyl-D-aspartate receptor mediated during epileptiform synaptic activity in the hippocampus. *British Journal of Pharmacology*, **91**: 815–22.

Babb, T. L. & Brown, W. J. (1986). Neuronal, dendritic and vascular profiles of human temporal lobe epilepsy correlated with cellular physiology in vivo. In *Basic Mechanisms of the Epilepsies: Advances in Neurology*, vol. 44, ed. A. V. Delgado-Escueta, A. A. Ward Jr, D. M. Woodbury & R. J. Porter, pp. 949–66. New York: Raven Press.

Babb, T. L., Kupfer, W. R., Pretorius, J. K., Crandall, P. H. & Levesque, M. F. (1991). Synaptic reorganization by mossy fibers in human epileptic fascia dentata. *Neuroscience*, **42**: 351–63.

Babb, T. L., Pretorius, J. K., Kupfer, W. R. & Crandall, P. H. (1989). Glutamate decarboxylase-immunoreactive neurons are preserved in human epileptic hippocampus. *Journal of Neuroscience*, **9**: 2562–74.

Bakst, I., Avendano, C., Morrison, J. H. & Amaral, D. G. (1986). An experimental analysis of the origins of somatostatin-like immunoreactivity in the dentate gyrus of the rat. *Journal of Neuroscience*, **6**: 1452–62.

Ben-Ari, Y. (1985). Limbic seizure and brain damage produced by kainic acid: mechanisms and relevance to human temporal lobe epilepsy. *Neuroscience*, **14**: 375–403.

Ben-Ari, Y., Tremblay, E., Ottersen, O. P. & Meldrum, B. S. (1980). The role of epileptic activity in hippocampal and 'remote' cerebral lesions induced by kainic acid. *Brain Research*, **191**: 79–97.

Ben-Ari, Y., Tremblay, E., Ottersen, P. & Naquet, R. (1979). Evidence suggesting secondary epileptogenic lesions after kainic acid: pretreatment with diazepam reduces distant but not local brain damage. *Brain Research*, **165**: 362–5.

Buzsáki, G., Freund, T. F., Bayardo, F. & Somogyi, P. (1989). Ischemia-induced changes in the electrical activity of the hippocampus. *Experimental Brain Research*, **78**: 268–78.

Chang, H. S., Steward, P. & Kassell, N. F. (1989). Decreases in excitatory transmission and increases in recurrent inhibition in the rat dentate gyrus after transient cerebral ischemia. *Brain Research,* 505: 220–4.

Cornish, S. M. & Wheal, H. V. (1989). Long term loss of paired pulse inhibition in the kainic acid lesioned hippocampus of the rat. *Neuroscience,* 28: 563–71.

Crain, B. J., Westerkam, W. D., Harrison, A. H. & Nadler, J. V. (1988). Selective neuronal death after forebrain ischemia in the Mongolian gerbil: a silver impregnation study. *Neuroscience,* 27: 387–402.

Cronin, J. & Dudek, F. E. (1988). Chronic seizures and collateral sprouting of dentate mossy fibres after kainic acid treatment in rats. *Brain Research,* 474: 181–4.

Cronin, J., Obenaus, A., Houser, C. & Dudek, F. E. (1992). Electrophysiology of dentate granule cells after kainate-induced synaptic reorganization of the mossy fibers. *Brain Research,* 573: 305–10.

Davenport, C. J., Brown, W. J. & Babb, T. L. (1990). Sprouting of GABAergic and mossy fiber axons in dentate gyrus following intra-hippocampal kainate in the rat. *Experimental Neurology,* 109: 180–90.

de Lanerolle, N. C., Kim, J. H., Robbins, R.J. & Spencer, D. D. (1989). Hippocampal interneuron loss and plasticity in human temporal lobe epilepsy. *Brain Research,* 495: 387–95.

Franck, J. E., Kunkel, D. D., Baskin, D. & Schwartzkroin, P. A. (1988). Inhibitory function in kainate-lesioned epileptogenic hippocampi: immunocytochemical, autoradiographic and physiologic characteristics. *Journal of Neuroscience,* 8:, 1991–2002.

Franck, J. E. & Roberts, D. L. (1991). Combined kainate and ischemia produces "mesial temporal sclerosis". *Neuroscience Letters,* 118: 159–64.

Franck, J. E. & Schwartzkroin, P. A. (1985). Do kainate-lesioned hippocampi become epileptogenic? *Brain Research,* 329: 309–13.

Gall, C. & Isackson, P. J. (1989). Limbic seizures increase neuronal production of messenger RNA for nerve growth factor in adult rat forebrain. *Science,* 245: 758–61.

Gall, C., Murray, K. & Isackson, P. J. (1991). Kainic acid-induced seizures stimulate increased expression of nerve growth factor mRNA in rat hippocampus. *Molecular Brain Research,* 9: 113–23.

Houser, C. R., Miyashiro, J. E., Swartz, B. E., Walsh, G. O., Rich, J. R. & Delgado-Escueta, A. V. (1990). Altered patterns of dynorphin immunoreactivity suggest mossy fiber reorganization in human hippocampal epilepsy. *Journal of Neuroscience,* 10: 267–82.

Imon, H., Mitani, A., Andou, Y., Arai, T. & Kataoka, K. (1991). Delayed neuronal death is induced without postischemic hyperexcitability: continuous multiple-unit recording from ischemic CA1 neurons. *Journal of Cerebral Blood Flow and Metabolism,* 11: 819–23.

Isackson, P. J., Huntsman, M. M., Murray, K. D. & Gall, C. M. (1991). BDNF mRNA expression is increased in adult rat forebrain after limbic seizures: temporal patterns of induction distinct from NGF. *Neuron,* 6: 937–48.

Ishizuka, N., Weber, J. & Amaral, D. G. (1990). Organization of intrahippocampal projections originating from CA3 pyramidal cells in the rat. *Journal of Comparative Neurology,* 295: 580–623.

Jensen, M., Lambert, J. D. C. & Johansen, F. F. (1991). Electrophysiological recordings from rat hippocampus slices following in vivo brain ischemia. *Brain Research,* 553: 166–75.

Johansen, F. F., Jorgensen, M. B. & Diemer, N. H. (1983). Resistance of hippocampal CA1 interneurons to 20 minutes of transient cerebral ischemia in the rat. *Acta Neuropathologica*, **61**: 135–40.

Johansen, F. F., Zimmer, J. & Diemer, N. H. (1987). Early loss of somatostatin neurons in dentate hilus after cerebral ischemia in the rat precedes CA1 pyramidal cell loss. *Acta Neuropathologica*, **73**: 110–14.

Lancaster, B. & Wheal, H. V. (1984). Chronic failure of inhibition of the CA1 area of the hippocampus following kainic acid lesions of the CA3/4 area. *Brain Research*, **295**: 317–24.

Laurberg, S. & Zimmer, J. (1981). Lesion-induced sprouting of hippocampal mossy fiber collaterals to the fascia dentata in developing and adult rats. *Journal of Comparative Neurology*, **200**: 433–59.

Masukawa, L. M., Higashima, M., Hart, G. J., Spencer, D. D. & O'Connor, M. J. (1991). NMDA receptor activation during epileptiform responses in the dentate gyrus of epileptic patients. *Brain Research*, **562**: 176–80.

Masukawa, L. M., Higashima, M., Kim, J. H. & Spencer, D. D. (1989). Epileptiform discharges evoked in hippocampal brain slices from epileptic patients. *Brain Research*, **493**: 168–74.

Morgan, J. I., Cohen, D. R., Hempstead, J. L. & Curran, T. (1987). Mapping patterns of c-*fos* expression in the central nervous system after seizure. *Science*, **237**: 192–7.

Nadler, J. V. & Cuthbertson, G. J. (1980). Kainic acid neurotoxicity toward hippocampal formation: dependence on specific excitatory pathways. *Brain Research*, **195**: 47–56.

Nadler, J. V., Evenson, D. A. & Smith, E. M. (1981). Evidence from lesion studies for epileptogenic and non-epileptogenic neurotoxic interactions between kainic acid and excitatory innervation. *Brain Research*, **205**: 405–10.

Nadler, J. V., Perry, B. W. & Cotman, C. W. (1978). Preferential vulnerability of hippocampus to intraventricular kainic acid. In *Kainic Acid as a Tool in Neurobiology*, ed. E. McGeer, J. Olney, & P. McGeer, pp. 219–37. New York: Raven Press.

Nadler, J. V., Perry, B. W. & Cotman, C. W. (1980*a*). Selective reinnervation of hippocampal area CA1 and the fascia dentata after destruction of CA3–CA4 with kainic acid. *Brain Research*, **182**: 1–9.

Nadler, J. V., Perry, B. W., Gentry, C. & Cotman, C. W. (1980*b*). Degeneration of hippocampal CA3 pyramidal cells induced by intracerebroventricular kainic acid. *Journal of Comparative Neurology*, **192**: 333–59.

Nadler, J. V., Perry, B. W., Gentry, C. & Cotman, C. W. (1980*c*). Loss and reacquisition of hippocampal synapses after selective destruction of CA3–CA4 afferents with kainic acid. *Brain Research*, **191**: 387–403.

Nakajima, S., Franck, J. E., Bilkey, D. & Schwartzkroin, P. A. (1991). Local circuit synaptic interactions between CA1 pyramidal cells and interneurons in the kainate-lesioned hyperexcitable hippocampus. *Hippocampus*, **1**: 67–78.

Onodera, H., Aoki, H., Yae, T. & Kogure, K. (1990). Post-ischemic synaptic plasticity in the rat hippocampus after long-term survival: histochemical and autoradiographic study. *Neuroscience*, **38**: 125–36.

Pokorný, J. & Schwartzkroin, P. A. (1991). Do hippocampal CA3 pyramidal cells project into the dentate hilus? *Society for Neuroscience Abstracts*, **17**: 126.

Pokorný, J., Schwartzkroin, P. A. & Franck, J. E. (1991). Physiologic and morphologic characteristics of granule cells from human epileptic hippocampus. *Epilepsia*, **32** (Suppl. 3): 67.

Pulsinelli, W. A., Brierley, J. B. & Plum, F. (1982). Temporal profile of neuronal damage in a model of transient forebrain ischemia. *Annals of Neurology*, **11**: 491–8.
Pulsinelli, W. A. & Buchan, A. M. (1988). The four-vessel occlusion rat model: method for complete occlusion of vertebral arteries and control of collateral circulation. *Stroke*, **19**: 913–14.
Ribak, C. E., Seress, L. & Amaral, D. G. (1985). The development, ultrastructure and synaptic connections of the mossy cells of the dentate gyrus. *Journal of Neurocytology*, **14**: 835–57.
Robbins, R. J., Brines, M. L., Kim, J. H., Adrian, T., de Lanerolle, N., Welsh, S. & Spencer, D. D. (1991). A selective loss of somatostatin in the hippocampus of patients with temporal lobe epilepsy. *Annals of Neurology*, **29**: 325–32.
Sater, R. A. & Nadler, J. V. (1987). On the relation between seizures and brain lesions after intracerebroventricular kainic acid. *Neuroscience Letters*, **84**: 73–8.
Scharfman, H. E. & Schwartzkroin, P. A. (1990a). Responses of cells of the rat fascia dentata to prolonged stimulation of the perforant path: sensitivity of hilar cells and changes in granule cell excitability. *Neuroscience*, **35**: 491–504.
Scharfman, H. E. & Schwartzkroin, P. A.(1990b). Consequences of prolonged afferent stimulation of the rat fascia dentata: epileptiform activity in area CA3 of hippocampus. *Neuroscience*, **35**: 505–17.
Schwartzkroin, P. A. & Haglund, M. M. (1986). Spontaneous rhythmic synchronous activity in epileptic human and normal monkey temporal lobe. *Epilepsia*, **27**: 523–33.
Simpson, L. H., Wheal, H. V. & Williamson, R. (1991). The contribution of non-NMDA and NMDA receptors to graded bursting activity in the CA1 region of the hippocampus in a chronic model of epilepsy. *Canadian Journal of Physiology and Pharmacology*, **69**: 1091–8.
Sloviter, R. S. (1987). Decreased hippocampal inhibition and a selective loss of interneurons in experimental epilepsy. *Science*, **235**: 73–6.
Sloviter, R. S. (1992). Possible functional consequences of synaptic reorganization in the dentate gyrus of kainate-treated rats. *Neuroscience Letters*, **137**: 91–6.
Sloviter, R. S. & Nilaver, G. (1987). Immunocytochemical localization of GABA-, cholecystokinin-, vasoactive intestinal polypeptide-, and somatostatin-like immunoreactivity in the area dentata and hippocampus of the rat. *Journal of Comparative Neurology*, **256**: 42–60.
Sloviter, R. S., Sollas, A. L., Barbara, N. M. & Laxer, K. D. (1991). Calcium-binding protein (Calbindin-D28K) and parvalbumin immunocytochemistry in the normal and epileptic human hippocampus. *Journal of Comparative Neurology*, **308**: 381–96.
Sutula, T., Cascino, G., Cavazos, J., Parada, I. & Ramirez, L. (1989). Mossy fiber synaptic reorganization in the epileptic human temporal lobe. *Annals of Neurology*, **26**: 321–30.
Tauck, D. L. & Nadler, J. V. (1985). Evidence of functional mossy fiber sprouting in hippocampal formation of kainic-acid treated rats. *Journal of Neuroscience*, **5**: 1016–22.
Turner, D. A. & Wheal, H. V. (1991). Excitatory synaptic potentials in kainic acid denervated rat CA1 pyramidal neurons. *Journal of Neuroscience*, **11**: 2786–94.

9

Sprouting as an underlying cause of hyperexcitability in experimental models and in the human epileptic temporal lobe

THOMAS P. SUTULA

Introduction

Epilepsy is a chronic disorder of the central nervous system characterized by paroxysmal excessive electrical activity and recurrent behavioral seizures. Epilepsy can develop at any time from infancy to old age as a manifestation of genetic, acquired, or degenerative diseases, but it also frequently develops in the absence of overt pathology. Epileptic disorders can be classified into distinct syndromes with specific etiologies and natural histories (Dreifuss *et al.*, 1985). For all of these reasons, epilepsy should not be considered as a single disorder, but as a heterogeneous condition defined by the common features of abnormal electrical activity and recurrent seizures.

The cellular and molecular events that play a role in the generation of seizures and epilepsy have been investigated in experimental models that are as varied and diverse as the clinical phenomena of epilepsy. For example, mechanisms of seizure generation have been studied with electrophysiological methods after *acute* induction of seizures by drugs that block inhibition, such as penicillin, bicuculline, or picrotoxin (Schwartzkroin & Prince, 1977; Prince, 1978; Hablitz, 1984; Gean & Shinnick-Gallagher, 1987). As the induced seizures cease when the convulsant drugs are withdrawn, the epileptic activity induced by these drugs is more appropriately considered as a model of seizure generation rather than epilepsy, a *chronic* condition characterized by recurrent seizures that usually occur sporadically and unpredictably over long intervals.

Epileptic phenomena have been studied in chronic experimental animal models that generate sporadic recurrent seizures, and thus more closely resemble the clinical features of epilepsy. In recent years, morphological and electrophysiological studies in these models have revealed long-lasting cellular alterations that may play a role in the generation of seizures and long-term consequences of epilepsy (Ben-Ari, 1985; Sloviter, 1985; Tauck & Nadler, 1985; Mody *et al.*, 1988; Sutula *et al.*, 1988; Cavazos & Sutula, 1990). In the kindling model of temporal lobe epilepsy, morphological studies have provided evidence of structural alterations in the neural circuitry of the hippocampus that develop in association with repeated seizures evoked by kindling. These alterations, which include progressive neuronal loss induced by repeated seizures, axon sprouting, and reorganization of synaptic connections (Sutula *et al.*, 1988; Cavazos & Sutula, 1990), have been observed in other experimental models of epilepsy (Stanfield, 1989; Golarai *et al.*, 1992), and also in the epileptic human temporal lobe (Represa *et al.*, 1989*a*; de Lanerolle *et al.*, 1989; Sutula *et al.*, 1989; Houser *et al.*, 1990).

The aim of this chapter is to review the available evidence that associates sprouting and structural plasticity with epileptic phenomena, to evaluate critically the more limited evidence about the possible functional consequences of axon sprouting and synaptic reorganization in hippocampal circuitry, and to identify some of the issues that need to be addressed in order to understand the significance and possible role of synaptic reorganization in epileptic disorders. This analysis also reviews how a series of experiments designed to identify the anatomical locus of alterations induced by kindling led to recognition of axon sprouting as a cellular phenomenon associated with epilepsy, and generated a conceptual strategy for analysis of putative cellular and molecular mechanisms in the kindling model and other chronic models.

The kindling phenomenon as a model of epilepsy

The conceptual impetus for the experiments that led to recognition of the association of axon sprouting with kindling had its origins in studies that attempted to identify the neural network that is altered during the development of kindled seizures. Kindling is the progression of behavioral and electrographic seizures induced by repeated activation of neural pathways that eventually results in the development of epilepsy (Goddard *et al.*, 1969; McNamara *et al.*, 1980). Kindled seizures can be induced by repeated activation with electrical or chemical stimulation that initially evokes only brief afterdischarges. With repeated activation, the evoked afterdischarges and behavioral seizures increase in duration and complexity, and eventually evolve into secondary generalized (class 5; Racine, 1972) seizures. The induced susceptibility to evoked seizures is permanent, and, with continued intermittent stimulation, spontaneous seizures eventually develop (Pinel & Rovner, 1978).

Kindling can be induced in a variety of species, including primates (Wada & Mizoguchi, 1984). The behavioral characteristics of kindled seizures resemble many features of human partial complex seizures (McNamara *et al.*, 1985). A variety of pathways in the central nervous system are susceptible to kindling (Goddard *et al.*, 1969). Hippocampal and limbic pathways that have been implicated by clinical, electro-encephalographic, and pathological observations in human epilepsy (Babb & Brown, 1987) are particularly susceptible to development of kindling in animal models. Many of the features of kindling are thus ideal as a chronic model of epilepsy.

Identifying transsynaptic changes induced by kindling

Goddard *et al.* (1969) suggested that kindling induced transsynaptic alterations in pathways beyond the focus of stimulation, as demonstrated by the observation that alterations induced by kindling survive lesions at the tip of the electrode at the primary stimulation site. Further direct evidence that kindling induced transsynaptic alterations was provided by Messenheimer *et al.* (1978), who demonstrated that, after kindling of the entorhinal cortex (EC) in rat, changes intrinsic to targets of the EC are sufficient to account for the kindling phenomenon. These studies relied on the previous observation that destruction of the ipsilateral perforant pathway from the EC to granule cells of the dentate gyrus (DG) is followed by sprouting of the normally sparse projection from the contralateral EC to ipsilateral DG (Steward *et al.*, 1974). Sprouting and synaptogenesis by contralateral surviving entorhinal neurons reaches a maximum at two weeks after the lesion, and results in reinnervation of the ipsilateral DG by sprouting contralateral axons and re-establishment of functional synaptic transmission in the denervated DG (Steward *et al.*, 1973, 1974, 1976; Cotman *et al.*, 1981).

After induction of kindling by EC stimulation in rat, Messenheimer *et al.* (1978) destroyed the site of stimulation in the EC by an electrolytic method, and studied the effect of the lesion on development of kindling by stimulation of the surviving contralateral EC. At two weeks after completion of kindling by ipsilateral EC stimulation, 5.2 stimulations of the contralateral EC were required to evoke a class 5 seizure. At two weeks after an ipsilateral EC lesion without prior ipsilateral kindling, 23.5 stimulations of the sprouted contralateral EC pathway were required to evoke a class 5 seizure. If the contralateral EC pathway was stimulated immediately after ipsilateral EC kindling and lesioning (prior to sprouting and reactive synaptogenesis by the surviving contralateral axons), 8.3 stimulations were required to evoke a class 5 seizure. In contrast, stimulation of the contralateral pathway two weeks after completion of kindling and EC lesioning (an interval that permits sprouting of the normally sparse pathway from the contralateral EC to the denervated dentate gyrus) evoked a class 5 seizure after only one or two stimulations. This series of observations demonstrated that kindling induced alterations in neural circuitry that is 'downstream' from the destroyed primary stimulation site, and suggests that sprouted fibers have gained access to neural circuitry that has been transsynaptically altered by kindling.

Criteria for evaluation of transsynaptic alterations as mechanisms of kindling

On the basis of these studies, the concept emerged that kindling induced long-lasting transsynaptic alterations in the neural network related to the site of stimulation. To begin to elucidate the cellular mechanisms that play a role in the development of kindling in this network, it would be desirable:

(1) To identify the specific pathways in the network that are transsynaptically altered during the development of kindling.
(2) To define the cellular and molecular alterations induced in pathways of the neural network that are transsynaptically altered during the development of kindling.
(3) To establish the relationship of these cellular and molecular alterations to the development, progression, and permanence of the evolving behavioral seizures.

These three steps form the guidelines of a strategy that can be used to begin to evaluate alterations induced by kindling stimulation as possible mechanisms of the kindling phenomenon in complex neural networks.

This strategy essentially defines spatial and temporal criteria that should be considered in the evaluation of cellular and molecular alterations as possible mechanisms of kindling in a neural network. Cellular and molecular alterations that are mechanisms of kindling should develop early in the course of kindling at sites in the network that are implicated in kindling development, progress with repeated seizures, and become permanent when the permanence of kindling is established. Alterations induced in remote circuitry that is not activated by kindling stimulation, or alterations induced in activated circuitry after establishment of kindled seizures, are unlikely to play a primary role in the development of kindling, and may be more likely to be reactive phenomena to the induced seizures, modulatory influences, or epiphenomena. Stimulation that induces kindling may also induce other changes that are unrelated to the development of permanent susceptibility to seizures, but may parallel kindling development.

Cellular and molecular alterations that develop in response to kindling stimulation and fulfill spatial and temporal requirements in the neural network should be further evaluated as potential mechanisms of kindling by additional experimental manipulations. Specifically, if cellular and molecular alterations develop at a critical locus in the neural network in a time course consistent with a role in the induction of kindling, prevention or blockade of those alterations should impede the development of kindled seizures. Conversely, enhancement or establishment of these alterations at this site prior to kindling stimulation should facilitate kindling development.

Many neurochemical and physiological alterations have been associated with kindling (McNamara, 1984), but its cellular and molecular mechanisms are still uncertain. The identity of the neural network that is altered by limbic kindling is still not well defined, and the cellular and molecular alterations induced in the neural network activated by kindling stimulation have been evaluated according to spatial and temporal criteria (as in steps (1), (2), and (3), above) in only a few circumstances.

The experiments of Messenheimer *et al.* implicated hippocampal circuitry as the sites of transsynaptic alterations induced by EC kindling, and were followed by a series of experiments on rats that more specifically identified the DG as the site of alterations that influenced the development of kindling (Dashieff & McNamara, 1982; Frush *et al.*, 1986; Sutula *et al.*, 1986; McNamara, 1988). These experiments led to the observation that axon sprouting and synaptic reorganization develop in the DG during kindling stimulation, and in association with seizures induced in other models of epilepsy. The analysis that follows evaluates axon sprouting and synaptic reorganization of the mossy fiber pathway in the DG as a possible cellular mechanism of seizure development in the neural network that is altered by limbic kindling.

The role of the dentate gyrus in the development and expression of kindling

The experiments of Messenheimer *et al.* (1978) implicated circuitry that is the target of entorhinal neurons as the site of transsynaptic alterations induced by kindling. The axons of entorhinal neurons project by the perforant path to granule cells of the DG. Axons of the granule cells, so-called mossy fibers, project to a diverse population of polymorphic neurons in the hilus of the DG, and to pyramidal neurons in CA3 (Swanson *et al.*, 1978).

The possibility that the DG is one component of the neural network that is altered by limbic kindling has been supported in several independent experiments that evaluated the effect of destruction of dentate granule cells on the development of kindling. After destruction of the DG by microinjection of colchicine, a relatively selective neurotoxin for granule cells of the DG (Goldschmidt & Steward, 1980), kindling can still be induced by EC stimulation, but about 40% more stimulations are required (Frush *et al.*, 1986; Sutula *et al.*, 1986). Destruction of the DG by colchicine (Dashieff & McNamara, 1982) or by microsectioning of perforant path axons from the EC (Savage *et al.*, 1985) also impairs the development of kindling in response to amygdala stimulation. Destruction of the DG *after* development of kindling by either EC or amygdala stimulation had no effect on the expression of kindled seizures (Dashieff & McNamara, 1982; Frush *et al.*, 1986; Sutula *et al.*, 1986).

The results of these studies demonstrated three important points about the role of the DG in the neural network that is altered by kindling:

(1) The DG is not required for the development of kindled seizures, as indicated by the failure of DG destruction or perforant path lesions to prevent the development of kindling. An intact perforant path from the EC to the DG is not required for either the development or expression of kindled seizures. Alternative projections from the EC that could include direct projections to the stratum moleculare of CA1 and CA3 (Steward & Scoville, 1976), rostrally directed projections to amygdala (Wyss, 1981) or olfactory areas (Haberly & Price, 1978), or antidromic activation of converging afferents to the EC (Krettek & Price, 1977), must be sufficient for induction of kindled seizures after DG destruction. These results, and the observations that both selective and non-selective lesions of the substantia nigra (McNamara, 1984) and piriform cortex (Racine *et al.*, 1988) also fail to prevent the development of kindling, support the view that the changes that underlie the development of kindled seizures are

distributed in multiple sites in the synaptic network related to the site of stimulation. It is probable that no single site is critical for the development of kindling. This view is consistent with the anatomical complexity of circuitry in the central nervous system.

(2) The DG is not required for the expression of kindled seizures or maintainence of the kindled state, as indicated by the failure of DG destruction after induction of kindling to prevent the expression of seizures in response to EC stimulation. Some of the EC projections remaining after DG destruction must also be sufficient for expression of kindled seizures. These results imply that the alterations that underlie the maintainence of the kindled state also reside in a distributed network of multiple pathways that are related to the site of stimulation. If trans-synaptic alterations induced by kindling are widely distributed in the neural network related to the stimulation site, it is likely that no single pathway will be critical for expression of the kindled state.

(3) Although the DG was not required for either the development or expression of kindled seizures, lesions of the DG were not without effect. An intact DG facilitated the emergence of kindled seizures in response to amygdala or EC stimulation. The DG is thus implicated as the site of alterations that influence the development of kindling in the neural network activated by stimulation of the amygdala or EC. The locus of the alterations in the DG could be intrinsic to granule cells, or could reside in any or all of the synapses of perforant path axons on granule cell dendrites, synapses of mossy fiber axons on their target neurons, or other cellular elements. These alterations influence only the development of kindling and are not required for the expression of the kindled state.

Facilitation of kindling after lesions of CA3/CA4

With a similar strategy, the effects of lesions of CA3 and polymorphic neurons in the hilus of the DG on development of kindling have also been assessed. The effects of kainic-acid-induced or electrolytic lesions of the CA3/hilar populations, the immediate synaptic targets of dentate granule cells, were strikingly different from effects of lesions of the DG. The CA3/hilar lesion produced a marked facilitation in the development of kindling by perforant path stimulation (Sutula *et al.*, 1987), amygdala stimulation, or hippocampal stimulation (Feldblum & Ackermann, 1987). This effect was particularly intriguing, since lesions of the hilar polymorphic neuronal population also induce synaptic reorganization of the mossy fiber pathway from granule cells of the DG (Nadler *et al.*, 1980*a*; Laurberg & Zimmer, 1981; see also Chapter 8, this volume).

Cell death of the hilar population results in degeneration of the commissural–associational pathway from the hilar neurons to the inner molecular layer of the DG (Nadler & Cuthbertson, 1980; Nadler *et al.*, 1980*b*), which is followed by axon sprouting of the mossy fiber pathway and reinnervation of the denervated zone in the inner molecular layer (Nadler *et al.*, 1980*a*; Laurberg & Zimmer, 1981). If mossy fiber synaptic reorganization increased recurrent excitation by positive feedback in the DG, it might be a factor in the facilitation of kindling after the lesion. The reorganization of the mossy fiber pathway is easily observed with the Timm method, a histochemical technique that identifies heavy metals, and selectively stains synaptic terminals of the mossy fibers due to their high content of zinc (Danscher, 1981; Frederickson *et al.*, 1984; Fig. 9.1) The Timm method permits identification of alterations in the distribution of mossy fiber synaptic terminals.

Axon sprouting and synaptic reorganization induced by kindling

Application of the Timm method to rats that received perforant path, amygdala, or olfactory bulb stimulation to induce kindled seizures revealed that the mossy fiber pathway undergoes reorganization of its synaptic connections during the development of kindling (Sutula *et al.*, 1988). As kindling was induced, Timm-stained granules that correspond ultrastructurally to mossy fiber synaptic terminals developed in the supragranular layer of the DG, where they were not normally found. These alterations, which most probaby develop by axon sprouting of the mossy fibers, were apparent early in the course of kindling before the induction of class 5 seizures, increased with repeated seizures, and were essentially permanent (Sutula *et al.*, 1988). Similar patterns of synaptic reorganization of the mossy fiber pathway have been observed in association with development of seizures in the *tg/tg* (*tottering*) strain of mice (Stanfield, 1989), and with repeated seizures evoked with pentylene-tetrazol (Golarai *et al.*, 1992). Other pathways of the hippocampal formation may undergo synaptic reorganization in association with the development of seizures, as indicated by alterations in the pattern of Timm histochemistry in the stratum moleculare of the CA1–subiculum transitional zone of limbic-kindled rats (Cavazos & Sutula, 1989), and in the stratum infrapyramidale of CA3 in Wistar rats kindled with amygdala stimulation (Represa *et al.*, 1989*a*).

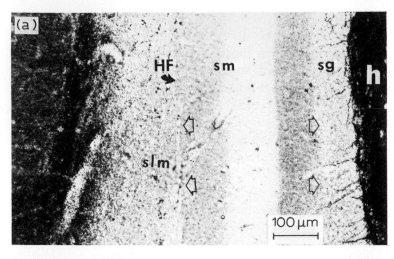

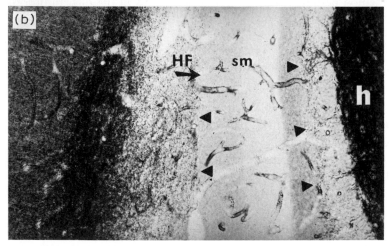

Fig. 9.1. Synaptic reorganization induced in the hippocampal formation by kindling. (a) A horizontal section of normal rat hippocampus and dentate gyrus (DG) stained with the Timm method. The area of dark staining in the hilus (h) of the DG is the normal site of synaptic termination of mossy fiber axons from granule cells in the stratum granulosum (sg). The normal pattern of staining in the stratum lacunosum–moleculare (slm) of the transitional area between CA1 and the subiculum is also demonstrated. Note the absence of dark staining granules in the supragranular region and slm region (open arrows). (b) A similar section from a rat that experienced 50 generalized tonic–clonic seizures evoked by kindling of the perforant path reveals dark granules that correspond ultrastructurally to synaptic terminals in the supragranular region of the DG and the slm region of the CA1–subiculum transition zone. In the DG these terminals most probably develop by axon sprouting and reorganization of the mossy fiber pathway. The cells of origin for the synaptic terminals in the CA1 region are not known. sm, stratum moleculare of the DG; HF, hippocampal fissure.

Axon sprouting and synaptic reorganization in human epilepsy

There is now also considerable evidence for synaptic reorganization in human epilepsy, as revealed by application of Timm histochemistry and other histological methods to the hippocampus and DG of patients who undergo temporal lobectomy for treatment of medically intractable epilepsy (de Lanerolle *et al.*, 1989; Represa *et al.*, 1989*b*; Sutula *et al.*, 1989; Houser *et al*, 1990). Alterations in the patterns of mossy fiber termination have been observed in the supragranular layer of the DG in both childhood (Represa *et al.*, 1989*b*) and adult epilepsies (Sutula *et al.*, 1989; de Lanerolle *et al.*, 1989; Houser *et al.*, 1990). In human epileptic tissue and after kindling, a variety of other histological markers of the mossy fiber pathway, such as dynorphin-A immunoreactivity (de Lanerolle *et al.*, 1989; Houser *et al.*, 1990) and high affinity kainic acid receptors (Represa *et al.*, 1989*a,b*), can be found in the supragranular layer of the DG, where they are not normally observed. The consistent observations of a variety of histological markers of the mossy fiber pathway in the supragranular layer is morphological evidence that this pathway undergoes axon sprouting and synaptic reorganization in association with epilepsy. Other pathways and neurotransmitter systems, such as the neuropeptide-Y system, also undergo synaptic reorganization in human temporal lobe epilepsy (de Lanerolle *et al.*, 1989). The similarity of the structural alterations in the mossy fiber pathway in both human epilepsy and a variety of animal models suggests the possibility that humans and animal experimental models may share common features, and that efforts to investigate the cellular and molecular mechanisms of synaptic rearrangements in the kindling model may be pertinent to human epilepsy.

Mossy fiber sprouting and synaptic reorganization as a possible mechanism of kindling

As indicated in the previous discussion, a variety of experimental studies have implictaed the DG as the site of alterations that influence the development of limbic kindling (Dashieff & McNamara, 1982; Frush *et al.*, 1986; Sutula *et al.*, 1986). What additional evidence can be considered with regard to the possibility that mossy fiber synaptic reorganization may be an alteration in the DG that plays a role in the induction and expression of kindling? Mossy fiber synaptic reorganization develops in the DG (a site implicated in the development of kindling) early in the course of kindling stimulation, in a time course consistent with axon sprouting, increases with the behavioral progression of kindling, and is essentially permanent. Mossy fiber synaptic reorganization in the DG thus fulfills at least some of the spatial and temporal requirements that might be expected for a possible cellular mechanism in the neural network activated by limbic kindling.

If synaptic reorganization of the mossy fiber pathway in the DG is one alteration that influences the development of kindling, it would be expected that experimental manipulations that induced synaptic reorganization of the pathway prior to kindling would facilitate emergence of kindled seizures. Lesions of the CA3 and hilar polymorphic population in the DG induced synaptic reorganization and also facilitated the development of kindling (Feldblum & Ackermann, 1987; Sutula *et al.*, 1987). Conversely, manipulations that block or prevent the development of mossy fiber synaptic reorganization would be expected to impair or delay the development of kindling. As already noted, lesions of the DG that prevent synaptic reorganization markedly impaired the development of kindling (Dashieff & McNamara, 1982; Frush *et al.*, 1986; Sutula *et al.*, 1986) These observations are consistent with the possibility that synaptic reorganization of the mossy fiber pathway may be a cellular rearrangement in the DG that influences the development of limbic kindling. The molecular events that underlie the synaptic reorganization in the DG may similarly be molecular mechanisms of kindling.

Although these observations are consistent with the possibility that synaptic reorganization might be a cellular mechanism of kindling, these experiments are *not* conclusive and do not constitute proof of the hypothesis. At least two major gaps in understanding currently limit further consideration of mossy fiber synaptic reorganization as a possible cellular mechanism of kindling. First, it is possible that synaptic reorganization is merely a reactive alteration that parallels or follows primary causal events that are responsible for the emergence of kindling with repeated stimulation. By this argument, the reorganization would be merely an epiphenomenon, and might have only limited functional impact on electrophysiological characteristics and information processing in the DG. Second, the functional consequences of synaptic reorganization of the mossy fiber pathway are at present uncertain. A major assumption of the hypothesis that synaptic reorganization is a mechanism for kindling and for facilitation of kindling after CA3/hilar lesions is that the rearrangement of connections in fact enhances synaptic transmission and excitability in hippocampal pathways. The difficulties presented by these issues, and some experimental approaches that might be considered in the effort to address them, are now discussed.

Assessing the functional significance of mossy fiber sprouting

If the sprouted mossy fiber axons form excitatory synapses on other granule cells, there are attractive reasons to speculate that reorganization of the mossy fiber pathway in the supragranular region of the DG leads to recurrent excitation by increasing positive feedback (Tauck & Nadler, 1985). However, the anatomical details of the synaptic rearrangements are at present not fully characterized. Although it is clear that many synaptic terminals of sprouted mossy fiber axons form asymmetric and thus putatively excitatory synapses on dendrites in the supragranular and inner molecular layer of the DG (Sutula et al., 1988), the identity of the postsynaptic structures is uncertain. In the case of mossy fiber axon sprouting after lesions induced by kainic acid, at least some of the synaptic terminals of the sprouted axons form synapses with dendrites of granule cells (Frotscher & Zimmer, 1983).

The functional consequences of synapse formation by sprouted axons on dendrites of granule cells or inhibitory interneurons would be very different (see Fig. 9.2). If the sprouted mossy fiber terminals form excitatory synapses on dendrites of other granule cells, functional synaptic transmission in these synapses would increase recurrent excitation among granule cells. This alteration might be important, as the normal granule cell population is notably lacking in both anatomical and electrophysiological evidence for recurrent excitatory circuitry. In contrast to pyramidal neurons, granule cells are normally quite resistant to burst discharge even when inhibition is blocked by bicuculline, picrotoxin, or penicillin (Fricke & Prince, 1984). One possible reason for the resistance of granule cells to burst discharge may be lack of intrinsic recurrent circuitry in the DG. If mossy fiber sprouting resulted in the development of recurrent excitatory circuitry, it might shift the balance of excitation/inhibition in favor of net excitation. Conversely, if the sprouted mossy fiber axons establish functional synaptic contacts on dendrites of inhibitory interneurons, the net effect of mossy fiber synaptic reorganization might be to increase inhibition (Fig. 9.2).

It is possible, if not likely, that terminals of sprouted mossy fiber axons could form synaptic contacts with dendrites of both granule cells and inhibitory interneurons (Ribak & Peterson, 1990). In this case, assessment of the functional outcome of the synaptic reorganization could be quite

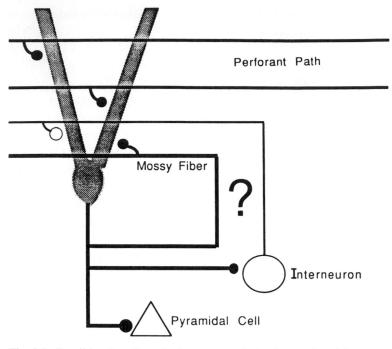

Fig. 9.2. Possible alterations in hippocampal circuitry induced by mossy fiber sprouting and synaptic reorganization. The mossy fiber axon from a schematically depicted dentate granule cell forms a synapse with a pyramidal neuron, and in addition sprouted axon collaterals may form autapses with the same granule cell, or synapses with other granule cells and inhibitory interneurons. The functional consequences of these possible alterations in circuitry on excitability would be very different.

complex, and might require quantitative determination of the frequency of mossy fiber terminal contacts on both granule cell dendrites and interneurons, as well as electrophysiological evaluation of the effects of these alterations in circuitry on individual granule cells and the granule cell population.

Is mossy fiber synaptic reorganization merely a reactive alteration, or does it actually contribute to the generation of seizures, and the development of kindling? In the kainic-acid-lesioned hippocampus of the rat, there is evidence that the density of the sprouted pathway appears to correlate with electrophysiological abnormality (Tauck & Nadler, 1985), and with the tendency to spontaneous seizure activity (Cronin & Dudek, 1988). Similarly, in the kindling model, mossy fiber synaptic reorganization becomes more prominent with repeatedly evoked seizures and the progression of kindling towards the stage of spontaneous seizures (Sutula *et al.*, 1988). These observations raise the possibility that synaptic reorganization may be contributing to abnormal excitability that results in spontaneous seizures, but are also consistent with the possibility that synaptic reorganization may merely be a reactive phenomenon resulting from repeated epileptic activity. As a first step to addressing this critical issue, it would be desirable to know the specific functional effects of mossy fiber synaptic reorganization in hippocampal circuitry.

Since the initial reports that linked axon sprouting and synaptic reorganization with development of epilepsy, there has been rapid progress in identification of morphological alterations in neural circuitry in association with both experimental and human epilepsy. However, assessment of the functional and electrophysiological effects of these morphological alterations has proceeded more slowly. The specific functional effects of mossy fiber sprouting are uncertain. In the normal rat, the mossy fiber pathway to pyramidal neurons in CA3 and polymorphic neurons in the hilus of the DG is excitatory (Deadwyler *et al.*, 1974). Activation of CA3 antidromically activates mossy fibers and normally evokes an extracellular field potential in the DG with a single population spike. In the kainic-acid-lesioned hippocampus, antidromic activation of the mossy fiber pathway evokes an abnormal multispike potential (Tauck & Nadler, 1985). This result is evidence for an association of mossy fiber synaptic reorganization with abnormal excitation. However, a variety of mechanisms, including decreases in inhibition as well as intrinsic cellular alterations in granule cells, could contribute to the generation of these epileptiform field potentials.

There is electrophysiological evidence that kindling induces long-lasting alterations in synaptic and intrinsic properties of granule cells of the DG. These alterations include the N-methyl-D-aspartate (NMDA)-mediated increases in synaptic transmission (Mody *et al.*, 1988) that are of particular interest, as the voltage dependence of NMDA-gated ion channels tends to amplify synaptic inputs. In the normal rat, NMDA receptors are present in the inner molecular layer, the dendritic region that receives the anomalous sprouted mossy fiber pathway induced by kindling (Monaghan *et al.*, 1983; Monaghan & Cotman, 1985; Cotman *et al.* 1987). These observations suggest the possibility that synapses in the inner molecular layer could be the site of functional alterations induced by kindling, but the specific contributions of the sprouted pathway to the generation of these functional alterations is currently uncertain.

Studies with current source density analysis have revealed that kindling induced abnormal inward membrane currents in the inner molecular and supragranular layer of the DG in the dendritic region that is the site of the sprouted mossy fiber pathway (Golarai & Sutula, 1990). These results are consistent with the possibility that the sprouted terminals might be contributing to net excitation in the supragranular layer of the DG, but do not distinguish between excitation of dendrites of granule cells or inhibitory interneurons. To define the effects of axon sprouting on electrophysiological and functional activity in hippocampal circuits, and to clarify the possible role of sprouting in the generation of epileptic events in the hippocampus, it will be necessary to design experiments that combine electrophysiological methods with anatomical assessment of the sprouted pathway.

Conclusions

This chapter has reviewed how experimental efforts to establish the identity of the anatomical network altered by limbic kindling led to recognition of the association of axon sprouting with the development of epilepsy. These experiments also generated criteria for the evaluation of morphological and physiological alterations induced by limbic stimulation in the neural network as possible cellular mechanisms of kindling. Axon sprouting and synaptic reorganization of the mossy fiber pathway were analyzed as cellular alterations that may play a role in the development and expression of kindled seizures.

The available data are consistent with the possibility that sprouting and synaptic reorganization could be cellular mechanisms that contribute to abnormal excitability and kindled seizures in hippocampal circuitry, but additional anatomical characterization of synaptic reorganization in the DG, as well as more specific electrophysiologcal evaluation of its functional effects, are required to test the hypothesis more rigorously. In particular, it will be necessary to determine more directly the effect of axon sprouting and synaptic reorganization on the properties of individual granule cells and the granule cell population, in experiments that evaluate directly the relationship of morphological alterations to electrophysiological properties.

More generally, the development of criteria for evaluation of cellular and molecular alterations in the neural network activated by kindling as possible mechanisms for kindled seizures provided a strategy that may be useful for in-vivo and in-vitro study of epileptic phenomena in other chronic models of the epilepsies.

References

Babb, T. J. & Brown, W. J. (1987). Pathological findings in epilepsy. In *Surgical Treatment of the Epilepsies*, ed. J. Engel, pp. 511–40. New York: Raven Press.

Ben-Ari, Y. (1985). Limbic seizure and brain damage produced by kainic acid: mechanisms and relevance to human temporal lobe epilepsy. *Neuroscience*, **14**: 375–43.

Cavazos, J. & Sutula, T. (1989). Morphological evidence for synaptic reorganization induced by kindling in the stratum moleculare of the CA1/subiculum transitional region of the rat hippocampal formation. *Society for Neuroscience Abstracts*, **15**: 454.

Cavazos, J. & Sutula, T. (1990). Progressive neuronal loss induced by kindling: a possible mechanism for mossy fiber synaptic reorganization and hippocampal sclerosis. *Brain Research*, **527**: 1–6.

Cotman, C., Monaghan, D., Ottersen, O. P. & Storm-Mathisen, J. (1987). Anatomical organization of excitatory amino acid receptors and their pathways. *Trends in Neurosciences*, 10: 273–80.

Cotman, C., Nieto-Sampedro, M. & Harris, E. (1981). Synapse replacement in the nervous system of adult vertebrates. *Physiological Reviews*, **61**: 684–784.

Cronin, J. & Dudek, F. E. (1988). Chronic seizures and collateral sprouting of dentate mossy fibers after kainic acid treatment in rats. *Brain Research*, **474**: 181–4.

Danscher, G. (1981). Histochemical demonstration of heavy metals – a revised version of the silver sulphide method suitable for both light and electron microscopy. *Histochemistry*, **71**: 1–16.

Dashieff, R. M. & McNamara, J. O. (1982). Intradentate colchicine retards the development of amygdala kindling. *Annals of Neurology*, **11**: 347–52.

de Lanerolle, N., Kim, J., Robbins, R. & Spencer, D. (1989). Hippocampal interneuron loss and plasticity in human temporal lobe epilepsy. *Brain Research*, **495**: 387–95.

Deadwyler, S. A., West, J. R., Cotman, C. & Lynch, G. (1974). A neurophysiological analysis of commissural projections to dentate gyrus of the rat. *Journal of Neurophysiology*, **38**: 167–83.

Dreifuss, F. E., Martinez-Lage, M., Roger, J., Seino, M. & Dam, M. (1985). Proposal for classification of epilepsies and epileptic syndromes. *Epilepsia*, **26**: 268–78.

Feldblum, S. & Ackermann, R. (1987). Increased susceptibility to hippocampal and amygdala kindling following intrahippocampal kainic acid. *Experimental Neurology*, **97**: 225–69.

Frederickson, C. J., Klitenick, M. A., Mauton, W. I. & Kirkpatrick, J. B. (1984). Cytoarchitectonic distribution of zinc in the hippocampus of man and the rat. *Brain Research*, **273**: 335–9.

Fricke, R. & Prince, D. (1984). Electrophysiology of dentate granule cells. *Journal of Neurophysiology*, **51**: 195–209.

Frotscher, M. & Zimmer, J. (1983). Lesion-induced mossy fibres to the inner molecular layer of the rat fascia dentata: identification of postsynaptic granule cells by the Golgi–EM technique. *Journal of Comparative Neurology*, **215**: 299–311.

Frush, D., Giacchino, J. & McNamara, J. (1986). Evidence implicating dentate granule cells in the development of entorhinal kindling. *Experimental Neurology*, **82**: 92–101.

Gean, P. & Shinnick-Gallagher, P. (1987). Picrotoxin induced epileptiform
activity in amygdaloid neurons. *Neuroscience Letters*, **73**: 149: 149–54.
Goddard, G., McIntyre, D. & Leech, C. (1969). A permanent change in brain
function resulting from daily electrical stimulation. *Experimental Neurology*,
25: 295–330.
Golarai, G., Cavazos, J. E. & Sutula, T. (1992). Activation of the dentate gyrus
by pentylenetetrazol evoked seizures induces mossy fiber reorganization.
Brain Research, **593**: 257–64.
Golarai, G. & Sutula, T. (1990). Perforant path evoked synaptic currents in the
dentate gyrus studied with current source density techniques after LTP and
kindling. *Society for Neuroscience Abstracts*, **16**: 1265.
Goldschmidt, R. & Steward, O. (1980). Preferential toxicity of colchicine for
granule cells of the dentate gyrus of the adult rat. *Proceedings of the
National Academy of Sciences, USA*, **77**: 3047–51.
Haberly, L. & Price, J. (1978). Association and commissural fiber systems of the
olfactory cortex in the rat. *Journal of Comparative Neurology*, **178**: 711–40.
Hablitz, J. (1984). Picrotoxin-induced epileptiform activity in hippocampus: role of
endogenous versus synaptic factors. *Journal of Neurophysiology*, **51**: 1011–27.
Houser, C., Miyashiro, J., Schwartz, B., Walsh, G., Rich, J. & Delgado-Escueta,
A. V. (1990). Altered patterns of dynorphin immunoreactivity suggest
mossy fiber reorganization in human hippocampal epilepsy. *Journal of
Neuroscience*, **10**: 276–82.
Krettek, J. E. & Price, J. L. (1977). Projections from the amygdaloid complex
and adjacent olfactory structures to the entorhinal cortex and to the
subiculum in the rat and cat. *Journal of Comparative Neurology*, **172**: 723–52.
Laurberg, S. & Zimmer, J. (1981). Lesion-induced sprouting of hippocampal
mossy fiber collaterals to the fascia dentata in developing and adult rats.
Journal of Comparative Neurology, **200**: 433–59.
McNamara, J. O. (1984). Role of neurotransmitters in seizure mechanisms in
the kindling model of epilepsy. *Federation Proceedings*, **43**: 2516–20.
McNamara, J. O. (1986). Kindling model of epilepsy. *Advances in Neurology*,
44, 303–18.
McNamara, J. O. (1988). Pursuit of the mechanisms of kindling. *Trends in
Neurosciences*, **11**: 33–6.
McNamara, J., Bonhaus, D., Shin, C., Crain, B. J., Gellman, R. L. & Giacchino,
J. L. (1985). The kindling model of epilepsy: a critical review. *CRC Critical
Reviews in Clinical Neurobiology*, **1**: 341–91.
McNamara, J. O., Byrne, M. C., Dashieff, R. M. & Fitz, J. (1980). The kindling
model of epilepsy: a review. *Progress in Neurobiology*, **15**: 139–59.
McNamara, J. O., Galloway, M. T., Rigsbee, L. & Shin, C. (1984). Evidence
implicating substantia nigra in regulation of kindled seizure threshold.
Journal of Neuroscience, **4**: 2410–17.
Messenheimer, J., Harris, E. W. & Steward, O. (1978). Sprouting fibers gain
access to circuitry transsynaptically altered by kindling. *Experimental
Neurology*, **64**: 469–81.
Mody, I., Stanton, P. & Heinemann, U. (1988). Activation of
N-methyl-D-aspartate receptors parallels changes in cellular and synaptic
properties of dentate granule cells after kindling. *Journal of
Neurophysiology*, **59**: 1033–54.
Monaghan, D. & Cotman, C. (1985). Distribution of N-methyl-D-aspartate-
sensitive L-[^{3}H]-glutamate-binding sites in rat brain. *Journal of
Neurosciences*, **5**: 2909–19.

Monaghan, D., Holets, V., Toy, D. & Cotman, C. (1983). Anatomical distributions of four pharmacologically distinct ^{3}H-L-glutamate binding sites. *Nature*, **306**: 176–8.

Nadler, J. V. & Cuthbertson, G. (1980). Kainic acid neurotoxicity toward the hippocampal formation: dependence on specific excitatory pathways. *Brain Research*, **195**: 47–56.

Nadler, J. V., Perry, B. & Cotman, C. (1980*a*). Selective reinnervation of hippocampal area CA1 and the fascia dentata after destruction of CA3–CA4 afferents with kainic acid. *Brain Research*, **183**: 1–9.

Nadler, J. V., Perry, B., Gentry, C. & Cotman, C. (1980*b*). Degeneration of hippocampal CA3 pyramidal cells induced by intraventricular kainic acid. *Journal of Comparative Neurology*, **192**: 333–59.

Pinel, J. P. & Rovner, L. (1978). Experimental epileptogenesis: kindling-induced epilepsy in rats. *Experimental Neurology*, **58**: 190–202.

Prince, D. (1978). Neurophysiology of epilepsy. *Annual Review of Neuroscience*, **1**: 395–415.

Racine, R. J. (1972). Modification of seizure activity by electrical stimulation. II. Motor seizure. *Electroencephalography and Clinical Neurology*, **32**: 281–94.

Racine, R., Paxinos, G., Mosher, J. M. & Kairess, E. W. (1988). The effects of various lesions and knife-cuts on septal and amygdala kindling in the rat. *Brain Research*, **454**: 264–74.

Represa, A., Le Gal La Salle, G. & Ben-Ari, Y. (1989*a*). Hippocampal plasticity in the kindling model of epilepsy in rats. *Neuroscience Letters*, **99**: 345–50.

Represa, A., Robain, O., Tremblay, E. & Ben-Ari, Y. (1989*b*). Hippocampal plasticity in childhood epilepsy. *Neuroscience Letters*, **99**: 351–5.

Ribak, C. E. & Peterson, G. M. (1991). Intragranular mossy fibers in rats form synapses with the somata and proximal dendrites of basket cells. *Hippocampus*, **1**: 355–64.

Savage, D. D., Rigsbee, L. C. & McNamara, J. O. (1985). Knife cuts of entorhinal cortex: effects on development of amygdaloid kindling and seizure-induced decrease of muscarinic cholinergic receptors. *Journal of Neuroscience*, **5**: 408–13.

Schwartzkroin, P. A. & Prince, D. (1977). Penicillin-induced epileptiform activity in the hippocampal in vitro preparation. *Annals of Neurology*, **1**: 463–9.

Sloviter, R. (1985). Decreases in hippocampal inhibition and a selective loss of interneurons in experimental epilepsy. *Science*, **235**: 73–6.

Stanfield, B. (1989). Excessive intra- and supragranular mossy fibers in the dentate gyrus of tottering (*tg/tg*) mice. *Brain Research*, **480**: 294–9.

Steward, O., Cotman, C. & Lynch, G. (1974). Growth of a new fiber projection in the brain of the adult rat: reinnervation of the dentate gyrus by the contralateral entorhinal cortex following ipsilateral entorhinal lesions. *Experimental Brain Research*, **20**: 45–66.

Steward, O. & Scoville, S. (1976). Cells of origin of entorhinal cortical afferents to the hippocampus and fascia dentata of the rat. *Journal of Comparative Neurology*, **169**: 347–69.

Steward, O., White, W. F., Cotman, C. & Lynch, G. (1976). Potentiation of excitatory synaptic transmission in the normal and in the reinnervated dentate gyrus of the rat. *Experimental Brain Research*, **26**: 423–41.

Steward, O., Cotman, C. & Lynch, G. (1973). Re-establishment of electrophysiologically functional entorhinal cortical input to the dentate gyrus deafferented by ipsilateral entorhinal lesions: innervation by the contralateral entorhinal cortex. *Experimental Brain Research*, **18**: 396–414.

Sutula, T., Cascino, G., Cavazos, J., Parada, I. & Ramirez, L. (1989). Mossy fiber synaptic reorganization in the epileptic human temporal lobe. *Annals of Neurology*, **26**: 321–30.

Sutula, T., Harrison, C. & Steward, O. (1986). Chronic epileptogenesis induced by kindling in the entorhinal cortex: the role of the dentate gyrus. *Brain Research*, **385**: 291–9.

Sutula, T., He, X., Cavazos, J. & Scott, G. (1988). Synaptic reorganization in the hippocampus induced by abnormal functional activity. *Science*, **239**: 1147–50.

Sutula, T., He, X. & Hurtenbach, C. (1987). Facilitation of kindling by CA3/CA4 lesions: evidence for epileptogenic potential of lesion-induced sprouting and synaptic reorganization. *Epilepsia*, **28**, 947.

Swanson, L. W., Wyss, J. & Cowan, W. M. (1978). An autoradiographic study of the organization of intrahippocampal association pathways in the rat. *Journal of Comparative Neurology*, **181**: 681–716.

Tauck, D. & Nadler, J. V. (1985). Evidence of functional mossy fiber sprouting in the hippocampal formation of kainic-acid treated rats. *Journal of Neuroscience*, **5**: 1016–22.

Wada, J. & Mizoguchi, T. (1984). Limbic kindling in the forebrain-bisected photosensitive baboon, *Papio papio*. *Epilepsia*, **25**: 278–87.

Wyss, J. (1981). An autoradiographic study of the efferent connections of the entorhinal cortex in the rat. *Journal of Comparative Neurology*, **199**: 495–51.

10

Rapidly recurring seizures and status epilepticus: ictal density as a factor in epileptogenesis

ERIC W. LOTHMAN, JANET L. STRINGER, and EDWARD H. BERTRAM

Introduction

The frequency with which seizures occur has received little attention as a factor in epileptogenesis. As a result, there is sparse information relating to the question of whether widely spaced seizures and status epilepticus activate the same pathophysiological processes or whether each is associated with its own particular set of events; it is also not known whether seizures and status epilepticus lead to the same acute and chronic sequelae. In addition, events involved in the progression from isolated seizures to status epilepticus have not been identified.

Over the past several years our laboratory has examined these questions. In order to have precise control over the site of origin and timing of seizures we have used electrical stimulation through electrodes stereotactically positioned in the hippocampal formation of rats. Our work has revealed that small differences in the timing of seizure recurrence can give rise to different sorts of epileptic response. As a consequence various models of epilepsy have emerged. Each is suited to investigate the questions germane to its own particular kind of epileptic condition. However, by comparing results among the models, a number of other broader issues can be explored. Much of our work has utilized awake animals, but we have also extended the models to rats anesthetized with urethane. This extension allows certain studies that are difficult or impossible to perform in the awake rat.

In order to utilize the electrical stimulation models presented here, there are a number of technical issues that must be dealt with. These issues are detailed in the Appendix at the end of this chapter.

323

Ictal density as a factor in epileptogenesis

On the basis of our own work as well as that of others, we have established a way reliably to trigger seizures rapidly from hippocampal stimulating electrodes (for details, see Appendix). To address the influence of the frequency of seizures (referred to below as ictal density) as a factor in epileptogenesis, we focused on the intertrain interval as the dependent experimental variable.

Although the intertrain interval can be varied over a wide range, two basic protocols were identified on the basis of responses (Fig. 10.1). These will be referred to as the continuous hippocampal stimulation (CHS) and the rapidly recurring hippocampal seizure (RRHS) protocols. The CHS protocol has been found to lead to an acute syndrome of self-sustaining limbic status epilepticus as well as a chronic syndrome of spontaneous, recurrent seizures. The RRHS protocol produces a rapid kindling that resembles kindling brought about by customary procedures, but takes place much more quickly. Rapid kindling leads to an enhancement in the severity of triggered seizures, but no spontaneous seizures occur.

Acute seizure responses – rapid kindling and status epilepticus

RRHS protocol

To examine RRHS studies, consider responses to 50 Hz/10 s suprathreshold stimuli delivered once every 5 min (Fig. 10.2(a)). With this paradigm, initial afterdischarges are short and the accompanying behavioral seizures are mild (class 0 or 1 on a conventional five-part kindling scoring system; Racine, 1972), but subsequently prolonged afterdischarge and kindled motor (behavioral classes 4–5) seizures appear. RRHS on subsequent test days shows that this enhanced responsiveness persists, even after several months without stimulation. Besides an enduring enhancement of epileptic responses, rapid kindling brought about by RRHS displays other features (such as transference) that characterize kindling brought about by traditional stimulus protocols. However, rapid kindling with stimuli over 5-min is erratic in that short afterdischarges and non-kindled motor responses are intermingled with kindled responses.

We then examined the effect of increasing the interval between stimuli, while retaining the other stimulus parameters in the RRHS protocol unchanged (Lothman *et al.*, 1985*b*, 1988a). In one experiment this change was instituted on the second or subsequent days of the study. Changing

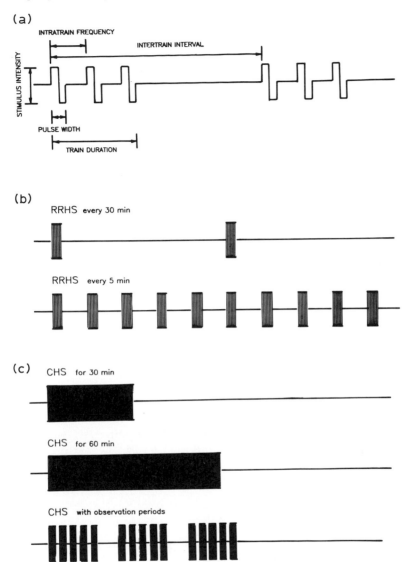

Fig. 10.1. Electrical stimulation protocols. (a) Parameters specifying characteristics of tetanic stimulus trains. Each train consists of three biphasic square wave pulses configured at a constant frequency and intertrain interval. (b) Rapidly recurring hippocampal seizure (RRHS) protocols, occurring at different intervals (see Fig. 10.2). (c) Continuous hippocampal stimulation (CHS) protocols. Two periods of continuous stimulation are illustrated for 30 min and 60 min, respectively. A 'continuous' hippocampal stimulation protocol with interspersed observation periods like that described by Lothman *et al.* (1989) is presented in C3; it included brief (1–5 s) observation periods between 10 s trains as well as long (1 min) stimulation-free intervals at the end of each 10 min epoch.

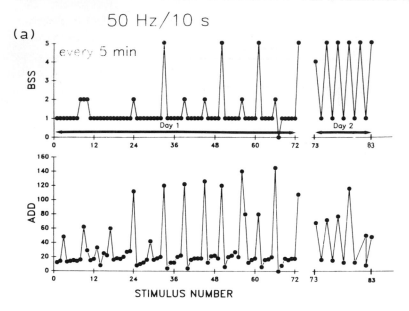

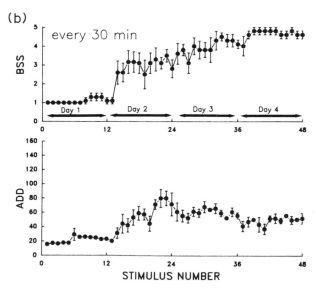

Fig. 10.2. Responses in RRHS protocols. Recurrent stimuli (50 Hz/10 s trains of 400 µA, 1 ms biphasic pulses) were given (a) every 5 min or (b) every 30 min. Behavioral seizure scores (BSS) and afterdischarge durations (ADD in seconds) are plotted against stimulus number (abscissae). Because of variability in responses among animals, data in (a) are from a single rat. With the longer intertrain interval (b) responses are much more homogeneous and data for a group ($n = 6$) of animals are given.

to an interstimulus interval of 30 min results in stable elicitation of kindled motor responses. As a result, this paradigm provides multiple ($\geqslant 16$ per day) stable, kindled responses that can readily be used to carry out time–action studies for various drugs (proconvulsants and anticonvulsants) or other experimental manipulations (Perlin *et al.*, 1987; Lothman *et al.*, 1988*b*).

In another experiment, we retained the previous stimulus parameters (50 Hz/10 s, suprathreshold trains), but set the interstimulus interval at 30 min at the outset of the RRHS protocol. This resulted in a smooth progressive kindling of both motor and electrographic responses, indistinguishable from that encountered with traditional kindling (Fig. 10.2(b)). With this protocol the first kindled responses were detected after an average of 19 stimuli, considerably fewer than are needed to kindle from the hippocampus with a traditional paradigm employing 60 Hz/1 s trains given once daily (Goddard *et al.*, 1969; see also studies reviewed by Lothman *et al.*, 1985*a*).

Thus, 10 s trains used in the RRHS protocol readily overcome the refractory process (adaptation) that causes 1 s trains to fail to trigger afterdischarge at short intervals (Goddard *et al.*, 1969; see also Appendix). Ten second trains are also more potent in triggering kindled responses than are 1 s trains, since intertrain intervals two to three times longer are needed for stable responses with the shorter stimulus duration. Yet, there is a limitation in the ability of the 10 s trains to overcome refractory processes after kindled responses, as they cannot elicit *motor* responses every 5 min.

CHS protocol

In another set of experiments (Lothman *et al.*, 1989), stimuli were kept as 50 Hz/10 s trains, but were moved even closer together so as to allow 0–5 s between trains, the CHS protocol. CHS establishes a condition of status epilepticus involving the hippocampus and associated limbic structures, as determined by electrographic recordings and 2-deoxyglucose autoradiography. We chose to call this syndrome self-sustaining limbic status epilepticus to underscore certain of its key aspects. The origins of the terms self-sustaining and status epilepticus are obvious. The descriptor 'limbic' points out which structures are most heavily involved, although non-limbic structures may be involved as well. Within the limbic system, the hippocampal formation is a major participant. The seizures persist after stimulation has stopped, and there is a stereotyped sequence of

Table 10.1. *Electrographic stages in CHS-induced self-sustaining limbic status epilepticus*

Stage 1: No paroxysmal activity or interictal spiking
Stage 2: Discrete ictal discharges
Stage 3: Continuous fast ictal activity
Stage 4: Intermittent seizures admixed with periodic epileptiform discharges
Stage 5: Periodic epileptiform discharges

electrographic events that progresses through five distinct stages (Table 10.1). It is important to note that the stages in the CHS model faithfully replicate electrographic stages of status epilepticus recorded in humans (Treiman *et al.*, 1990). CHS of ≥30 min duration is needed to establish self-sustaining limbic status epilepticus, which may last up to 24 h. Naive rats and those previously made 'epileptic' by kindling are equally likely to develop status epilepticus with CHS.

The main behavioral accompaniments of CHS-induced status epilepticus are similar to classes 1–2 seizures in kindling (head and facial movements, inattention to environmental stimuli). A few convulsions similar to stage 3–5 seizures in kindling occur intermittently in some animals. During self-sustaining limbic status epilepticus behavioral seizure activity ceases long before electrographic seizures stop (Lothman *et al.*, 1989).

Chronic epileptic sequelae

Another consequence of CHS-induced self-sustaining limbic status epilepticus is recurrent, spontaneous seizures, detected with implanted hippocampal electrodes one month or more after CHS (Lothman *et al.*, 1990) and which persists for at least 14-months, the longest period so far studied (E. W. Lothman & E. H. Bertram, unpublished results). In rats that received RRHS, either at an interstimulus rate of once every 5 or every 30 min, we have not detected any such chronic, spontaneous seizures. The possibility remains that with more intensive monitoring such events might be found. In any case, the propensity for chronic spontaneous seizures is greater after CHS than after RRHS. Thus, the RRHS and CHS protocols lead to different chronic sequelae. With RRHS there is an enhanced responsiveness of triggered seizures; a syndrome of chronic, spontaneous seizures follows CHS.

Because the RRHS and CHS protocols differ only with respect to intertrain interval (being identical for all other stimulus parameters), it follows that the ictal density of the two protocols is the critical factor in influencing the type of response encountered. This point can be best evaluated by comparing electrographic responses from the RRHS and CHS protocols. Consider first acute responses. With RRHS, afterdischarges lengthen up to a certain limit. If the responses are spaced out far enough ($\geqslant 30$ min intertrain interval), stable, recurrent, serial kindled seizures are produced with each stimulus. If the stimulus frequency is fast enough (e.g. every 5 min), certain refractory processes serve to intermix kindled and non-kindled responses. Yet epileptiform activity retains constant electrographic features and remains stimulus locked. In contrast, CHS provokes epileptiform activity that is self-sustaining and evolves through several electrographic stages. With respect to chronic effects, CHS establishes a condition of spontaneous, recurrent seizures whereas RRHS does not.

Mechanisms of critical ictal density

Several hypothetical schemes can be offered to account for these different responses (Fig. 10.3). In the first scheme, there is a build-up of an epileptogenic factor in proportion to the duration of triggered seizure activity until a critical threshold is exceeded, after which self-perpetuating, spontaneous epileptic discharges persist. In the second, the activation of an epileptogenic factor depends on the duration of triggered seizure activity exceeding critical length. In the third, each seizure leads to a fixed amount of change and the appearance of self-sustaining discharges happens when the cumulative alteration exceeds a threshold. In the fourth, there may be a critical period late in a seizure or just after a seizure that only closely spaced stimuli (either by virtue of a short intertrain interval or by the lengthening of seizures 'moving' this sensitive period closer to the next stimulus) activate. These four schemes are not mutually exclusive. In addition, it is possible that different mechanisms can be invoked for each scheme, and one mechanism may account for acute findings and another for chronic findings.

To address the question of whether a critical ictal density could be identified, we further varied the frequency of trains but kept other stimulus parameters constant. While all possible interstimulus intervals between the every 5-min RRHS and every few seconds CHS protocols presented above have not been explored, we have determined that a rate of once

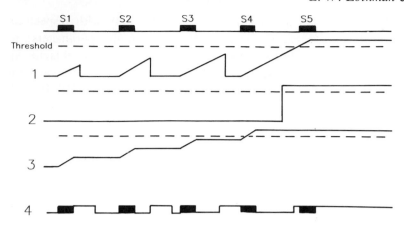

Fig. 10.3. Possible ways in which recurrent seizures may activate processes critical for the development of self-sustaining status epilepticus. Top line indicates when stimuli (S) are given. Although not shown, it should be recognized that seizures will lengthen. Below are four theoretical schemes discussed in text.

every 3-min gives a typical RRHS response while a rate of once every 30 s leads to self-sustaining limbic status epilepticus (Fig. 10.4). Of note also is the fact that 30 min, the length of time determined to be critical for establishing self-sustaining limbic status epilepticus with immediately juxtaposed stimulus trains (see above) was also sufficient when the 'CHS' was 'broken' into more widely separate stimuli. Our typical 6 h, every 5 min, RRHS protocol delivers 72 stimuli. The tightly packed (one train every 10–15 s) 30 min CHS protocol delivers 120 stimuli, while the loosely packed (one train every 30 s) 30 min CHS protocol delivers 60 stimuli. Even though one could attribute the difference between the response to the tightly packed CHS protocol and that to the RRHS protocol to a larger number of stimuli in the former, the findings with the loosely packed CHS protocol exclude this possibility. One can also exclude the expression of kindled motor seizures as a factor. Even in animals that have had several hundred serial kindled motor seizures (elicited with the every 30 min RRHS protocol), self-sustaining limbic status epilepticus did not develop. Thus, we believe that critical criteria for eliciting self-sustaining limbic status epilepticus are the occurrence of multiple closely spaced electrographic seizures *and* that this persists for 30 min or more. This observation not only has clinical relevance (Lothman, 1990), but also has implications for studying mechanisms.

Interestingly the every 30 s protocol also showed lengthening of

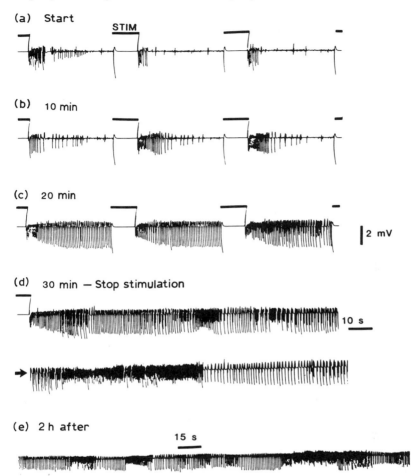

Fig. 10.4. Induction and progression of self-sustaining limbic status epilepticus. Recordings from bipolar electrode stereotactically positioned in the hippocampus and also used to deliver recurrent (every 30 s) stimulus trains (50 Hz, 10 s duration, 400 μA biphasic pulses), as indicated by STIM marks. Time during the CHS protocol is indicated above each line. A total of 30 min of CHS was provided, during which seizures progressively lengthened and eventually became self-sustaining. Electrographic activity in (d) to (e) is stage 4 (see Table 10.1).

triggered afterdischarges like that with the kindling of RRHS (Fig. 10.4). This finding indicates that rapid kindling and establishment of self-sustaining limbic status epilepticus are not mutually exclusive. Of course, this finding does not determine to what degree rapid kindling and self-sustaining limbic status epilepticus share common mechanisms.

The network responsible for epileptic responses in hippocampal stimulation models

To define the functional anatomy of the epileptic conditions established with the CHS and RRHS protocols, experiments employing 2-deoxyglucose autoradiography were carried out. The strategy was to use the autoradiographic findings to direct subsequent studies that were aimed at defining specific types of alteration through the use of electrophysiological, biochemical, pharmacological, and anatomical techniques.

Autoradiographs obtained with RRHS (Lothman *et al.*, 1985a), both before and after rapid kindling, displayed comparably increased glucose utilization bilaterally throughout Ammon's horn (CA3 and CA1). Before kindling, glucose metabolism in the dentate gyrus with seizures was no different from the control (non-seizure) state. After kindling, glucose utilization was increased in this structure, but was still below that in the cornu Ammonis. The transition from the non-kindled to the kindled state was accompanied by more extrahippocampal structures with increased glucose utilization. An implication of these findings is that the dentate gyrus is important in the expression of kindled responses and somehow promotes the propagation of seizures from the hippocampus proper to extrahippocampal regions (see e.g. Chapter 9, this volume).

Autoradiographs obtained during CHS-induced self-sustaining limbic status epilepticus (VanLandingham & Lothman, 1991) also showed bilateral increases of glucose utilization in the cornu Ammonis. The changes on the stimulated and unstimulated sides were equal and were greater than those associated with RRHS. Glucose metabolism was also increased in the dentate gyrus in CHS-induced self-sustaining limbic status epilepticus to a greater degree than in RRHS, so that it equalled the increased glucose utilization in the hippocampus proper. In addition, after CHS there were profound increases in glucose utilization in parahippocampal structures, such as the subiculum, parasubiculum, and entorhinal cortex, and in various other limbic (e.g., amygdala) and extralimbic (e.g. thalamus, substantia nigra) structures. These data indicate that alterations take place not only in the hippocampal formation (cornu Ammonis and dentate gyrus) but also in other closely linked structures.

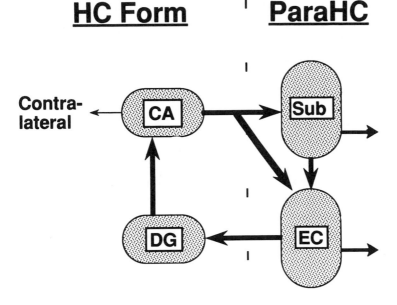

Fig. 10.5. Functional anatomy of circuits important in recurrent hippocampal seizures. Anatomical connections between the hippocampal formation (HC Form, consisting of the dentate gyrus (DG) and cornu Ammonis (CA)) and parahippocampal structures (ParaHC, including the subiculum (Sub) and entorhinal cortex (EC)) form a functional loop, the hippocampal–parahippocampal circuit, that appears to play a role in RRHS and CHS responses as discussed in the text.

The dentate gyrus as a control point for seizures in the hippocampal-parahippocampal loop

It is particularly interesting to note the changes in the parahippocampal structures mentioned above. These regions receive afferents from the hippocampus and, in turn, project back to the hippocampus by way of the perforant pathway, which synapses in the dentate gyrus (Fig. 10.5). Accordingly, a possible feedback loop exists by which hippocampal seizures can be reinforced. Thus, even though the RRHS and CHS protocols stimulate the hippocampus proper, they lead to activation of the dentate gyrus. The 2-deoxyglucose experiments reviewed above suggest that the dentate gyrus operates as a critical control point for epileptogenesis in the hippocampal formation. After kindling, the seizure-associated changes in the dentate gyrus are greater than before; with CHS-induced seizures they are even greater. One way that this could come about is that the dentate gyrus normally serves a gating function, restricting the flow of epileptic activity in the hippocampal–parahippocampal loop (see Fig.

10.5), whereas under conditions of enhanced epileptogenesis, it would operate to support or even amplify seizure activity. Previously we introduced this concept in our studies where recurrent seizures were induced in the entorhinal cortex or perforant pathway (Collins *et al.*, 1983*b*).

Investigating cellular and synaptic processes involved in regulation of seizures by the dentate gyrus

For the reasons just presented, our attention was drawn to the dentate gyrus as an important control point in epileptogenesis. In the cornu Ammonis, even though the CA3 region seems important in generating *interictal* discharges, it is the CA1 region that is critical in generating *ictal* discharges, at least in the mature brain (McBain *et al.*, Chapter 14, this volume; Jensen & Yaari, 1988; Traynelis & Dingledine, 1988). The situation may be different in immature brain (Swann *et al.*, 1988; Swann *et al.*, Chapter 6, this volume). Therefore we elected also to examine the CA1 region of the hippocampus.

To examine cellular and synaptic processes in the CA1 and dentate gyrus in the CHS and RRHS models, we chose electrophysiological recordings. Major experimental advantages of the hippocampal formation in this regard relate to its anatomy. Principal cells (pyramidal cells in the hippocampus proper (cornu Ammonis) and granule cells in the dentate gyrus) constitute the majority of neurons and are arranged in distinct, restricted laminae. Interneurons, while far fewer in number, are also certainly quite important functionally. Yet positioning a microelectrode at various sites along the somato-dendritic domain of principal cells in the hippocampal formation is a practical means of assessing the operation not only of the principal cells but also the interneurons. Obviously intracellular recordings would provide quite important information, either with stimuli that activate large populations of presynaptic terminals or with dual intracellular recordings that activate a single presynaptic cell. However, extracellular recordings in the hippocampal formation are also quite a powerful electrophysiological tool because the laminar anatomy gives rise to large, reproducible, graded population responses (population excitatory postsynaptic potentials and population spikes). Single and paired stimulus paradigms, used to activate various combinations and sequences of afferents innervating the principal cells, can be employed to assess the potency of excitatory and inhibitory processes (Fig. 10.6).

Other technical details should be mentioned. Microelectrode recordings

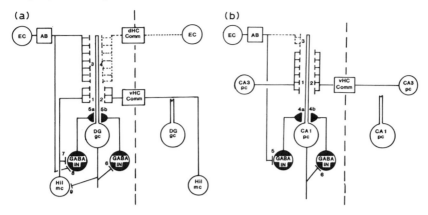

Fig. 10.6. Functional circuitry of dentate gyrus (DG) and CA1 region. Excitatory and inhibitory connections onto (a) DG granule cells (gc) and (b) CA1 pyramidal cells (pc). The midline is indicated by long dashed line, transecting dorsal hippocampal commissure (dHC Comm) and ventral hippocampal commissure (vHC Comm). Anatomically sparse and/or functionally weak inputs indicated by short dotted lines. Note prominent bilateral commissural and associational inputs from hilar mossy cells (Hil mc) onto DG gc ((a):1 and 2). In contrast, the input from entorhinal cortex (EC) is predominantly through the ipsilateral angular bundle (AB) to DG gc ((a):3) and only a sparse input comes from the contralateral side ((a):4). Both ipsilateral ((b):1) and contralateral ((b):2) CA3 pc have heavy projections onto CA1 pc. There is also an input from the ipsilateral EC onto CA1 pc ((b):3), but this does not seem to participate in the generation of seizures (see the text and Stringer & Lothman, 1989c). GABAergic interneurons (GABA IN) project inhibitory terminals onto DG gc ((a):5a and 5b) and onto CA1 pc ((b):4a and 4b). GABA IN may be activated either by feedback ((a):6, (b):6) or feedforward ((a):7, (a):8; (b)5) modes. Hilar mc are also excited by collaterals from DG gc, thereby providing feedback excitation that interacts with feedback inhibition.

can be made in the hippocampal formation of awake rats. However, there are additional confounding issues for the RRHS and CHS protocols. First, convulsions are especially prone to produce artifacts and to dislodge electrodes. Second, there are reasons for using glass instead of the metal microelectrodes that are customarily employed in electrophysiology studies in awake rats. Third, for proper recording of population responses, it is desirable to control the position of the tips of electrodes with a resolution of $\leqslant 10\ \mu m$. Recently we have been able to overcome all these difficulties and record with precisely positioned glass microelectrodes in awake animals during RRHS, but these experiments are difficult and time consuming. The majority of our work took another approach, using rats anesthetized with urethane.

To determine chronic changes brought about by the CHS and RRHS protocols, we enacted these protocols in awake animals and then, after an appropriate 'recovery' period, studied the animals under urethane anesthesia. These data were compared to control animals that had electrodes implanted but did not have seizures. With these experiments, as with all chronic studies, there is the issue of what is the proper recovery time. If recording is done too early, one may be detecting transient rather than enduring alterations. We dealt with this possibility by standardly carrying out our studies with a recovery time of one month (time since last seizure with RRHS and time since end of self-sustaining limbic status epilepticus with CHS). Additional analyses were done in fewer animals at earlier (one to two weeks) and later (several months) times for both RRHS and CHS studies, assuming that if no differences were detected at these points from the one month studies the alterations were permanent.

To determine acute changes, we relied on the fact that both the CHS and RRHS protocols established the desired conditions in a matter of hours. Accordingly, measurements could be made in the same animal before, during, and after establishing the desired epileptiform conditions. It has been determined that in urethane-anesthetized animals results with the CHS and RRHS protocols are, with respect to electrographic responses, comparable to those in awake animals. Motor convulsions are blocked, but electrographic seizures in the hippocampal formation and related limbic structures persist. When RRHS are elicited in urethane-anesthetized rats, there is a brisk electrographic kindling of afterdischarges, recorded in CA1 and in the dentate gyrus, manifested by three-fold or more lengthening of afterdischarge over the course of 20–30 stimuli (Kapur *et al.*, 1989*c*; Stringer & Lothman, 1989*c*; Kapur & Lothman, 1990). In urethane-anesthetized rats, CHS induces a condition of spontaneous epileptiform discharges, but it is less robust and shorter-lived than in awake rats (Kapur & Lothman, 1989; Stringer & Lothman, 1989*a*). In addition, in anesthetized rats there is characteristically a 'quiescent period' between the end of CHS and the appearance of the spontaneous discharges. This quiescent period allows electrophysiological measurements of changes leading up to the appearance of spontaneous epileptiform activity without those discharges actually complicating the measurements.

Maximal dentate activation – a substrate for enhanced epileptic responses

To study mechanisms we used the stimulating and recording arrangements summarized in Fig. 10.7. Stimulating electrodes were placed in the angular bundle (AB) and the regio inferior (RI). Recordings were made with glass

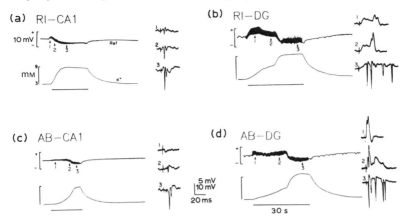

Fig. 10.7. Maximal activation in CA1 and dentate gyrus. Each panel consists of chart tracings registering DC potential (top) and $[K^+]_o$ (below) responses to a stimulus train (10 Hz). In each panel the stimulus site (either the contralateral regio inferior (RI) or the ipsilateral angular bundle (AB)) is given first and the recording site (either in the stratum pyramidale of the CA1 or the stratum granulosum of the dentate gyrus (DG)) second. The stimulation is indicated by lines below $[K^+]_o$ traces. Calibrations are given in (a). For each panel the right-hand inserts present oscilloscope traces obtained at times indicayed on DC chart recordings. Calibration for these oscilloscope traces given between (c) and (d); horizontal, 20 ms throughout; vertical 5 mV in (a) and (c); 10 mV in (b) and (d).

micropipettes (in most cases potassium-sensitive microelectrodes) positioned either in the stratum pyramidale of the CA1 region or the stratum granulosum of the dentate gyrus (Stringer & Lothman, 1989c; Stringer *et al.*, 1989). Using the population spikes, DC steady potential changes and, extracellular potassium concentration ($[K^+]_o$) responses, tetanic stimuli were employed to identify conditions of 'maximal activation' at the two recording sites (Fig. 10.7). Maximal activation in CA1 showed a brisk, smooth build-up, and was seen with frequencies of 10–100 Hz with RI stimuli. Maximal dentate activation (MDA) was demarcated by a *delayed* DC shift, 'secondary' rise in $[K^+]_o$, and extremely large amplitude (20–40 mV) population spikes and was activated over a narrow (10–40 Hz) intratrain frequency range. MDA from RI and AB stimulation were identical. Maximal activation of CA1 with AB stimulation was delayed, indicating that it was 'gated' by prior MDA. Identical patterns of maximal activation were found when the RI stimulation was ipsilateral to the recording sites.

The role MDA plays in the responses observed in CA1 was further examined by using intraparenchymal colchicine injections selectively to lesion dentate granule cells (Stringer *et al.*, 1989). Such lesions abolished MDA and caused maximal activation of CA1 to be unsustained, the response failing at about the time MDA would normally have been expected.

Several other features of MDA are noteworthy. We have determined that MDA occurs in awake animals and hence is not an artifact of urethane anesthesia. Furthermore, in awake animals there is a strong correlation between the length of MDA and motor kindling. Moreover, MDA can be activated by stimuli that repeatedly elicit amygdala afterdischarges. Under these conditions, electrographic and motor kindling take place only *after* MDA has appeared (Stringer *et al.*, 1991).

Other information about MDA has been obtained in urethane-anesthetized animals. Under anesthesia, MDA is elicited only with long duration (≥ 5 s) stimulus trains, as would be predicted by its latency (Fig. 10.8). MDA also has an interesting relationship to afterdischarges (Figs. 10.8 and 10.9). Short duration (1–2 s), high frequency (50–100 Hz) trains can elicit afterdischarges, but the corresponding afterdischarge thresholds are several times higher than in the awake animal (J. M. Williamson and E. W. Lothman, unpublished results). At sufficient intensity, long duration trains provide a type of afterdischarge different from those elicited by

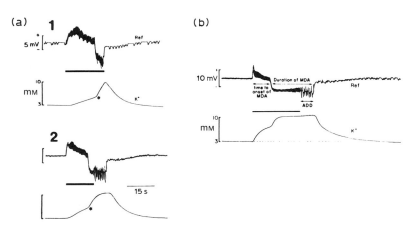

Fig. 10.8. Maximal dentate activation parameters and association with afterdischarges. Stimulation and recording as in Fig. 10.7(b), except that stimulation is to ipsilateral regio inferior and the intratrain frequency is 20 Hz. In (a):1 (stimulus intensity 100 µA) maximal dentate activation (MDA) takes place but remains stimulus-locked so that there is no afterdischarge; in (a):2 (stimulus intensity 650 µA) MDA persists after the stimulus is over, giving rise to an afterdischarge. (b) MDA parameters are defined, including time to onset of MDA, duration of MDA, and afterdischarge duration (ADD).

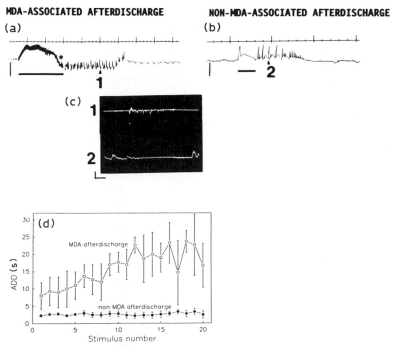

Fig. 10.9. Different types of hippocampal afterdischarges. Recordings obtained in the stratum granulosum of the dentate gyrus in response to stimulation of the contralateral regio inferior. (a) and (b) Chart recordings. Calibration: vertical, 5 mV; horizontal, see second marks above (a) and (b). (a) Stimulation (12 s, 20 Hz, 100 μA, indicated by line below tracing) produces MDA that persists after train to cause MDA-associated afterdischarge. (b) Stimulus (2 s, 100 Hz, 1000 μA) elicits no MDA, but a non-MDA associated afterdischarge develops. Oscilloscope tracing obtained at times 1 (a) and 2 (b) are presented in (c). Calibration: vertical, 7 mV; horizontal, 50 ms. (d) Lengths (ordinate, mean ± s.e.m.) of MDA-associated afterdischarges (open circles, $n = 6$ experiments) and non-MDA-associated afterdischarges (closed circles, $n = 5$ experiments) when repeatedly elicited (abscissa) are shown. Note that MDA-associated afterdischarges are longer and show robust lengthening in comparison to non-MDA-associated afterdischarges.

short duration high frequency trains. The afterdischarges triggered by long duration trains have a greater duration and involve continuation of MDA processes beyond the stimulus. In contrast to those for short duration trains, the afterdischarge thresholds for long duration stimuli were not different between awake and urethane-anesthetized animals (Kapur *et al.*, 1989*c*).

These two kinds of afterdischarge also differ markedly in their response to repeated stimuli. MDA-associated afterdischarges display a robust

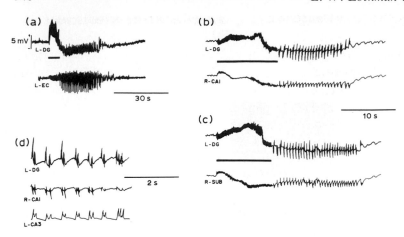

Fig. 10.10. Reverberatory epileptiform activity in hippocampal–parahippocampal circuits in association with maximal dentate activation. (a) to (c) Stimuli were given to the right regio inferior (line below top trace) and recordings were obtained from the stratum granulosum of the left dentate gyrus (DG, top trace) and from other regions as indicated. (d) Faster speed recording of MDA-associated afterdischarge. Calibration: vertical 5 mV, see (a); horizontal, see 30 s (a), 10 s (b) and (c) and 2 s (d) bars. EC, entorhinal cortex; SUB, subiculum.

lengthening upon repetition, whereas afterdischarges not involving MDA do not (Fig 10.9). During MDA-associated afterdischarges, epileptiform activity is synchronized not only in the hippocampal formation, but also in other structures that comprise the hippocampal–parahippocampal loop (Fig. 10.10).

Because of its distinct morphology (Fig. 10.8), MDA can be quantified by several parameters (Stringer & Lothman, 1989c). The time to onset of MDA is an index of how readily MDA is initiated. The duration of MDA is an index of the self-sustaining tendency of MDA. Another measure of this tendency involves the observation that in naive animals the stimulus intensity just sufficient to provoke MDA does not cause an afterdischarge. Rather, MDA ceases when the train is discontinued (Fig. 10.8). However, when the intensity is increased, MDA-associated afterdischarges appear. Accordingly, the ratio of thresholds (for MDA production: MDA-associated afterdischarge production) is a quantitative means for studying MDA.

MDA thus delineates when the dentate gyrus switches from a gating mode, which restricts the flow of epileptiform activity into the hippocampal formation, to a mode that sustains epileptiform activity (Stringer & Lothman, 1989c; Stringer et al., 1989). In the context of the hippocampal–

parahippocampal loop, MDA indicates when reverberatory, self-reinforcing seizures are occurring in this circuit. In addition, MDA is quite 'plastic'. MDA parameters distinguish between 'epileptic conditions' (Stringer & Lothman, 1989*c*). Chronically kindled animals (studied one month after their last seizure) have significantly longer durations of MDA than do naive animals. In naive animals the threshold for MDA afterdischarges is six times higher than the threshold for MDA without afterdischarges; in chronically kindled animals the two thresholds are equal. These alterations are also detected just after (one to two hours) completion of a three hour RRHS protocol in a urethane-anesthetized animal.

Thus, MDA appears to be intimately involved in rapid kindling brought about by RRHS. MDA-associated afterdischarges monitor the course of electrographic kindling, and MDA parameters demarcate a kindled state, measured either just after rapid kindling or at some time later. Whether the same mechanisms are involved in the change of MDA parameters at acute and chronic time points remains to be determined. Because of the difference in the responses of the two types (MDA associated and non-MDA associated) of afterdischarges to repetitive stimuli (see above), MDA also seems to be a potential substrate for rapid kindling of hippocampal seizures.

The relationship between MDA and CHS responses has been studied in urethane-anesthetized rats (Stringer & Lothman, 1989*a*). As mentioned above, the responses under urethane anesthesia are less dramatic than in awake animals. At the outset of CHS there is a sustained seizure that lasts for several minutes. For the remainder of the CHS period, 'cyclic' seizures are noted, each lasting for 30–60 s. These cyclic seizures are associated with MDA. Immediately after CHS, spontaneous epileptiform activity persists for up to 90 min. This activity has features of non-MDA-associated afterdischarges. A quiescent period follows, with no spontaneous discharges. Spontaneous seizure activity returns an average of two hours after termination of CHS. Again, this activity typically has features of non-MDA-associated afterdischarges. Only occasionally are paroxysms with MDA features detected, and in these cases the discharges are notably longer. Autoradiographs, using ^{3}H-labelled 2-deoxyglucose, obtained at this time with the CHS model, in urethane-anesthetized rats do not show increased glucose utilization in the dentate gyrus or parahippocampal structures. This contrasts to autoradiographs obtained in awake animals at a comparable time after CHS in which these structures were labeled.

From these findings, it can be hypothesized that MDA plays an important role in the development of CHS-induced limbic status epilepticus. The following scheme is suggested for the observations on CHS responses in urethane-anesthetized rats. During CHS (as with RRHS), the elicitation of MDA allows recurrent seizures at high frequency. The long duration stimulus trains employed in the RRHS and CHS protocols permit the ready elicitation of MDA. Even though spontaneous epileptiform activity develops in the wake of the recurrent seizures, it is not sufficient to show progressive enhancement, evolving through various stages, or even to become self-sustaining. In contrast, in the awake animal, spontaneous MDA supports self-sustaining seizures in the hippocampus and associated structures.

Changes of inhibition in the dentate gyrus influence epileptic responses

It is now clear that GABA-mediated inhibition in the hippocampus and presumably elsewhere in the forebrain, is quite complex (Andersen *et al.*, 1969; Alger & Nicoll, 1982; Buzsáki, 1984; Bormann, 1988; Dichter, 1988; Lacaille & Schwartzkroin, 1988*a,b*; Nicoll & Dutar, 1989). Much evidence indicates that there are diverse types of inhibitory interneurons, that they can be activated both in a feedforward as well as a feedback fashion, and that there are at last two classes of GABA receptors ($GABA_A$ and $GABA_B$). Our laboratory chose to examine long-lasting changes in GABAergic inhibition as a factor in the epileptic conditions brought about by RRHS and CHS. Recognizing the complexity of GABA-mediated inhibition, we elected first to examine inhibition exerted through $GABA_A$ receptors. A paired-pulse procedure was developed that took into account both the time between the two stimuli and stimulus strength as factors in inhibition (Kapur *et al.*, 1989*c*; Stringer & Lothman, 1989*a*). The procedure also focused on the feedback mode of activation of inhibitory interneurons, although some degree of feedforward activation could not be excluded. This procedure has now been used to analyze the effects of the RRHS and CHS protocols on the potency of GABAergic inhibition in the dentate gyrus and in CA1. Our findings, along with complementary data from other laboratories are summarized in Table 10.2. The results deal with enduring changes and not with the transient suppression of GABA-mediated inhibition that individual seizures cause (Ben-Ari *et al.*, 1979; Kapur *et al.*, 1989*c*; McCarren & Alger, 1985).

Findings are most complete for CA1. RRHS leads to a diminution of GABAergic inhibition, first detectable after completion of the protocol (Kapur *et al.*, 1989*c*), and also chronically after a seizure-free interval

Table 10.2. *Changes of paired-pulse inhibition in stimulation models.*

	CA1		Dentate gyrus	
	Acute	Chronic	Acute	Chronic
RRHS/kindling	↓[a]	↓[b]	↑[c]	↑[d]
CHS/status epilepticus	↓↓[e]	↓↓[f]	↓↓[g]	↓↓[h]

↓, some decrease; ↓↓ large decrease; ↑ some increase.
[a] Kapur *et al.*, 1989*c*; Kapur & Lothman, 1990.
[b] Kapur *et al.*, 1989*a,b*.
[c] Stringer & Lothman, 1989*b*.
[d] Tuff *et al.*, 1983; de Jonge & Racine, 1987.
[e] Kapur & Lothman, 1990.
[f] Lothman *et al.*, 1990.
[g] R. A. Pearce and E. W. Lothman, unpublished results.
[h] J. Kapur and E. W. Lothman, unpublished results; Sloviter, 1983, 1987.

greater than a month (Kapur *et al.*, 1989*b*). Biochemical studies indicate that chronic change involves a dysfunction of GABAergic interneurons (Kapur *et al.*, 1989*a*). The exact nature of this dysfunction and whether the mechanisms underlying the chronic changes relate to mechanisms underlying the acute changes are issues that remain to be determined. Both in our hands and in other laboratories (Kamphuis, 1988; Kapur *et al.*, 1989*a,b*), traditional kindling has also been associated with a diminution of GABA-mediated inhibition in the CA1 region.

CHS leads also to a diminution of GABA-mediated inhibition in CA1, both shortly after completion of the protocol and chronically, several months after dissipation of CHS-induced self-sustaining limbic status epilepticus. In both instances, the changes are much larger than those resulting from the RRHS protocol. We have postulated that the larger diminution of GABA-mediated inhibition that is seen after CHS than after RRHS may be related to the fact that spontaneous seizures are seen in the former condition but not in the latter (Kapur & Lothman, 1989; Lothman *et al.*, 1990). A number of mechanisms could account for the decrement in GABA-mediated inhibition brought about by CHS, including a destruction of inhibitory interneurons, a diminution in their ability to synthesize and/or release GABA, or their disconnection from afferent activation. Which ones are involved remain to be determined.

Observations made in the dentate gyrus are particularly interesting because the CHS and RRHS protocols cause opposite changes in the potency of GABA-mediated inhibition. After RRHS, there is an *enhancement* of inhibition (Stringer & Lothman, 1989*b*). Others have found the same after traditional kindling (Tuff *et al.*, 1983; de Jonge & Racine, 1987). Recently we determined that in the quiescent period after CHS there is a diminution of GABA-mediated inhibition in the dentate gyrus (R. A. Pearce and E. W. Lothman, unpublished results). Chronically ($\geqslant 1$ month) after self-sustaining limbic status epilepticus GABA-mediated inhibition is markedly diminished (R. A. Pearce and E. W. Lothman, unpublished results). Both the observations made acutely and those made chronically after CHS are identical with the results of Sloviter (1983, 1987), who used an electrical stimulus protocol like CHS to model status epilepticus. As for the changes in CA1, the mechanisms underlying the acute and chronic changes in the dentate gyrus have yet to be determined.

Speculations on local circuit alterations in the CHS and RRHS models

In the following we consider mechanisms behind the findings just presented. To account for the acute changes seen after RRHS and CHS, a fragile interneuron hypothesis may be put forward (cf. Fig. 10.6). The key features of this hypothesis are that interneurons are especially vulnerable to the effects of seizures and that the type of vulnerable interneuron differs between the CA1 region and the dentate gyrus. Because of the nature of the stimulus trains used in the RRHS and CHS protocols, one could argue that the changes are the results of the stimulus rather than the seizures they induce. No direct experimental evidence is available on this point. However, as reviewed above, comparable changes in inhibition are detected after traditional kindling stimuli (60 Hz/1 s trains) as after RRHS. Consequently, for the purposes of this discussion it seems appropriate to implicate the seizures. A third component of the hypothesis is that the 'wiring diagram' of the CA1 region contains only inhibitory (GABAergic) interneurons, whereas that of the dentate gyrus contains both inhibitory (GABAergic) and excitatory (hilar mossy cells) interneurons. It is recognized that the wiring diagram can be considered to be oversimplified for the dentate gyrus, given the wealth of neuro-anatomical data suggesting a wide diversity in the morphology and immunohistochemistry of hilar interneurons (Amaral, 1978; Sloviter & Nilaver, 1987).

First consider applications of the hypothesis to the CA1 region. Since they are the only sort of interneuron, GABAergic cells would seem to be vulnerable. Electrophysiological work by Miles & Wong (1987*a,b*) indicates that this type of cell is indeed vulnerable and would begin to dysfunction quickly when exposed to rapidly recurring seizure activity. Our biochemical studies (Kapur *et al.*, 1989*a*) also are consistent with this idea. Since this is the only type of interneuron dysfunction response possible, the same qualitative effect would follow RRHS or CHS, and the more profound disturbance of GABAergic inhibition after the latter could be attributed to the cells experiencing more total seizure activity, to the proximity of seizures, or to both factors (cf. Fig. 10.3).

Next consider the dentate gyrus. In this case the excitatory interneurons (hilar mossy cells) are preferentially vulnerable. The work of Scharfman & Schwartzkroin (1988, 1989, 1990) supports this assumption. Since both types of interneuron are activated in a feedback mode (through collaterals from the dentate granule cells), they normally exert a mixture of excitatory and inhibitory inputs into granule cells. Removal of some or all of the feedback excitatory input, as in the case of preferential dysfunction of excitatory interneurons after recurrent seizures, would be expressed as an increase in paired-pulse inhibition. This sequence would explain the findings of paired-pulse inhibition detected in the dentate gyrus after RRHS. In the extreme, with eradication of all feedback excitatory input to granule cells, the system becomes like the 'more simplified' scheme considered above for CA1.

One can then consider the consequence of impairing the function of the feedback inhibitory circuit in the dentate gyrus. As in CA1, such a deterioration would promote epileptogenesis. Less deterioration would be expected to have a milder influence, serving to allow paroxysms to persist longer once they were initiated. More severe deterioration would exert a stronger influence, perhaps even participating in the initiation or sustenance of paroxysms. In this way, CHS could first lead to an augmentation of paired-pulse inhibition and then a diminution. So far, our experiments have detected only the latter, but this result could be attributed to the timing of the test after CHS. Alternatively, a critical ictal density could account for damage to inhibitory interneurons. In CA1 the inhibitory interneuron damage would come about with more widely spaced seizures (RRHS), whereas in the dentate damage to the inhibitory interneuron would take place only with CHS.

How can one explain the selective vulnerability proposed above? A number of possibilities exist, including different patterns of innervation of the interneurons, differences in the sensitivities of the cells to neurotoxins such as glutamate or quinolinic acid (as determined by dissimilarities in types or densities of receptors on the interneurons), differences in abilities of interneurons to buffer intracellular Ca^{2+} (Meldrum, 1983; Sloviter, 1989), differences in the abilities of interneurons to regulate phosphorylation of receptors (Stelzer *et al.*, 1988), differences in second-messenger systems in interneurons, or differences in the ability of interneurons to sustain high energy phosphates under demands of recurrent seizures. Morphological studies indicate that recurrent seizures, both those of status epilepticus as well as the more widely spaced seizures of kindling, are associated with loss of neurons and sprouting (R. S. Sloviter, personal communication; Sutula *et al.*, 1988; E. W. Lothman & J. M. Williamson, unpublished results). These observations raise a number of other possible mechanisms that could account for the changes after RRHS and CHS. For example, if RRHS caused a selective dropout of excitatory interneurons, subsequent sprouting of granule cell terminals in response to this loss might hyperinnervate GABAergic interneurons, further potentiating paired-pulse inhibition. On the other hand, such sprouting might form synapses on adjacent granule cells setting up a condition of hyerpexcitability through recurrent excitatory feedback.

It is most likely that if the morphological mechanisms just mentioned are involved, they are associated with chronic changes. However, the time course of the sprouting has not yet been worked out. Biochemical mechanisms are more likely to underlie acute changes, and it is possible that rapidly developing changes might be reversible, so that function may be restored, at least in part, to its normal condition. It is possible also that the progression of events might be arrested, leading to chronic dysfunction. Achieving the former would provide information especially useful in dealing with status epilepticus in its emergent presentation; achieving the latter would provide a potential means for modifying the chronic pathophysiology that exists in the epileptic brain, even between seizures. To reach these goals properly will require a thorough interplay of physiological and anatomical investigations.

Acknowledgments

This work was supported in part by grants NS21671, NS25605, and NS01324 from the NINDS. Much of the work reported here was done in collaboration with John Williamson, Jaideep Kapur, Jon Perlin, and Jon Bekenstein. We express our gratitude to Rose Powell for assistance in preparing the manuscript.

Appendix: Electrical stimulation and models of epilepsy

Advances of electrical stimulation-induced models of epilepsy

A number of models rely on chemical agents to elicit epileptiform discharges, and they are discussed elsewhere in this book (see Chapters 2 and 8). Although we began our studies (Lothman & Collins, 1981; Collins *et al.*, 1983*b*; Westbrook & Lothman, 1983) on limbic seizures with 'chemoconvulsants' we subsequently shifted to electrical stimulation because of a number of advantages that this approach offers.

First, electrical stimulation can be delivered either through widely separated macroelectrodes to activate epileptiform discharges throughout the brain (thereby triggering *generalized* seizures) or through closely spaced microelectrodes to activate epileptiform discharges at a chosen site (thereby triggering *focal* seizures). An example of the former is maximal electroshock through corneal electrodes or a pair of skull electrodes to trigger generalized convulsions; examples of the latter are kindling through electrodes placed in a limbic site or electrical stimulation of the neocortex, producing models of complex partial and simple partial seizures, respectively.

Second, as regards stimulus intensity, electrical stimulation is arguably more precise than is pharmacological stimulation. For experiments with systemic administration of chemoconvulsants there are the issues of: (a) how much of the agent passes from the blood to the brain (blood–brain barrier) (e.g. Simon *et al.*, 1982; Zucker et al., 1983); (b) whether seizures change the blood–brain barrier; and (c) how brain concentrations of a chemoconvulsant change over time. Focal administration of chemoconvulsants into selected brain areas is prone to inconsistencies. In some cases the problem can be as mundane as a clogged cannula. Other cases prove enigmatic in that the injections appear to go well, but the typical response is not obtained. In our hands, electrical stimulation has proven more reliable for consistently producing focal seizures than focal injections of drugs into the brain, and afterdischarge thresholds can be readily used to exclude 'bad preparations'. With focal drug injections, even with precise drug deliveries, one must contend with gradients of chemoconvulsant radiating from the injection site and the decline of tissue concentrations of the injected drug over time.

Third, with electrical stimulation the experimenter has accurate control over the timing and occurrence of seizures. Since the stimulus can be turned on and off precisely, stimulus pulses can be delivered for a discrete and fixed time interval and removed, and endogenous epileptogenic processes then observed. In contrast, a chemoconvulsant is present until it is cleared, and this clearance is slow in comparison to the step-function that can be achieved with electrical stimulation. To capitalize fully on this advantage of electrical stimulation attention must be paid to issues of stimulating and recording. We employ an electronic switch that allows us to deliver a stimulus train through an electrode and then record through that electrode just after the stimulus, thereby readily discerning local afterdischarges of the site of stimulation (Lothman *et al.*, 1985*b*). Repeated or prolonged administration of chemical agents introduces the possibilities of tolerance or desensitization.

Fourth, even though electrical stimuli are relatively short and discrete, under the right circumstances they can lead to long-lasting or even permanent epileptiform responses. Perhaps the most familiar of such enduring alterations is the kindled state, which was identified over two decades ago (Goddard *et al.*, 1969).

Fifth, chemoconvulsants also may exert neurotoxic actions separate from their epileptogenic actions (Lothman & Collins, 1981; Collins *et al.*, 1983*a*; Sloviter, 1983). This neurotoxic action may, in turn, confound interpretations. The use of electrical stimulation avoids such neurotoxic complications.

Selection of stimulus parameters

The types of electrical stimulation effective in triggering epileptiform activity are all 'tetanic' stimulus trains. Accordingly, experimental protocols involving such stimuli must be specified by a number of parameters (Fig. 10.1(a)). There is precedent for considering stimulus intensity as an index of epileptogenicity. For example, afterdischarge thresholds, the amount of current necessary for a particular type of electrical stimulus train to elicit a self-sustaining electrographic seizure (afterdischarge), has been used to assess how readily a particular site of the brain develops seizures and how much of an anti-epileptic effect a given dose of drug exerts (Moshé *et al.*, 1981; Löscher & Schmidt, 1988). As is discussed below, a number of other stimulus parameters can be altered as independent experimental variables, looking for their influence on epileptogenicity. This breadth contrasts with chemoconvulsants, which may be varied with respect to only dose given and, under some circumstances, number of doses given.

There is also the question of where to stimulate. In theory any of a number of cortical and subcortical sites could be deemed worthy of study. In the past decade, several structures have been suggested to be critical for *generalized* seizures (Gale, 1988; Miller & Ferrendelli, 1988), but only a few have been studied to any degree with seizures elicited with electrical stimulation. The other major category of seizures, partial seizures, are well suited to study with electrical stimulation, since they depend on discharges originating at a discrete focus. The material presented above deals exclusively with models of epilepsy established with focal stimulation of the hippocampus. The degree to which the findings obtained with our 'hippocampal models' holds for stimulation at other sites, either in the limbic system or elsewhere, remains to be determined.

There were several reasons for focusing on seizures triggered with focal hippocampal stimulation. Previously we had studied the effects of systemic (intravenous) kainic acid (Lothman & Collins, 1981). A pattern of gradually intensifying seizures was found; it began in the hippocampus and then spread progressively to extrahippocampal structures. Interestingly, the augmentation of seizure activity occurred when brain levels of kainic acid were falling. This result suggested that repetitive seizures in the hippocampus were especially potent in activating 'positive feedback processes' that intensified subsequent epileptiform responses.

In addition, there were clinical and experimental reasons behind our selecting the hippocampus for study. A number of observations indicate that the hippocampus is important in epileptogenesis in human patients (Engel, 1987; Falconer, 1978; Sagar & Oxbury, 1987; Wieser, 1988, 1989). In the majority of complex partial seizure patients that have depth electrodes placed, the hippocampus seems to be the primary site of seizure initiation. Removal of the hippocampus in selected epileptic patients can prevent subsequent seizures. Often patients with epilepsy have a distinct neuropathology – hippocampal sclerosis (see Chapters 8 and 9, this volume). The marked tendency of the hippocampus for seizures was well established in experimental animals many years ago (Green, 1964). Even when isolated as slices in vitro, the hippocampus is inclined to epileptiform activity. Furthermore, because of its anatomical features, the hippocampus is especially well suited for a variety of neurobiological studies, including morphology, biochemistry, and physiology.

Having chosen the site for stimulation, we then addressed the question of what type of stimulation should be given. For electrical stimuli to trigger seizures effectively, they must be configured as trains or tetani. While several parameters must be specified (Fig. 10.1), they can be lumped together as determining three critical stimulus features: type of pulse, configuration of pulses within a train, and disposition of trains over time. The proper selection of stimulus parameters is not trivial. As discussed in the text, different selections lead to profoundly different experimental results, either qualitatively (presence or absence of certain findings) or quantitatively (speed of obtaining a particular response or its stability). Our selections of stimulus parameters for the CHS and RRHS protocols were arrived at through a combination of empiric testing and reviewing the work of others.

For all of the work presented here we have used biphasic square wave pulses of regulated currents. We have reasoned that, compared to regulated voltage pulses, current pulses would provide more consistent results among animals, that biphasic pulses would be less prone to charge build-up, and that, compared to ramps or sine waves, square waves would be more effective. While we have not carried out an exhaustive analysis, it has been determined that pulses of 0.3–1.0 ms (for each phase) are effective in the models under consideration. Standardly we employ 0.5 ms pulses.

In order to select stimulus intensities, we have used afterdischarge threshold as an index of stimulus effectiveness. We determined the influence of train duration (0.5–10 s), intratrain frequency (10–100 Hz), and pulse width (0.5–1.0 ms) on afterdischarge thresholds (for details, see Lothman & Williamson, 1992). Suffice it to say here that afterdischarge thresholds were inversely proportional to train duration, intratrain frequency, and pulse width. Pulse width exerted only a minor influence while the other two parameters had a marked influence. Above certain values (train duration $\geqslant 2$ s, intratrain frequency > 20 Hz) afterdischarge thresholds converged (Fig. 10.11). Thus, one can select a variety of stimuli that are 'matched' with respect to afterdischarge thresholds, even though they differ with respect to other parameters. The stimulation models presented above employ suprathreshold stimuli, with current intensities set several times above afterdischarge threshold. Because of the information just presented, suprathreshold stimuli can also be matched.

As a result of our kainic acid work, we became interested in determining the effects of rapidly recurring seizures in the hippocampus, but triggered with electrical stimuli. Findings from prior work with the kindling model were relevant. First, the intensification of motor and electrographic seizure activity with kainic acid bore a resemblance to kindling brought about by recurrent electrical stimuli (Goddard *et al.*, 1969; McNamara *et al.*, Chapter 1, this volume). Second, in the course of their studies on kindling, previous workers had made several observations about the ability of electrical stimuli to elicit a second seizure soon after an initial seizure and to elicit reliably a series of seizures at short intervals. Although often referred to as 'inhibition', 'refractory processes' seems a more appropriate phrase to describe these phenonema.

When traditional kindling stimuli (60 Hz/1 s trains to the amygdala) were given more rapidly than every 20 min, they soon failed to trigger afterdischarge, a process that was called adaptation (Goddard *et al.*, 1969). Mucha & Pinel (1977) studied the effect of changing the interval between such traditional

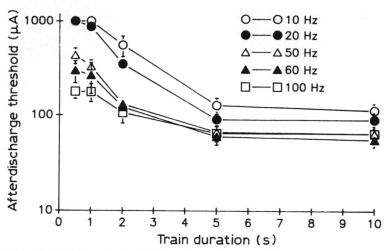

Fig. 10.11. Influence of train duration and intratrain frequency on afterdischarge thresholds. Afterdischarge thresholds for stimuli delivered to bipolar electrodes in the hippocampus were determined in seven animals with an incremental method (Lothman *et al.*, 1985*b*). Amount of current (ordinate, mean ± s.e.m.) needed to produce an afterdischarge is plotted for trains of various lengths (abscissa). Afterdischarge thresholds for different intratrain frequencies indicated by various symbols. Pulse width of 1 ms for all stimuli. If no afterdischarge was obtained by 1000 μA (*n* = 7 for 10 Hz and 20 Hz tests), this value was used in the analysis.

kindling stimuli in amygdala-kindled rats. They determined that there was an interval of 60–90 min after a kindled *motor* seizure before another kindled *motor* seizure could be triggered. There was a shorter interval of about 39 min before another *afterdischarge* could be triggered. Sainsbury *et al.* (1978) obtained the same results when the stimulus site was moved to the hippocampus.

With these points in mind, we carried out a systematic investigation of the stimulus parameters needed to trigger afterdischarge in the hippocampus at a rate of once every few minutes. To summarize the findings, consider one stimulus frequency (50 Hz) and compare the effects of short (1 s) versus long duration (10 s) trains. The amounts of current needed to elicit an afterdischarge were comparable with 50 Hz/1 s and with 50 Hz/10 s trains. However, the afterdischarges triggered by the long duration stimulus trains had markedly different response properties than those triggered by the short duration trains. With short duration trains, there was a long refractory period; they could not be repeated more often than every 60–90 min with the current set at afterdischarge thresholds. If the current was set several times above the afterdischarge threshold, the short duration stimuli could not drive after-discharges faster than every 30 min without the afterdischarge soon failing. These findings were the same as the adaptation mentioned above. In contrast, the long duration stimuli could repetitively drive seizures every few minutes, even with the stimulus intensity set just (10 μA) above the afterdischarge threshold.

One explanation for the greater efficacy of the long duration over the short duration trains could be related to a larger net number of stimuli delivered. To

Table 10.3. *Influence of stimulus parameters on rapid kindling*

Stimulus train: frequency (Hz)/duration (s)	Number of stimuli to first kindled motor seizure
100/10	19.4 ± 2.1 (n = 8)
50/10	19.5 ± 3.3 (n = 6)
20/10	11.0 ± 2.1 (n = 7)
100/2	19.7 ± 2.4 (n = 6)

n, no. of rats; stimuli values are means ±S.E.M.

assess the effect of pulse number and train duration on rapid kindling, we compared rapid kindling (see above) in four groups of rats that received suprathreshold stimulus trains every 30 min, 12 stimuli per day for four consecutive days. Stimulus trains for the four groups were: (a) 100 Hz/10 s; (b) 50 Hz/10 s; (c) 20 Hz/10 s; and (d) 100 Hz/2 s. By the end of the fourth day, all animals gave kindled responses to each stimulus. All of the 10 s trains gave as fast or faster kindling than occurred with the 2 s train (Table 10.3). Moreover, the speed of kindling did not correlate with the number of pulses. In fact, for the 10 s trains, the fastest kindling was seen with the stimulus with the fewest number of pulses. For the stimuli that were matched with respect to number of stimuli (20 Hz/10 s and 100 Hz/2 s trains), the longer duration kindled almost twice as fast. Thus, intratrain frequency is an important factor.

References

Alger, B. E. &Nicoll, R. A. (1982). Feedforward dendritic inhibition in rat hippocampal pyramidal cells studied in vitro. *Journal of Physiology*, **328**: 105–23.

Amaral, D. G. (1978). A Golgi study of cell types in hilar region of the hippocampus in the rat. *Journal of Comparative Neurology*, **32**: 851–914.

Andersen, P., Gross, G. N., Lømo, T. & Sveen, O. (1969). Participation of inhibitory and excitatory interneurones in the control of hippocampal cortical output. In *The Interneuron*, ed. M. A. B. Brazier, pp. 415–65. Berkeley and Los Angeles: University of California Press.

Ben-Ari, Y., Krnjević, K. & Reinhardt, W. (1979). Hippocampal seizures and failure of inhibition. *Canadian Journal of Physiology and Pharmacology*, **57**: 1462–6.

Bormann, J. (1988). Electrophysiology of $GABA_A$ and $GABA_B$ receptors subtypes. *Trends in Neuroscience*, **11**: 112–16.

Buzsáki, G. (1984). Feed-forward inhibition in the hippocampal formation. *Progress in Neurobiology*, **22**: 131–53.

Collins, R. C., Lothman, E. W. & Olney, J. W. (1983a). Status epilepticus in the limbic system: biochemical and pathological changes. In *Advances in Neurology*, vol. 34 *Status Epilepticus*, ed. A. V. Delgado-Escueta, C. G. Wasterlain, D. M. Treiman & R. J. Porter, pp. 277–87. New York: Raven Press.

Collins, R. C., Pearse, R. G. & Lothman, E. W. (1983*b*). Functional anatomy of limbic seizures: focal discharges from medial entorhinal cortex in rat. *Brain Research*, **280**: 25–40.

de Jonge, M. & Racine, R. J. (1987). The development and decay of kindling-induced increases in paired-pulse depression in the dentate gyrus. *Brain Research*, **412**: 318–28.

Dichter, M. A. (1988). Modulation of inhibition and the transition to seizures. In *Mechanisms of Epileptogenesis – The Transition to Seizure*, ed. M. A. Dichter, pp. 169–82. New York: Plenum Press.

Engel, J., Jr (1987). *Surgical Treatment of the Epilepsies*. New York: Raven Press.

Falconer, M. A. (1978). Mesial temporal (Ammon's horn) sclerosis as a common cause of epilepsy: aetiology, treatment, and prevention. *Lancet*, **ii**, 767–70.

Gale, K. (1988). Anatomical and neurochemical substrates of clonic and tonic seizures. In *Mechanisms of Epileptogenesis – Transition to Seizure*, ed. M. A. Dichter, pp. 111–52. New York: Plenum Press.

Goddard, G. V., McIntyre, D. C. & Leech, C. K. (1969). A permanent change in brain functioning resulting from daily electrical stimulation. *Experimental Neurology*, **25**, 295–330.

Green, J. D. (1964). The hippocampus. *Physiological Reviews*, **44**: 561–605.

Jensen, M. S. & Yaari, Y. (1988). The relationship between interictal and ictal paroxysms in an in vitro model of focal hippocampal epilepsy. *Annals of Neurology*, **24**: 591–8.

Kamphuis, W. (1988). Kindling epileptogenesis in CA1 area of the rat hippocampus. Doctoral thesis, University of Amsterdam.

Kapur, J., Bennett, J. P., Jr, Wooten, G. F. & Lothman, E. W. (1989*a*). Evidence for a chronic loss of inhibition in the hippocampus after kindling: biochemical studies. *Epilepsy Research*, **4**: 100–8.

Kapur, J. & Lothman, E. W. (1989). Loss of inhibition precedes delayed spontaneous seizures in the hippocampus after tetanic electrical stimulation. *Journal of Neurophysiology*, **61**: 427–34.

Kapur, J. & Lothman, E. W. (1990). NMDA receptor activation mediates the loss of GABAergic inhibition induced by recurrent seizures. *Epilepsy Research*, **5**: 103–11.

Kapur, J., Michelson, H. B., Buterbaugh, G. G. & Lothman, E. W. (1989*b*). Evidence for a chronic loss of inhibition in the hippocampus after kindling: electrophysiology studies. *Epilepsy Research*, **4**: 90–9.

Kapur, J., Stringer, J. L. & Lothman, E, W. (1989*c*). Evidence that repetitive seizures in the hippocampus cause a lasting reduction of GABAergic inhibition. *Journal of Neurophysiology*, **61**: 417–26.

Lacaille, J.-C. & Schwartzkroin, P. A. (1988*a*). Stratum lacunosum–moleculare interneurons of hippocampal CA1 region. I. Intracellular response characteristics, synaptic responses, and morphology. *Journal of Neuroscience*, **8**: 1400–10.

Lacaille, J.-C. & Schwartzkroin, P. A. (1988*b*). Stratum lacunosum–moleculare interneurons of hippocampal CA1 region. II. Intrasomatic and intradendritic recordings of local circuit interactions. *Journal of Neuroscience*, **8**: 1411–24.

Löscher, W. & Schmidt, D. (1988). Which animal models should be used in the search for new antiepileptic drugs? A proposal based on experimental and clinical considerations. *Epilepsy Research*, **2**: 145–81.

Lothman, E. W. (1990). The biochemical basis and pathophysiology of status epilepticus. *Neurology*, **40** (Suppl 2): 13–23.

Lothman, E. W., Bertram, E. H., Bekenstein, J. W. & Perlin, J. B. (1989). Self-sustaining limbic status epilepticus induced by "continuous" hippocampal stimulation: electrographic and behavioral characteristics. *Epilepsy Research*, **3**: 107–19.

Lothman, E. W., Bertram, E. H., Kapur, J. & Stringer, J. L. (1990). Recurrent spontaneous hippocampal seizures in the rat as a chronic sequela to limbic status epilepticus. *Epilepsy Research*, **6**: 110–18.

Lothman, E. W. & Collins, R. C. (1981). Kainic acid induced limbic seizures: metabolism, behavioral, electroencephalographic and neuropathological correlates. *Brain Research*, **218**: 299–318.

Lothman, E. W., Hatlelid, J. M. & Zorumski, C. F. (1985a). Functional mapping of limbic seizures originating in the hippocampus: a combined 2-deoxyglucose and electrophysiologic study. *Brain Research*, **360**: 92–100.

Lothman, E. W., Hatlelid, J. M., Zorumski, C. F., Conry, J. A., Moon, P. F. & Perlin, J. B. (1985b). Kindling with rapidly recurring hippocampal seizures. *Brain Research*, **360**: 83–91.

Lothman, E. W., Perlin, J. B. & Salerno, R. A. (1988a). Response properties of rapid recurring hippocampal seizures in rats. *Epilepsy Research*, **2**: 356–66.

Lothman, E. W., Salerno, R. A., Perlin, J. B. & Kaiser, D. L. (1988b). Screening and characterization of antiepileptic drugs with rapidly recurring hippocampal seizures. *Epilepsy Research*, **2**: 367–79.

Lothman, E. W. & Williamson, J. N. (1992). Influence of electrical stimulus parameters on afterdischarge thresholds in the rat hippocampus. *Epilepsy Research*, in press.

McCarren, M. & Alger, B. E. (1985). Use dependent depression of IPSPs in rat hippocampal pyramidal cells in vitro. *Journal of Neurophysiology*, **53**: 557–71.

Meldrum, B. S. (1983). Metabolic factors during prolonged seizures and their relation to nerve cell death. In *Advances in Neurology*, vol. 34, ed. A. V. Delgado-Escueta, C. G, Wasterlain, D. M. Treiman & R. J. Porter, pp. 261–76. New York: Raven Press.

Miles, R. & Wong, R. K. S. (1987a). Latent synaptic pathways revealed after tetanic stimulation in the hippocampus. *Nature*, **329**: 724–6.

Miles, R. & Wong, R. K. S. (1987b). Inhibitory control of local excitatory circuits in the guinea-pig hippocampus. *Journal of Neurophysiology*, **388**: 611–29.

Miller, J. W. & Ferrendelli, J. A. (1988). Brainstem and diencephalic structures regulating experimental generalized (pentylenetetrazol) seizures in rodents. In *Current Problems in Epilepsy*, vol. 6 *Anatomy of Epileptogenesis*, ed. B. S. Meldrum, J. A. Ferrendelli & H. G. Wieser, pp. 57–70. London: John Libbey.

Moshé, S. L., Sharpless, N. S. & Kalan, J. (1981). Kindling in developing rats: variability of afterdischarge thresholds with age. *Brain Research*, **211**: 190–5.

Mucha, R. F. & Pinel, J. P. J. (1977). Postseizure inhibition of kindled seizures. *Experimental Neurology*, **54**: 266–82.

Nicoll, R. A. & Dutar, P. (1989). Physiological roles of $GABA_A$ and $GABA_B$ receptors in synaptic transmission in the hippocampus. In *Allosteric Modulation of Amino Acid Receptors: Theoretical Implications*, ed. E. A. Barnard & E. Costa, pp. 195–204. New York: Raven Press.

Perlin, J. B., Lothman, E. W. & Geary, W. A., II (1987). Somatostatin augments the spread of limbic seizures from the hippocampus. *Annals of Neurology*, **21**: 475–580.

Racine, R. J. (1972). Modification of seizure activity by electrical stimulation. II. Motor seizure. *Electroencephalography and Clinical Neurophysiology*, **32**: 281–94.

Sagar, H. J. & Oxbury, J. M. (1987). Hippocampal neuron loss in temporal lobe epilepsy: correlation with early childhood convulsions. *Annals of Neurology*, **22**: 334–40.

Sainsbury, R. S., Bland, B. H. & Buchan, D. H. (1978). Electrically induced seizure activity in the hippocampus: time course for postseizure inhibition of subsequent kindled seizures. *Behavioral Biology*, **22**: 479–88.

Scharfman, H.E. & Schwartzkroin, P. A. (1988). Electrophysiology of morphologically identified mossy cells of the dentate hilus in guinea pig hippocampal slices. *Journal of Neuroscience*, **8**: 3812–21.

Scharfman, H. E. & Schwartzkroin, P. A. (1989). Protection of dentate hilar cells from prolonged stimulation by intracellular calcium chelation. *Science*, **246**: 257–60.

Scharfman, H. E. & Schwartzkroin, P. A. (1990). Responses of cells of the rat fascia dentata to prolonged stimulation of the perforant path: sensitivity of hilar cells and changes of granule cell excitability. *Neuroscience*, **35**: 49–504.

Simon, R. P., Benowitz, N. L., Bronstein, J. & Jacob, P. (1982). Increased brain uptake of lidocaine during bicuculline-induced status epilepticus in rats. *Neurology*, **32**: 196–9.

Sloviter, R. S. (1983). "Epileptic" brain damage in rats induced by sustained electrical stimulation of the perforant path. I. Acute electrophysiological and light microscopic studies. *Brain Research Bulletin*, **10**: 675–97.

Sloviter, R. S. (1987). Decreased hippocampal inhibition and a selective loss of interneurons in experimental epilepsy. *Science*, **235**: 73–6.

Sloviter, R. S. (1989). Calcium-binding protein (calbindin-D_{28K}) and paravalbumin immunocytochemistry: localization in the rat hippocampus with specific reference to the selective vulnerability of hippocampal neurons to seizure activity. *Journal of Comparative Neurology*, **280**: 183–96.

Sloviter, R. S. & Nilaver, G. (1987). Immunocytochemical localization of GABA-, cholecystokinin-, vasoactive intestinal polypeptide-, and somatostatin-like immunoreactivity in the area dentata and hippocampus of the rat. *Journal of Comparative Neurology*, **256**: 42–60.

Stelzer, A., Kay, A. R. & Wong, R. K. S. (1988). GABA-receptor function in hippocampal cells is maintained by phosphorylation factors. *Science*, **241**: 339–41.

Stringer, J. L. & Lothman, E. W. (1989*a*). Model of spontaneous hippocampal epilepsy in the anesthetized rat: electrographic, $[K^+]_o$, and $[Ca^{2+}]_o$ response patterns. *Epilepsy Research*, **4**: 177–86.

Stringer, J. L. & Lothman, E. W. (1989*b*). Repetitive seizures cause an increase in paired-pulse inhibition in the dentate gyrus. *Neuroscience Letter*, **105**: 91–5.

Stringer, J. L. & Lothman, E. W. (1989*c*). Maximal dentate activation: characteristics and alterations after repeated seizures. *Journal of Neurophysiology*, **62**: 136–43.

Stringer, J. L., Williamson, J. M. & Lothman, E. W. (1989). Induction of paroxysmal discharges in the dentate gyrus: frequency dependence and relationship to afterdischarge production. *Journal of Neurophysiology*, **62**: 126–35.

Stringer, J. L., Williamson, J. M. & Lothman, E. W. (1991). Maximal dentate activation is produced by amygdala stimulation in unanesthetized rats. *Brain Research*, **542**: 336–42.

Sutula, T., Xiao-Xian, H., Cavazos, J. & Scott, G. (1988). Synaptic reorganization in the hippocampus induced by abnormal functional activity. *Science*, **239**: 1147–50.

Swann, J. W., Brady, R. J., Smith, K. L. & Pierson, M. G. (1988). Synaptic mechanisms of focal epileptogenesis in the immature nervous system. In *Disorders of the Developing Nervous System: Changing Views on Their Origins, Diagnoses, and Treatments*, ed. J. W. Swann & A. Messer, pp. 19–49. New York: Alan R. Liss.

Traynelis, S. F. & Dingledine, R. (1988). Potassium-induced spontaneous electrographic seizures in the rat hippocampal slice. *Journal of Neurophysiology*, **59**: 259–76.

Treiman, D. M., Walton, N. Y. & Kendrick, C. (1990). A progressive sequence of electroencephalographic changes during generalized convulsive status epilepticus. *Epilepsy Research*, **5**: 49–60.

Tuff, L. P., Racine, R. J. & Damec, R. (1983). The effects of kindling on GABA-mediated inhibition in the dentate gyrus of the rat. I. Paired pulse depression. *Brain Research*, **277**: 79–90.

VanLandingham, K. E. & Lothman, E. W. (1991). Self-sustaining limbic status epilepticus. I. Acute and chronic metabolic studies – limbic hypermetabolism and cortical hypometabolism. *Neurology*, **41**: 1942–9.

Westbrook, G. L. & Lothman, E. W. (1983). Cellular and synaptic basis of kainic acid-induced hippocampal epileptiform activity. *Brain Research*, **273**: 97–109.

Wieser, H.G. (1988). EEG studies, origin and patterns of spread. In *Current Problems in Epilepsy*, vol. 6 *Anatomy of Epileptogenesis*, ed. B. S. Meldrum, J. A. Ferrendelli & H. G. Wieser, pp. 139–54. London: John Libbey.

Wieser, H. G. (1989). The phenomenology of limbic seizures. In *Current Problems in Epilepsy*, vol. 3 *The Epileptic Focus*, ed. H. G. Wieser, E.-J. Speckmann & J. Engel Jr, pp. 113–36. London: John Libbey.

Zucker, D. K., Wooten, G. F & Lothman, E. W. (1983). Blood–brain barrier changes with kainic acid-induced limbic seizures. *Experimental Neurology*, **79**, 4223.

Section 3

'Normal' brain mechanisms that support epileptiform activities

Introduction

In Section 1 of this volume, many current concepts in epilepsy research were discussed within the context of intact animal models. In Section 2, the emphasis was on insights from the in-vitro examination of tissue from such models. In this last section, the experimental 'model' begins with normal tissue. The investigators have asked, 'What are the basic cellular properties, present in normal cells and tissue, that could contribute to the generation of abnormal activity?' These studies provide a lexicon of the 'mights' and 'coulds' with respect to various forms of epileptiform activities.

The discussions presented in this section provide examples of a variety of different levels of analysis. In the chapters by Wilson & Bragdon (Chapter 11) and by Connors & Amitai (Chapter 12), the emphasis is on local circuitry (the connectivity between neural elements) and a consideration of which elements are critical for the generation of abnormal activities. Connors & Amitai pursue this issue by examining the properties of a given cell type as it relates to the generation of epileptiform activities within the circuit. In Chapter 14 (McBain *et al.*) the focus is on the influence of the extracellular milieu surrounding neurons – how changes in that environment might lead to the transformation from normal to abnormal activities, even in the absence of specific abnormalities within given cell populations. Chapter 13 (Wong & Miles) is devoted to the analysis of the critical GABA transmitter/receptor system. GABA (γ-aminobutyric acid), as the primary inhibitory neurotransmitter in the forebrain, maintains normal excitability in the face of many excitatory factors. Wong & Miles show how the function of the GABA system can be modulated by a variety of influences, not restricted to the loss of GABAergic neurons. Finally, Speckmann & Walden (Chapter 15) describe work on voltage-dependent calcium channels, an example of a voltage-dependent current that may contribute significantly to the development of hyperexcitability.

The analyses at each level help to increase our understanding of how epileptiform activity develops, is maintained, and spreads. Each analysis is an extension of prior work carried out in vivo and in in-vitro preparations from chronic models. For example, the circuitry required for the development and spread of epileptiform activities in intact animals has been discussed at some length (e.g. McNamara *et al.* (Chapter 1), Gale (Chapter 2), Jobe *et al.* (Chapter 3) and Moshé (Chapter 5)). In Section 3, however, the *microcircuitry* receives primary attention. In particular, local synaptic interaction in neocortical and limbic system structures are examined to answer such questions as, 'What parts of the systems are low threshold, and function as trigger elements?' In hippocampus, the role of trigger element has been long attributed to the CA3 pyramidal cells – a hypothesis based on the fact that spontaneous synchronous burst discharge can be established in CA3, even when it is isolated from the rest of the hippocampal slice (whereas CA1 requires input from CA3 to establish synchronized bursts, and the dentate gyrus shows little bursting; Mesher & Schwartzkroin, 1980; Miles *et al.*, 1984). Connors & Amitai (Chapter 12) describe an 'intrinsically bursting' cell type in the neocortex that may play a role similar to that of CA3 cells in the hippocampus, or that of deep cells in pyriform cortex described by Hoffman & Haberly (1991). The intrinsic nature of these cells appears to be an important contributor to the establishment of synchronized bursting in these regions. Another apparent requirement in such a population is for a certain degree of synaptic interaction among neurons, such that discharge of one (or a small number of) cell(s) enlists the activity of its neighbors. In the hippocampus, excitatory interconnections between CA3 pyramidal cells have been established experimentally (MacVicar & Dudek, 1980; Miles & Wong, 1986), and our understanding further refined by the development of computer models incorporating that interaction (Traub & Miles, 1991). Given the presence of these bursting cells, and the occurrence of excitatory interactions among them in normal tissue, it may actually seem somewhat surprising that epileptiform discharge is not a 'normal' characteristic of such cell populations.

A number of hypotheses have been offered to account for the development of discharging cell populations, and many of them have studied in-vitro models. Recent work has focused particularly on the role of N-methyl-D-aspartate (NMDA) receptors. Much is now known about the various factors that regulate the efficacy of NMDA receptors – its voltage-dependent blockade by magnesium (Mayer et al., 1984; Nowak et al., 1984), and modulation by glycine (Kleckner & Dingledine, 1988), zinc (Westbrook & Mayer, 1987), and polyamines (Williams et al., 1990). The high level of interest in this receptor–channel complex is based, at least in part, on the fact that the open channel admits calcium into the cell (Dingledine, 1983), where it initiates a number of critical intracellular processes. In many models of epileptiform activity, the development of abnormal bursting activity seems very much dependent on the involvement of NMDA receptors. For example, in the low magnesium model used by a number of laboratories (see e.g. Anderson et al., 1986; Stanton et al., 1987), spontaneous synchronous burst discharge in hippocampal pyramidal cell populations is sensitive to NMDA antagonists such as MK-801. That finding suggests that it is the opening of NMDA channels, by relieving the magnesium blockade, that facilitates epileptiform activity. However, using other means to produce epileptiform discharge (for example, by reducing inhibition with a GABA antagonist) investigators have found a smaller NMDA dependency (Kohr & Heinemann, 1989). We might speculate that the blockade of GABA inhibitory postsynaptic potentials (IPSPs) leads to the facilitation of NMDA channel function, since depolarized cells (i.e., cells that are no longer hyperpolarized by GABA) would show a less effective magnesium blockade of the NMDA channel. However, NMDA blockers are not very effective in antagonizing epileptiform events produced by GABA blockers such as penicillin and bicuculline. In contrast, blockers of voltage-dependent calcium channels have been reported to antagonize bursting activity in these GABA blockade models (Aicardi & Schwartzkroin, 1990; Straub et al., 1990; Chapter 15, this volume).

Studies in normal slices have been quite important for investigating not only issues related to intrinsic cell properties, but also matters of circuitry. In particular, studies of the local circuitry, and of the connections between a target structure and its afferent sources, can be valuable in determining the basis for development of hyperexcitability. However, investigation of these relationships often requires an examination of circuitry that is somewhat broader than that which is found in a simple hippocampal or neocortical slice. It is therefore not surprising that recent efforts have been made to enlarge the extent of the in-vitro preparation to include additional circuitry that might be critical in conferring hyperexcitable sensitivity on target tissues. A number of investigations have now focussed specifically on the relationship between entorhinal cortex and hippocampus. Studies (Stanton et al., 1987; Wilson et al., 1988; Jones & Lambert, 1990 see also

Chapter 11, this volume) have found that interactions between these two regions modulate their discharge patterns. This circuitry is especially interesting for examining the mechanisms underlying interictal versus ictal activities; Wilson & Bragdon's in-vitro studies provide insight into previous clinical observations that suggest that seizures and interictal spiking are, in fact, mutually exclusive (Gotman & Marciani, 1985) (i.e., that there is not a good correlation – or perhaps a negative correlation – between seizure occurrence and frequency of interictal bursting). An understanding of the relationship between generators of interictal and ictal activity is a critical one, since mapping of interictal events is sometimes used to define epileptic foci in the clinical setting (Engel, 1989, p. 8). The in-vitro studies suggest that different brain regions may be responsible for initiation of these two types of epileptiform activity (an observation also made in some cases with position emission tomography imaging; Engel *et al.*, 1982). Resection of foci based on localization of interictal activity may effectively reduce seizures, not because the seizure focus has been removed, but because the circuitry required for generation of this complex pattern of activity has been interrupted or reduced below a critical level.

Support for this point of view, that different regions are preferentially involved in ictal versus interictal activity, comes not only from extended circuitry studies in vitro but also from the work on 'simple' hippocampal slices. For example, as described in Chapter 14 on the effects of high potassium levels on hippocampal discharge, the CA3 region appears to be uniquely designed for synchronized burst discharge (i.e., interictal spiking), whereas CA1 (and entorhinal cortex) appears more likely to be involved in seizure generation. That CA3 should show such characteristics is consistent with the finding that CA3 shows a relatively high degree of recurrent excitatory connectivity among pyramidal cells, but also a powerful inhibitory local circuitry that curtails the duration of the bursts. Thus, in CA3, the 'interictal' burst appears to be a reflection of the interaction mediated by excitatory local circuitry, the intrinsic properties of CA3 pyramidal cells, powerful hyperpolarizing influences, and the extracellular milieu.

If circuitry is important, we might well ask how much of the circuit is necessary to produce epileptiform activity – and what forms of activity remain as the circuit is reduced (as may occur in surgical resections of epileptic foci). Work in in-vitro slices suggests that synchronized bursting activity can be developed in rather small pieces of tissue (e.g., see Chapter 12 (neocortex) and Chapter 13 (hippocampus)). This 'minimal aggregate' appears to be sufficient to support interictal-type discharge, but larger regions may be required for generating ictal-like events. Also, the size of the 'minimal aggregate' depends critically on which cell types are included. This issue is illustrated by Haberly and colleagues in their studies of pyriform cortex (Tseng & Haberly, 1989; Hoffman & Haberly, 1991). Although cells in the deep endopyriform nucleus appear to be capable of generating 'interictal' burst discharge, seizure activity appears to depend on the interaction/connection of endopyriform nucleus and deep pyriform cortical pyramidal cells.

The question of how interictal activity is 'transformed' into ictal discharge has long been a key issue in epilepsy research. Just as much of the early work on interictal burst discharge involved studies of GABAergic IPSPs, current hypotheses to explain the interictal-to-ictal transition now also focus on GABA-related mechanisms. The nature of the GABAergic influence, however, has become considerably more complex, given our new understanding of GABA receptors and their modulation. Conventionally, GABA responses have been viewed as chloride-mediated IPSPs that hyperpolarize target neurons. This hyperpolarizing response, mediated by a receptor complex that has many modulation sites (Olsen, 1981; Barnard et al., 1987) (e.g., by benzodiazepines, β-carbolines, etc.) and a variety of 'blocking' sites (e.g., by bicuculline at the GABA receptor itself, or picrotoxin at a site associated with the chloride channel), is not the only effect produced when GABA is applied to central nervous system neurons. Activation of the $GABA_A$ receptor produces depolarizations as well as hyperpolarizations, the former apparently a function of a 'reversed' chloride gradient in the cell (Thompson et al., 1988) (i.e., high intracellular chloride, resulting in chloride efflux when the GABA-gated channel is opened). This depolarizing $GABA_A$ response is seen frequently in immature cortical neurons (Mueller et al., 1984; Luhmann & Prince, 1991) and may account for some aspects of the hyperexcitability of immature tissue. In some sense, even the GABA depolarization may be viewed as inhibitory, since there is a large conductance 'shunt' associated with this depolarizing response. Both hyperpolarizing and depolarizing GABA postsynaptic potentials can serve to synchronize cell populations. Clearly, however, there is a qualitative difference between 'inhibition' produced by hyperpolarizing versus depolarizing $GABA_A$ IPSPs. Wong and colleagues (see Chapter 13, this volume) have shown that there is a variety of means for modulating the efficacy of the $GABA_A$ receptor. Repetitive activation of the receptor with the agonist, as may occur when inhibitory neurons fire repetitively, may lead to a loss of inhibitory efficacy on the postsynaptic cell (McCarren & Alger, 1985). Receptor desensitization and changes in chloride gradient have been explored as underlying bases for these changes (Thompson & Gähwiler, 1989a). Changes in GABA inhibitory efficacy can lead to important effects on the excitability of the system. Indeed, GABAergic IPSPs have been shown to be quite labile in response to repetitive activation of cortical cell populations, as may occur during epileptiform discharge. Chagnac-Amitai & Connors (1989) have shown that even a small percentage change in GABA inhibition can have profound effects on neocortical epileptogenesis, and computer models of hippocampal epileptogenicity are consistent with that demonstration (Traub *et al.*, 1987). These changes in GABAergic inhibition may be the key to an explanation of how repetitive discharge patterns give rise to ictal discharge. Further, there appears to be a significant increase in excitatory postsynaptic potential frequency prior to seizure initiation (Traub & Dingledine, 1990), an observation that is consistent with (but not necessarily causally related to) loss of IPSP efficacy prior to ictal onset.

The loss of inhibitory effects – and the transition between interictal and ictal activities – may depend on even more complex GABAergic mechanisms. The $GABA_B$ receptor is now receiving significant attention for its potential role in control of excitability (Bowery *et al.*, 1990). Activation of $GABA_B$ receptors on cortical neurons produces a rather profound hyperpolarizing effect postsynaptically (Newberry & Nicoll, 1984). Further, data are accumulating that suggest that activation of presynaptic $GABA_B$ receptors results in a reduction of transmitter release, which may be critical to the issue's discharge propensity (Thompson & Gähwiler, 1989b). Activation of $GABA_B$ function in some regions appears to have a clear, pro-seizure effect, whereas its blockade leads to increased inhibitory strength (Mott *et al.*, 1989, 1990). Intuitively, it would seem that presynaptic $GABA_B$ receptors, to have a specialized excitatory or inhibitory effect, must be preferentially localized to either inhibitory or excitatory terminals. For example, activation of presynaptic $GABA_B$ receptors on GABAergic neurons (Misgeld *et al.*, 1989) might well result in a reduction in GABA release, resulting in a more hyperexcitable population; $GABA_B$ inhibition of excitatory neurotransmitter release would have the opposite effect. The differential presynaptic localization of $GABA_B$ receptors on identified cell populations is still to be determined.

Since $GABA_B$ inhibition is mediated not by chloride flux, but by an increase in potassium conductance, the efficacy of this inhibition may also be sensitive to the level of extracellular potassium. It has been known for many years that potassium may play an important role in determining the excitability of a cell population. Early studies showed that epileptiform activity can be induced by bathing central nervous system tissue in artificial cerebrospinal fluid containing high concentrations of potassium (Zuckermann & Glaser, 1970). Using ion-sensitive microelectrodes, investigators have demonstrated significant changes in local extracellular potassium concentrations during burst discharge (Fisher et al., 1976; Heinemann et al., 1977; Hablitz & Heinemann, 1987). These changes are of a magnitude that could affect cell excitability in a number of ways: by depolarizing cell membrane potential, by decreasing the efficacy of potassium dependent potentials (e.g., $GABA_B$ IPSPs, and various afterhyperpolarizing potentials), by depolarizing terminals to produce more transmitter release, etc. Indeed, one hypothesis explaining development of the epileptic focus is that hyperexcitability results from the abnormal function of glia (Pollen & Trachtenberg, 1970) that are unable to provide adequate buffering of the extracellular potassium environment. The view that extracellular potassium is important in the *generation* of seizure activity fell into disfavor when it was discovered (with ion-sensitive microelectrodes) that the transient changes in extracellular potassium associated with bursting activity appeared to be a *result*, not a cause, of neuronal bursting. However, more recent studies have suggested that small steady-state changes in extracellular potassium may have an important effect, particularly in the transition between interictal and ictal activities. The increase in excitatory synaptic activity reported to precede afterdischarge activity (Traub & Dingledine, 1990), and the loss of IPSP hyperpolarizations and of afterhyperpolarizations (Dichter et al., 1972) may be attributed to a rise in extracellular potassium. In immature tissue, extracellular potassium regulation appears to be relatively poorly developed (Haglund & Schwartzkroin, 1990), a factor that may help to explain the seizure propensity of immature brains (Moshé et al., 1983; Hablitz, 1987). It is clear also that potassium channel blockers such as 4-aminopyridine (4-AP) can produce epileptiform activity when applied to cortical and hippocampal tissues (Perreault & Avoli, 1989). Dingledine and collaborators have also shown that changes in extracellular space – which would certainly exaggerate the effect of extracellular potassium – is characteristic of those brain regions that are particularly seizure prone (e.g., CA1 versus CA3) (McBain et al., 1990). Finally, data are accumulating from molecular biological studies that suggest that potassium channel function may play a critical role in seizure generation. For example, one potassium channel in *Drosophila* gives rise to a behavioral phenotype that has seizure-like aspects (the *shaker* mutant; Papazian *et al.*, 1987; Baker & Salkoff, 1990). Other potassium channels, primarily delayed rectifiers, have been cloned from mouse brain (Chandy *et al.*, 1990), and may be involved in seizure-like behaviors in some mouse mutants.

Aside from the potassium channels, the cellular 'pores' that have received most attention in recent years in epilepsy research are the calcium channels (Hess, 1990; Miller, 1991). As discussed previously, several different channels have been identified, and conventionally grouped into three primary types (Nowycky *et al.*, 1985): a transient T-type channel, the L-type channel, and an N-type channel. Evidence for a fourth (P-type) calcium channel has now emerged from toxin studies on cerebellar Purkinje cells (Llinas *et al.*, 1989). Relatively little is known about the functional role of N-type channels in the mammalian central nervous system neurons, although investigators have suggested that it is the predominant calcium channel type in presynaptic terminals. The T-type channel is widespread, but is perhaps most dominant in thalamic neurons. Inactivation of the T-type channel at near resting levels, and the requirement for membrane hyperpolarization to relieve this inactivation, are peculiarly adapted for a contribution toward rhythmic activity (McCormick & Pape, 1990), especially when a large population of such cells receives the output from a single hyperpolarizing influence (i.e., reticular thalamic neuron input to thalamic relay cells; Steriade *et al.*, 1985). Prince and colleagues have found that the T-type channnel is sensitive to ethosuximide, a drug also clinically effective in treating spike-and-wave (absence) activity (Coulter *et al.*, 1989). Thus, it seems likely that these T-type channels are important in the generation of the rhythmic activity that characterizes this type of epilepsy. In contrast, the L-type channel, which is sensitive to dihydropyridines, activates at relatively depolarized thresholds, and stays open for long periods of time (if the cell remains depolarized) (Hess, 1990). It is thought that these channels may be involved in the calcium-mediated bursts that are characteristic of CA3 pyramidal neurons. Catteral and colleagues have recently localized L-type channels to the proximal dendritic regions of pyramidal and granule cells of the hippocampus (Westenbroek *et al.*, 1990). A number of laboratories have suggested that L-type channel blockers may be effective in blocking epileptiform activities (e.g. Meyer *et al.*, 1990; see Chapter 15, this volume).

As is the case for potassium, the cause/effect involvement of calcium in epileptogenesis is complex. It appears that there is significant calcium influx into many neurons when the cells are active; that is, calcium comes into the cell when the cells are depolarized – but calcium does not cause cell depolarization de novo. In this sense, calcium does not appear to play a direct epileptogenic role. However, its role in maintaining burst activity is sufficiently important that various calcium channel antagonists have been studied in clinical trial (Overweg et al., 1986). Perhaps more important, the entry of high levels of calcium into neurons may have serious consequences for the potentiation of synaptic potentials. Long-term potentiation (LTP) phenomena, and perhaps kindling also (see Section I), appear to be dependent on calcium entry (Heinemannn & Hamon, 1986; Malenka et al., 1989). Calcium-binding proteins are common features of cortical neurons, and may be modified by the level of activity within a cell population (Baimbridge et al., 1985); the calcium currents in such cells may show parallel shifts (Mody et al., 1990). Indeed, some cell populations that are deficient in parvalbumin and calbindin are also particularly sensitive to excitotoxic injury (Sloviter, 1987). That high levels of intracellular calcium may lead to cell damage is widely accepted, and calcium channel blockers have been found to be effective in blocking neuronal injury in the cortex and hippocampus, for example in ischemia (Choi & Rothman, 1990). Interestingly, the ischemic patterns of cell loss are similar to those seen in epileptic brain (Franck & Roberts, 1990; Chapter 8, this volume). The source of the calcium rise that leads to such effects is often unclear, since release from intracellular stores, entry through ligand-gated (e.g., NMDA) channels, and entry through voltage-dependent channels (such as the L-type channel) could all contribute.

In searching for cellular factors that might contribute to epileptiform activity, investigators have identified many attributes of normal cell activity. Modulation of transmitter effects, of voltage-gated channels, and of cell electrical properties, involves processes that presumably occur continually during normal brain function. This plasticity allows the cortex to 'learn from experience' and alter the discharge properties of key elements. Current data suggest that the same *plastic* mechanisms may be involved in epileptogenicity – that risk of epileptiform activity is the price we have had to pay for a nervous system that is so adaptive.

References

Aicardi, G. & Schwartzkroin, P. A. (1990). Suppression of epileptiform burst discharges in CA3 neurons of rat hippocampal slices by the organic calcium channel blocker, verapamil. *Experimental Brain Research*, **81**: 188–296.

Anderson, W. W., Lewis, D. V., Swartzwelder, H. S. & Wilson, W. A. (1986). Magnesium-free medium activates seizure-like events in the rat hippocampal slice. *Brain Research*, **398**: 215–19.

Baimbridge, K. G., Mody, I. & Miller, J. J. (1985). Reduction of rat hippocampal calcium-binding protein following commissural, amygdala, septal, perforant path and olfactory bulb kindling. *Epilepsia*, **26**: 460–5.

Baker, K. & Salkoff, L. (1990). The *Drosophila shaker* gene codes for a distinctive K$^+$ current in a subset of neurons. *Neuron*, **2**: 129–40.

Barnard, E. A., Darlison, M. G. & Seeburg, P. (1987). Molecular biology of the GABA$_A$ receptor: the receptor/channel superfamily. *Trends in Neurosciences*, **10**: 502–9.

Bowery, N. G., Bittinger, H. & Olpe, H.-R. (eds.) (1990). *GABA$_B$ Receptors in Mammalian Function*. Chichester: John Wiley.

Chagnac-Amitai, Y. & Connors, B. W. (1989). Horizontal spread of synchronized activity in neocortex and its control by GABA-mediated inhibition. *Journal of Neurophysiology*, **61**: 747–58.

Chandy, G. Williams, C. B., Spencer, R. H., Aguilar, B. A., Ghahshani, S., Tempel, B. L. & Gutman, G. A. (1990). A family of three mouse potassium channel genes with intronless coding regions. *Science*, **247**: 973–5.

Choi, D. W. & Rothman, S. M. (1990). The role of glutamate neurotoxicity in hypoxic-ischemic neuronal death. *Annual Review of Neuroscience*, **13**: 171–82.

Coulter, D. A., Huguenard, J. R. & Prince, D. A. (1989). Characterization of ethosuximide reduction of low-threshold calcium current in thalamic neurons. *Annals of Neurology*, **25**: 582–93.

Dichter, M. A., Herman, C. J. & Selzer, M. (1972). Silent cells during interictal discharges and seizures in hippocampal penicillin foci. Evidence for the role of extracellular K$^+$ in the transition from the interictal state to seizures. *Brain Research*, **48**: 173–83.

Dingledine, R. (1983). *N*-methyl aspartate activates voltage-dependent calcium conductance in rat hippocampal pyramidal cells. *Journal of Physiology*, **343**: 385–405.

Engel, J., Jr (1989). *Seizures and Epilepsy*. Philadelphia: F. A. Davis Co.

Engel, J., Jr, Kuhl, D. E., Phelps, M. E. & Crandall, P. H. (1982). Comparative localization of epileptic foci in partial epilepsy by PET and EEG. *Annals of Neurology*, **12**: 529–37.

Fisher, R. S., Pedley, T. A., Moody, W. J., Jr & Prince, D. A. (1976). The role of extracellular potassium in hippocampal epilepsy. *Archives of Neurology*, **33**: 76–83.

Franck, J. E. & Roberts, D. L. (1990). Combined kainate and ischemia produces 'mesial temporal sclerosis'. *Neuroscience Letters*, **118**: 159–63.

Gotman, J. & Marciani, M. G. (1985). Electroencephalographic spiking activity, drug levels, and seizure occurrence in epileptic patients. *Annals of Neurology*, **17**: 597–603.

Hablitz, J. J. (1987). Spontaneous ictal-like discharges and sustained potential shifts in the developing rat neocortex. *Journal of Neurophysiology*, **58**: 1052–65.

Hablitz, J. J. & Heinemann, U. (1987). Extracellular K$^+$ and Ca^{2+} changes during epileptiform discharges in the immature rat neocortex. *Developmental Brain Research*, **36**: 299–303.

Haglund, M. M. & Schwartzkroin, P. A. (1990). Role of Na,K pump potassium regulation and IPSPs in seizures and spreading depression in immature rabbit hippocampal slices. *Journal of Neurophysiology*, **63**: 225–39.

Heinemann, U. & Hamon, B. (1986). Calcium and epilepsy. *Experimental Brain Research*, **65**: 1–10.

Heinemann, U., Lux, H. D. & Gutnick, M. J. (1977). Extracellular free calcium and potassium during paroxysmal activity in the cerebral cortex of the cat. *Experimental Brain Research*, **27**: 237–43.

Hess, P. (1990). Calcium channels in vertebrate cells. *Annual Review of Neuroscience*, **13**: 337–56.

Hoffmann, W. H. & Haberly, L. B. (1991). Bursting-induced epileptiform EPSPs in slices of piriform cortex are generated by deep cells. *Journal of Neuroscience*, **11**: 2021–31.

Jones, R. S. G. & Lambert, J. D. C. (1990). The role of excitatory amino acid receptors in the propagation of epileptiform discharges from the entorhinal cortex to the dentate gyrus in vitro. *Experimental Brain Research*, **80**: 310–22.

Kleckner, N. W. & Dingledine, R. (1988). Requirement for glycine in activation of NMDA-receptors expressed in *Xenopus* oocytes. *Science*, **241**: 835–7.

Kohr, G. & Heinemann, U. (1989). Effects of NMDA-antagonists on picrotoxin-, low Mg^{2+}- and low Ca^{2+}-induced epileptogenesis and on evoked changes in extracellular Na^+ and Ca^{2+} concentrations in rat hippocampal slices. *Epilepsy Research*, **4**: 187–200.

Llinas, R., Sugimori, M., Lin, J.-W. & Cherksey, B. (1989). Blocking and isolation of a calcium channel from neurons in mammals and cephalopods utilizing a toxin fraction (FTX) from funnel-web spider poison. *Proceedings of the National Academy of Sciences, USA*, **86**, 1689–93.

Luhmann, H. J. & Prince, D. A. (1991). Postnatal maturation of the GABAergic system in rat neocortex. *Journal of Neurophysiology*, **65**: 247–63.

MacVicar, B. A. & Dudek, F. E. (1980). Local synaptic circuits in rat hippocampus: interactions between pyramidal cells. *Brain Research*, **184**: 220–3.

Malenka, R. C., Kauer, J. A., Perkel, D. J. & Nicoll, R. A. (1989). The impact of postsynaptic calcium on synaptic transmission – its role in long-term potentiation. *Trends in Neurosciences*, **12**: 444–50.

Mayer, M. L., Westbrook, G. L. & Guthrie, P. B. (1984). Voltage-dependent block by Mg^{2+} of NMDA responses in spinal cord neurones. *Nature*, **309**: 261–3.

McBain, C. J., Traynelis, S. F. & Dingledine, R. (1990). Regional variation of extracellular space in the hippocampus. *Science*, **249**: 674–7.

McCarren, M. & Alger, B. E. (1985). Use-dependent depression of IPSPs in rat hippocampal pyramidal cells in vitro. *Journal of Neurophysiology*, **53**: 557–71.

McCormick, D. A. & Pape, H.-C. (1990). Properties of a hyperpolarization-activated cation current and its role in rhythmic oscillation in thalamic relay neurons. *Journal of Physiology*, **431**: 291–318.

Mesher, R. A. & Schwartzkroin, P. A. (1980). Can CA3 epileptiform discharge induce bursting in normal CA1 hippocampal neurons? *Brain Research*, **183**: 472–6.

Meyer, F. B., Anderson, R. E. & Sundt, T. M., Jr (1990). Anticonvulsant effects of dihydropyridine Ca^{2+} antagonists in electrocortical shock seizures. *Epilepsia*, **31**: 68–74.

Miles, R. & Wong, R. K. S. (1986). Excitatory synaptic interactions between CA3 neurones in the guinea-pig hippocampus. *Journal of Physiology*, **373**: 397–418.

Miles, R., Wong, R. K. S. & Traub, R. D. (1984). Synchronized after-discharges in the hippocampus: contribution of local synaptic interaction. *Neuroscience*, **12**: 1179–89.

Miller, R. J. (1991). The control of neuronal Ca^{2+} homeostasis. *Progress in Neurobiology*, **37**: 255–85.

Misgeld, U., Müller, W. & Brunner, H. (1989). Effects of (−) baclofen on inhibitory neurons in the guinea pig hippocampal slice. *Pflügers Archiv*, **414**: 139–44.

Mody, I., Reynolds, J. N., Salter, M. W., Carlen, P. L. & MacDonald, J. F. (1990). Kindling-induced epilepsy alters calcium currents in granule cells of rat hippocampal slices. *Brain Research*, **531**: 88–94.

Moshé, S. L., Albala, B. J., Ackermann, R. F. & Engel, J., Jr (1983). Increased seizure susceptibility of the immature brain. *Developmental Brain Research*, **7**: 81–5.

Mott, D. D., Bragdon, A. C. & Lewis, D. V. (1990). Phaclofen antagonizes post-tetanic disinhibition in the rat dentate gyrus. *Neuroscience Letters*, **110**: 131–6.

Mott, D. D., Bragdon, A. C., Lewis, D. V. & Wilson, W. A. (1989). Baclofen has a proepileptic effect in the rat dentate gyrus. *Journal of Pharmacology and Experimental Therapeutics*, **249**: 721–5.

Mueller, A. L., Taube, J. S. & Schwartzkroin, P. A. (1984). Development of hyperpolarizing inhibitory postsynaptic potentials and hyperpolarizing responses to γ-aminobutyric acid in rabbit hippocampus studied in vitro. *Journal of Neuroscience*, **4**: 860–7.

Newberry, N. R. & Nicoll, R. A. (1984). Direct hyperpolarizing action of baclofen on hippocampal pyramidal cells. *Nature*, **308**: 450–2.

Nowak, L., Bregostovski, P., Ascher, P., Hebert, A. & Prochiantz, A. (1984). Magnesium gates glutamate-activated channels in mouse central neurones. *Nature*, **307**: 462–5.

Nowycky, M. C., Fox, A. P. & Tsien, R. W. (1985). Three types of neuronal calcium channels with different calcium agonist sensitivity. *Nature*, **316**: 440–3.

Olsen, R. W. (1981). The GABA postsynaptic membrane receptor–ionophore complex. *Molecular Cellular Biochemistry*, **39**: 261–79.

Overweg, J., Ashton, D., deBeukelaar, F., Binnie, C. D. & Wauquier, A. (1986). Add-on therapy in epilepsy with calcium entry blockers. *European Neurology*, **25** (Suppl. 1): 93–101.

Papazian, D. M., Schwartz, T. L., Tempel, B. L., Jan, Y. N. & Jan, L. Y. (1987). Cloning of genomic and complementary DNA from *shaker*, a putative potassium channel gene from *Drosophila*. *Science*, **237**: 749–53.

Perreault, H. P. & Avoli, M. (1989). Effects of low concentrations of 4-aminopyridine on CA1 pyramidal cells of the hippocampus. *Journal of Neurophysiology*, **61**: 953–90.

Pollen, D. A. & Trachtenberg, M. C. (1970). Neuroglia: gliosis and focal epilepsy. *Science*, **167**: 1252–3.

Sloviter, R. S. (1987). Decreased hippocampal inhibition and a selective loss of interneurons in experimental epilepsy. *Science*, **235**: 73–6.

Stanton, P. K., Jones, R. S. G., Mody, I. & Heinemann, U. (1987). Epileptiform activity induced by lowering extracellular $[Mg^{2+}]_0$ in combined hippocampal–entorhinal cortex slices: modulation by receptors for norepinephrine and N-methyl-D-aspartate. *Epilepsy Research*, **1**: 53–62.

Steriade, M., Deschenes, M., Domich, L. & Mulle, C. (1985). Abolition of spindle oscillations in thalamic neurons disconnected from nucleus reticularis thalami. *Journal of Neurophysiology*, **54**: 1473–97.

Straub, H., Speckmann, E.-J., Bingmann, D. & Walden, J. (1990). Paroxysmal depolarization shifts induced by bicuculline in CA3 neurons of hippocampal slices: suppression by the organic calcium antagonist verapamil. *Neuroscience Letters*, **111**, 99–101.

Thompson, S. M., Deisz, R. A. & Prince, D. A. (1988). Relative contributions of passive equilibrium and active transport to the distribution of chloride in mammalian cortical neurons. *Journal of Neurophysiology*, **60**: 105–24.

Thompson, S. M. & Gähwiler, B. H. (1989a) Activity-dependent disinhibition. II. Effects of extracellular potassium, furosemide, and membrane potential on E_{Cl^-} in hippocampal CA3 neurons. *Journal of Neurophysiology*, **61**: 512–22.

Thompson, S. M. & Gähwiler, B. H. (1989b) Activity-dependent disinhibition. III. Desensitization and $GABA_B$ receptor-mediated presynaptic inhibition in the hippocampus in vitro. *Journal of Neurophysiology*, **61**: 524–33.

Traub, R. D. & Dingledine, R. (1990). Model of synchronized epileptiform bursts induced by high potassium in the CA3 region of the rat hippocampal slice: role of spontaneous EPSPs in initiation. *Journal of Neurophysiology*, **64**: 1009–18.

Traub, R. D. & Miles, R. (1991). *Neuronal Networks of the Hippocampus.* Cambridge: Cambridge University Press.

Traub, R. D., Miles, R. & Wong, R. K. S. (1987). Models of synchronized hippocampal bursts in the presence of inhibition. I. Single population events. *Journal of Neurophysiology*, **58**: 730–51.

Tseng, G.-F. & Haberly, L. B. (1989). Deep neurons in piriform cortex. II. Membrane properties that underlie unusual synaptic responses. *Journal of Neurophysiology*, **62**: 386–400.

Westbrook, G. L. & Mayer, M. L. (1987). Micromolar concentrations of Zn^{2+} antagonize NMDA and GABA responses of hippocampal neurones. *Nature*, **328**: 640–3.

Westenbroek, R. E., Ahlijanian, M. K. & Catterall, W. A. (1990). L-type calcium channels are clustered at the base of major dendrites in hippocampal pyramidal neurons. *Nature*, **347**: 281–4.

Williams, K., Dawson, V. L., Romano, C., Dichter, M. A. & Molinoff, P. B. (1990). Characterization of polyamines having agonist, antagonist, and inverse agonist effects at the polyamine recognition site of the NMDA receptor. *Neuron*, **5**: 199–208.

Wilson, W. A., Swartzwelder, H. S., Anderson, W. W. & Lewis, D. V. (1988). Seizure activity in vitro: a dual focus model. *Epilepsy Research*, **2**: 289–93.

Zuckermann, E. C. & Glaser, G. H. (1970). Activation of experimental epileptogenic foci. Action of increased K^+ in extracellular spaces of brain. *Archives of Neurology*, **23**: 358–64.

11

Brain slice models for the study of seizures and interictal spikes

WILKIE A. WILSON and ANDREW BRAGDON

Introduction

One of the most interesting and controversial aspects of epilepsy research is the relationship between interictal spikes and seizures. Do these phenomena result from the same epileptogenic processes? What does the presence of interictal spikes tell us about conditions in the neuronal network expressing them? How do these two phenomena respond to pharmacological treatments? Does the presence of interictal spiking alter the probability of the network undergoing seizure activity? These and many other long-standing questions remain unresolved.

Our purpose in writing this chapter is not to answer these questions, but to point to model systems in which the relationship between interictal activity and seizures can be explored. Here we describe brain slice preparations in which the slices are subjected to repetitive electrical stimulation. The stimulation transforms the networks so that they exhibit hyperexcitable behavior that is quite similar to the interictal and ictal discharges seen in vivo. We compare stimulation models to a model that utilizes low magnesium artificial cerebrospinal fluid (ACSF) to produce seizure-like activity and epileptiform bursts. We aim to illustrate not only the techniques for implementing such stimulation models, but to offer some sense of the potential rewards and pitfalls that accompany their use.

Definition of terms

First we need to define the electrophysiological phenomena that are discussed below. It is important to remember that the activity observed in brain slices is just that – it is limited by the small network that is present in the recording chamber, and is not a perfect mirror of what goes on in vivo. However, since the brain slice preparations are used as models of in-vivo epileptiform activity, the terminology should relate the events in the slice to those seen clinically or with in-vivo experiments.

In this chapter we use *epileptiform burst* (EB) to refer to the coordinated discharge of a population of neurons lasting 10–200 ms. EBs can be either spontaneous or they can be produced in response to stimulation of the network (triggered EBs). Extracellular recordings of this activity usually show multiple population spikes superimposed on an excitatory post-synaptic potential (EPSP). This is the in-vitro correlate of the interictal spike.

We also need to define what we mean by 'seizures in slices'. 'Seizure' usually refers to a behavioral event, seen in vivo, that is accompanied by organized electrical activity. Since brain slices cannot exhibit behavior, those of us who work with in-vitro preparations are often criticized for referring to seizures in slices. However, the slice models we discuss here do exhibit electrical activity that closely resembles that recorded during behavioral seizures; thus we feel that it is reasonable to believe that the in-vivo activity is based on the same mechanisms that are seen in-vitro. We therefore call 'seizure-like activity' seen in brain slices electrographic seizures or EGSs.

Finally, we need to define the term 'epileptogenesis'. This term has been used in a number of ways, but here we use it to refer to a form of neuroplasticity in which there is a transformation of the neural networks. Thus, we use epileptogenesis to indicate the *process by which a network acquires the ability to express epileptiform activity*, either spontaneously or under stimulation; and, this transformation is *long lasting*, at least for the life of the slice.

For epilepsy, the most studied form of epileptogenesis is the kindling model of seizures. This in-vivo model (see Chapter 1, this volume) is a now classic example of this process of epileptogenesis. Brief electrical stimulations, which initially have little effect on the animal, produce progressively larger and larger responses; eventually the animal exhibits full seizures in response to the same stimulus that initially produced little activity. It is this model of epileptogenesis that inspired our studies in tissue slices in vitro.

Rationale for inducing epileptogenesis by stimulation: studies in slices

Given all of the readily available chemicals that are known convulsants, what is the advantage of using an electrical stimulation technique to induce epileptiform behavior in brain slices? Electrical stimulation offers two primary benefits that chemical treatments do not now offer. First, it allows the genesis of EBs and EGSs without completely overwhelming an inhibitory or excitatory system, yet it mimics the brain activity seen during a seizure. Second, electrical stimulation allows the gradual development of epileptiform activity (epileptogenesis), since the hyperexcitability increases with each stimulation.

What could one expect to gain from a model of epileptogenesis? Primarily, there is the opportunity to study the mechanisms that produce the gradual transformation of the network from normality to hyperexcitability. As is discussed later, there is emerging evidence that epileptogenesis may be pharmacologically separable from seizure expression; i.e., some drugs can suppress the ability of the network to be transformed into a hyperexcitable state, while others do not suppress the transformation but do suppress the epileptiform activity once it is established.

Our first reason for using stimulation models was the ability to induce epileptiform activity without markedly perturbing any known excitatory or inhibitory systems. To us, this offers the clear advantage that all of the neurotransmitter systems are functioning and are thus subject to pharmacological manipulation. Consider, for example, models in which GABA (γ-aminobutyric acid)-mediated inhibition is blocked. There is no doubt that these models are very useful for a variety of studies, but do they give us a true picture of the effects of drugs that might potentiate GABA-mediated activity? Similar concerns would apply to models in which potassium currents are suppressed. One could not examine the network responses to any pharmacological agent that might utilize or modify the behavior of those channels.

Finally, there are the advantages of any brain slice preparation. The brain slices provide a limited neuronal network, so whatever activity is seen must be originating from that network and is not projected from some other unknown site. Moreover, whatever changes underlie the epileptogenesis are certainly within the slice and not in some remote, but connected, network. Finally, the environment of the slice is easily changed to modify the ionic and gas content of the extracellular fluid; and it is easy to achieve known drug levels in the extracellular environment.

Limitations of the models

A clear limitation of any slice model is the loss of neuronal circuitry that slicing produces. First, there is the obvious lack of the *extrinsic* inputs to the hippocampal formation. Whatever modulatory action these circuits may have is missing, yet these could be critical for the expression of the actions of some agents. So, the lack of effect of a chemical on a brain slice model does not necessarily mean that there will be a lack of effect in vivo.

Another potential limitation is the damage to the intrinsic circuitry within the hippocampal formation that slicing produces, including the loss of intrinsic inhibitory and excitatory connections that may run out of the plane of the slice.

Finally, the cutting of brain slices, and the unavoidable crushing and twisting of the tissue, leads to significant cell death. In fact, it is amazing that after about an hour the slices recover sufficiently to display more-or-less normal electrophysiological responses. Most surprising of all, they retain the ability to show remarkable plasticity, which is really the heart of epileptogenesis. However, in the preparation process, there is not only the frank destruction of some neurons, but the release of intracellular matter and transmitter, which may have prolonged effects on slice physiology. So, all of the studies with these models are done in the context of a limited neuronal network that has been subjected to considerable trauma.

Development of the models

Our studies of interictal-like activity and electrographic seizures has evolved over the past seven years. The models have grown from a simple stimulation routine that produced only epileptiform bursting to a complex model in which spontaneous electrographic seizures can be inhibited or triggered by interictal-like bursting. In the following sections we review the development of the various models and consider the strengths and limitations of each of them.

Slice stimulation: a model for producing epileptiform bursts

The first stimulation model we identified was a procedure for inducing epileptiform bursts in hippocampal slices (Stasheff *et al.*, 1985). We stumbled upon this model in the process of giving stimulus trains to induce long-term potentiation in area CA3 of the hippocampus. Several minutes after a particularly strong stimulus train, we noticed that spontaneous epileptiform bursting had developed (Fig. 11.1). This activity strongly resembled the interictal spiking seen in various models of epilepsy, including in-vivo kindling. Thus, we reasoned that the procedure of giving very strong stimulus trains to brain slices might be an

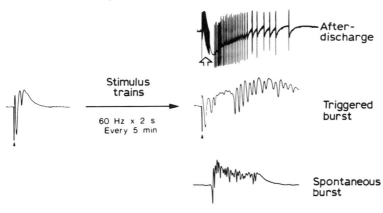

Fig. 11.1. The initial model of stimulus-train-induced bursting (STIB) produced three types of activity illustrated here. Stimulus trains were given every 5 min, and the activity seen here is an extracellular recording from the CA3 stratum pyramidale. First, afterdischarges (top) were seen after each stimulus train (open arrowhead). This is a particularly robust example; often the afterdischarges consisted of only two or three bursts. In the middle trace is an example of a triggered burst that was provoked by a single stimulus to the stratum radiatum of CA3. The bottom trace is a spontaneous burst recorded from the same area. For comparison, a normal field in response to a single pulse (arrowhead) is shown at the left. Figs. 11.1 to 11.6 all use Sprague–Dawley rats aged 21–30 days.

in-vitro technique for producing epileptiform activity that was analogous to in-vivo kindling.

For an electrophysiological model to be maximally useful it should reliably produce a robust and consistent signal. Our most important criterion was the stability of the slices. We put considerable effort therefore toward ensuring that our slices were physiologically stable, i.e., that they would not produce epileptiform bursting just by sitting in the recording chamber without stimulation. First, we set the ionic components of the ACSF closer to those measured in vivo and thus to values consistent with lack of hyperexcitability. We set the extracellular potassium at 3.3 mM (rather than the then-typical level of 5 mM), the calcium level at 1.8 or 1.3 mM, and the magnesium concentration at 1.2 mM. Second, we considered the effects of slice thickness. Although there was some concern that thicker slices would become hypoxic because of the difficulty of oxygen diffusion into the center of a thick slice, we wanted to preserve as many of the inhibitory connections in the slice as possible. Since many inhibitory interneuron axons do not run in the same plane as the slice, we reasoned that thicker slices would contain more inhibitory influences.

We settled on a slice thickness of 625 μm. In comparison to the more common thickness of 400 μm, this setting yielded slices that had less tendency to exhibit spontaneous multiple population spikes in area CA3.

We feel that to have consistent results with stimulation models, it is crucial to restrict variability in animal age and/or size. As we discuss later, full electrographic seizure activity can be seen far more easily in young (age 22–30 days) rats than in older animals. For the original model of epileptiform bursting, we used rats of from 40 to 60 days of age. These older animals were markedly more resistant to epileptogenesis.

Finally, we suspect that the location of the hippocampal slice along the septo-temporal axis of the hippocampus is important. Using ACSF with elevated potassium concentration to induce epileptiform bursting, we have shown that burst frequency varies markedly among the slices (Bragdon *et al.*, 1986). The more temporal the slice, the higher the burst frequency. It is quite important to recognize this source of variability if burst frequency is measured as part of a study. By restricting the location of the slices, one can have less variation in the 'control' condition, and fewer experiments are required in order to see a treatment difference. In our experiments we usually restrict the study to slices from the middle third of the hippocampus.

Although we have studied some of the possible variables in this model, neither we nor others have done a full parametric study of it. For example, we set the stimulus arbitrarily to be 60 Hz for 2 s at twice the stimulus intensity necessary to evoke the maximum orthodromic population spike. We have never systematically explored the use of stimuli of different intensities, different frequencies, or different durations. Also, there has not been a full study of the effects of different concentrations of various ions on the rate of induction of bursting or the burst frequency. We suspect that changing any of these parameters might certainly change the model in a quantitative manner, although we have no reason to believe that any such changes would produce qualitative differences.

So what can we learn from a slice stimulation model that exhibits epileptiform bursting? We feel that it is of great value to have the opportunity to watch epileptogenesis occur over a short, but controllable, period in a network that is very simple compared to the intact central nervous system. What changes occur in the network that allow the bursting to occur? What neurotransmitters mediate this neuroplasticity? What are their second messengers? How much of the network is required for epileptogenesis? What cells are altered in the process? Each of these questions has been long standing in epilepsy research, and, to the extent that a slice model is representative of the intact brain, these questions can be addressed with relative ease in such a model.

Such a stimulation model may be of use in understanding the relationship between interictal spikes and seizures. Later in the chapter we discuss an extension of this model to yield full electrographic seizures (EGSs), and we describe some recent experiments that explore the relationship between them and epileptiform bursting. However, first we review a different model of EGSs in slices and describe the clear relationship between interictal-like discharges and EGSs in that model.

The interaction between epileptiform bursting and seizure-like events: low magnesium ACSF

As we studied the pharmacology of the process of epileptogenesis it became clear that N-methyl-D-aspartate (NMDA) receptors were required for genesis of the hyperexcitability, and we wanted to enhance NMDA function as much as possible. To do this, we omitted magnesium ions from our ACSF (0 Mg^{2+} ACSF), since they are well known to block the NMDA channels when cells are hyperpolarized. To our surprise, the hippocampal slices exposed to this 0 Mg^{2+} ACSF produced organized seizure-like activity (Anderson *et al.*, 1986). Figure 11.2 shows that, unlike the constant, repetitive, epileptiform bursting seen in the stimulus train model described above, the EGSs seen in magnesium-deficient medium were organized into phases of activity that closely resembled the components of EGSs recorded in vivo.

As we studied the EGSs in this environment, we noticed a rather stereotypical pattern to the evolution and decay of the EGSs. First, when the slices were exposed to 0 Mg^{2+} ACSF, epileptiform bursting would occur for a number of seconds. These bursts would resemble the vigorous EBs seen in many models exhibiting 'interictal-like' spiking. Then the intensity of the bursting would increase, there would be a negative shift of the extracellular potential, and the firing rate would increase dramatically. During this early phase of firing, the extracellular recordings at the cell body layer of CA3 showed simple negative deflections occurring at rates of up to 15 Hz. After a few seconds, the activity would change to prolonged, clustered bursts of population spikes; then activity would cease for periods ranging from 3 to 20 min. The cycle would then repeat.

As we watched the progression of this activity, we saw that the quiet period between seizures became shorter and shorter, and the seizures were

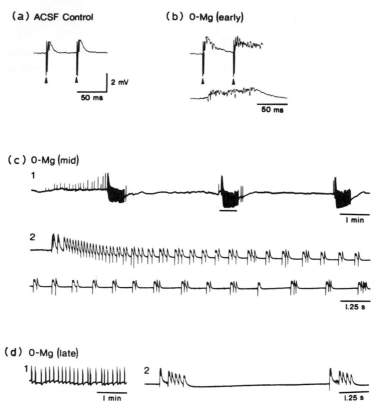

Fig. 11.2. The effects of ACSF with no added magnesium (0 Mg^{2+} ACSF). All traces are extracellular recordings from the stratum pyramidale of CA3 (Sprague–Dawley rats, aged 21–30 days). (a) The response to a pair of stimuli to the stratum radiatum. (b) The early response (after about 30 min of lowered magnesium) to the same stimulus. The lower trace shows a spontaneous burst. (c) Trace 1 shows a series of electrographic seizures; trace 2 shows an enlargement of the middle seizure (bar). (d) The conversion from seizures to spontaneous bursting as the slice remains in the low magnesium solution. Lines 1 and 2 are slow and fast traces of EB activity. (From Anderson *et al.*, 1986.)

eventually replaced by constant epileptiform bursts. At this point, no seizures could be evoked by any kind of stimulation. Apparently, the EBs had rendered the slice incapable of expressing seizures. This was the first indication that constant interictal-like activity could suppress seizures in this model.

To test whether the EBs were indeed responsible for suppressing the EGSs, we used the GABA$_B$ agonist baclofen to inhibit the EBs. Previous studies have shown that baclofen was remarkably effective at suppressing

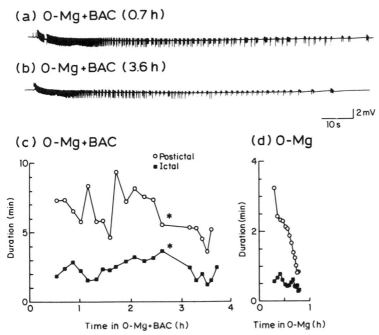

(a) O-Mg+BAC (0.7 h)

(b) O-Mg+BAC (3.6 h)

2mV
10s

(c) O-Mg+BAC

o Postictal
■ Ictal

(d) O-Mg

Duration (min)

Time in O-Mg+BAC (h)

Time in O-Mg (h)

Fig. 11.3. Baclofen prevents the transition from EGSs to spontaneous epileptiform bursting: (a) and (b) a typical experiment. Extracellular recordings from CA3 early and late in the exposure to 0 Mg^{2+} ACSF. (c) and (d) Graphs of the postictal and ictal periods with and without baclofen (2 µM). The ictal period is the time between the first and last discharge of the EGS (duration). The postictal period is the period between the last discharge of one EGS and the discharge of the subsequent EGS (i.e., the interval between EGSs). At the asterisk a 25 s period of epileptiform bursting occurred, but the EGSs resumed after that event. (From Swartzwelder *et al.*, 1987.)

spontaneous and triggered EBs without suppressing normal function. The results using baclofen were startling. Baclofen suppressed the spontaneous EBs, and allowed the EGSs to return vigorously (Swartzwelder *et al.*, 1987). As seen in Fig. 11.3, baclofen also allowed the expression of EGSs for several hours longer than would have occurred in 0 Mg^{2+} ACSF alone.

Then, to test whether the effects of baclofen were mediated through EB suppression or by some other mechanism, we mimicked EBs by repeated field stimulation pulses and found that the EGSs were suppressed. Even strong stimulus trains could not evoke EGSs in these conditions.

This led us to see whether we could make the EGSs reappear by suppressing EBs in another way. We hypothesized that lowering the extracellular potassium and raising the extracellular calcium would suppress EBs and permit the EGSs to reappear. Of course, this would depend upon the EGSs not being blocked by these ionic manipulations. To test this hypothesis, slices were bathed in 0 Mg^{2+} ACSF. We waited until the EGSs were replaced by EBs. Then we lowered the extracellular potassium to 1.5 mM and raised the extracellular calcium to 3 mM. In response to these changes, the EBs disappeared and the EGSs were restored (Bragdon et al., 1992).

We were fascinated to find that the EBs and the EGSs had different sites of initiation. Our slices contained significant amounts of entorhinal cortex, and thus we have a more extensive network than is often present in hippocampal slices. We found that the EBs clearly began in CA3; however, the EGSs started in the entorhinal cortex and spread throughout the slice (Wilson et al., 1988; Bragdon et al., 1992; see also Lewis et al., 1990). The relationship between the EBs and the EGSs was complex, but quite interesting. EBs arose in CA3 and were projected to entorhinal cortex. When EBs were infrequent, they triggered EGSs in the entorhinal cortex, which in turn drove seizures in the hippocampus. When EBs were frequent, they suppressed EGSs in the entorhinal cortex, apparently by causing the entorhinal circuits to fire too frequently. Selectively interrupting the pathway from the hippocampus via CA1 to the entorhinal cortex, while preserving the pathway from the entorhinal cortex through the dentate gyrus to the hippocampus, rendered the EBs from CA3 incapable of suppressing seizure activity in entorhinal cortex or hippocampus (Bragdon et al., 1992).

These data suggest a possible new principle for the relationship between EBs and EGSs, namely, that EBs and EGSs can arise in separate, mutually interactive, locations. Moreover, although EBs can trigger EGSs, their main effect may be to suppress seizures arising in their target areas. Thus, interictal spikes in humans may have a suppressive effect on seizure discharges.

What are the interictal spikes doing to inhibit the expression of EGSs? We do not know for certain. However, we do have one clue. Lewis et al. (1989) pretreated rats with pertussis toxin to suppress G-protein-dependent processes. Then they prepared hippocampal slices from these rats and exposed the slices to 0 Mg^{2+} ACSF. Under these conditions, there were frequent spontaneous EBs coexisting with EGSs. The tendency for the EBs to suppress the EGSs was markedly reduced. It was clear that some pertussis-toxin-sensitive process was mediating the suppression of the EGSs by the EBs. The pertussis effect was not complete because, during prolonged exposure to 0 Mg^{2+} ACSF, the EGSs eventually disappeared.

However, for long periods, the interictal bursting could coexist with EGSs.

It is not known which pertussis-sensitive mechanisms are important, how the EBs activate them, and how they suppress EGSs. However, this experiment illustrates the opportunities provided by an in-vitro model in which EBs interact with EGSs. Such a model offers multiple ways to analyze the relationship between interictal events and seizures and can make possible a detailed pharmacological analysis of the mechanisms of their interaction.

Electrographic seizures in normal ACSF: triggering and suppression by epileptiform bursting

The experiments using 0 Mg^{2+} ACSF revealed two important aspects about the slice preparation. First, they revealed that slices can have organized, repeatable discharges that closely resemble seizures in vivo. Second, they showed that interictal-like bursts of activity can suppress such discharges and render the network incapable of expressing full seizures.

Is it important that slices can have seizures? We believe so, because it indicates that whatever mechanisms underlie the genesis and expression of this complex electrical behavior, these mechanisms reside completely in the relatively restricted area of the slice. We do not have to be concerned that the activity we see in the hippocampus is simply a reflection of something going on in another area projecting to it. We know that whatever neurophysiological alterations accompany seizure genesis, they exist in the section of brain that is in the chamber. Since epilepsy is often considered to be a complex disorder involving numerous brain nuclei and pathways, it is useful to know that the patterned activity of a seizure can be generated in so simple a preparation. The fact that epileptiform bursting can suppress this activity indicates that there may be some important control points or processes in the network that serve an 'anticonvulsant' function. Again, it is encouraging to know that these must also exist in the confines of the slice itself.

Producing EGSs by lowering magnesium was useful, but this did not represent the normal physiological state of the central nervous system; we wanted therefore to find a model in which EGSs could be expressed without ionic alterations or addition of toxins. Electrical stimulation again provided this.

When we originally developed stimulus-train-induced bursting, we observed that accompanying the development of EBs, there was the development of afterdischarges following the stimulus trains (Fig. 11.1). For these studies most of the rats we had used were more than 40 days old. However, our studies with low magnesium indicated that younger animals gave better seizures. We then explored the afterdischarges following stimulus trains in young animals, aged 21–30 days.

Giving stimulus trains to hippocampal slices from these young animals resulted in the 'kindling' of profound electrographic seizures (Stasheff *et al.*, 1989). As shown in Fig. 11.4, the first stimulus train often produced a brief afterdischarge, but it did not resemble a full EGS. However, the trains were given every 10 min; after no more than ten trains the afterdischarges had developed into full EGSs that were quite similar from train to train. The afterdischarges were virtually identical with those seen in 0 Mg^{2+} ACSF. They could last up to 2 min, and they had strong and separable tonic and clonic phases. Most important, we were able to demonstrate that once the network was stimulated a sufficient number of times, the EGSs showed a stereotypical patterned discharge; i.e., they exhibited 'all-or-none' behavior (Anderson *et al.*, 1990).

By all-or-none behavior, we mean that the EGSs were not proportional to the stimulus intensity. We varied the duration of the stimulus train, and in each slice detected a sharp threshold for triggering the EGSs. Once a threshold stimulus was given, the EGSs were fully expressed, and further lengthening of the stimulus train produced no significant enhancement of the EGSs. This is illustrated in Fig. 11.5. This indicated that the afterdischarges we observed were not simply a momentary enhancement of excitability produced by the stimulus train, but represented a transformation of the network to express an organized patterned discharge.

We have begun to investigate whether epileptiform bursting can suppress EGSs in this model. Usually, the induction of EGSs is accompanied by the occurrence of some spontaneous epileptiform bursting. These bursts usually last for less than 50 ms, often resemble large extracellular EPSPs with no or few population spikes, and are certainly not nearly as robust as the bursts seen in 0 Mg^{2+} ACSF. These minor bursts do not prevent the EGSs, and, although we have not done quantitative studies, they do not appear to have much of a suppressive effect. Thus, minor EBs in normal ACSF do not appear to alter EGSs that are driven by strong stimulus trains. However, we are now finding that stronger interictal bursts can suppress these EGSs.

We have observed that application of the $GABA_A$ antagonist bicuculline produces extremely strong EBs in these slices, and these EBs can suppress

Train No.

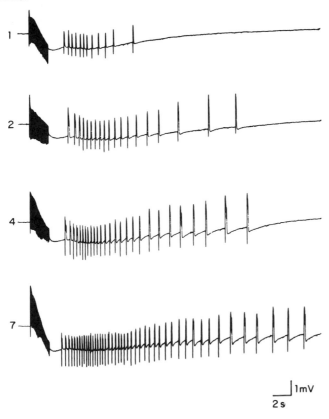

Fig. 11.4. The gradual development of EGS following stimulus trains to slices of the stratum radiatum of CA3. These are extracellular recordings taken from an electrode placed in slices of the stratum pyramidale of CA3. Note the gradual development of a rapid firing (tonic) phase early in the EGS.

the EGSs. These bursts can last more than 200 ms, and often consist of multiple firings of population spikes at the cell body layer throughout the duration of the burst. When these EBs were present, there was a marked reduction in the duration of the triggered EGSs, and especially strong suppression of the tonic phase of firing (Barr & Wilson, 1991).

We tested whether the suppression of the EGSs was caused by the presence of the EBs or simply by some pharmacological effect of the bicuculline. Again, as in the $0 \ Mg^{2+}$ ACSF experiments, we blocked the spontaneous activity with baclofen. As we saw previously, the full EGSs

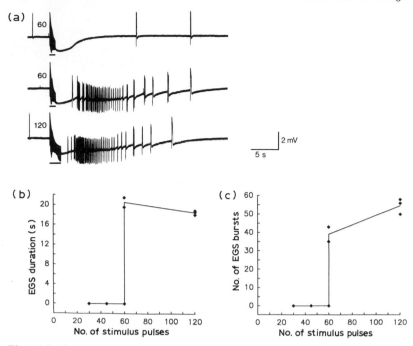

Fig. 11.5. An example of the threshold characteristics of EGSs. These are extracellular recordings from slices of the stratum pyramidale of CA3 following induction of EGSs. In (a) the threshold is shown to be just at 60 stimulus pulses for a 60 Hz train. The first trace shows that a train of 60 pulses at 60 Hz does not elicit an EGS in the slice, while the second trace, taken a few minutes later, shows that the same train does produce an EGS. (b) and (c) Plots of EGS duration and the number of bursts as a function of the number of stimulus pulses in the 60 Hz train. Note the virtually all-or-nothing characteristic. Data from a typical experiment. (From Anderson *et al.*, 1990.)

returned with the cessation of the interictal-like bursting. Moreover, in the presence of the baclofen and bicuculline, we stimulated the slice to mimic spontaneous bursting, and the EGSs were again suppressed. Thus it appears that interictal-like firing in normal ACSF can suppress EGSs *if* the bursting is sufficiently strong.

   One of our concerns is that, while we are able to study triggered EGSs easily, we do not have a good model of spontaneous EGSs in normal ACSF. In our routine experiments, we apply a substantial stimulus to evoke an EGS. A typical threshold stimulus train would be 60 Hz for 0.5 s at a current that was twice that needed to evoke the maximum orthodromic population spike. So, like in-vivo kindling, it has been difficult to push the network to spontaneous seizures. A slice model of stimulus-induced

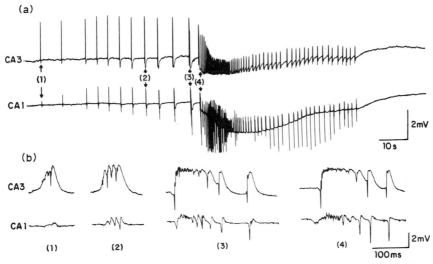

Fig. 11.6. Spontaneous seizures induced by repeated stimulus trains in the hippocampal slice. (a) The two records labeled CA3 and CA1 were recorded simultaneously from stratum pyramidale during the evolution of a spontaneous seizure. The epileptiform bursts were initially of very low amplitude in area CA1, but increased in size during the transition to the EGS. The negative DC shift during the EGSs and the division into tonic and clonic phases can be seen clearly. (b) The expanded traces are seen, correlating with the numbered bursts in (a). Burst 1 is the first in the series, and it begins in CA3. Burst 2 shows a shorter latency and greater amplitude in CA3. Burst 3 shows almost no latency from CA3 to CA1 and contains afterdischarges. Burst 4 begins the EGS and now note that it appears to begin in CA1. (From Lewis & Wilson, 1990.)

spontaneous seizures would be important in determining how spontaneous EBs might modify the network either to suppress or to evoke EGSs.

In a few cases, we have been fortunate to have slices showing spontaneous EGSs in normal ACSF (Fig. 11.6; Lewis & Wilson, 1990). As we have worked with the model, we have begun to find that, after repeated stimulus trains, some slices will exhibit spontaneous EGSs. This is especially true of slices from animals ranging from 15 to 25 days of age. In slices with spontaneous EGSs, we have observed that the EGSs are apparently triggered by the spontaneous interictal-like activity. Once stable EGSs are seen in the slice, the stimulations are stopped. There is then a quiet period, followed by a slow onset of EBs. The EBs increase in duration and frequency, and finally an EGS begins. After the EGS, there is a quiet period, and then the cycle repeats. In several slices that did not show consistent spontaneous EGSs, we could mimic spontaneous

EBs by using stimulus pulses every second. This would often produce a similar build-up of activity that eventually led to an EGS.

So, in this case the interictal-like spontaneous bursts led the network into EGSs. This suggests that there can be a 'pro-epileptic' role for interictal spikes if the network is in such a condition that a build-up of this activity can trigger a seizure.

Conclusion

Is interictal activity pro- or anti-epileptic? It seems to depend on the state of the network. Apparently, if the interictal activity is very strong and if the underlying pacemakers for it are hard to inhibit, then persistent bursting can suppress EGSs. How they do it is not at all clear. On the other hand, if the EGSs are easy to trigger, if the bursting is strong, and if the pacemaker for it is inhibited for a while after the EGS, then the EBs can apparently build up and develop into a full EGS.

It is clear from these models that one can use in-vitro preparations to study electrographic seizures and interictal-like bursts in the same neural network. Considering the damage done during slicing, the loss of inputs from other networks, and the modified physiological environment, the fact that seizure-like activity can be induced and expressed tells us that the mechanisms underlying this must be quite resilient. Furthermore, a network does not have to remain totally intact to support a seizure.

One could argue that this is a very hopeful situation for those who want to understand and ameliorate seizure disorders. Whatever physiological mechanisms underlie epilepsy, at least some of them can likely be revealed by studying brain slices in vitro. This study should be facilitated now that we have models expressing both interictal-like bursts and electrographic seizures.

Finally, the models are clearly sensitive to the developmental stage of the animal. While this means one has to be rigorous in controlling for animal age, it also means that these models can be used to study the role of developmental changes in regulating seizure susceptibility. As more is understood about why young animals are so vulnerable to seizures, we know more how to suppress and potentially to reverse epileptogenesis.

References

Anderson, W. W., Lewis, D. V., Swartzwelder, H. S. & Wilson, W. A. (1986). Magnesium-free medium activates seizure-like events in the rat hippocampal slice. *Brain Research*, **398**: 215–19.

Anderson, W. W., Stasheff, S. F., Swartzwelder, H. S. & Wilson, W. A. (1990). Regenerative, all-or-none electrographic seizures in the rat hippocampal slice in Mg-free and physiological medium. *Brain Research*, **532**: 288–98.

Barr, D. S. & Wilson, W. A. (1991). Bicuculline-induced interictal bursting decreases the duration of stimulus-induced ictal bursting in the rat hippocampal slice. *Society for Neuroscience Abstracts*, **17**: 1441.

Bragdon, A. C., Kojima, H. & Wilson, W. A. (1992). Suppression of interictal bursting in hippocampus unleashes seizures in entorhinal cortex: a paradoxical pro-epileptic effect of lowering $[K^+]_o$ and raising $[Ca^{2+}]_o$. *Brain Research*, in press.

Bragdon, A. C., Taylor, D. M. & Wilson, W. A. (1986). Potassium-induced epileptiform activity in area CA3 varies markedly along the septotemporal axis of the rat hippocampus. *Brain Research*, **378**: 169–73.

Lewis, D. V., Jones, L. S. & Mott, D. D. (1990). Hippocampal epileptiform activity induced by magnesium-free medium: differences between areas CA1 and CA2-3. *Epilepsy Research*, **6**: 95–101.

Lewis, D. V., Jones, L. S. & Swartzwelder, H. S. (1989). The effects of baclofen and pertussis toxin on epileptiform activity induced in the hippocampal slice by magnesium depletion. *Epilepsy Research*, **4**: 109–18.

Lewis, D. V. & Wilson, W. A. (1990). Spontaneous electrographic seizures in the hippocampal slice: an *in vitro* model for the study of the transition from interictal bursting to ictal activity. In *Kindling 4*, ed. J. A. Wada, pp. 11–19. New York: Plenum Press.

Stasheff, S. F., Anderson, W. W., Clark, S. & Wilson, W. A. (1989). NMDA antagonists differentiate epileptogenesis from seizure expression in an *in vitro* model. *Science*, **245**: 648–51.

Stasheff, S. F., Bragdon, A. C. & Wilson, W. A. (1985). Induction of epileptiform activity in hippocampal slices by trains of electrical stimuli. *Brain Research*, **344**: 296–302.

Stasheff, S. F. & Wilson, W. A. (1990). Increased ectopic action potential generation accompanies epileptogenesis *in vitro*. *Neuroscience Letters*, **111**: 144–50.

Swartzwelder, H. S., Lewis, D. V., Anderson, W. W. & Wilson, W. A. (1987). Seizure-like events in brain slices: suppression by interictal activity. *Brain Research*, **410**: 362–6.

Wilson, W. A., Swartzwelder, H. S., Anderson, W. W. & Lewis, D. V. (1988). Seizure activity in vitro: a dual focus model. *Epilepsy Research*, **2**: 289–93.

12

Generation of epileptiform discharge by local circuits of neocortex

BARRY W. CONNORS and YAEL AMITAI

Introduction

So many books have been written on epilepsy that it may seem rash to add
another . . .
(Jackson, 1874)[1]

The neuronal essence of seizures is exceptionally synchronous activity.
Cortical neurons performing normal tasks tend to fire with relatively low
synchrony (Abeles, 1982), but during a seizure the activity of affected
neurons is abruptly usurped. The kernel of this idea was suggested by
John Hughlings Jackson in the nineteenth century; however, the pathological changes that allow hypersynchrony, and the mechanisms that
mediate it, are still elusive (Dichter & Ayala, 1987). Synchrony necessarily
requires interactions between neurons, and the most obvious substrate
for interaction is synaptic circuitry. Here, we focus on the neurons and
circuitry involved in epileptiform activity within the neocortex. The
justification for another discourse on the subject is recent research that
suggests specific circuit-oriented mechanisms for epileptogenesis.

We begin with a brief description of our experimental model, essentially
just an isolated fragment of neocortex in a controlled environment. Our
concern is the minimum amount of tissue necessary for epileptiform
activity, and in the cerebral cortex that turns out to be a surprisingly
small volume. Next we describe the context for seizures, namely for
neurons, synapses and circuits in the neocortex, and describe their
characteristics. Then we investigate hypersynchronous activity itself,
beginning with the phenomena and mechanisms of its initiation, and

---

[1] Quotations of John Hughlings Jackson were taken from the compilation of Taylor (1931).

continuing with the modes of its propagation. We conclude with specific hypotheses about certain forms of synchronous activity in the neocortex. The principal conclusion is that, at most only a few thousand specific neocortical neurons, from one layer (layer 5), are sufficient to initiate, generate and propagate epileptiform activity.

The experimental model

This is the case of a boy who has fits when his head is touched. The case is in many respects very like that of a guinea-pig rendered 'epileptic' by some operation...
(Jackson, 1886)

Our experimental model is completely defined by two manipulations: a small slice of neocortex (about 400 µm thick) is isolated in a specified environment, and its major system of synaptic inhibition is depressed pharmacologically. The advantages of this in-vitro approach include an exquisite degree of control over a small piece of cortical circuitry, and an ability to observe the components of the system in sharp detail. A potential drawback is complacency; it is easy to forget that each fragment of cortex is normally surrounded by a myriad of influences from the rest of the brain, and that it may behave differently in its minimal in-vitro milieu. However, our goal is to isolate and understand a small but fundamental aspect of the problem of epilepsy, and brain slice methods have facilitated this.

The sundry methods of preparing, maintaining and recording from neocortical slices in-vitro have been extensively described (Connors *et al.*, 1982; Connors & Gutnick, 1984*a*; Stafstrom *et al.*, 1984; Thomson, 1986; Hablitz, 1988). Our own rendition is not exceptional. It includes putting the slices (usually derived from the somatosensory area of rats or guinea pigs) at the chamber's gas/liquid interface (Connors *et al.*, 1982), maintaining them at about 34 °C, and using intracellular and extracellular recording, intracellular injections of dye, micropressure ejection of substances, and fine dissection of the slices to isolate layers and pathways.

Compromising synaptic inhibition is one of the most common methods of inducing experimental seizures (Avoli, 1988). It is most easily accomplished pharmacologically. The major inhibitory neurotransmitter in cortex is γ-aminobutyric acid (GABA; Nicoll *et al.*, 1990). Drugs that antagonize receptors for GABA were used to produce experimental epilepsy even before it was understood that they were GABA antagonists;

the most notable example is the antibiotic penicillin (Prince, 1969). In our recent studies we have continued this tradition, substituting well-characterized antagonists of the GABA$_A$ receptor–channel complex (such as bicuculline and its congeners) for the ill-defined drugs of old. It is reasonable to ask why we have stubbornly persisted in studying this aged seizure model, when so many others have been introduced. The answer is that disinhibition is still the best-defined of all the experimental manipulations that produce seizures. The GABA$_A$ system is one of the most ubiquitous and comprehensively understood transmitter systems in the brain, and the drugs available to manipulate it are among the most specific in neuropharmacology (Olsen & Venter, 1987). Many of these drugs are potent convulsants, while others are among the most clinically useful of anticonvulsants (Macdonald, 1989). There is also diverse evidence that the GABA$_A$ system may be very sensitive to brain state and pathology, and even a slight change of its inhibitory efficacy leads to profound changes in cortical excitability (Prince et al., 1990). Also, changes in cortical GABA cells, synapses and receptors have been associated with various chronic models of animal (Ribak, 1991) and human (Lloyd et al., 1986) epilepsy. By contrast, almost all other seizure models work via poorly defined, indirect, or completely unknown cellular and molecular mechanisms. Despite our emphasis on inhibition and epilepsy, we nevertheless recognize that the underlying pathology in various types of seizure disorders is very likely to involve many cellular and neurotransmitter mechanisms.

As presented here, the model of disinhibited neocortical slices takes two major forms: GABA$_A$ receptors are either strongly antagonized (high dose experiments), or only slightly antagonized (low dose experiments). The former use bicuculline or picrotoxin concentrations of about 50 to 100 μM, which essentially eliminates GABA$_A$-mediated inhibition, while the latter use doses of about 0.5 to 1.5 μM, which reduce inhibition by about 10–20% (for references, see Chagnac-Amitai & Connors, 1989a). High dose experiments are presumably simpler to interpret, since the major form of cortical inhibition is essentially eliminated. However, low dose experiments are probably closer to some clinical reality; they have the added advantage of better defining the differences in epileptogenicity between cortical layers and areas.

The disinhibited cortical slice is intended primarily to mimic partial (or focal) epilepsy, seizures that clearly begin within the cortex because of some localized pathology. However, it is reasonable to take a broader view. Some of the mechanisms revealed here may have significance to generalized epilepsies as well. Certain of these idiopathic clinical syndromes may arise from a global cortical pathology that results in a slight reduction in inhibitory strength, due to downregulation of receptors, loss of inhibitory neurons or alteration in GABA biosynthesis for example. As described in Initiation of epileptiform discharge, below, a slightly disinhibited slice of cortex exhibits discrete areas of hyperexcitability, perhaps because of regional differences in the density of certain types of neuron, or synaptic connectivity. One might explain focal phenomena such as auras, or specific afferent stimuli that precipitate seizures (reflex seizures), as the consequence of hyperexcitable hot spots in an otherwise diffusely disinhibited cortex, and the development over time of preferential pathways of seizure spread. Direct tests of these possibilities will be, to say the least, difficult.

Neurons, synapses and circuits of neocortex

We must notice what the normal function of nerve tissue is. Its function is to store up and expend force.
(Jackson, 1873)

Many excellent volumes have recently reviewed the structure and function of the neocortex (see e.g., Jones & Peters, 1984a,b, 1991; White & Keller, 1989), but none has provided a comprehensive treatment of its cellular physiology. There is no space to redress that problem here (for reviews of selected topics, see Connors & Gutnick, 1984a, 1990; McCormick, 1989a; Douglas & Martin, 1990); however, it is worth describing some of the more salient physiology because of its fundamental importance to epileptogenesis.

The neurons

The classification of neocortical neurons has been a biological cottage industry for over a century. With the addition of each new neurotechnology, more weight has been added to the view that neocortex has two major types of neuron, which are concisely (though simplistically) described in either structural terms (spiny cells and smooth cells; cf. Douglas & Martin, 1990), or their respective functional equivalents (excitatory cells and inhibitory cells). The two types differ sharply in anatomy, physiology, chemistry, and synaptic connections. Excitatory (spiny) cells are mostly pyramidal neurons, with a relatively large, polarized apical dendrite and, of course, high densities of dendritic spines.

Their axons almost always leave the cortex to connect with various parts of the central nervous system, but not before sending collaterals that make numerous connections within the cortex itself. The somas of spiny cells lie in layers 2 to 6. The transmitter released by their axons has an excitatory action. By contrast, dendrites of the inhibitory (smooth) cells have a large variety of patterns, but they have no apical dendrite and relatively few spines. Smooth cells can be found from layer 1 to the white matter. Their axons almost never leave the cortex, and the primary transmitter they release is GABA. Within these two classes of cells, many subclasses have been proposed. However, multidisciplinary descriptions of the subclasses are very incomplete, nomenclature is inconsistent, and a general consensus has not emerged. Among the smooth cells, the most widely accepted subtypes are identified by the connections of their axons (Martin, 1984): thus, axoaxonic cells make synapses only onto the initial segments of pyramidal cells, basket cells synapse onto the somas and main dendrites of pyramidal cells, and double bouquet cells may inhibit other smooth cells (Somogyi & Cowey, 1981).

Classically, neurons have been categorized by their morphology, but physiological criteria have also proven very useful. Often, the anatomy and physiology of neurons within a neuronal structure show striking correlations (see e.g., Sterling, 1990). Recent electrophysiological studies have revealed that the intrinsic membrane properties of neocortical neurons are systematically diverse (for a review, see Connors & Gutnick, 1990). The most distinctive difference is, not surprisingly, between the spiny cells and the smooth cells. Hints of this came initially from extracellular studies in vivo (Mountcastle *et al.*, 1969; Simons, 1978), where variations were seen in the shapes of individual action potentials. The large majority of cells had relatively broad action potentials (termed regular spikes), while occasional cells produced only 'thin' or 'fast' spikes. Subsequent intracellular studies in vitro using injections of dye into single cells showed that regular-spiking (RS) cells were inevitably spiny pyramidal cells, whereas fast-spiking (FS) cells were smooth cells with the size and dendritic patterns of GABAergic interneurons (Fig. 12.1(a) and (b); McCormick *et al.*, 1985; Naegle & Katz, 1990). Huettner & Baughman (1988) showed, in tissue-cultured neocortical neurons, that RS cells generated synaptic responses with excitatory glutaminergic characteristics, and FS cells produced inhibitory postsynaptic potentials (IPSPs) with GABAergic pharmacology. RS and FS cells also generate distinctive temporal patterns of repetitive firing; RS cells strongly adapt during prolonged current pulses, whereas FS cells undergo little or no adaptation.

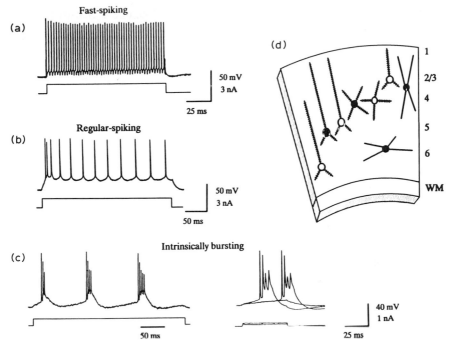

Fig. 12.1. Diversity of intrinsic firing patterns in neocortical neurons. (a) Fast-spiking (FS) neurons have relatively brief action potentials, and can fire at exceptionally high frequencies with little or no adaptation. FS neurons are smooth or sparsely spined neurons, and probably correspond to GABAergic interneurons. (b) Regular-spiking (RS) neurons have more prolonged action potentials, and can fire at relatively high frequencies for only two or three spikes before showing strong adaptation. RS cells correspond to subclasses of pyramidal cells or spiny stellate cells. (c) Intrinsically bursting (IB) cells generate clusters of spikes rather than more continuous trains. With prolonged stimuli, some cells can generate a rhythmic series of bursts (left). The threshold reponse is usually a burst of spikes (right: responses to three current steps superimposed). (d) Schematic summary of the correlations between intrinsic firing patterns and morphological classes of neocortical neurons. Filled cells are smooth, GABAergic neurons with FS properties, located in all layers; open cells are RS neurons, whose somata can be found in layers 2 through 6; shaded cells are IB neurons, whose somata are found only in layer 4 or 5. WM, white matter. (Adapted from Connors & Gutnick, 1990.)

It seems therefore that the two cell types transform synaptic input into spike output very differently. Strict equivalence between RS and spiny cells, and between FS and smooth cells, must be considered tentative. Recent evidence from the hippocampus suggests that there may be subtypes of smooth GABAergic neurons with intrinsic firing properties more similar to RS neurons than to FS neurons (Lacaille & Schwartzkroin, 1988).

The structural diversity of spiny neurons might also be expected to yield a variety of biophysical fingerprints. This was, in fact, clearly shown in pioneering studies of fast and slow pyramidal tract cells of the cat (Takahashi, 1965; Calvin & Sypert, 1976). Studies in vitro have extended the early observations, and provided direct morphological information about cells with particular firing properties. The finding most relevant to this discussion is that, while most spiny cells have properties that conform more or less to the RS definition, a subset of spiny neurons can generate bursts of spikes, either individually or in rhythmic, repeated patterns (Fig. 12.1(c)). The latter, which we call intrinsically bursting (IB) neurons (Connors *et al.*, 1982; McCormick *et al.*, 1985), are mostly pyramidal cells with somas restricted to layers 4 and 5 (however, cf. Foehring & Wyler, 1990; Montoro *et al.*, 1988). By contrast, RS and FS cells are encountered in all laminae (Fig. 12.1(d)).

At least some of the subtypes of spiny cell physiology appear to have distinctive morphological correlates. The most obvious is the laminar position of the soma; however, there are more subtle features as well. Two recent studies have compared neurons within layer 5 (Fig. 12.2;

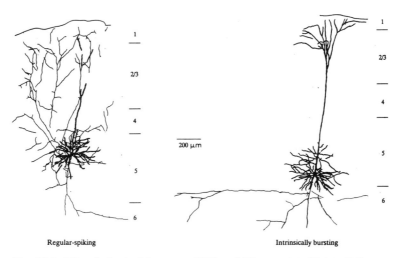

Regular-spiking   Intrinsically bursting

Fig. 12.2. Morphological features of RS and IB neurons of layer 5. In general, IB neurons have relatively larger somata and more profusely branching apical dendrites than do RS cells. IB neurons tend to send horizontally directed axonal collaterals that remain restricted to layers 5 and 6. By contrast, most RS cells send extensive branching collaterals into supragranular layers. (Adapted from Chagnac-Amitai *et al.*, 1990.)

Chagnac-Amitai *et al.*, 1990; Mason & Larkman, 1990). Both found that IB cells are relatively large pyramidal neurons with a robust apical dendrite that branches profusely in layer 1. RS cells with somas in layer 5 are, by contrast, smaller and have fewer and thinner apical dendrites. The most interesting difference is that axon collaterals of the IB cells arborize primarily in layers 5 and 6, while those of the RS cells innervate mainly the upper cortical layers (Chagnac-Amitai *et al.*, 1990). These differences in intracortical connectivity suggest differences in function within the local circuit. An interesting question is whether the RS and IB cells of layer 5 also project to different subcortical sites. The peculiar physiology of IB neurons, together with their anatomy and restricted location, have suggested some unique roles for them in the generation of synchronized activity in both normal and epileptiform neocortex (see below).

Another interesting physiological property that may be restricted to the spiny cells of layer 5 is the ability to generate prolonged and stable patterns of rhythmic firing (Agmon & Connors, 1989; Silva *et al.*, 1991). Some layer 5 pyramidal cells will elicit epochs of single spikes or repeated bursts (Fig. 12.1(c), left) when triggered within a narrow membrane voltage range around $-60\,mV$. The basal frequencies of rhythmic firing are typically 5–12 Hz in different neurons.

The synapses

Many potential neurotransmitters, including neuroactive peptides, have been identified in the cerebral cortex during the last decade (for reviews, see Jones & Peters, 1984*a,b*; Nicoll *et al.*, 1990), and for almost all of them more than one receptor type has been identified. Immunocytochemical and autoradiographic techniques show further that the transmitters and their receptors are distributed in laminar patterns, which can vary dramatically from one cortical area to the other (Lidow *et al.*, 1989). The chemical anatomy of neocortex is impressively complex; however, most of the rapid neuronal interactions in the cortex are mediated by only two simple amino acids: glutamic acid (or possibly aspartic in some synapses) and GABA. The former are utilized as excitatory transmitters, and the latter is recognized to be the main inhibitory neurotransmitter.

The neurotransmitter roles of glutamate and GABA on pyramidal cells are each mediated by two major receptor types, which are pharmacologically distinct and linked to different ion channels. Excitatory responses (EPSPs) are generated by two major classes of receptor, those most sensitive to the agonist _N_-methyl-D-aspartate (NMDA receptors) and those less sensitive (non-NMDA receptors). In cerebral cortex, the non-NMDA receptors appear to generate faster, non-voltage-dependent responses, whereas responses mediated by NMDA receptors are slower and are strongly voltage dependent (Thomson, 1986; Bekkers & Stevens, 1989; Sutor & Hablitz, 1989_a_,_b_; LoTurco _et al._, 1990). Inhibitory responses (IPSPs) on pyramidal cells are mediated by both $GABA_A$ and $GABA_B$ receptors. The former activate fast, large conductance, chloride-selective conductances, and the latter open much slower, smaller, potassium-selective conductances (Connors _et al._, 1988; McCormick, 1989_b_). There is also good evidence for $GABA_B$ receptors on presynaptic terminals in cortex, where they may mediate a suppression of transmitter release (Howe _et al._, 1987; Deisz & Prince, 1989).

The availability of relatively specific antagonists of each transmitter receptor type is now allowing a detailed chemical dissection of cortical function. However, what we know about the mechanisms of neurotransmitters in cerebral cortex comes almost exclusively from studies of particular subsets of pyramidal neurons, mostly in hippocampus (Nicoll _et al._, 1990). By contrast, almost nothing is known about the physiology of synapses on GABAergic interneurons. The few studies that have succeeded in directly measuring from them indicate that they may have a very different complement of postsynaptic receptors, compared to spiny cells (McCormick & Prince, 1986; Madison & Nicoll, 1988). We also know very little about the generality of synaptic processes among different pyramidal cells. While basic membrane mechanisms may be relatively uniform in cortex, the spatial distribution of receptors, channels, and synapses on each cell provides opportunity for significant diversity between neuronal populations.

The local synaptic circuitry

For present purposes it is the neuronal connections within the cortex (rather than between cortex and other brain structures) that are of primary interest. In fact, the major input to each cortical area is from _other_ cortical areas, and there are also very numerous connections within each area. By one estimate (Douglas & Martin, 1990), 90% of the excitation onto each pyramidal cell is provided by intracortical axons, presumably from other spiny cells. Unfortunately, while the organization of inputs and outputs for many cortical areas is reasonably well understood, the patterns of local intracortical connections are very sketchy. The characteristics of local connections are central to an understanding of seizures. It is generally true that the axonal connections from each cortical spiny neuron are strikingly divergent. Each pyramidal cell may receive about 10^4 excitatory synapses (Peters, 1987), but the number of synaptic contacts between two individual pyramids is probably very small. Hard data on this point are as sparse as the synapses themselves, and limited to only a few types of neuron, but they indicate that the number of contacts per cell pair is generally one or at most a few (Gabbot *et al.*, 1987). This anatomy is reflected in the small size of the synaptic effect of one spiny cell upon another; estimates from dual somatic recordings range from a few microvolts to about 2 mV, with a modal value of about 0.1 mV (Komatsu *et al.*, 1988; Thomson *et al.*, 1988). This implies that there must be enormous summation of converging synaptic input to generate significant output from pyramidal cells.

The internal architecture of the neocortex is characterized by two major organizational features: horizontal lamination and vertical columnation. Simple histology reveals that the laminae arise from the size and packing density of their neuron cell bodies. More elegant methods show that each layer possesses a specific combination of inputs, outputs, and intrinsic connections. The strengths of vertical connections (between layers) has long been emphasized by the anatomy and physiology (Lorente de Nó, 1938; Hubel & Wiesel, 1977; Mountcastle, 1979; DeFilipe & Jones, 1988). The vertical connections comprise the extended apical dendrites of pyramidal cells that span layers, and both excitatory and inhibitory axons with a predominant vertical orientation. Strong radial interactions are the basis for the notion of the cortical column, which emphasizes the similarity of neuronal function along the vertical dimension.

The major intracortical pathways have been summarized in a minimalist 'canonical model' by Douglas & Martin (1990; Fig. 12.3(a)). The model applies generally to all cortical areas, and contains three populations of cells: the smooth inhibitory cells, and two groups of spiny cells (those from layer 4 and above, and those from below layer 4). The spiny cells are segregated because of distinct differences in their output targets. The most relevant feature in the context of epileptogenesis is the extensive interconnectedness of all three populations of neurons. Indeed, every possible intergroup and intragroup connection is represented. On the basis of our research on rodent SI neocortex, we suggest a complicating addition to the canonical model that incorporates a population of IB cells from layers 4 and 5 (Fig. 12.3(b)). The details of our modifications are discussed in Initiation of epileptiform discharge, below.

(a)   (b)

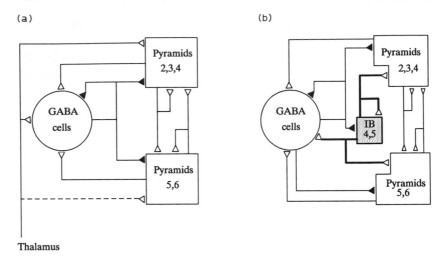

Thalamus

Fig. 12.3. A canonical neocortical circuit. (a) Circuit suggested by Douglas & Martin (1990) to be generally applicable to all cortical areas so far examined. The key features include reciprocal excitation among pyramidal cells both within and between layers, and both feedforward and feedback GABAergic inhibition to all cells, smooth and spiny. Excitatory synapses are represented by open triangles, inhibitory synapses by closed triangles. (b) Modified canonical model, which includes a population of IB pyramidal neurons within layers 4 and 5. The neurons within the IB network are assumed to be strongly interconnected, and in turn strongly to excite the other three classes of neuron. Connections from non-IB pyramidal cells back to the IB cells are likely, but not illustrated.

While the importance of vertical organization is not in dispute, much work has also revealed extensive horizontal connections within neocortex (see e.g., Gilbert & Wiesel, 1983). Neurons within layers 2 through 6 make both near (10 s to 100 s of micrometers) and distant (millimeters to centimeters) connections to other cortical neurons. These connections are not made haphazardly, nor are the patterns symmetric or uniform. Most are excitatory; axonal domains of inhibitory cells tend to be relatively more restricted. The patterns of horizontal connections reveal themselves in interesting ways during the propagation of epileptiform activity (see pp. 409–15).

Experimental epileptiform discharge

Epileptic discharges are occasional, abrupt, and excessive discharges of parts of the cerebral hemisphere (paroxysmal discharges).
(Jackson, 1876)

One approach to an analysis of epileptogenesis is to divide the problem into two somewhat arbitrary components: the initiation of synchronous discharge, and its subsequent propagation. This has heuristic value: it simplifies, and it follows the clinical wisdom that a partial seizure originates (initiates) within a very circumscribed focus of cortex and either remains confined there, or spreads (propagates) to new areas. There is also evidence that the two processes have some mechanistic differences. As we show below, initiation can begin within a single cortical layer, but it proceeds very rapidly in the vertical dimension to encompass all other layers. Propagation implies movement in the horizontal dimension. Thus, initiation and propagation of synchronous discharge will engage the two major dimensions of intracortical organization: columnar (vertical) and horizontal, respectively. We begin by summarizing the phenomenology of epileptiform discharge in neocortex in vitro, then describe the mechanisms of initiation and propagation in detail.

In the spirit of simplification, we look at only the most elementary forms of epileptiform activity. These are usually manifest as large, monophasic events that are often compared to the interictal (or between-seizure) spikes recorded from the electroencephalograms (EEGs) of many epileptic patients. Representative epileptiform events are illustrated (Fig. 12.4, top) by field potential recordings from a cortical slice treated with a high dose of bicuculline. Several characteristics justify the designation 'epileptiform'. First, the events are extremely large in amplitude and duration; such prolonged potentials are never seen under control conditions, even when electrical stimuli are relatively very strong. Second, the events are essentially all-or-none; they exhibit a sharp threshold for activation, and take only one form. Third, when evoked by a small electrical stimulus, the latency of the events is extremely variable from trial-to-trial; variability is especially pronounced near threshold. Fourth, there is extremely high synchrony in the timing of events across neurons (Gutnick *et al.*, 1982*a*). These characteristics apply literally to events under high dose GABA$_A$ antagonist conditions. However, under low dose conditions the events tend to be smaller and shorter, their shapes may vary from trial-to-trial, and due to intermittent propagation failures synchrony across a slice of cortex may be less than complete (Fig. 12.4, bottom). Most interestingly, the synaptic manifestations of the synchronous event may differ dramatically from one cell to another (see next section).

It is worth asking how closely our model of interictal spikes resembles a characteristic of clinical epilepsy. Perhaps most importantly, interictal spikes themselves appear to be highly correlated with epilepsy. In studies

50 μM Bicuculline

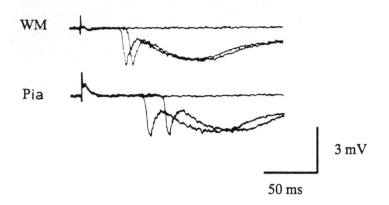

WM

Pia

3 mV

50 ms

0.8 μM Bicuculline

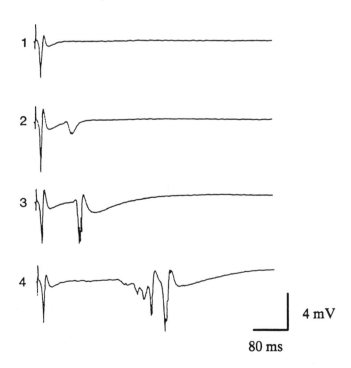

1

2

3

4

4 mV

80 ms

of the EEGs of non-epileptic patients only about 1.5–2.2% showed focal 'spikes' or 'sharp waves'; conversely, the large majority of patients showing focal EEG spikes also had behavioral seizures (for a review, see Pedley, 1984). Interictal spikes of seizure patients may be very variable in size and waveform, even from the same scalp location on a single subject. They may also arise from a variety of different sites within a small cortical locus. In this way they may more closely resemble the experimental epileptiform events induced in the presence of inhibition (low dose experiments), rather than the more robust and stable events generated in its absence.

Initiation of epileptiform discharge

Probably, few cells are abnormally highly unstable; in severe seizures the sudden and excessive discharge of those highly unstable cells overcomes, it is supposed, the resistance of healthy cells in physiological connection with those highly unstable.
(Jackson, 1881)

A basic problem of epilepsy research is the mechanism(s) of neuronal synchronization: what processes can suddenly convert the cortex from its normal, relatively desynchronized, modes to the uniquely correlated states of seizures? Neuronal synchrony, in particular rhythmic synchrony, is a classic experimental and theoretical problem in neurobiology (Cohen *et al.*, 1988). It is very clear that nervous systems have evolved many different ways to generate and regulate the synchrony of activity within pools of neurons. Two basic concepts are widespread. They are by no means mutually exclusive. The simplest is the notion that one neuron (or a small

Fig. 12.4. Epileptiform field potentials from layers 2 and 3 of disinhibited slices of neocortex. In the presence of high doses of bicuculline (top traces), which virtually eliminate $GABA_A$-mediated inhibition, epileptiform events are stereotyped regardless of the pathway by which they are evoked, and they have very variable latencies. By contrast, at bicuculline levels that are near the threshold for allowing epileptiform activity (bottom traces) synchronized events are much more variable in size, shape, and duration. Traces in high [bicuculline] consist of superimposed responses evoked by consecutive shocks to either the underlying white matter (WM) or the overlying pial edge. Stimuli were just suprathreshold intensity; note that the short-latency field potentials are consistent from trial-to-trial, but differ with stimulus site. Epileptiform events vary in latency, but are consistent in shape. Responses in low [bicuculline] are from four consecutive shocks evoked from the white matter; stimulus amplitude was slightly incremented between responses 1 and 2, and kept constant from 2 to 4. (High [bicuculline] traces are from Connors, 1984; low [bicuculline] traces are from Chagnac-Amitai & Connors, 1989*b*.)

number of tightly coupled neurons) acts as the pacemaker for a synaptically connected population of passive followers. Several invertebrate systems seem to use this mechanism to generate patterned synchrony for loco-motion, feeding, heartbeat and similar rhythmic behaviors (Getting, 1989). In its purest form the pacemaker is the master clock for the entire system; it derives its basic activity pattern solely from intrinsic sources, notably its various membrane currents. Control of synchrony can be achieved by directly modulating the activity of the pacemaker neuron, or by changing the efficacy of the pacemakers's synaptic coupling to its followers. Alternatively, synchronous activity can arise in a pool of neurons devoid of pacemakers. For this to work, there must be some strong form of neuronal interaction (usually via synapses), and a particular balance of intrinsic excitability, probability and quality of connections, and timing. Synchrony in the absence of individual pacemakers is, necessarily, an emergent property of the neural network. However, these two mechanisms of synchrony are caricatures of most real systems. It seems likely that most vertebrate neural systems incorporate features of both: networks of pacemaker neurons interacting, sometimes reciprocally, with networks of followers. Epileptiform synchrony in neocortex may also be such a hybrid system. Stated simply, the proposal is that a particular population of neurons, located primarily within layer 5, acts as the initiator for epileptiform activity, which is then projected upon the other neurons of the cortex. The most distinguishing feature of the initiator cells is their unusually high intrinsic excitability. We suggest that IB neurons are the primary initiators. The rest of this section presents evidence that bears upon this hypothesis.

Middle layer initiation

A variety of experimental studies in vitro and in vivo suggests that neocortical layers 4 and/or 5 are especially epileptogenic. These results are summarized in Table 12.1. The earliest evidence came from studies in vivo, in which the $GABA_A$ antagonists bicuculline or penicillin were microinjected into different layers of rat parietal cortex (Lockton & Holmes, 1983), cat visual cortex (Chatt & Ebersole, 1982; Ebersole & Chatt, 1986) or rabbit visual or motor cortex (Pockberger *et al.*, 1984*b*). Layers 4 and/or 5 proved the most sensitive to the convulsant properties of these drugs, a finding confirmed in slices in vitro (Connors, 1984). Layer 4 or 5 is also where epileptiform activity often begins. With epicortical application of penicillin, current-source density (CSD) analysis revealed

Table 12.1. *Experimental evidence implicating layers 4 and 5 in the initiation of epileptiform discharge*

Finding	Layer implicated	Species/area	Model	Ref.
Highest convulsant sensitivity	4	Cat area 17	Penicillin, bicuculline	1
Highest convulsant sensitivity	4	Rat MI	Penicillin	2
Highest convulsant sensitivity	4/5	Guinea pig SI	Bicuculline	3
Highest convulsant sensitivity	4/5	Rabbit VI, MI	Penicillin	4
First current sink	4/5	Guinea pig SI	High [bicuculline]	3
First current sink	4/5	Rabbit VI, MI	Penicillin	4
Lowest threshold to glutamate	4/5	Guinea pig SI	High [bicuculline]	3
Highest sensitivity to GABA	4/5	Rat SI	Bicuculline	5
First reduction of $[Ca^{2+}]_o$	3/4	Rat SI	Penicillin	6
Specific site of synchronized excitation	4/5	Rat SI	Low [bicuculline]	7
Isolated layer is epileptogenic	5	Rat SI	Low [bicuculline]	5
Isolated layer is epileptogenic	5	Rat SI	Low $[Mg^{2+}]_o$	8

References: 1, Ebersole & Chatt, 1986; 2, Lockton & Holmes, 1983; 3, Connors, 1984; 4, Pockberger *et al.*, 1984*b*; 5, Telfeian *et al.*, 1990; 6, Pumain *et al.*, 1983; 7, Chagnac-Amitai & Connors, 1989*b*; 8, Silva & Connors, 1990.

that earliest epileptiform current sinks (i.e., current leaving the extracellular space to enter cells) occurred in layer 5 (Pockberger *et al.*, 1984*a*). Each epileptiform spike in a penicillin focus is accompanied by a transient reduction in $[Ca^{2+}]_o$ as Ca^{2+} flows into massively activated voltage- and transmitter-gated membrane channels (Heinemann *et al.*, 1977). Pumain *et al.* (1983) showed that the latency of the drop in $[Ca^{2+}]_o$ is shortest in layer 3 and the border zone of layer 4. CSD analysis in bicuculline-treated neocortical slices showed the earliest sinks invariably centered 900–1100 μm below the pia, corresponding to layer 4 and superficial 5 (Connors, 1984). Also, when focal applications of L-glutamate were used to trigger epileptiform events in slices, these same layers had by far the lowest thresholds (Connors, 1984).

There are clearly some differences in the particular cortical layers implicated by these investigations; layers 3, 4, and 5 have all been named. Some, but not all, of this can be attributed to variations in the species, models or methods, but it is worth remembering the basic cellular structure of the neocortex. Connections in the vertical direction are extremely heavy, and the majority of pyramidal cells send a large apical dendrite from their soma to layer 1. This will lead to a vertical smearing of electrically measured activities, ion changes and chemical sensitivities, because the cells themselves, and their activities, are distributed across the layers.

A more direct implication of layer 5 has been provided by experiments on neocortical slices treated with picrotoxin (Gutnick *et al.*, 1982*b*), low concentrations of bicuculline (Telfeian *et al.*, 1990) or media containing low $[Mg^{2+}]_o$ (Silva *et al.*, 1991). The last of these conditions results in spontaneous, repetitive, synchronous events that apparently depend upon enhanced activation of NMDA receptors (Sutor & Hablitz, 1989*b*; Thompson, 1986). In each of these, microdissection of the slices showed that only fragments containing layer 5 could sustain robust epileptiform activity. Slice fragments without layer 5 could not produce such activity; conversely, fragments of layer 5 alone were fully capable of it. Thus, layer 5 is both necessary and sufficient for generating synchronized activity, whether it is induced by reduced inhibition or increased excitation.

Considering this assortment of evidence, it is hard to escape the conclusion that the neuronal circuits within layer 5 (and perhaps 4) play a central role in the initiation of certain forms of epileptiform activity. The next obvious question is, what distinguishes the excitability of these layers from the others?

Role of intrinsic membrane properties

As described in Neurons, synapses and circuits of neocortex, above, some of the neurons in layers 4 and 5 (but apparently not other layers) have distinctive membrane properties that allow them to generate bursts of rhythmic activity. Therein lies a striking correspondence: the IB cells and the site of epileptiform initiations are in the same place. This suggests an obvious hypothesis: that some forms of synchronized activity in the neocortex are initiated by interconnected networks of IB neurons (Gutnick *et al.*, 1982*a*; Connors, 1984; Connors & Gutnick, 1984*b*). To be compelling, however, more evidence than this simple correlation is necessary. For example, it has been proposed that intrinsically bursting neurons are responsible for the extreme epileptogenicity of the CA3 region of hippo-campus (Schwartzkroin & Prince, 1979; Traub & Wong, 1982; Wong & Traub, 1983). Direct support was provided by experiments in vitro, where the electrical stimulation of a single CA3 neuron was often sufficient to trigger a full-blown, synchronized epileptiform event (Miles & Wong, 1983). Similar attempts in neocortex have consistently failed (B. W. Connors and Y. Amitai, unpublished results). This finding by itself does not doom the hypothesis for neocortex, since it may take the simultaneous firing of more than one IB cell to do the job. However, it does force the use of other, less direct tests of the hypothesis.

Some of the supporting evidence is circumstantial. When inhibition is strongly suppressed by high doses of bicuculline (Gutnick *et al.*, 1982*a*) or picrotoxin (Hablitz, 1988), all neocortical neurons display prolonged depolarizing events, arising largely from excitatory synaptic currents. Many IB cells generate short-latency, non-synaptic events (namely action potentials) that precede the epileptiform synaptic events (Gutnick & Friedman, 1986). This is consistent with the IB initiator hypothesis, since in principle it should be possible to detect some cells generating intrinsic events before widespread synchrony occurs.

Stronger support for the role of IB cells as initiators was provided by recordings made from slices bathed in threshold doses of bicuculline or bicuculline methiodide (0.8–1.0 μM). At these concentrations, $GABA_A$-mediated inhibition is still largely intact (Chagnac-Amitai & Connors, 1989*a*). Synchronous epileptiform events were evoked by electrically stimulating layer 6, and paroxysmal events were identified by large, all-or-none extracellular field potentials that propagated horizontally for variable distances up to several millimeters (Fig. 12.4, bottom). When recording was done intracellularly, the character of the synchronous activity varied greatly from cell to cell. The key finding was that the type of synchronized synaptic activity correlated closely with the intrinsic membrane properties of the recorded neuron. Thus, in phase with each field event, most RS cells of all layers were very strongly *inhibited*, whereas all IB cells demonstrated robust *excitation* with little detectable inhibition (Fig. 12.5; Chagnac-Amitai & Connors, 1989*b*). This correlation held even within layer 5 itself. The FS cells, which are presumed to be inhibitory interneurons, were also synchronously excited. This is consistent with their role as mediators of synchronous IPSPs on RS cells. The important conclusion is that, of all the cells that were capable of excitatory output, only the IB cells actually produced substantial output. The rest of the neurons were actively inhibited. This is strong

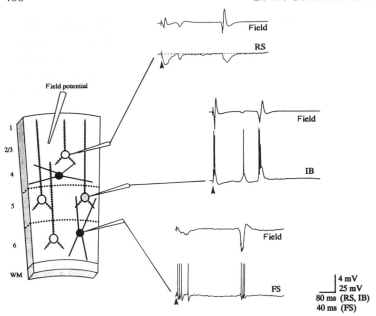

Fig. 12.5. Synchronized epileptiform events in the presence of inhibition. Neo-cortical slices were bathed in a dose of bicuculline ($0.9 \mu M$) that reduced GABAergic inhibition by no more than about 20%. The schematic diagram shows the experimental arrangement: field potentials were recorded in layers 2/3, while a simultaneous intracellular recording was obtained from an RS, IB or FS type of neuron in layers 2 through 6 (see Fig. 12.1 for explanation of shading). The dotted lines represent the minimal piece of cortex necessary to generate epileptiform activity. Stimuli were applied to the deep aspect of layer 6. Representative responses are shown to the right. In phase with the epileptiform events recorded extracellularly, most RS cells generated synaptic responses that were over-whelmingly inhibitory. This was true even in layer 5. IB cells of layers 4 and 5, on the other hand, generated strongly excitatory responses that were synchronized with the field potentials. FS cells also generated synchronized excitatory responses. (Data are modified from Chagnac-Amitai & Connors, 1989*b*.)

support for labeling the IB cells as the initiators, and leads inevitably to the question 'What property of the IB cells confers upon them the central role in synchronous activity?'

Figure 12.3(b) shows our modification of the canonical model proposed by Douglas & Martin (1990), which simply adds a new neuronal population, the IB cells. The IB group is derived from the original two populations of spiny cells, hence the bites taken from their corners. The IB cells are given the same basic intrinsic connections as the other spiny cells, since the electrophysiology shows they can be both excited and inhibited synaptically (McCormick *et al.*, 1985). But is this what makes them such exquisite initiators of epileptiform activity? Their most obvious distinction is embodied in their name; they have the ability to generate a relatively large excitatory output (the burst) with a very small increment in stimulus intensity (Figure 12.1(c)). This trait alone might, all other things being equal, make such a cell type especially epileptogenic. However, other characteristics may also contribute. Preliminary study of the local connections onto IB cells suggests that they may receive weaker GABAergic inhibition than do RS cells of the same, and other, layers (Silva *et al.*, 1991). It is also possible that IB cells have uncommonly strong interconnections among themselves; this would greatly facilitate their ability to synchronize their activity. The intracortical axonal arborizations of IB cells are consistent with this possibility (Fig. 12.2; Chagnac-Amitai *et al.*, 1990). It is also interesting that IB cells of rat SI were found to have a significantly lower probability of receiving direct thalamic input than were RS cells of the same layer (Agmon & Connors, 1992), indicating some specificity to the connections of the two cell types. There are no data available on the relative neurotransmitter sensitivities of IB versus RS neurons. Further work is clearly necessary to define the place of IB cells in the neocortical circuit.

Minimal epileptogenic aggregate

Several investigations have tried to define the minimal epileptogenic population in the cortex. That is, how small can an epileptic focus be? Studies of cat primary visual cortex suggested that this might be a volume as modest as a single cortical column containing only cells with the same orientation and ocular dominance (Gabor *et al.*, 1979; Reichenthal & Hocherman, 1979; Gabor & Scobey, 1980). The contention was that such a column, which might be only about 125 μm in diameter, could *independently* generate synchronized spike activity when treated with focal epicortical penicillin. Ebersole & Chatt (1986) went further, and suggested that a single layer (layer 4) within one column of cat visual cortex might constitute the critical mass for epileptogenesis. The dimensions implied by these studies are very uncertain because of the variable and unknown gradients of applied convulsant concentration, and imprecision in mapping the boundaries of epileptiform activity. It is also unclear what role is played by the surrounding, non-epileptogenic, cortex in the behavior of the focus in vivo. Nevertheless, these studies hinted that an unexpectedly small piece of neocortex can generate highly synchronized discharges.

Recent experiments in vitro show directly that single cortical layers can support impressive epileptiform activity. When slices (400 μm thick) were either treated with bicuculline (Gutnick *et al.*, 1982*b*; Telfeian *et al.*, 1990) or bathed in a solution with a low concentration of magnesium (Silva & Connors, 1990) they generated highly synchronized discharges even when vertical cuts reduced them to slivers 1 mm wide. These slivers were further reduced with cuts made in the horizontal dimension; in both models a cortical fragment containing no more than layer 5 was sufficient to support fully synchronized discharges (Fig. 12.5, dotted lines). Conversely, fragments containing layers 1 through 4, or layer 6 plus the white matter, were much less epileptogenic. In the case of the low magnesium model a fragment less than 1 mm wide, 0.4 mm deep, and the thickness of layer 5 was sufficient to sustain spontaneous, synchronized, rhythmic events of several seconds duration (Silva & Connors, 1990). Remarkably, the somas and basal dendrites of these neurons retain essentially normal electrophysiological activity even in the absence of most of their apical dendrites (Telfeian *et al.*, 1990). Such a fragment of layer 5 contains, very roughly, 5000 pyramidal neurons (cf. Peters, 1985), suggesting that the minimal epileptogenic aggregate is at least this small. If only the IB cells are relevant to actual initiation, then it is likely that no more than half this number of neurons is necessary. This compares well with studies of disinhibited hippocampal slices, which suggest that no more than about 1000 pyramidal cells of the CA3 area are needed to produce seizure-like activity (Miles *et al.*, 1983).

Propagation of epileptiform discharge

To speak figuratively, this 'mad part' compels many collateral 'sane' cells . . . to cooperate in its occasional and sudden excesses.
(Jackson, 1890)

An insidious characteristic of seizures is that, although they may begin as a very small focus of abnormal activity, they can sometimes propagate and eventually usurp normal functions over most, or even all, of the cortex. In the previous section we proposed that the initiation focus can be as small as a fragment of layer 5, that is, about 0.2 mm^3. If this happens in vivo it implies that propagation must occur in both the vertical and horizontal dimensions. Most studies of propagation have been concerned with relatively gross patterns of seizure movement in the horizontal direction, i.e. movement from one large cortical area to another on the scale of many millimeters and up to centimeters. Spatial resolution has traditionally been limited by the use of relatively large surface electrodes, placed imprecisely or at a long distance from the cortex, and by the inability to isolate functionally the activity of one region, or layer, of cortex from adjacent ones. More recently, the mechanisms of propagation have been examined at a finer anatomical level by using innovations such as vertical electrode arrays, optical recording and cortical slices in vitro. In this section we summarize observations on the phenomena and mechanisms of propagation on a smaller scale, 10 s to 100 s of micrometers, and within and between single cortical layers and columns.

Vertical propagation

Since the traditional (and still prevailing) view is that neocortex is dominated by vertical connections between neurons, through both axonal projections and dendritic spread, it is not surprising that the vertical propagation of synchronized activity is very rapid. Nevertheless, little is known about the pathways and mechanisms of radial seizure spread. The extensive overlap of vertical neuronal elements makes their specific study especially difficult. Anatomical studies provide the best clues. If it is accepted that a network of IB cells is the site of epileptiform initiation, then it follows that excitation spreads vertically via their axon collaterals, either directly or indirectly. Since IB cells seem to make extensive connections within layers 5 and 6 (Chagnac-Amitai *et al.*, 1990), spread within infragranular layers is straightforward. Electrophysiological measurements, however, demonstrate rapid and very powerful spread to supragranular layers (see e.g., Gutnick *et al.*, 1982*b*; Connors, 1984; Pockberger *et al.*, 1984*b*; Goldensohn & Salazar, 1986; Schroeder *et al.*, 1990), perhaps via those IB collaterals that do turn upward (Chagnac-Amitai *et al.*, 1990), or perhaps via disynaptic connections with non-IB cells within deeper layers. The vertical spread of synchronized inhibition is more easily explained. Anatomical studies consistently demonstrate extensive, vertical, intralaminar projections of GABAergic neurons (Somogyi *et al.*, 1983; Kisvarday, 1987). Still, this is admittedly too much speculation for comfort, and only further study of vertical propagation will provide the remedy.

Horizontal propagation

Both clinical and experimental observations have shown that epileptic activity propagates horizontally over preferred routes, rather than along strictly concentric pathways (Petsche *et al.*, 1974; Kooi *et al.*, 1978). The prevailing explanation has been that the preferred pathways reflect something about the directions and strengths of excitatory connections between areas. However, other interpretations are possible. For example, if the general excitability of neurons (determined by either intrinsic membrane properties or efficacy of synaptic inhibition) differed regionally, propagation might be biased. No study has attempted to correlate the spatial patterns of intercortical connections, as determined anatomically, with the spatial patterns of propagation in the same brain. The precise cellular factors governing propagation remain obscure, although modeling studies of hippocampal networks have provided some insight (Traub et al., 1987).

Long slices of disinhibited neocortex provide a high resolution view of horizontal propagation. When $GABA_A$ receptors are strongly blocked with bicuculline, synchronized discharges can be evoked by a weak electrical stimulus from any site on the slice. Following rapid vertical propagation, each discharge propagates away from the stimulus site in both horizontal directions at a mean velocity (measured over several millimeters of cortex) of about 60–90 mm/s (Chervin et al., 1988). This is relatively slow compared even to the thinnest central unmyelinated axons, which conduct at about 100 mm/s (Foster et al., 1982); while available data on the velocities of intracortical axons are very sparse, they begin at 0.3 m/s and range up to 32 m/s (Waxman & Swadlow, 1977). Clearly, we must look to some form of network-dependent activity to account for the limiting factor in epileptiform propagation, even in the absence of inhibition.

The complexity of propagation is underscored by its spatial and temporal pattern. Using pairs of recording electrodes spaced 100–200 μm apart (Fig. 12.6(a)), Chervin et al. (1988) estimated the local velocity of propagation at close intervals across various types of neocortex. The measurements showed that velocity was stable over time, but very variable over space. Examples from SI cortex of rat (Figure 12.6(b)) and V1 cortex of cat show that the synchronized discharges did not move smoothly, but in fits and starts. The spatial frequencies of the velocity, illustrated as power spectra (Fig. 12.6(c)), yielded prominent peaks at about 1/mm. When the propagation patterns were compared for the two directions across these same pieces of cortex they were often negatively correlated, i.e., the points on the cortex where propagation was fastest from medial to lateral were most likely to be the points where it was slowest from lateral to medial. Finally, the spatial patterns of propagation varied from one area of cortex to another; in fact, within V1 of the rat propagation

(a)

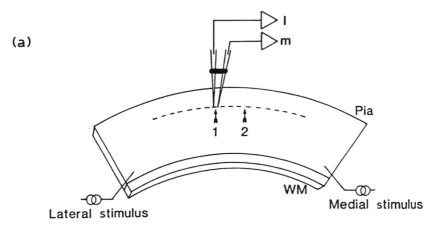

(b)

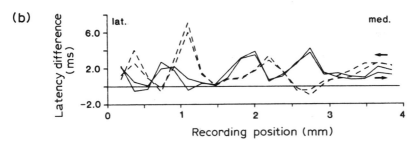

(c)

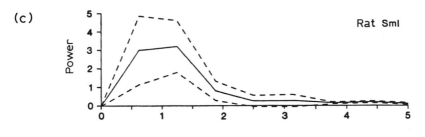

Rat SmI

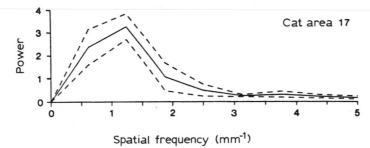

Cat area 17

Spatial frequency (mm⁻¹)

(For caption, see overleaf)

patterns were conspicuously stable until discharges approached the border between V1 and adjacent secondary visual areas, where there were consistently sharp changes.

The phenomenology of horizontal propagation in the absence of inhibition suggests that it is primarily determined by the spatial patterns of excitatory connectivity, and that those patterns are very variable between and within cortical areas. Several arguments support this. First, the propagation velocity in different directions across single points was often anticorrelated (Fig. 12.6(b)), implying that variations in velocity cannot be due simply to local differences in excitability. A relatively more/less excitable area of cortex would be expected to speed/slow propagation in both directions. Second, the dominant spatial frequency is similar in two very different types of neocortex, SI of rat and V1 of cat. Anatomically, the dominant periodicities in rat SI are the barrels, which are roughly cylindrical domains of high stellate cell density in layer 4 (Welker & Woolsey, 1974). In the cat the dominant pattern is that of the ocular dominance and orientation columns (Hubel & Weisel, 1963; Lowel et al., 1987). However, while the 1 mm periodicity of epileptiform propagation closely fits the column periodicity of cat V1, it is significantly longer than the spacing of even the largest barrels in the rat SI. Third, discharges occasionally *jumped* across a region of cortex before propagating backward into it, implying a spatially discontinuous and elongated substrate.

Fig. 12.6. Periodicity and directionality of horizontally propagating discharges. (a) Schematic arrangement. Slices were bathed in 10 μM bicuculline, and epileptiform events similar to those in Fig. 12.4 (top) were evoked with shocks to either corner of the slice. A pair of extracellular electrodes was fixed at an intertip distance of 80–170 μm, and moved along a horizontal line in stepwise intervals of 100–180 μ. The propagation velocity of the epileptiform event was estimated from the difference in the latencies of its arrival at the two electrodes. (b) Propagation patterns for a representative slice of rat SI cortex. Latency difference is plotted against distance along the horizontal dimension. Dashed lines are for events propagating from medial-to-lateral, continuous lines for events going in the opposite direction. Data are mean values for two sets of measurements made about 90 min apart, and illustrate the temporal stability of the patterns. The most interesting features are the inhomogeneity of the propagation velocities, and the generally anticorrelated velocities of propagation in opposite directions across each part of the cortex; i.e., those spots where the event travels fastest in one direction tend to be the spots where the event travels slowest in the opposite direction. med., medial. (c) The dominant spatial frequencies of the propagation patterns are centered at about 1/mm in both rat SI cortex (Sm1) and cat V1 cortex (area 17). Graphs plot power spectra derived from data of the type shown in (b). Continuous lines plot the mean, and dashed lines the S.D., for six experiments in the rat and four in cat. (Modified from Chervin et al., 1988.)

Fourth, the lack of clear periodicity and directionality in at least one cortical area (rat V1) suggests that the primary determinant of local propagation patterns is not a consistent feature of cortex, but varies from one cytoarchitectonic area to the other.

Chervin *et al.* (1988) proposed a simple model of horizontal connectivity to account for the nature of propagation. A cartoon representation of some of these ideas, combined with the notion of laminar specificity of initiation, is illustrated in Fig. 12.7(a). Inhibition is neglected, since it is assumed to be virtually absent in high bicuculline concentrations. The important feature of the model is that either the mean length or density of horizontal connections from each narrow column of cortex is allowed to vary periodically across the wider expanse of cortex. Connections from each particular cortical column are directionally symmetric. With the assumption that the velocity of propagation into a region is dependent upon the density of connections leading into it, the model reproduces the periodicity and directionality of the propagation velocity. Jumping of discharges was not modeled, but presumably feedforward excitatory connections with patchy discontinuities could mediate this. Patchy connections have been seen in anatomical studies of a wide range of species and neocortical areas, including rodent barrel cortex (Gilbert & Wiesel, 1983; Chapin *et al.*, 1987; Bernardo *et al.*, 1990).

It is likely that GABAergic inhibition is prominent even in very epileptogenic areas of cortex. Considering the ubiquity of inhibitory synapses on cortical neurons, it is also likely that inhibition plays a modulating role in epileptiform propagation. This suspicion is borne out by studies of cortical slices in low bicuculline concentrations (Chagnac-Amitai & Connors, 1989*a*; Telfeian *et al.*, 1990). When drug concentrations were just high enough to evoke epileptiform activity (0.4–1.0 µM), propagation was very variable both temporally and spatially. Synchronized discharges did not necessarily propagate across the entire slice, but often failed consistently or intermittently at particular sites. Propagation was often much better in one direction than another. Discharges could be reflected from particular sites back toward (or even past) their area of initiation, often leading to very complicated waveforms recorded from certain points along the cortex (e.g., Fig. 12.4, trace 4). As described in the preceding section, intracellular recordings from RS cells confirmed that synchronized inhibition was a prominent feature of cortical activity under these conditions (Fig. 12.5).

Studies of seizure foci in situ have shown that synchronous inhibition often dominates the area surrounding a focus center (Prince, 1968; Dichter

(a)   No GABA$_A$ inhibition:

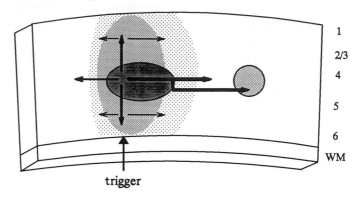

(b)   GABA$_A$ inhibition:

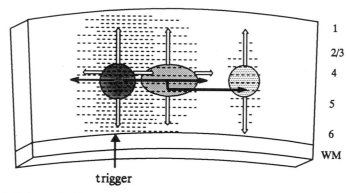

Fig. 12.7. Schematic diagrams of the intracortical flow of activity during epileptiform discharges in (a) the absence and (b) the presence of GABA$_A$-mediated inhibition. Shaded regions represent areas of net synchronous excitation; dashed areas net synchronous inhibition. Filled arrows are excitatory connections; open arrows are inhibitory. (a) In the absence of significant inhibition, the main features are initiation within middle layers, subsequent spread to upper and lower layers, strong asymmetries in horizontal propagation, and a tendency occasionally to jump ahead due to patchy excitatory connections. (b) In the presence of strong (i.e., only slightly compromised) inhibition, excitation in pyramidal cells is confined largely to the IB neurons of middle layers. These preferentially project synchronous excitation via horizontal connections in layer 5, and disynaptic inhibition to layers above and below, as well as horizontally. For more details, see the text.

& Spencer, 1969; Ayala *et al.*, 1970). It was proposed that surround inhibition served to constrain the propagation of the seizure into uninvolved areas. This basic idea must also incorporate the vertical propagation of activity, since a synchronous inhibitory surround can clearly extend above, below, and even within a single layer of epileptiform activity (Elger & Speckmann, 1983; Chagnac-Amitai & Connors, 1989*b*; Goldensohn & Salazar, 1986; Schwartzkroin & Haglund, 1986). Figure 12.7(b) illustrates hypothesized flow of epileptiform activity in the presence of strong cortical inhibition.

Recent studies have demonstrated that synaptic inhibition is relatively fragile; its efficacy may decline with repetitive activation (McCarren & Alger, 1985; Huguenard & Alger, 1986; Prince *et al.*, 1990), allowing the inhibitory barriers around a focus to dissolve. It is also now clear that GABA$_A$ receptors may be under the control of a variety of modulatory systems, both via extracellular ligand sites on the GABA receptor and phosphorylation intracellularly (Olsen & Venter, 1987; Sigel & Baur, 1988; Stelzer *et al.*, 1988). Some of the most useful anticonvulsant agents (including barbiturates and benzodiazepines) act by generally enhancing the efficacy of GABA$_A$-mediated chloride channels (Macdonald, 1989). The emerging view is that cortical inhibition is an extremely dynamic system whose effectiveness may be varied over a wide range. Small alterations to it may dramatically change the probability that a behaviorally insignificant focus will generalize into a major seizure.

Conclusions and speculations

Before describing our researches apropos of Ferrier's experiments we will remark that the idea put forward by Wilks, Hughlings Jackson, and others, of localizing epilepsy in the cortical layer of the brain is not new ... It will be shown further on that this theory is unsustainable.
(Dupuy)[1]

Hypotheses should usually be presented with caution, and some humility. We best remember Hughlings Jackson for those few of his ideas that still conform to our own. But Jackson also espoused notions, such as his views on the evolution and dissolution of the nervous system, that were on the intellectual fringe even a century ago, and earn him only obscure footnotes today (unfortunately for the memory of Dupuy, he chose the wrong

[1] Quoted by Jackson in 1874 (see Taylor, 1931, p. 164).

Jacksonian theory to attack). With all of this in mind, we make the following specific suggestions:

(1) Only a slight (about 10–20%) reduction of the normal level $GABA_A$-mediated inhibition is necessary to allow propagating epileptiform activity in the neocortex.

(2) Under some conditions, notably when inhibition is suppressed or NMDA receptor efficacy is enhanced, epileptiform discharges arise first within layer 5. The neurons of layer 5 are both necessary and sufficient to generate epileptiform activity under threshold convulsant conditions.

(3) A subpopulation of spiny neurons, the IB cells, can act as the initiator of epileptiform discharge. This occurs by dint of their unique intrinsic excitability and synaptic interconnections.

(4) The initiating cells can project a hypersynchronous barrage of EPSPs upon other neurons of a local area of cortex. If the general efficacy of GABAergic inhibition is high, this results in a domination of synchronous inhibition of spiny cells in all layers; if inhibition is badly impaired, synchronous excitation overwhelms activity in all cells.

(5) The preferred pathways for horizontal propagation of epileptiform activity are the excitatory axon collaterals of layer 5. The spatial and temporal patterns of propagation will primarily reflect the properties of these pathways, and the inhibitory circuitry they engage. However, under intense epileptiform conditions collateral axons of any layer can mediate propagation.

These hypotheses are concrete and testable. To date, most of the research supporting them has been done in rodent cortex. Their generality and their relevance to human seizure conditions are unknown. But with the recent increase in the application of cellular methods to human epileptic tissue (Schwartzkroin & Prince, 1976; Prince & Wong, 1981; Schwartzkroin & Knowles, 1984; Avoli & Olivier, 1989; McCormick, 1989*b*; Foehring & Wyler, 1990), answers should soon be forthcoming.

Acknowledgments

We thank our colleagues Aric Agmon, Larry Cauller, Ron Chervin, Mike Gutnick, Dave McCormick, Pam Pierce, David Prince, Laurie Silva, Albert Telfeian, and Mike Wehr for their invaluable contributions to the research presented here. We are also grateful for the vital support of the NIH and the Klingenstein Foundation.

References

Abeles, M. (1982). *Local Cortical Circuits: An Electrophysiological Study*. New York: Springer-Verlag.

Agmon, A. & Connors, B. W. (1989). Repetitive burst-firing neurons in the deep layers of mouse somatosensory cortex. *Neuroscience Letters*, **99**: 137–41.

Agmon, A. & Connors, B. W. (1992). Correlation between intrinsic firing patterns and thalamocortical synaptic responses of neurons in mouse barrel cortex. *Journal of Neuroscience*, **12**: 319–29.

Avoli, M. (1988). GABAergic mechanisms in epileptic seizures. In *Neurotransmitters and Cortical Function. From Molecules to Mind*, ed. M. Avoli, T. A. Reader, R. W. Dykes & P. Gloor, pp. 187–206. New York: Plenum Press.

Avoli, M. & Olivier, A. (1989). Electrophysiological properties and synaptic responses in the deep layers of the human epileptogenic neocortex in vitro. *Journal of Neurophysiology*, **61**: 589–606.

Ayala, G. F., Matsumoto, H. & Gumnit, R. J. (1970). Excitability changes and inhibitory mechanisms in neocortical neurons during seizures. *Journal of Neurophysiology*, **33**: 73–85.

Bekkers, J. M. & Stevens, C. F. (1989). NMDA and non-NMDA receptors are co-localized at individual excitatory synapses in cultured rat hippocampus. *Nature*, **341**: 230–3.

Bernardo, K. L., McCasland, J. S., Woolsey, T. A. & Stominger, R. N. (1990). Local intra- and interlaminar connections in mouse barrel cortex. *Journal of Comparative Neurology*, **291**: 231–55.

Calvin, W. H. & Sypert, G. W. (1976). Fast and slow pyramidal tract neurons, an intracellular analysis of their contrasting repetitive firing properties in the cat. *Journal of Neurophysiology*, **39**: 420–34.

Chagnac-Amitai, Y. & Connors, B. W. (1989a). Horizontal spread of synchronized activity in neocortex, and its control by GABA-mediated inhibition. *Journal of Neurophysiology*, **61**: 747–58.

Chagnac-Amitai, Y. & Connors, B. W. (1989b). Synchronized excitation and inhibition driven by intrinsically bursting neurons in neocortex. *Journal of Neurophysiology*, **62**: 1149–62.

Chagnac-Amitai, Y., Luhmann, H. J. & Prince, D. A. (1990). Burst generating and regular spiking layer 5 pyramidal neurons of rat neocortex have different morphological features. *Journal of Comparative Neurology*, **296**: 598–613.

Chapin, J. K., Sadeq, M. & Guise, J. L. U. (1987). Corticocortical connections within the primary somatosensory cortex of the rat. *Journal of Comparative Neurology*, **263**: 326–46.

Chatt, A. B. & Ebersole, J. S. (1982). The laminar sensitivity of cat striate cortex to penicillin-induced epileptogenesis. *Brain Research*, **241**: 382–7.

Chervin, R. D., Pierce, P. A. & Connors, B. W. (1988). Periodicity and directionality in the propagation of epileptiform discharges across neocortex. *Journal of Neurophysiology*, **60**: 1695–713.

Cohen, A. H., Rossignol, S. & Grillner, S. (eds.) (1988). *Neural Control of Rhythmic Movements.* New York: John Wiley.

Connors, B. W. (1984). Initiation of synchronized neuronal bursting in neocortex. *Nature,* **310**: 685–7.

Connors, B. W. & Gutnick, M. J. (1984*a*). Neocortex: cellular properties and intrinsic circuits. In *Brain Slices.* ed. R. Dingledine, pp. 313–39. New York: Plenum Press.

Connors, B. W. & Gutnick, M. J. (1984*b*). Cellular mechanisms of neocortical epileptogenesis in an acute experimental model. In *Electrophysiology of Epilepsy,* ed. P. Schwartzkroin & H. Wheal, pp, 79–105. New York: Academic Press.

Connors, B. W. & Gutnick, M. J. (1990). Intrinsic firing patterns of diverse neocortical neurons. *Trends in Neurosciences,* **13**: 99–104.

Connors, B. W., Gutnick, M. J. & Prince, D. A. (1982). Electrophysiological properties of neocortical neurons in vitro. *Journal of Neurophysiology,* **48**: 1302–20.

Connors, B. W., Malenka, R. C. & Silva, L. R. (1988). Two inhibitory postsynaptic potentials, and $GABA_A$ and $GABA_B$ receptor-mediated responses in neocortex of rat and cat. *Journal of Physiology,* **406**: 443–68.

DeFelipe, J. & Jones, E. G. (1988). *Cajal on the Cerebral Cortex,* pp. 557–622. New York: Oxford University Press.

Deisz, R. A. & Prince, D. A. (1989). Frequency-dependent depression of inhibition in guinea-pig neocortex in vitro by $GABA_B$ receptor feed-back on GABA release. *Journal of Physiology,* **412**: 513–41.

Dichter, M. A. & Ayala, G. F. (1987). Cellular mechanisms of epilepsy: a status report. *Science,* **237**: 157–64.

Dichter, M. A. & Spencer, W. A. (1969). Penicillin-induced interictal discharges from the cat hippocampus. II. Mechanisms underlying origin and restriction. *Journal of Neurophysiology,* **32**: 663–87.

Douglas, R. J. & Martin, K. A. C. (1990). Neocortex. In *The Synaptic Organization of the Brain,* ed. G. M. Shepherd, pp. 389–438. New York: Oxford University Press.

Ebersole, J. S. & Chatt, A. B. (1986). Spread and arrest of seizures: the importance of layer 4 in laminar interactions during neocortical epileptogenesis. In *Advances in Neurology,* vol. 44, eds. A. V. Delgado-Escueta, A. A. Ward Jr, D. M. Woodbury & R. J. Porter, pp. 515–58. New York: Raven Press.

Elger, C. E. & Speckmann, E.-J. (1983). Penicillin-induced epileptic foci in the motor cortex: vertical inhibition. *Electroencephalography and Clinical Neurophysiology,* **56**: 604–22.

Foehring, R. C. & Wyler, A. R. (1990). Two patterns of firing in human neocortical neurons. *Neuroscience Letters,* **14**: 279–85.

Foster, R. E., Connors, B. W. & Waxman, S. G. (1982). Rat optic nerve: electrophysiological, pharmacological and anatomical studies during development. *Developmental Brain Research,* **3**: 371–86.

Gabbot, P. L. A., Martin, K. A. C. & Whitteridge, D. (1987). Connections between pyramidal neurons in layer 5 of cat visual cortex (area 17). *Journal of Comparative Neurology,* **259**: 364–81.

Gabor, A. J. & Scobey, R. P. (1980). The physiological basis of epileptogenic neural aggregates. *Trends in Neuroscience,* **4**: 210–21.

Gabor, A. J., Scobey, R. P. & Wehrli, C. J. (1979). Relationship of epileptogenicity to cortical organization. *Journal of Neurophysiology*, **42**: 1609–25.

Getting, P. (1989). Emerging principles governing the operation of neural networks. *Annual Review of Neuroscience*, **12**: 185–204.

Gilbert, C. D. & Wiesel, T. N. (1983). Clustered intrinsic connections in cat visual cortex. *Journal of Neuroscience*, **3**: 1116–33.

Goldensohn, E. S. & Salazar, A. M. (1986). Temporal and spatial distribution of intracellular potentials during generation and spread of epileptogenic discharges. In *Advances in Neurology*, vol. 44, ed. A. V. Delgado-Escueta, A. A. Ward Jr, D. M. Woodbury & R. J. Porter, pp. 559–82. New York: Raven Press.

Gutnick, M. J., Connors, B. W. & Prince, D. A. (1982a). Mechanisms of neocortical epileptogenesis in vitro. *Journal of Neurophysiology*, **48**: 1321–35.

Gutnick, M. J. & Friedman, A. (1986). Synaptic and intrinsic mechanisms of synchronization and epileptogenesis in vitro. *Experimental Brain Research Supplement*, **14**: 327–35.

Gutnick, M. J., Grossman, Y. & Carlen, P. (1982b). Epileptogenesis in subdivided neocortical slices. *Neuroscience Letters Supplement*, **10**: S226.

Hablitz, J. J. (1988). Spontaneous ictal-like discharges and sustained potential shifts in the developing rat neocortex. *Journal of Neurophysiology*, **58**: 1052–65.

Heinemann, U., Lux, H. D. & Gutnick, M. J. (1977). Extracellular free calcium and potassium during paroxysmal activity in the cerebral cortex of cats. *Experimental Brain Research*, **27**: 237–43.

Howe, J. R., Sutor, B. & Zieglgansberger, W. (1987). Baclofen reduces postsynaptic potentials of rat neocortical neurones by actions other than its hyperpolarizing action. *Journal of Physiology*, **384**: 539–69.

Hubel, D. H. & Wiesel, T. N. (1963). Shape and arrangement of columns in the cat's striate cortex. *Journal of Physiology*, **165**: 559–68.

Hubel, D. H. & Wiesel, T. N. (1977). Functional architecture of macaque monkey visual cortex. *Proceedings of the Royal Society of London, Series B*, **198**: 1–59.

Huettner, J. E. & Baughman, R. W. (1988). The pharmacology of synapses formed by identified corticocollicular neurons in primary culture of rat visual cortex. *Journal of Neuroscience*, **8**: 160–75.

Huguenard, J. R. & Alger, B. E. (1986). Whole-cell voltage clamp study of the fading of GABA-activated currents in acutely dissociated hippocampal neurons. *Journal of Neurophysiology*, **56**: 1–18.

Jones, E. G. & Peters, A. (eds.) (1984a) *Cerebral Cortex*, vol. 1 *Cellular Components of the Cerebral Cortex*. New York: Plenum Press.

Jones, E. G. & Peters, A. (eds.) (1984b). *Cerebral Cortex*, vol. 2 *Cortical Function*. New York: Plenum Press.

Jones, E. G. & Peters, A. (eds.) (1991). *Cerebral Cortex*, vol. 9 *Normal and Altered States of Function, Including Hippocampus*. New York: Plenum Press.

Kisvarday, Z. F., Martin, K. A. C., Friedlander, M. J. & Somogyi, P. (1987). Evidence for interlaminar inhibitory circuits in the striate cortex of the cat. *Journal of Comparative Neurology*, **260**: 1–19.

Komatsu, Y., Nakajima, S., Toyama, K. & Fetz, E. (1988). Intracortical connectivity revealed by spike-triggered averaging in slice preparations of cat visual cortex. *Brain Research*, **442**: 359–63.

Kooi, K. A., Tucker, R. P. & Marshall, R. E. (1978). *Fundamentals of Electroencephalography*, 2nd edn. New York: Harper & Row.

Lacaille, J.-C. & Schwartzkroin, P. A. (1988). Stratum lacunosum-moleculare interneurons of hippocampal CA1 region. I. Intracellular response characteristics, synaptic responses, and morphology. *Journal of Neuroscience*, **8**: 1400–10.

Lidow, M. S., Goldman-Rakic, P. S., Gallager, D. W., Geschwind, D. H. & Rakic, P. (1989). Distribution of major neurotransmitter receptors in the motor and somatosensory cortex of the rhesus monkey. *Neuroscience*, **32**: 609–27.

Lloyd, K. G., Bossi, L., Morselli, P. L., Munari, C., Rougier, M. & Loiseau, H. (1986). Alterations of GABA-mediated synaptic transmission in human epilepsy. In *Advances in Neurology*, vol. 44, ed. A. V. Delgado-Escueta, A. A. Ward Jr, D. M. Woodbury & R. J. Porter, pp. 1033–44. New York: Raven Press.

Lockton, J. W. & Holmes, O. (1983). Penicillin epilepsy in the rat: the responses of different layers of the cortex cerebri. *Brain Research*, **259**: 79–89.

Lorente de Nó, R. (1938). The cerebral cortex: architecture, intracortical connections and motor projections. In *Physiology of the Nervous System*, ed. J. F. Fulton, pp. 291–339. London: Oxford University Press.

LoTurco, J. J., Mody, I. & Kriegstein, A. R. (1990). Differential activation of glutamate receptors by spontaneously released transmitter in slices of neocortex. *Neuroscience Letters*, **114**: 265–71.

Lowel, S., Freeman, B. & Singer, W. (1987). Topographic organization of the orientation column system in large flat-mounts of the cat visual cortex. A 2-deoxyglucose study. *Journal of Comparative Neurology*, **255**: 401–15.

Macdonald, R. L. (1989). Antiepileptic drug actions. *Epilepsia*, **30** (Suppl. 1): S19–S28.

Madison, D. V. & Nicoll, R. A. (1988). Enkephalin hyperpolarizes interneurones in the rat hippocampus. *Journal of Physiology*, **398**: 123–301.

Martin, K. A. C. (1984). Neuronal circuits in the cat striate cortex. In *Cerebral Cortex*, vol. 2 *Functional Properties of Cortical Cells*, ed. E. G. Jones & A. Peters, pp. 241–78. New York: Plenum Press.

Mason, A. Larkman, A. (1990). Correlations between morphology and electrophysiology of pyramidal neurons in slices of rat visual cortex. II. Electrophysiology. *Journal of Neuroscience*, **10**: 1415–28.

McCarren, M. & Alger, B. E. (1985). Use-dependent depression of IPSPs in rat hippocampal pyramidal cells in vitro. *Journal of Neurophysiology*, **53**: 557–71.

McCormick, D. A. (1989*a*). Cholinergic and noradrenergic modulation of thalamocortical processing. *Trends in Neurosciences*, **12**: 215–21.

McCormick, D. A. (1989*b*). GABA as in inhibitory neurotransmitter in human cerebral cortex. *Journal of Neurophysiology*, **62**: 1018–27.

McCormick, D. A., Connors, B. W., Lighthall, J. W. & Prince, D. A. (1985). Comparative electrophysiology of pyramidal and sparsely spiny stellate neurons of the neocortex. *Journal of Neurophysiology*, **54**: 782–806.

McCormick, D. A. & Prince, D. A. (1986). Mechanisms of action of acetylcholine in the guinea-pig cerebral cortex in vitro. *Journal of Physiology*, **375**: 169–94.

Miles, R. & Wong, R. K. S. (1983). Single neurones can initiate synchronized population discharge in the hippocampus. *Nature*, **306**: 371–3.

Miles, R., Wong, R. K. S. & Traub, R. D. (1983). Synchronized afterdischarges in the hippocampus: contribution of local synaptic interaction. *Neuroscience*, **12**: 1179–89.

Montoro, R. J., Lopez-Barneo, J. & Jassik-Gerschenfeld, A. (1988). Differential burst-firing modes in neurons of the mammalian visual cortex in vitro. *Brain Research*, **460**: 168–72.

Mountcastle, V. B. (1979). An organizing principle for cerebral function: the unit module and the distributed system. In *The Neurosciences, Fourth Study Program*, ed. F. O. Schmitt & F. G. Worden, pp. 21–42. Cambridge, MA: MIT Press.

Mountcastle, V. B., Talbot, W. H., Sakata, H. & Hyvarinen, J. (1969). Cortical neuronal mechanisms in flutter-vibration studied in unanaesthetized monkeys. Neuronal periodicity and frequency discrimination. *Journal of Neurophysiology*, **32**: 452–84.

Naegele, J. R. & Katz, L. C. (1990). Cell surface molecules containing N-acetylgalactosamine are associated with basket cells and neurogliaform cells in cat visual vortex. *Journal of Neuroscience*, **10**: 540–57.

Nicoll, R. A., Malenka, R. C. & Kauer, J. (1990). Functional comparison of neurotransmitter receptor subtypes in mammalian central nervous system. *Physiological Reviews*, **70**: 513–65.

Olsen, R. & Venter, J. C. (eds.) (1987). *Benzodiazepine/GABA Receptors and Chloride Channels: Structural and Functional Properties.* New York: Alan R. Liss.

Pedley, T. A. (1984). Epilepsy and the human electroencephalogram. In *Electrophysiology of Epilepsy*, ed. P. Schwartzkroin & H. Wheal, pp. 1–30. New York: Academic Press.

Peters, A. (1985). The neuronal composition of area 17 of rat visual cortex. III. Numerical considerations. *Journal of Comparative Neurology*, **238**: 263–74.

Peters, A. (1987). Number of neurons and synapses in primary visual cortex. In *Cerebral Cortex*, vol. 6 *Further Aspects of Cortical Function, Including Hippocampus*, ed. A. Peters & E. G. Jones, pp. 267–94. New York: Plenum Press.

Petsche, H., Prohaska, O., Rappelsburger, P., Vollmer, R. & Kaiser, A. (1974). Cortical seizure patterns in a multidimensional view: the information content of equipotential maps. *Epilepsia*, **15**: 439–63.

Pockberger, H., Rappelsburger, P. & Petsche, H. (1984a). Penicillin-induced epileptic phenomena in the rabbit's neocortex. I. The development of interictal spikes after epicortical application of penicillin. *Brain Research*, **309**: 247–60.

Pockberger, H., Rappelsburger, P. & Petsche, H. (1984b). Penicillin-induced epileptic phenomena in the rabbit's neocortex. II. Laminar-specific generation of interictal spikes after the application of penicillin to different cortical depths. *Brain Research*, **309**: 261–9.

Prince, D. A. (1969). Microelectrode studies of penicillin foci. In *Basic Mechanisms of the Epilepsies*, ed. H. H. Jasper, A. A. Ward & A. Pope, pp. 320–8. Boston: Little, Brown.

Prince, D. A. (1968). Inhibition in 'epileptic' neurons. *Experimental Neurology*, **21**: 307–21.

Prince, D. A., Deisz, R. A., Thompson, S. M. & Chagnac-Amitai, Y. (1990). Functional alterations in GABAergic inhibition during activity. In *Neurotransmitters in Epilepsy*, eds. G. Avanzini et al., pp. 47–57. New York: Demos.

Prince, D. A. & Wong, R. K. S. (1981). Human epileptic neurons studied in vitro. *Brain Research*, **210**: 323–33.

Pumain, R., Kurcewicz, I. & Louvel, J. (1983). Fast extracellular calcium transients: involvement in epileptic processes. *Science*, **222**, 117–79.

Reichenthal, E. & Hocherman, S. (1979). A critical epileptic area in the cat's cortex and its relation to cortical columns. *Electroencephalography and Clinical Neurophysiology*, **47**: 147–52.

Ribak, C. E. (1991). Epilepsy and cortex. In *Cerebral Cortex*, vol. 9 *Normal and Altered States of Function, Including Hippocampus*, ed. E. G. Jones & A. Peters, pp. 427–84. New York: Plenum Press.

Schroeder, C. E., Tenke, C. E., Givre, S. J., Arezzo, J. C. & Vaughan, H. G. (1990). Laminar analysis of bicuculline-induced epileptiform activity in area 17 of the awake macaque. *Brain Research*, **515**: 326–30.

Schwartzkroin, P. A. & Haglund, M. M. (1986). Spontaneous rhythmic synchronous activity in epileptic human and normal monkey temporal lobe. *Epilepsia*, **27**: 523–33.

Schwartzkroin, P. A. & Knowles, W. D. (1984). Intracellular study of human epileptic cortex: in vitro maintenance of epileptiform activity? *Science*, **223**: 709–12.

Schwartzkroin, P. A. & Prince, D. A. (1976). Microphysiology of human cerebral cortex studied in vitro. *Brain Research*, **115**: 497–500.

Schwartzkroin, P. A. & Prince, D. A. (1979). Penicillin-induced epileptiform activity in the hippocampal in vitro preparation. *Brain Research*, **147**: 117–30.

Sigel, E. & Baur, R. (1988). Activation of protein kinase C differentially modulates neuronal Na^+, Ca^{2+}, and γ-aminobutyrate type A channels. *Proceedings of the National Academy of Sciences, USA*, **85**: 6192–6.

Silva, L. R., Amitai, Y. & Connors, B. W. (1991). Intrinsic oscillations of neocortex generated by layer 5 pyramidal neurons. *Science*, **251**: 432–5.

Silva, L. R. & Connors, B. W. (1990). Layer 5 neurons can initiate NMDA-dependent, 4–7 Hz synchronized rhythms in neocortex. *Society for Neuroscience Abstracts*, **16**: 1134.

Simons, D. J. (1978). Response properties of vibrissa units in rat SI somatosensory neocortex. *Journal of Neurophysiology*, **41**: 798–820.

Somogyi, P. & Cowey, A. (1981). Combined Golgi and electron microscopic study on the synapses formed by double bouquet cells in the visual cortex of the cat and monkey. *Journal of Comparative Neurology*, **195**: 547–66.

Somogyi, P., Cowey, A., Kisvarday, Z. F., Freund, T. F. & Szentagothai, J. (1983). Retrograde transport of γ-amino-[H^3]butyric acid reveals specific interlaminar connections in the striate cortex of monkey. *Proceedings of the National Academy of Sciences, USA*, **80**: 2385–9.

Stelzer, A., Kay, A. R. & Wong, R. K. S. (1988). $GABA_A$-receptor function in hippocampal cells is maintained by phosphorylation factors. *Science*, **242**: 339–41.

Sterling, P. (1990). Retina: In *The Synaptic Organization of the Brain*, ed. G. M. Shepherd, pp. 389–438. New York: Oxford University Press.

Stafstrom, C. E., Schwindt, P. C., Flatman, J. A. & Crill, W. E. (1984). Properties of subthreshold response and action potential recorded in layer V neurons from cat sensorimotor neocortex in vitro. *Journal of Neurophysiology*, **52**: 244–63.

Sutor, B. & Hablitz, J. (1989a). EPSPs in rat neocortical neurons in vitro. I. Electrophysiological evidence for two distinct EPSPs. *Journal of Neurophysiology*, **61**: 607–20.

Sutor, B. & Hablitz, J. (1989b). EPSPs in rat neocortical neurons in vitro. II. Involvement of *N*-methyl-D-aspartate receptors in the generation of EPSPs. *Journal of Neurophysiology*, **61**: 621–34.

Takahashi, K. (1965). Slow and fast groups of pyramidal tract neurons and their respective membrane properties. *Journal of Neurophysiology*, **28**: 908–24.

Taylor, J. (ed.) (1931). *Selected Writings of John Hughlings Jackson*, vol. 1 *On Epilepsy and Epileptiform Convulsions*. London: Hodder & Stoughton.

Telfeian, A. E., Wehr, M. S. & Connors, B. W. (1990). Layer 5 is the preferred pathway for horizontal propagation of epileptiform discharges in neocortex. *Society for Neuroscience Abstracts*, **16**: 21.

Thomson, A. M. (1986). A magnesium-sensitive post-synaptic potential in rat cerebral cortex resembles neuronal responses to N-methylaspartate. *Journal of Physiology*, **370**: 531–49.

Thomson, A. M., Girdlestone, D. & West, D. C. (1988). Voltage-dependent currents prolong single-axon postsynaptic potentials in layer III pyramidal neurons in rat neocortical slices. *Journal of Neurophysiology*, **60**: 1896–907.

Traub, R. D., Knowles, W. D., Miles, R. & Wong, R. K. S. (1987). Models of the cellular mechanism underlying propagation of epileptiform activity in the CA2–CA3 region of the hippocampal slice. *Neuroscience*, **21**: 457–70.

Traub, R. D. & Wong, R. K. S. (1982). Cellular mechanism of neuronal synchronization in epilepsy. *Science*, **216**: 745–7.

Waxman, S. G. & Swadlow, H. A. (1977). The conduction properties of axons in central white matter. *Progress in Brain Research*, **8**: 297–324.

Welker, C. & Woolsey, T. A. (1974). Structure of layer IV in the somatosensory cortex of the rat: description and comparison with the mouse. *Journal of Comparative Neurology*, **158**: 437–54.

White, E. L. & Keller, A. (1989). *Cortical Circuits: Synaptic Organization of the Cerebral Cortex – Structure, Function and Theory*. Boston, MA: Birkhäuser.

Wong, R. K. S. & Traub, R. D. (1983). Synchronized burst discharge in the hippocampal slice. I. Initiation in the CA2–CA3 region. *Journal of Neurophysiology*, **49**: 459–71.

13

Study of GABAergic inhibition and GABA$_A$ receptors in experimental epilepsy

ROBERT K. S. WONG and RICHARD MILES

Introduction

Interictal spikes, identifiable as sharp transient deflections (30–50 ms) in electroencephalographic recordings, are electrographic markers of epilepsy (Pedley, 1984). Recordings during epileptic surgery operations show that up to 50% of cells exhibit burst discharge in the focus during interictal spikes (Wyler & Ward, 1981). These studies demonstrate directly that synchronized burst firing in populations of cortical neurons sustains the epileptiform activity. Clearly, information concerning the mechanisms underlying synchronized burst discharge are of fundamental importance to the understanding of epileptogenesis.

That GABAergic (GABA is γ-aminobutyric acid) inhibitory transmission regulates epileptiform activity is indicated by the action of several convulsant compounds. Analogues of interictal spikes can be produced experimentally with agents such as penicillin, bicuculline, and picrotoxin. These agents are all potent blockers of GABA$_A$ receptor function (see e.g., Macdonald, 1984). We have asked how a block of GABA$_A$ receptors can give rise to synchronized population discharges in cortical neurons.

This chapter describes the application of two in-vitro preparations from guinea pig in studies to assess the role of GABAergic inhibition in the control of epileptiform discharges. In hippocampal slices we have used dual recordings to examine, at the unitary level, synapses involved in the generation of recurrent inhibition and excitation. Acutely dissociated hippocampal neurons have allowed a detailed examination of intracellular regulation of the efficacy of GABA$_A$ receptors. The account is based primarily on our own experiments using the hippocampal slice and dissociated cell preparations. These data have allowed us to construct a computer model, consisting of up to 9000 cells (Traub et al., 1989), simulating the collective behavior of the network. Two important questions emerge from these studies: (a) what are the cellular and synaptic mechanisms underlying the interictal spike and (b) how does GABAergic inhibition control epileptiform activities?

Cellular and synaptic mechanisms underlying the interictal spike

Our simulation studies emphasized the role of recurrent excitatory synapses for the generation of interictal spikes. Pyramidal cells in the CA3 region are connected by axon collateral synapses. Neuronal activities are transmitted via these synapses to produce mutual excitation. Two further properties of these connections are: (a) that single pyramidal cells make contact with more than one postsynaptic cell, and (b) that the synaptic connections between pyramidal cells are sufficiently strong that spiking activities in the presynaptic neuron can elicit firing in postsynaptic cells. The simulations show that activity in one pyramidal cell can set up a propagating excitatory wave via the recurrent axons, and recruits a rapidly enlarging population into the interictal event (Fig. 13.1).

Experiments were carried out in the slice preparation to assess the validity of some of the assumptions of the model. Using paired intracellular recordings, the properties of the excitatory synaptic connections between CA3 cells have been characterized (Miles & Wong, 1986) and are described briefly later in the chapter.

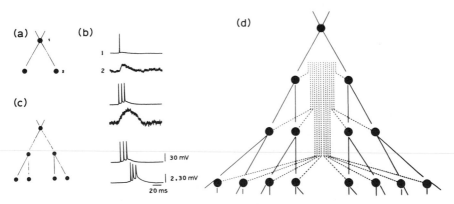

Fig. 13.1. Propagation of excitatory bursting through the hippocampal network. (a) Schematic of connectivity in the CA3 region. (b) Intracellular recordings from two monosynaptically connected cells (those labeled 1 and 2, for example, in (a)). A burst in cell 1 produced summed EPSPs in 2. The summed EPSPs can trigger burst firing. (c) If a presynaptic cell burst can induce a burst in postsynaptic cells, and the connection between cells shows divergence, then an increasing number of neurons can be driven into activity. (d) The model for an interconnected group of CA3 pyramidal cells. Each pyramidal cell contacts four postsynaptic cells.

GABAergic inhibition regulates epileptiform discharges

According to the scheme shown in Fig. 13.1, synchronized discharges are sustained by interconnections between CA3 pyramidal cells. Experimentally, epileptiform discharges are expressed when GABAergic inhibition is blocked. Together, these data suggest that the recurrent inhibitory circuit somehow suppresses the spread of excitation among CA3 pyramidal cells (Schwartzkroin & Prince, 1978; Miles & Wong, 1987a).

Recurrent inhibitory circuits were first examined in vivo by Kandel *et al.* (1961) and Andersen *et al.* (1963). They showed that powerful and prolonged inhibitory postsynaptic potentials (IPSPs) were activated by antidromic stimulation of pyramidal cells. Two processes are involved in generating recurrent inhibition: (a) pyramidal cells excite local GABAergic cells; (b) these in turn inhibit pyramidal cells. Recent studies show that inhibitory cells located in the stratum pyramidale have low firing thresholds, and pyramidal cells elicit large, unitary excitatory postsynaptic potentials (EPSPs) that can induce action potentials in inhibitory cells (Knowles & Schwartzkroin, 1981; Miles & Wong, 1984; Lacaille & Schwartzkroin, 1988). The latency between pre- and postsynaptic action potentials can be as short as 2–3 ms, and the probability of spike transmission can be as high as 0.6. Additional results demonstrated that the strong connection between pyramidal and inhibitory cells allows single action potentials in the pyramidal cell to activate a disynaptic IPSP in other pyramidal cells with latencies as short as 3–5 ms, with a probability of occurrence of about 0.3 (Miles, 1990). These results emphasize the strength and thus the functional significance of recurrent inhibitory connections.

Recurrent inhibition may prevent the spread of epileptiform discharge in the CA3 population in two ways. First, it prevents the recruitment of intrinsic burst discharges of pyramidal cells by the EPSPs. Previous studies show that hippocampal pyramidal cells possess an assembly of ionic conductances that, when activated upon depolarization, produces a burst firing pattern (Hablitz & Johnston, 1981; Wong & Prince, 1978, 1981). The intrinsic excitability of individual pyramidal cells is also greatly enhanced by the presence of multiple burst initiation sites in the dendrites in addition to the somatic initiation site (Wong *et al.*, 1979). Brief depolarizations of the soma or dendrites of pyramidal cells (and in particular CA3 cells) frequently elicit bursts of three to four action potentials of durations (20–40 ms) that outlast the stimulus. Orthodromic stimulation evokes an EPSP–IPSP sequence in pyramidal cells. The IPSP is timed to suppress burst firing. Thus, the recruitment of recurrent IPSPs during the spread of excitation between CA3 pyramidal cells blocks burst firing in individual cells and thereby arrests the spread of the excitatory wave.

A second way by which GABAergic inhibition regulates epileptiform discharge results from the extensive divergence of projections of single inhibitory interneurons onto pyramidal cells (Traub *et al.*, 1989). A single GABAergic neuron innervates up to 200 pyramidal cells. Thus, recruitment of inhibition in the initial phase of the synchronized discharge should dampen the excitability of a larger population of pyramidal cells, including those further downstream from the initially excited group. Consequently, the probability of eliciting burst firing in these pyramidal cells is reduced. With strong inhibitory synapses, the spread of burst firing will be arrested and the epileptiform discharge prevented (see e.g., Miles & Wong, 1987*a*).

Properties of the recurrent synapses

Experiments and simulations described above suggest that detailed studies of recurrent synapses can illuminate the basic mechanisms of epileptogenesis. The hippocampal slice preparation is an ideal model for studying recurrent excitatory and inhibitory synapses at the unitary level. The connections are intrinsic, contained within the in-vitro preparation, and one can expect a significant preservation of their anatomical and physiological properties. In contrast, results derived from studies in cultured preparations of dissociated neurons suggest that synapses between neurons may have developed abnormally. For example, the number of terminals per synaptic contact (Pun *et al.*, 1986), unitary PSP conductance (Segal & Barker, 1984; Forsythe & Westbrook, 1988), and miniature excitatory postsynaptic current amplitude (Bekkers & Stevens, 1990) may be abnormally large in cultured neurons.

Afferent synapses such as the Schaffer collateral projection to CA1 neurons have been examined by stimulating electrically in a region of the slice, and monitoring intracellular responses in a single neuron. This approach is difficult to use in the study of recurrent synapses embedded in a single restricted region. Synaptic connectivities should be characterized at the unitary level to provide essential information. For example, by observing the fluctuations in the size of the unitary events, information regarding the number of release sites at the synapse as well as the number of postsynaptic channels activated by transmitter released from a single release site can be estimated. Furthermore, analysis of unitary events allows questions such as the following to be assessed. Can spiking activities from a single cell drive postsynaptic cells to fire? What is the divergent and convergent connectivity pattern formed by a single cell to the population?

Four approaches have been used to define the properties of unitary synaptic events in the hippocampus. First, a weak stimulus may activate only one or a few similar cells or afferent fibers (MacNaughton et al., 1981; Turner, 1988). Unitary properties of synaptic connections can be inferred from characteristics of 'minimal' events, i.e., threshold events activated by the stimulus in an all-or-none fashion. However, it remains unclear whether these events result from the activation of the same presynaptic cell and whether apparent transmission failures represent a failure to activate the cell. Second, focal glutamate application can excite, in an asynchronous fashion, somata of spatially restricted cell groups, while not activating passing axons (Christian & Dudek, 1988). Correlating postsynaptic events with extracellular spikes from neurons in the region of glutamate application enhances the reliability of the technique (Jankowska & Roberts, 1972). The asynchronized activation of neurons by glutamate should also be helpful in resolving unitary events (Yamamoto, 1982). Third, spontaneous synaptic events recorded intracellularly could also provide useful information on aspects of transmitter release and receptor pharmacology (Brown et al., 1979; Collingridge et al., 1984; Cotman et al., 1986). Spontaneous events may also be recorded in conditions where spiking is blocked using tetrodotoxin so that the properties of a single quantum can be studied. A major drawback of these approaches is that synaptic events originating from different classes of presynaptic cells cannot be readily separated. In the fourth approach, pre- and postsynaptic cells can be recorded simultaneously in the slice preparation. Synaptic events can be unequivocally attributed to a single cell whose physiological properties can also be assessed. This method provides direct and precise information; however, the success rate of this approach is low.

In the following, unitary properties of excitatory and GABAergic synapses are presented. The information was obtained primarily from experiments using paired intracellular recordings of CA3 cells.

Unitary inhibitory events

We have used simultaneous intracellular recordings to study properties of synapses made by inhibitory cells located in the CA3 region. IPSPs generated by these inhibitory cells in CA3 pyramidal cells have a mean amplitude that ranged between 0.3 and 2.6 mV at postsynaptic potentials between -60 and -70 mV. The amplitude of these unitary events is considerably larger than that recorded in motoneurons (up to 0.4 mV). The difference may be explained by the larger input resistance of pyramidal cells (20–40 Ω, compared to 2–5 Ω for motoneurons). More recent work (Miles, 1990) suggests that unitary IPSPs initiated by these inhibitory cells are mediated exclusively by chloride ion fluxes. However, IPSPs evoked by strong afferent stimuli consist of an additional late GABA$_B$-mediated component (Newberry & Nicoll, 1984). Information on unitary GABA$_B$-mediated events remains limited (Lacaille & Schwartz-kroin, 1988).

Paired recordings are also crucial to characterize the presynaptic neuron. Hippocampal inhibitory cells are often assumed to have firing patterns and membrane properties that are common and distinct from those of pyramidal cells. For example, the inhibitory neurons shown by Knowles & Schwartzkroin (1981) and Lacaille *et al.* (1987) in the CA1 stratum pyramidale region of the hippocampus were spontaneously active and had pronounced spike afterhyperpolarizations. The postsynaptic response to repetitive action potential firing (50–100 Hz) in these neurons is a slow hyperpolarization of about 2–4 mV rather than a rapidly rising synaptic potential. Exploration in the CA3 stratum pyramidale region revealed that cells with this firing pattern are indeed inhibitory. However, other cells that initiate monosynaptic IPSPs have a different firing pattern not dissimilar from that of pyramidal cells (Miles & Wong, 1984).

Properties of inhibitory neurons in the stratum lacunosum–moleculare region of CA1 have also been studied (Lacaille & Schwartzkroin, 1988). These inhibitory cells differ from those located close to the stratum pyramidale in firing pattern, source of excitatory input, and possibly in postsynaptic receptors. Single action potentials in the inhibitory cell did not evoke measurable events; however, summed IPSPs of peak amplitude about 1 mV were activated by repetitive presynaptic firing.

Unitary excitatory events

Recurrent synapses between CA3 cells can also be examined using paired intracellular recordings (MacVicar & Dudek, 1980). The time course of these EPSPs is slow and variable. Their time to peak was 8–15 ms, the peaks can be prolonged, and are often followed by an undershoot. The quantal amplitude (q) was measured to be about 0.5 mV and the mean number of quanta of transmitter released (m) was in the range 1–5, on the basis of estimations using the variance technique or on synaptic transmission failure. This value for m is small compared to that of other synapses (frog neuromuscular junction 200–300 and about 10 000 at the squid giant synapse; for a review, see McLachlan, 1978). The data suggest that either the release probability is low in CA3 cells or that a limited number of release sites (terminals) exist at synapses between CA3 pyramidal cells. Indeed, morphological data from the neocortex show that one pyramidal cell makes no more than five contacts on a postsynaptic cell (Kisvarday *et al.*, 1985) suggesting that m may in fact be low for recurrent synapses between cortical pyramidal cells and, by analogy, perhaps hippocampal cells. Studies using the paired recording approach showed that larger unitary EPSPs (up to 3 mV) can be detected in the immature rat hippocampus (Smith *et al.*, 1988).

Our studies also show that despite the small value of m, depolarizations mediated by recurrent synapses are effective in triggering firing in postsynaptic cells. Previous studies show that the pyramidal cells in CA3 region generate burst firing patterns (Wong & Prince, 1978, 1979; Hablitz & Johnston, 1981). Our results show that a burst in the presynaptic cell can cause postsynaptic cells to burst. Further, the axon of a presynaptic cell appears to diverge and excite about 20 follower cells (Kay *et al.*, 1986). Thus, the conditions predicted by simulation are confirmed. One cell can generate EPSPs that drive more than one postsynaptic cell to fire and thereby contribute to the propagation of synchronized discharge.

Recent studies suggest that GABAergic inhibition in the hippocampus may show use-dependent plasticities. Specifically, our experimental results suggest that repetitive afferent stimulation reduces the efficacy of GABAergic inhibition (Miles & Wong, 1987*b*). Using the slice preparation we obtained intracellular recordings from a pair of cells in the CA3 region of the hippocampus. These cells showed no synaptic interaction. Tetani were applied to the mossy fibers, an afferent system to the region. Following tetanization, activity in one of the recorded cells began to produce polysynaptic EPSPs in the other cell. Additional data revealed that disynaptic IPSPs activated by one pyramidal cell to the other, via intercalating GABAergic neurons, were suppressed following tetani. The results demonstrated that within a recurrently connected population, disinhibition caused previously non-communicating members to become connected by recurrent synapses via polysynaptic pathways. Possible modifiable sites include:

(1) Pyramidal cell to GABAergic cell excitatory synapse.

(2) Intrinsic excitability of GABAergic cells.
(3) The inhibitory synapses between GABAergic cells and pyramidal cells.

Sites 1 and 3 can be further divided into pre- and postsynaptic regions.

Isolated cells and studies on GABA$_A$ receptor properties

Using the acutely dissociated cell preparation, we have recently begun to examine the modifiability of GABA receptors in adult guinea pig hippocampal pyramidal cells (site 3). GABA$_A$ responses progressively decreased in amplitude (run down) following breakthrough of the cell membrane by the recording pipette during whole-cell patch-clamp recording experiments. The run down was not caused by desensitization. When ATP and Mg^{2+} together with the 'fast' Ca^{2+} buffer (BAPTA) were included in the patch pipette solution, GABA$_A$ responses stabilized. This suggests that the GABA$_A$ receptor must be phosphorylated to remain functional. The phosphorylation process, which confers stability on the functional state of the receptor, is counteracted by a dephosphorylation process activated by elevation of intracellular Ca^{2+} (Stelzer *et al.*, 1988; Chen *et al.*, 1990).

Measurement of intracellular calcium in isolated cells using the Fura-2 imaging technique demonstrates the significance of calcium-dependent GABA$_A$ receptor function. The experiments show that extremely long-lasting gradients of Ca^{2+} were induced in the apical dendrites of the cells after brief (1–3 s) local application of either glutamate or NMDA. These gradients were sustained by continuous influx of Ca^{2+} into the dendrites. The appearance of a longlasting Ca^{2+} gradient generally required a priming or conditioning stimulation with the excitatory agonist. The sustained gradients, but not the immediate transient response to agonists, were prevented by prior treatment of cells with sphingosine, possibly via the blockade of kinase C action (Connor *et al.*, 1988).

The usefulness of the isolated cell preparation in the study of intracellular control of GABA$_A$ receptor function has been significantly enhanced with the recent development of an intracellular perfusion system that allows substances to be added to or removed from the intracellular space of a 'patched' isolated cell. The experimental arrangement for intracellular perfusion is shown in Fig. 13.2.

Various intracellular solutions can be placed in containers connected to a common pressurized chamber. An outlet from the chamber feeds into a valve. A thin tube leads from the output of the valve into the pipette,

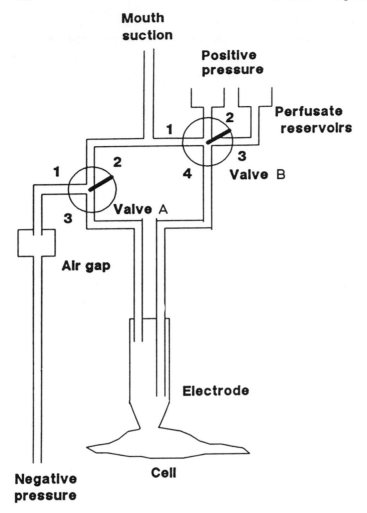

Fig. 13.2. Recording arrangement for switching intracellular perfusion solutions during whole-cell recording. Outlets 2 and 3 of valve A and 1 and 4 of valve B were connected during attempts to form high-resistance seals through suction applied by mouth. After cell penetration, outlets 1 and 3 of A and 2 (or 3) and 4 of B were connected. Positive pressure was applied at position 4 of B and negative pressure was applied at position 3 of A to facilitate the influx and efflux of solutions at the tip of the pipette.

extending close to the tip. Efflux is achieved through another tube that is connected to a column of water to generate negative pressure. In a typical experiment outlets 2 and 3 of valve A and 1 and 4 of valve B are first connected during attempts to form high resistance seals through mouth suction. After cell penetration, outlets 1 and 3 of A and 2 (or 3) and 4 of B are connected. Positive pressure applied at position 4 of B will force the solution into the pipette, and negative pressure applied at 3 of A will facilitate solution efflux. Solutions can be perfused at 0.2 to 0.4 ml/min through the recording pipette. Effects of different agents introduced into the cell can be detected 3–5 min after a switch.

By using the intracellular perfusion system, we have carried out experiments to characterize further the regulation of $GABA_A$ receptor function by the phosphorylation–dephosphorylation process (Chen *et al.*, 1990). The results show that run-down of the $GABA_A$ response caused by the absence of intracellular ATP is reversible, suggesting that the loss of the response is not due to a catabolic process but instead is consistent with the involvement of a phosphorylation–dephosphorylation process. We also have attempted to stabilize $GABA_A$ receptor function by strengthening the phosphate bond of the substrate protein against hydrolysis. The ATP analogue, ATPγS, is useful for this purpose because the thiophosphate group donated by this nucleotide is resistant to enzyme hydrolysis (Eckstein, 1985) so that dephosphorylation proceeds more slowly than it does when the phosphate group is donated by ATP. The data revealed that $GABA_A$ response run-down proceeded slowly when ATP was substituted by ATPγS.

In summary, our studies support the following scheme for $GABA_A$ receptor function:

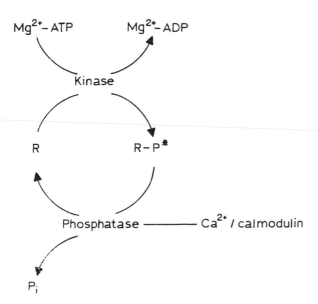

Three essential features predicted by the hypothesis are: (a) the $GABA_A$ receptor protein or a closely associated protein can exist in either dephospho- or phosphorylated forms; (b) the presence of a protein kinase, which catalyzes the conversion of the substrate protein from dephospho- to phosphorylated form; and (c) the existence of a phosphoprotein phosphatase, which catalyzes the reverse reaction. Additional data revealed that the phosphatase is activated by elevations of intracellular $[Ca^{2+}]$, suggesting that calcineurin is the phosphatase involved. At present, the identity of the kinase remains unclear. Additional experiments are needed to assess the physiological significance of the intracellular site regulating the $GABA_A$ response.

Conclusion

Previous studies have emphasized the importance of $GABA_A$ receptors in the control of epileptogenesis. In-vitro slice experiments have shown that synaptic inhibition mediated by $GABA_A$ receptors is labile and attenuates following repetitive stimulation. Additional experiments, carried out in isolated cells, suggest that the newly discovered intracellular regulation site for the $GABA_A$ receptor may have a role in facilitating plastic changes in synaptic inhibition and may be a site of vulnerability for epileptogenesis.

References

Andersen, P., Eccles, J. C. & Løyning, Y. (1963). Recurrent inhibition in the hippocampus with identification of inhibitory cells and its synapses. *Nature*, **198**: 540–2.

Bekkers, J. M. & Stevens, C. F. (1990). Presynaptic mechanisms for long-term potentiation in the hippocampus. *Nature*, **346**: 724–9.

Brown, T. H., Wong, R. K. S. & Prince, D. A. (1979). Spontaneous miniature synaptic potentials in hippocampal neurons. *Brain Research*, **177**: 194–9.

Chen, Q. X., Stelzer, A., Kay, A. R. & Wong, R. K. S. (1990). $GABA_A$ receptor function is regulated by phosphorylation in acutely dissociated guinea-pig hippocampal neurones. *Journal of Physiology*, **420**: 207–21.

Christian, E. P. & Dudek, F. E. (1988). Characteristics of local excitatory circuits studied with glutamate microapplications in the CA1 area of rat hippocampal slices. *Journal of Neurophysiology*, **59**: 90–109.

Collingridge, G. L., Gage, P. W. & Robertson, B. (1984). Inhibitory postsynaptic currents in rat hippocampal CA1 neurons. *Journal of Physiology*, **356**: 551–64.

Connor, J. A., Wadman, W. J., Hockberger, P. E. & Wong, R. K. S. (1988). Sustained dendritic gradients of Ca^{2+} induced by excitatory amino acids in CA1 hippocampal neurons. *Science*, **240**: 649–53.

Cotman, C. W., Flatman, J. A., Ganong, A. & Perkins, M. N. (1986). Effects of excitatory amino acid antagonists on evoked and spontaneous excitatory potentials in guinea pig hippocampus. *Journal of Physiology*, **378**: 403–15.

Eckstein, F. (1985). Nucleoside phosphorothioates. *Annual of Biochemistry*, **54**: 367–402.

Forsythe, I. D. & Westbrook, G. L. (1988). Slow excitatory postsynaptic currents mediated by *N*-methyl-D-aspartate receptors on cultured mouse central neurons. *Journal of Physiology*, **396**: 515–33.

Hablitz, J. J. & Johnston, D. (1981). Endogenous nature of spontaneous bursting in hippocampal pyramidal neurons. *Cellular and Molecular Neurobiology*, **1**: 325–34.

Jankowska, E. & Roberts, W. J. (1972). Synaptic action of single interneurones mediating Ia inhibition of motoneurones. *Journal of Physiology*, **222**: 623–42.

Kandel, E. R., Spencer, W. A. & Brinkley, F. J. (1961). Electrophysiology of hippocampal neurons. I. Sequential invasion and synaptic organization. *Journal of Neurophysiology*, **24**: 225–58.

Kay, A. R., Miles, R. & Wong, R. K. S. (1986). Intracellular fluoride alters the kinetic properties of calcium currents facilitating the investigation of synaptic events in hippocampal neurons. *Journal of Neuroscience*, **6**: 2915–20.

Kisvarday, Z. F., Martin, K. A. C., Whitteridge, D. & Somogyi, P. (1985). Synaptic connections of intracellularly filled clutch cells: a type of small basket cell in the visual cortex of the cat. *Journal of Comparative Neurology*, **241**: 111–37.

Knowles, W. D. & Schwartzkroin, P. A. (1981). Local circuit interactions in hippocampal brain slices. *Journal of Neuroscience*, **1**: 318–22.

Lacaille, J. C., Mueller, A. L., Kunkel, D. D. & Schwartzkroin, P. A. (1987). Local circuit interactions between oriens–alveus interneurons and CA1 pyramidal cells in hippocampal slices: electrophysiology and morphology. *Journal of Neuroscience*, **7**: 1979–93.

Lacaille, J. C. & Schwartzkroin, P. A. (1988). Stratum lacunosum–moleculare interneurons of hippocampal CA1 region. II. Intrasomatic and intradendritic recordings of local circuit synaptic interactions. *Journal of Neuroscience*, **8**: 1411–24.

Macdonald, R. L. (1984). Anticonvulsant and convulsant drug actions on vertebrate neurones in primary dissociated cell culture. In *Electrophysiology of Epilepsy*, ed. P. A. Schwartzkroin & H. Wheal, pp. 351–87. London: Academic Press.

MacVicar, B. A. & Dudek, F. E. (1980). Local synaptic circuits in rat hippocampus: interactions between pyramidal cells. *Brain Research*, **184**: 220–3.

McLachlan, E. M. (1978). The statistics of transmitter release at chemical synapses. In *International Review of Physiology, Neurophysiology III*, ed. R. Porter, pp. 49–116. Baltimore, MD: University Park Press.

McNaughton, B. L., Barnes, C. A. & Andersen, P. (1981). Synaptic efficacy and EPSP summation in granule cells of rat fascia dentata studied in vitro. *Journal of Neurophysiology*, **46**: 952–66.

Miles, R. (1990). Synaptic excitation of inhibitory cells by single CA3 pyramidal cells of the guinea-pig in vitro. *Journal of Physiology*, **428**: 61–77.

Miles, R. & Wong, R. K. S. (1984). Unitary inhibitory synaptic potentials in the guinea-pig hippocampus in vitro. *Journal of Physiology*, **356**: 97–113.

Miles, R. & Wong, R. K. S. (1986). Excitatory synaptic interactions between CA3 neurones in the guinea-pig hippocampus. *Journal of Physiology*, **373**: 397–418.

Miles, R. & Wong, R. K. S. (1987*a*). Inhibitory control of local excitatory circuits in the guinea-pig hippocampus. *Journal of Physiology,* **388**: 611–29.

Miles, R. & Wong, R. K. S. (1987*b*). Latent synaptic pathways revealed after tetanic stimulation in the hippocampus. *Nature,* **329**: 724–6.

Newberry, N. R. & Nicoll, R. A. (1984). A bicuculline resistant inhibitory postsynaptic potential in rat hippocampal pyramidal cell in vitro. *Journal of Physiology,* **348**: 239–54.

Pedley, T. A. (1984). Epilepsy and the human electroencephalogram. In *Electrophysiology of Epilepsy,* ed. P. A. Schwartzkroin & H. Wheal, pp. 1–30. London: Academic Press.

Pun, R. Y. K., Neal, E. A., Guthrie, P. B. & Nelson, P. G. (1986). Active and inactive central synapses in cell culture. *Journal of Neurophysiology,* **6**: 1242–56.

Schwartzkroin, P. A. & Prince, D. A. (1978). Cellular and field potential properties of epileptogenic hippocampal slices. *Brain Research,* **147**, 117–30.

Segal, M. & Barker, J. L. (1984). Rat hippocampal neurons in culture: voltage clamp analysis of inhibitory synaptic connections. *Journal of Neurophysiology,* **52**: 469–87.

Smith, K. L., Turner, J. & Swann, J. W. (1988). Paired intracellular recordings reveal mono- and poly-synaptic excitatory interactions in immature hippocampus. *Society for Neuroscience Abstracts,* **14**: 883.

Stelzer, A., Kay, A. R. & Wong, R. K. S. (1988). $GABA_A$-receptor function in hippocampal cells is maintained by phosphorylation factors. *Science,* **241**: 339–41.

Traub, R. D., Miles, R. & Wong, R. K. S. (1989). Model of the origin of rhythmic population oscillations in the hippocampal slice. *Science,* **243**: 1319–25.

Traub, R. D. & Wong, R. K. S. (1982). Cellular mechanism of neuronal synchronization in epilepsy. *Science,* **216**: 745–7.

Turner, D. A. (1988). Waveform and amplitude characteristics of evoked responses to dendritic stimulation of CA1 guinea pig pyramidal cells. *Journal of Physiology,* **395**: 419–39.

Wong, R. K. S. & Prince, D. A. (1978). Participation of calcium spikes during intrinsic burst firing in hippocampal neurons. *Brain Research,* **159**: 385–90.

Wong, R. K. S. & Prince, D. A. (1979). Dendritic mechanisms underlying penicillin-induced epileptiform activity. *Science,* **204**: 1228–31.

Wong, R. K. S. & Prince, D. A. (1981). Afterpotential generation in hippocampal pyramidal cells. *Journal of Neurophysiology,* **45**: 86–97.

Wong, R. K. S., Prince, D. A. & Basbaum, A. I. (1979). Intradendritic recordings from hippocampal neurons. *Proceedings of the National Academy of Sciences, USA,* **76**: 986–90.

Wyler, A. R. & Ward, A. A., Jr (1981). Neurons in human epileptic cortex. Response to direct cortical stimulation. *Journal of Neurosurgery,* **55**: 904–8.

Yamamoto, C. (1982). Quantal analysis of excitatory postsynaptic potentials induced in hippocampal neurons by activation of granule cells. *Experimental Brain Research,* **46**: 170–6.

14

High potassium-induced synchronous bursts and electrographic seizures

CHRISTOPHER J. McBAIN,
STEPHEN F. TRAYNELIS, and
RAYMOND DINGLEDINE

Introduction

Recent studies have shown that properly cut hippocampal slices contain sufficient circuitry and cellular elements to sustain electrographic seizure activity with a duration of a minute or more. The 'high-K' model of hypersynchronous, epileptiform activity is produced by elevation of the extracellular potassium ion concentration ($[K^+]_o$) bathing the hippocampal slice. The resulting activity has several unique features. At least two distinct types of epileptiform event arise when $[K^+]_o$ is raised from 3.5 to 7–8.5 mM, with the concentration of $[Ca^{2+}]_o$ and $[Mg^{2+}]_o$ maintained nominally at 1.5 mM. So-called interictal bursts, defined as a rapid and brief depolarization of the neuronal membrane coincident with a burst of action potentials, arise predominantly in the CA3b or CA3c subfield and propagate synaptically to CA1 pyramidal cells. In addition, electrographic seizures (often referred to as ictal events) with both tonic- and clonic-like components, appear in, and are restricted to, the CA1 subfield. Thus, the elevation of $[K^+]_o$ permits the study of both spontaneous interictal activity and electrographic seizures proper in a relatively intact system *without* the requirement of electrical stimulation of afferent pathways. Perhaps the most potentially relevant and exciting feature of this model is that interictal bursts originating in hippocampal CA3 precipitate periods of intense, focal seizure activity in CA1. This relationship between the different types of high $[K^+]_o$-induced epileptiform activity presents a good opportunity to study the mechanisms of the transition between interictal and ictal activity, as it occurs in CA1 pyramidal cells. In this review, we address several characteristics of the high-K model, and attempt to relate them to those mechanisms that are potentially involved in seizure initiation and maintenance.

Overview

Interictal bursts

Following the elevation of $[K^+]_o$ interictal burst firing occurs in all hippocampal pyramidal subfields (Fig. 14.1). Extracellularly recorded population spikes are coincident with a sudden paroxysmal depolarizing shift (PDS) and thus, similar to other models discussed in this book, represent the synchronous discharge of a large aggregate of neurons (Rutecki *et al.*, 1985; Korn *et al.*, 1987). Interictal activity is typically 50–100 ms in duration occurring at a frequency of ∼1 Hz. The burst initiation site within hippocampal slices bathed in high $[K^+]_o$ is typically subfield CA3b/c (cf. $GABA_A$ antagonist-induced bursts originate in CA2; Knowles *et al.*, 1987), and interictal events then propagate to all other pyramidal subfields except the CA4 region. Simultaneous recordings from both CA1 and CA3 subfields reveal that interictal activity is synchronous in these regions. Sectioning of the Schaffer collateral afferent pathway, however, eliminates bursting activity in CA1 (Fig. 14.2), demonstrating that those bursts arising in CA1 (followers) are synaptically driven by CA3 (pacemakers).

Electrographic seizures

In approximately 20% of slices showing interictal activity, electrographic seizures recur spontaneously and exclusively in the CA1 region (Fig. 14.1). CA1 electrographic seizures contain components reminiscent of electrical discharges recorded in vivo during tonic–clonic motor seizures (Matsumoto & Ajmone-Marsan, 1964a,b). The tonic phase typically lasts 1–10 s and consists of a sustained depolarization during high frequency spike-firing of CA1 pyramidal cells. It is associated with a negative extracellular potential in the cell layer that is presumably linked to activity-dependent increases in $[K^+]_o$. The clonic phase lasts tens of seconds and is composed of paroxysmal bursts with afterdischarges in pyramidal cells. The seizure interval is approximately 3 min. While both the tonic phase and each clonic discharge of the seizure are triggered synaptically by a CA3 interictal burst, the frequency and amplitude of the CA3 interictal bursts do not change. Thus resulting electrographic seizures remain focal in nature in that they do not reinvade the CA3 region (see Fig. 14.1(b)), suggesting that the interictal spike generator can be anatomically distinct from the seizure zone yet be crucially involved in seizure generation. Sectioning of the Schaffer collateral afferent pathway eliminates seizure

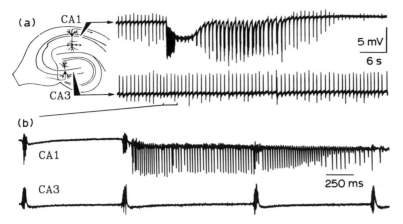

Fig. 14.1. Depolarization and burst firing of CA1 and CA3 pyramidal neurons during an electrographic seizure from a slice bathed in 8.5 mM $[K^+]_o$. (a) Schematic representation of the recording array within a transverse hippocampal slice. Simultaneous extracellular recordings from both CA1 and CA3 subfields during a seizure are also shown. (b) Expansion of CA1 tonic phase and CA3 interictal bursts shown in (a). Note that the interictal bursts in CA3 proceed unchanged during a CA1 seizure. (From Traynelis & Dingledine, 1989*b*.)

occurrence without affecting interictal bursting in CA3 (Fig. 14.2(b)). Subsequent replacement of the synaptic input by periodic electrical stimulation of the stratum radiatum, patterned to mimic interictal burst input, re-establishes recurring seizure activity (Fig. 14.2(c)), which confirms the controlling role of CA3 interictal input to seizure generation in the CA1 region. CA1 electrographic seizures but not CA3 interictal bursts are readily abolished by the *N*-methyl-D-aspartate (NMDA) receptor antagonist D-APV (D-2-amino-5-phosphonovaleric acid; Traynelis & Dingledine, 1988). In 53% of those slices generating interictal activity but not spontaneous seizures, a brief period of hypoxia (5–60 s) can lead to a single electrographic seizure restricted to area CA1, whereas CA3 continues to show only interictal activity (Kawasaki *et al.*, 1990). In their appearance, site of origin, dependence on the elevation of extracellular potassium and dependence on CA3 burst input, hypoxia-induced CA1 seizures appear similar to spontaneously occurring seizures.

Which actions of increased $[K^+]_o$ contribute to epileptiform activity?

Small changes in $[K^+]_o$ have, perhaps, more actions on neuronal function than changes of any of the other major extracellular ions. With only a

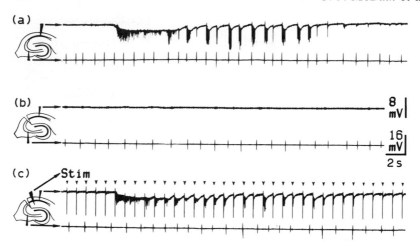

Fig. 14.2. CA3 interictal bursts synaptically trigger CA1 electrographic seizures. (a) Simultaneous extracellular recordings from the CA1 (top trace) and CA3 (bottom trace) regions during spontaneous seizure activity. Note that in this slice CA1 interictal bursts are barely distinguishable. (b) Electrodes were withdrawn from the slice, and a microlesion was made as indicated, followed by electrode replacement. Spontaneous interictal bursts continued in the CA3 region; however, seizures were abolished in the CA1 region. (c) Electrical stimulation of the Schaffer commissural input (55/min) to the CA1 region in the form of short trains of current pulses, patterned to mimic interictal input, re-established CA1 electrographic seizures. Each train consisted of five current pulses (75 µA, 100 µs) over a period of 35 ms. (From Traynelis & Dingledine, 1988.)

few exceptions (activation of electrogenic Na^+,K^+-ATPase and axonal conduction block), the events subsequent to increased $[K^+]_o$ are excitatory. It therefore should be no surprise that a number of investigators have expanded upon different predicted consequences of increased $[K^+]_o$ to formulate hypotheses of the mechanisms contributing to abnormal neuronal excitability and seizure generation (Green, 1964; Fertziger & Ranck, 1970; Dichter *et al.*, 1972; Traynelis & Dingledine, 1988; Haglund & Schwartzkroin, 1990). As space does not permit us to review comprehensively the actions of increased $[K^+]_o$ on neurophysiology, we consider here three important categories of the excitatory actions of K^+.

Reduced K^+ driving force

The most obvious action of increased $[K^+]_o$ is a reduction of the electromotive force that drives transmembrane K^+ current. For example, an increase in $[K^+]_o$ from 3.5 to 8.5 mM would cause a depolarizing shift in E_K of 23 mV (assuming a constant $[K^+]_i$). For K^+ conductances that exhibit a linear current–voltage relationship near the resting potential, this shift in the K^+ driving force should cause a reduction of outward (hyperpolarizing) K^+ currents. Such changes in driving force for K^+ currents have a wide variety of excitatory actions. A positive shift of E_K depolarizes hippocampal CA1 and CA3 pyramidal cells (Alger *et al.*, 1983; McBain & Dingledine, 1992), which brings the membrane potential closer to spike threshold, and can potentially activate voltage-regulated conductances (see e.g., Nowak *et al.*, 1984). One additionally might predict that increased $[K^+]_o$ would reduce the action potential threshold, a possibility consistent with an observed decrease of this parameter in CA1 pyramidal cells exposed to the K^+-channel blocker 4-aminopyridine (Perreault & Avoli, 1989). A decreased K^+ driving force will also decrease the repolarizing component of action potentials mediated by both I_A and I_C (Storm, 1987), and the afterhyperpolarization (AHP) that appears to terminate bursts of action potentials carried by I_C (Alger & Williamson, 1988) and I_{AHP} (Pennefather *et al.*, 1985; Lancaster & Adams, 1986). The reduction of the repolarizing conductance of action potentials increases action potential duration, which might enhance the influx of Ca^{2+} into the synaptic terminal. In addition, a reduction of the non-inactivating M-current, responsible for spike train accommodation (Halliwell & Adams, 1982), will favour prolonged periods of repetitive firing. All of these effects could promote the progression of single action potentials to multi-spike events, or increase the duration of bursts of action potentials. One further effect of a decreased K^+ driving force would be a decrease in the amplitude of slow $GABA_B$ inhibitory postsynaptic potentials (IPSPs) (Newberry & Nicoll, 1984).

Impaired GABA_A receptor-mediated inhibition

An indirect excitatory action of increased $[K^+]_o$ involves the impairment of postsynaptic, recurrent $GABA_A$ receptor-mediated inhibition (Korn *et al.*, 1987). The elevation of $[K^+]_o$ from 3.5 to 8.5 mM is known to produce a 9 mV depolarizing shift in the fast Cl^--mediated IPSP reversal potential, in hippocampal CA3 pyramidal cells (Korn *et al.*, 1987; see also Alger & Nicoll, 1983). This K^+-induced reduction in IPSP amplitude is not accompanied by any reduction in inhibitory synaptic conductance and consequently is dissimilar to block by $GABA_A$ antagonists. Rather, the shift of the reversal potential suggests that increased $[K^+]_o$ produces a decrease in the electromotive driving force for $GABA_A$ receptor-mediated

Cl⁻ currents, presumably via a redistribution of Cl^- across the plasma membrane and an increase in $[Cl^-]_i$ (see Misgeld et al., 1986). The mechanism by which increased $[K^+]_o$ could elevate $[Cl^-]_i$, however, is still somewhat speculative. Possible explanations include K^+-induced alterations of K^+, Cl^- cotransport mechanisms, or Donnan equilibrium forces, as originally predicted by Fertziger & Ranck (1970).

K^+-induced glial swelling

Potassium is released into the extracellular space with each action potential, and $[K^+]_o$ appears to fluctuate during normal neuronal function (see e.g., Heinemann & Lux, 1977; Hounsgaard & Nicholson, 1983). A key role for glial cells in clearing K^+ that accumulates in the extracellular space as a result of neuronal firing is now firmly established (for a review, see Walz, 1989). This action of glial cells presumably prevents the disruption of normal neuronal function that would occur as a result of the excitatory actions of elevated $[K^+]_o$ (see above). Yet, it seems that the various mechanisms that glial cells possess to clear excessive extracellular K^+ also render these cells susceptible to osmotically induced swelling when $[K^+]_o$ becomes too high (Bourke & Nelson, 1972; Ransom et al., 1985; Walz, 1989; McBain et al., 1990). Glial cell swelling will consequently lead to a reduction in the extracellular space. While there is little doubt that K^+ can cause glial swelling, there remain at least two important questions: (a) what glial regulatory processes are responsible for glial swelling (see Dietzel et al., 1989) and (b) what is the threshold level of $[K^+]_o$ necessary to induce glial swelling and the consequent decrease in the extracellular space? The first question is difficult to address, since different clearance mechanisms operate at different $[K^+]_o$. Nevertheless, there appear to be two primary means by which increases in $[K^+]_o$ can lead to increased intraglial osmolality and subsequent swelling (Fig. 14.3). First, K^+ can move across glial plasma membranes via passive diffusion through K^+ channels that are open at the resting membrane potential (see Walz, 1989), active transport via Na^+,K^+ ATP-ase (Ballanyi et al., 1987), and an amiloride-sensitive K^+,Cl^- cotransport system (Kimelberg & Frangakis, 1985; Walz & Mukerji, 1988). Second, the uptake of excessive K^+ by glia is accompanied by spatial redistribution of K^+ through glial processes and gap junctions, driven by potential and concentration gradients (see Dietzel et al., 1989). As K^+ moves effectively through the glial syncytium from areas of high concentration to those of low, a counter-current is generated in the

K- INDUCED GLIAL SWELLING

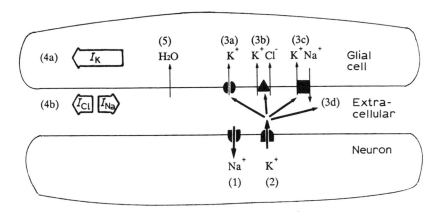

Fig. 14.3. Potassium movement in glial cells. Three compartments are depicted: intraneuronal (bottom), extracellular (middle), and intra-glial (top). The net movement of Na^+ across neuronal membranes during action potentials (1) results in K^+ efflux (2) into the extracellular space. K^+ can move via several paths (3), four of which are shown: (a) K^+ enters glial cells through open K^+ channels; (b) K^+ is actively transported via a K^+,Cl^--cotransport system; (c) K^+ is a substrate for Na^+,K^+-ATPase; (d) K^+ can diffuse passively in the extracellular space. During intense neuronal firing, K^+ can accumulate in glia at sites bordering excitable membranes. The open arrow (4a) within the glial compartment illustrates a current generated as K^+ effectively moves down an electrochemical gradient from areas of high concentration through processes and coupled glia to areas of low concentration. This current induces a counter-current (4b) in the extracellular space (open arrows) carried by Na^+ moving towards, and Cl^- moving away from the active site, proportional to their respective mobilities. Since only about half of the potassium ions removed from the extracellular space are replaced by Na^+, and a roughly equal number of chloride ions move away, an osmotic gradient exists at the original site of K^+ accumulation. The K^+,Cl^- cotransport augments this osmotic gradient, and (5) water enters the glial cells as swelling ensues.

extracellular fluid carried by Na^+ towards, and Cl^- away from, the site where $[K^+]_o$ first increased. Since positive ions carry only about half of the countercurrent, the K^+ ions removed at the site of the initial disturbance are only approximately half-replaced by Na^+, further sustaining the osmotic gradient. It is crucial to know the threshold level(s) of K^+ that will induce significant water movement into glia, in order to judge the relevance of glial swelling to neuronal function in normal and pathological situations. Yet, whereas radiotracer studies suggest that swelling occurs as $[K^+]_o$ reaches roughly 10 mM (Bourke & Nelson, 1972;

see also Walz, 1989), few studies to date have been directed at determining whether extracellular volume fraction is altered by moderate and graded changes in $[K^+]_o$ (see pp. 448–52).

Relative importance of the different actions of K^+ to epileptiform activity

The quantitative evaluation of different K^+-clearing mechanisms is confounded by the lack of basic information about how neurons and glia respond electrically and metabolically to complex changes in ions and increased energy demands. Thus, we can make only a few qualitative arguments as to the relative importance of the various above-mentioned actions of increased $[K^+]_o$. First, impaired inhibition in high $[K^+]_o$ by itself is insufficient to account for the high frequency of spontaneous interictal-type bursts that occur among CA3 pyramidal cells (Chamberlin & Dingledine, 1988). Second, the insensitivity of the frequency of spontaneous *interictal* bursts to hyperosmotic expansion of the extracellular space (Traynelis & Dingledine, 1989a) suggests that the excitatory actions of reduced extracellular space do not contribute to the initiation of these hypersynchronous bursts of action potentials. In contrast, the observation of an increase in tissue resistance immediately prior to seizure initiation, and the ability of hyperosmotic expansion of the extracellular space to suppress seizure occurrence, together suggest that high $[K^+]_o$-induced reductions of the extracellular space are *critically* involved in the conversion of abnormal, hypersynchronous synaptic input into electrographic seizures (Traynelis & Dingledine, 1988, 1989a).

Why is burst firing initiated preferentially in the CA3 area?

It is important to note that CA1 pyramidal cells bathed in high $[K^+]_o$, in spite of having a low seizure threshold, are very reluctant to generate spontaneous synchronous bursts when isolated from the CA3 region (e.g. Fig. 14.2(b)). What explains this striking difference between CA3 and CA1 regions? In principal the more pronounced tendency to generate synchronous bursts in CA3 could be due to a higher density of ion channels or electrical junctions that promote burst firing, and also due to recurrent excitatory synaptic connections. The ability of CA3 pyramidal cells to fire intrinsic bursts has often been commented on (see e.g., Wong *et al.*, 1979; Bilkey & Schwartzkroin, 1990). This intrinsic bursting property may well contribute to the tendency towards synchronous interictal activity of the CA3 region under some conditions, even though intrinsic bursting is not a prominent feature of CA3 neurons in high [K$^+$]. Other work favors the original suggestion (Ayala *et al.*, 1973) that recurrent excitatory collateral pathways within the CA3 region (which appear sparse in CA1) contribute greatly to its propensity to generate synchronous bursts (Miles & Wong, 1987; Christian & Dudek, 1988).

One feature characteristic of CA3 pyramidal neurons is their constant bombardment by both EPSPs and IPSPs, some of which are probably due to the firing of presynaptic neurons (Miles & Wong, 1986), although others probably result from random release of transmitter quanta (Brown *et al.*, 1979). Several lines of evidence support the contention that each interictal burst is triggered by an EPSP cascade that grows rapidly to recruit the whole pyramidal cell population. First, the probability of observing an EPSP in an individual pyramidal cell is not constant but instead rises just before burst onset. For example, in the results of the CA3 pyramidal cell experiment given in Fig. 14.4, EPSP occurrence was monitored during 41 spontaneous bursts. Forty-five EPSPs (of >1 mV amplitude) occurred in the 50 ms intervals just preceding each burst, compared to only 13 in the intervals 250–300 ms before each of the same bursts. When this analysis was carried out for 11 spontaneously bursting cells in 8.5 mM [K$^+$]$_o$, the probability of observing an EPSP rose from 0.22 ± 0.04 in the 250–300 ms period before each burst, to 0.60 ± 0.10 in the 50 ms interval immediately preceding each burst (Chamberlin *et al.*, 1990). Second, submaximal concentrations of the AMPA (α-amino-3-hydroxy-5-methyl-4-isoxazole propionic acid) receptor antagonist, CNQX (6-cyano-7-nitro-quinoxaline-2,3-dione), which decreases EPSP amplitude, can abolish or slow the frequency of spontaneous bursts (Chamberlin *et al.*, 1990). These findings are compatible with the idea that random firing of a few CA3 neurons in high [K$^+$]$_o$ synaptically entrains the pyramidal cell population via recurrent excitatory pathways. Each pyramidal cell connects to about 20 other pyramidal neurons (Miles *et al.*, 1988), and this degree of divergence is important for ensuring the rapid spread of activity out of the small group of activated neurons. The reduced inhibition caused by the depolarizing shift in E_{IPSP} (see above) would be expected to accentuate excitatory coupling among CA3 cells (Miles & Wong, 1987), since individual EPSPs should be more effective in the absence of recurrent inhibitory potentials. The increased rate of EPSPs leading up to each burst could simply reflect increased firing of CA3 pyramidal neurons as they emerge from the AHP of the previous burst.

The critical role of recurrent synaptic excitation for initiation of spontaneous bursts is also supported by a computer simulation of the CA3

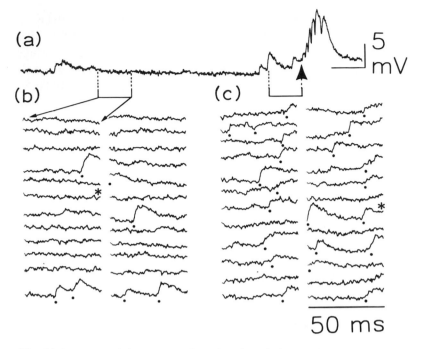

Fig. 14.4. Increased frequency of EPSPs just before a burst. (a) Intracellular recording from a CA3 neuron bathed in 8.5 mM $[K^+]_o$. The dashed vertical lines denote 50 ms intervals 0–50 and 250–300 ms before the PDS onset (arrowhead). Note that action potentials were suppressed by inclusion of QX-314 in the recording electrode, so that only the depolarizing wave underlying the burst appears. (b) For the same cell as in (a) 24 sample traces of 50 ms intervals 250–300 ms before each PDS. (c) For the same cell, 24 traces of intervals 0–50 ms before the PDS. The sweeps marked by asterisks are expansions of segments of the sweep in (a). The small dots mark the foot of each EPSP > 1 mV in amplitude. Notice that more EPSPs were seen in the 0–50 ms intervals (c) than in 250–300 ms intervals before each PDS. The mean interburst interval for this cell was 909 ms. The time calibration in (a) is 50 ms. (From Chamberlin et al., 1990.)

region. This model (Miles et al., 1988) was modified to include four additional features: the absence of intrinsic burst firing, a depolarizing shift in E_K and E_{IPSP}, the existence of spontaneous EPSPs not triggered by a presynaptic action potential, and a steady depolarization of pyramidal cells (Traub & Dingledine, 1990). The model generates spontaneous interictal bursts at intervals of 1.0–1.5 s and, importantly, synchronous bursts are immediately preceded by barrages of EPSPs in individual pyramidal cells. This can be appreciated from Fig. 14.5, in which the population spiking behavior is monitored during the recovery period from

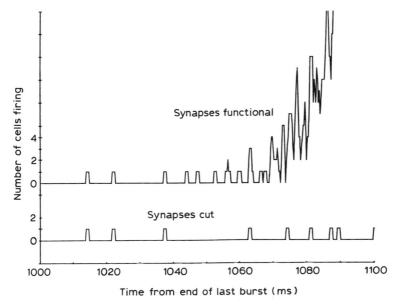

Fig. 14.5. The role of spontaneous EPSPs in the synchronization process in a computer model of the CA3 region bathed in high $[K^+]_o$ is to trigger firing in a very small number of cells. To show this, the number of cells firing in the initial stages of a burst is plotted (upper trace, Synapses functional). The run is then repeated with identical parameters and connectivity; but, just after the previous burst, all synaptic connections were cut (lower trace, Synapses cut). In the lower trace, all cell firing is due to spontaneous EPSPs only. Note that in the lower trace, only one cell at a time fires. The build-up of synchrony (upper trace) therefore results from cooperative interactions, not from wearing off of the AHP or from the bias currents alone. The take-off point in the upper trace is hard to define precisely, but it seems to involve four or fewer cells. Such cells would be hard to find experimentally. (From Traub & Dingledine, 1990.)

the preceding burst under two conditions: (a) recurrent synapses remain intact as usual between bursts, and (b) all excitatory collaterals are severed just after the previous burst terminates. Although the latter manipulation is impossible to carry out experimentally, it demonstrates that, in the computer model, the enhanced cell firing leading up to burst onset is synaptically driven rather than being a result of the declining AHP and steady depolarizing current imposed on the neurons. With synaptic connections cut, the low rate of background firing continues monotonously. With synaptic connections intact, however, as the AHP wears off sporadic firing in a few cells leads explosively to the next population burst.

This computer model is in agreement also with several other observations made in hippocampal slices subjected to elevated $[K^+]_o$. For example, bursts are abolished by a partial block of EPSPs, and burst duration is increased and frequency decreased when fast synaptic inhibition is blocked. Thus, both experimental results and simulations support the idea that recurrent excitatory pathways in CA3 play a major role in initiating synchronous bursts in high $[K^+]_o$, and that spontaneous EPSPs, coupled with a steady pyramidal cell depolarization, can provide the necessary driving force. Furthermore, it seems likely that spontaneous EPSPs are similarly important for initiation of spontaneous bursts in other in-vitro models such as hippocampal slices treated with $GABA_A$ receptor blockers (Miles & Wong, 1986; Chapter 13, this volume) or 4-aminopyridine (Ives & Jefferys, 1990). Once a population of neurons becomes entrained into burst initiation, however, other excitatory processes (e.g., electrical field interactions) assume a major task of further synchronizing the pyramidal cell population into the familiar 'ringing' field burst (Dudek *et al.*, 1986).

Why are seizures restricted to the CA1?

One of the most intriguing aspects of the high-K model is the propensity of the CA1 area to generate spontaneous seizure activity, yet only in the presence of a synchronous synaptic 'drive' from CA3 neurons. Moreover, the CA3 region shows a reluctance to generate seizures, and continues to generate only the brief interictal activity during intense CA1 seizures. Let us consider four possible properties of CA1 that may underlie this area's selective vulnerability to seizure generation.

The extracellular volume fraction

Reductions in extracellular space have a number of excitatory actions. Two experimental observations suggest that the extracellular environment is dynamically involved in seizure initiation in hippocampal slices maintained in high $[K^+]_o$. First, measurements of tissue electrical resistance (usually between two tungsten electrodes placed in the tissue) are dominated by current flow in the extracellular compartment and hence permit an indirect estimation of changes in the extracellular volume (Holsheimer, 1987). Electrical resistance measurements of the hippocampal slice demonstrated that tissue resistance increases in the CA1 stratum pyramidale immediately prior to, and during, seizure activity (Fig. 14.6). The magnitude of tissue resistance increase was small in comparison to that which occurred during spreading depression (Fig. 14.6(b)). Second,

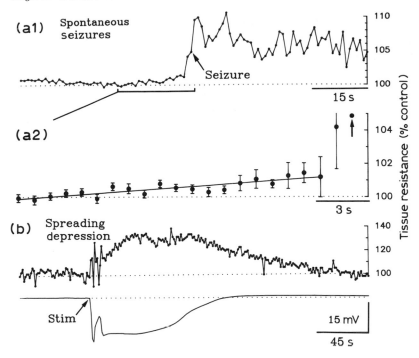

Fig. 14.6. Tissue resistance rises before and during electrographic seizures. (a1) Tissue resistance was sampled at 1 Hz in 12 slices over a total of 286 seizures, and the resulting arrays of measured values were averaged to produce a composite plot. The ordinate represents a percentage of the value 20 s before seizure onset; the arrow indicates the time of seizure occurrence, determined to within ± 1 s. (a2) The expansion of the 20 s period immediately preceding seizure onset illustrates a gradual and significant increase in resistance, suggesting that extracellular space might decrease prior to seizure initiation. The line represents linear regression over these 20 values; s.e.m. is shown as error bars. For comparison, traces in (b) illustrate tissue resistance and field potential measured during spreading depression produced by <1 s orthodromic stimulation (100 Hz; 100 µA; see arrow) in a single slice. Again resistance is referenced to its value 20 s prior to spreading depression onset. Time course of spreading depression is coincident with the negative shift in the DC potential (lower); tissue resistance in this slice (upper) rose to a ceiling of ~130% control. (From Traynelis & Dingledine, 1989a.)

the introduction of media made hyperosmotic by a variety of structurally unrelated carbohydrates (e.g., sucrose, mannitol, dextran) that largely remain restricted to the extracellular space reversibly abolished seizure activity but not CA3 interictal activity; such manipulations also reduced tissue resistance, suggesting that their actions may be linked to the expansion of the extracellular space (Traynelis & Dingledine, 1989a).

Analysis of the diffusion profiles of an iontophoretically introduced impermeant quaternary ammonium ion, measured with a nearby ion-sensitive microelectrode, allows the direct measurement of the extracellular volume fraction (EVF) of the brain slice (Nicholson & Phillips, 1981). With this technique, we have demonstrated that the CA1 stratum pyramidale possesses an exceptionally low EVF compared to all other regions of the hippocampus tested (Fig. 14.7; McBain *et al.*, 1990). CA1 stratum pyramidale exhibited an EVF of 0.12, while the EVF of CA3 and dentate was considerably higher – 0.18 and 0.15, respectively. It is likely that fundamental differences in extracellular space will influence each region's excitability, and also their response to pathological situations such as hypoxia (see below). Interestingly, synchronous activity generated in the absence of synaptic transmission is reminiscent of the tonic-like component of electrographic seizures (Jefferys & Haas, 1982; Taylor & Dudek, 1982; Snow & Dudek, 1984). The relative susceptibility of the three hippocampal subregions (CA1 > dentate gyrus > CA3) is inversely related to their EVF. It is likely that the reduced extracellular space will result in stronger ephaptic interactions in CA1 than in CA3. Furthermore, when $[K^+]_o$ was raised from 3.5 to 8.5 mM we found that the EVF was reversibly reduced by 30% (Fig. 14.7(c)), suggesting that K^+-induced changes in EVF do occur at concentrations of K^+ that are physiologically (and pathologically) relevant. This observation is consistent with both the increase in tissue resistance during seizure activity, and the observed block of seizure initiation by hyperosmotic agents. This K^+-induced reduction in EVF is due presumably to glial cell expansion as well as the possible swelling of neurons (see Dietzel *et al.*, 1989).

One intriguing ramification of the CA1 region's intrinsically low EVF might be a modification of the manner in which the tissue responds to and accommodates hypoxia and ischemia. The restricted EVF of CA1 probably contributes to the greater rate of rise of $[K^+]_o$ observed during hypoxia-induced seizures observed in CA1 compared to CA3 (Kawasaki *et al.*, 1990). In addition, some of the excitatory actions of reduced

Fig. 14.7. Regional variation of extracellular volume fraction. (a) Schematic to show the electrode array and recording sites (filled dots) within the hippocampal slice. Iontophoretic and sensing electrodes were positioned parallel to the cell layer at a depth of 150 μm. (b) Comparison of tetramethyl ammonium (TMA^+) diffusion profiles during a 50 s iontophoretic application of TMA^+, in agar, and in stratum pyramidale of both CA1 and CA3. TMA^+ was applied between 20 and 70 s from the start of the trial. Dots represent the measured extracellular TMA^+, whereas the continuous lines show theoretical curves based on the mean

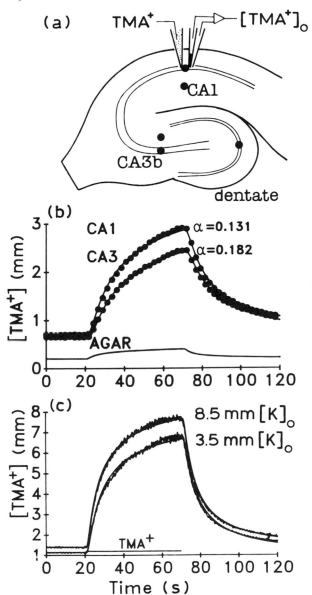

parameters from three trials. The steeper rise and the larger increase for the curve obtained in CA1 indicate a smaller volume fraction in this area. The extracellular volume fraction (α) is shown beside each trace. (c) A comparison of TMA$^+$ diffusion profiles in 3.5 and 8.5 mM [K$^+$]$_o$ demonstrates a 34% reduction within the stratum pyramidale of CA1 (α is reduced from 0.121 to 0.079). The superimposed smoothed curves represent theoretical diffusion curves calculated from the specific parameter obtained from the experiment. (From McBain *et al.*, 1990.)

extracellular volume fraction should compromise the tissue's ability to resist hypoxic damage, by increasing neuronal firing and metabolic demand at the very time when the energy supply is limited. Swelling observed in some isolated glial cell preparations is known to lead to the release of neuroactive substances (e.g., glutamate, aspartate, and taurine) as part of the process of regulatory volume decrease (Gilles, 1987); swollen astrocytes may be an additional source of release for glutamate and aspartate (Kimelberg *et al.*, 1990). Interstitial glutamate is already known to become elevated during experimental ischemia (Benveniste *et al.*, 1984); if tissue swells in response to the elevated $[K^+]$ observed during hypoxia, the concentration of neurotransmitters in the interstitial space could become elevated further. Such rises in the interstitial concentrations of transmitters such as glutamate and glycine could lead to larger tonic activation of NMDA receptors (see e.g., Sah *et al.*, 1989), which could exacerbate hypoxia-mediated neuronal damage. Thus, the combination of an already low EVF and the observed marked response of the CA1 region to an elevation in $[K^+]_o$ can help to explain the historically observed vulnerability of CA1 neurons to cell damage during hypoxia (Kawasaki *et al.*, 1990).

Density of NMDA receptors

The susceptibility of the CA1 region to seizure generation is correlated with the distribution of NMDA receptors. Indeed, on the basis of NMDA displaceable $[^3H]$ glutamate binding, the highest levels of NMDA binding sites within the central nervous system are within the strata radiatum and oriens of the hippocampal CA1 area and the inner portions of the dentate gyrus molecular layer (for a review, see Cotman *et al.*, 1987). It has been estimated that $\sim 80\%$ of the glutamate binding sites in area CA1 represent NMDA receptors (Cotman *et al.*, 1987). Within the rest of the hippocampus moderate levels of NMDA-binding sites are found in the strata oriens and pyramidale of CA3 and the outer molecular layer of the dentate gyrus; the stratum lucidum and dentate hilus have the lowest NMDA receptor density.

NMDA receptors can be activated synaptically via the Schaffer collateral–commissural pathway, since presumably the excitatory transmitters released on to the pyramidal cells bind to both AMPA and NMDA receptors (Forsythe & Westbrook, 1987; Bekkers & Stevens, 1989). The relative contribution of each receptor type to the synchronous burst thus depends on the circuitry engaged and the degree to which the voltage-dependent blockade of the NMDA channel by Mg^{2+} is relieved. Cutting the Schaffer collateral input to the CA1, or perfusion with the NMDA receptor antagonist D-APV, prevents both spontaneous (Traynelis & Dingledine, 1988) and hypoxia-induced seizures in high $[K^+]_o$ (Kawasaki *et al.*, 1990; see also Onodera *et al.*, 1986), implicating NMDA receptor activation in both initiation and maintenance of CA1 seizure activity in high-K and hypoxia-induced seizures. Conversely, the lack of effect of NMDA receptor antagonists on CA3 interictal frequency is consistent with a low NMDA receptor density in this area and the independence of burst initiation on NMDA receptors.

Na^+,K^+-ATPase activity

The CA1 region has a lower Na^+,K^+-ATPase activity than does CA3 (Haglund *et al.*, 1985; Haglund & Schwartzkroin, 1990). Furthermore, throughout development and maturation Na^+,K^+-ATPase activity increases in both regions, but remains consistently higher in the CA3 region. The resistance of the CA3 region to both seizure activity and a similar phenomenon described by Haglund & Schwartzkroin (1990) can possibly be attributed to this region's more effective $[K^+]_o$ regulation, secondary to Na^+,K^+-ATPase and perhaps a larger EVF. The Na–K pump probably plays a more important role in the prevention of seizure initiation (and spreading depression; Haglund & Schwartzkroin, 1990) in the CA3 than the CA1 region. Furthermore, a compromise in the Na–K pump activity could have a larger effect on the presynaptic terminal than on cell bodies. This is because the large surface-to-volume ratio of presynaptic terminals will limit the terminal's ability to buffer increases in $[K^+]_o$, and may contribute to an increased release of neurotransmitter (Haglund & Schwartzkroin, 1990). Possible involvement of Na^+,K^+-ATPase in human epilepsy remains an intriguing possibility, in the light of a decrease in Na^+,K^+-ATPase activity in human epileptic foci (Rapport *et al.*, 1985).

Effects of an elevated pH

It is now established that neuronal activity produces stereotyped alkaline and acid shifts in the brain interstitial space (see Chesler, 1990). Stimulation of the Schaffer collateral pathway in hippocampal slices bathed in 3.0 mM K^+ results, in addition to fast and slow acid changes, in an apparent alkaline shift that can reach 0.2 pH units in the CA1 area (Chesler, 1990;

Carlini & Ransom, 1986). The pH rise in CA1 was up to five times that observed in the dentate gyrus (no measurements were made in CA3) and is consistent with a restricted EVF. These exaggerated CA1 extracellular pH shifts in high K^+ could be particularly relevant to the onset and termination of seizures in area CA1. Indeed, systemic respiratory alkalosis has long been associated with a predisposition to seizure (see Chesler, 1990). In slices of cingulate cortex, extracellular alkalosis can induce epileptiform activity that is blocked by NMDA receptor antagonists (Aram & Lodge, 1987). Perhaps the link between the observed pH shifts and excitability rests with the recently reported proton inhibition of NMDA receptors (Traynelis & Cull-Candy, 1990). NMDA receptor responses on cerebellar granule cells were selectively inhibited by protons with an IC_{50} that is close to physiological pH, implying that NMDA receptors are not fully active under normal conditions.

Selective vulnerability

It seems more than coincidental that so many properties that have excitatory consequences are restricted to CA1 and that historically the CA1 region is recognized to be extremely susceptible to damage in several pathological situations. For example, CA1 cells are particularly susceptible to damage caused by ischemia or hypoxia in humans (Brierly & Graham, 1984) and in rats (Onodera *et al.*, 1986). Likewise recovery from synaptic transmission failure after hypoxia is less complete in CA1 than in the dentate gyrus (Aitken & Schiff, 1986). Sclerosis of the horn of Ammon is a degeneration of pyramidal neurons in most pyramidal subfields after severe epilepsy. The pattern of hippocampal cell loss after seizures is variable, but the CA1 region is always prominently involved, especially when seizures are accompanied by hypoxia (Meldrum *et al.*, 1974; Dam, 1980). It is likely that the factors that predispose the CA1 area to develop seizures are also responsible for the neuropathology often associated with this region.

How well does the high-K model approximate events in situ?

It still remains somewhat unclear which, if any, in-situ seizure states are accurately modeled by high $[K^+]_o$ seizures. In any event, once a seizure is initiated by any means, the rise in $[K^+]_o$ that occurs within seconds would be expected to maintain or prolong the seizure. In this sense consideration of the multiple excitatory feedback loops set up by a rise in

$[K^+]_o$ contributes to our understanding of events that occur during seizures.

A clear rise in $[K^+]_o$ can be recorded just before seizure onset in a variety of in-vitro models, including low $[Ca^{2+}]_o$ (Yaari *et al.*, 1986), hypoxia (Kawasaki *et al.*, 1990) and 4-aminopyridine (Perreault & Avoli, 1989); in addition, spontaneous seizure-like activity occurs in neocortical and hippocampal slices from neonatal rats bathed in $GABA_A$ antagonists when $[K^+]_o$ is 5.0–6.25 mM (Swann & Brady, 1984; Hablitz, 1987). Furthermore, intraventricular injection of potassium triggers seizures in unrestrained cats (Feldberg & Sherwood, 1957). Indeed, the threshold $[K^+]_o$ for hippocampal seizures in situ was calculated to be between 5.4 and 8.1 mM (Zuckermann & Glaser, 1968), very similar to that which causes electrographic seizures in rat hippocampal slices, but higher than the 'normal' range within which $[K^+]_o$ fluctuates. The excitatory effects of increased $[K^+]_o$ are intensified, however, by a slight fall in $[Ca^{2+}]_o$ (Yaari *et al.*, 1986; Traynelis & Dingledine, 1989*b*), which suggests that a moderate increase in $[K^+]_o$ accompanying interictal spikes in situ might be sufficient to trigger seizures if the concentration of divalent cations were reduced simultaneously.

Whether a rise in $[K^+]_o$ presages or only follows seizure onset in situ has been difficult to determine. Stimulus-evoked seizures in rat hippocampi are preceded by a rise in $[K^+]_o$ to about 8 mM (Somjen & Giacchino, 1985), but earlier attempts to demonstrate a rise in $[K^+]_o$ leading up to spontaneous seizures in other in-situ models have failed (see e.g., Moody *et al.*, 1974; Fisher *et al.*, 1976). One obvious difference between in-situ models and the high $[K^+]_o$ model is that the baseline $[K^+]_o$ in situ in the interictal periods is not noticeably elevated by treatments (e.g., application of GABA receptor blockers) that induce periodic seizures. Although it remains possible that seizures are precipitated in all models by local elevations in $[K^+]_o$, which could go unnoticed if the K^+-sensing electrode were not precisely positioned (cf. Somjen & Giacchino, 1985), a convincing temporal link between high $[K^+]_o$ seizures in vitro and events during spontaneous tonic–clonic seizures in most acute models of epilepsy has not been demonstrated.

Two pathological situations deserve attention as the more likely in-situ analogues of high $[K^+]_o$ seizures, namely status epilepticus and hypoxic seizures. During status epilepticus, seizures occur at intervals of as short as several minutes, similar to the observed frequency in hippocampal slices (Traynelis & Dingledine, 1988). Moreover, the repeated seizure episodes in status epilepticus would be expected to elevate the interstitial $[K^+]_o$

and perhaps decrease $[Ca^{2+}]_o$, both of which would make the tissue more prone to seizure. Seizures that occur during the onset of, or recovery from, hypoxia (Solomon *et al.*, 1983) may also be caused by the gradual rise in $[K^+]_o$ known to occur in brain tissue subjected to ischemia or hypoxia (Hansen, 1977). Indeed, brief bouts of hypoxia (5–60 s) can trigger electrographic seizures with typical tonic and clonic components in the CA1 region of hippocampal slices perfused with 8.5 mM $[K^+]_o$ (Kawasaki *et al.*, 1990).

Unresolved issues

The high-K model has been fruitful in permitting the study of the interictal to ictal transition and in defining those changes that lead up to spontaneous seizures. However, several important issues remain unanswered.

(1) Do the rises in $[K^+]_o$ described here occur in situ in other animal models?

(2) Is there a single event that precipitates the cascade of events known to underlie seizure activity? This can be answered only by better temporal resolution of those mechanisms involved.

(3) Which of the many consequences of an increase in $[K^+]_o$ are most critical for seizure activity? Figure 14.8 incorporates a number of the effects of increased $[K^+]_o$ into a scheme to emphasize the positive feedback mechanisms that can lead to further elevations of $[K^+]_o$ and increases in neuronal excitability and eventually to seizure initiation.

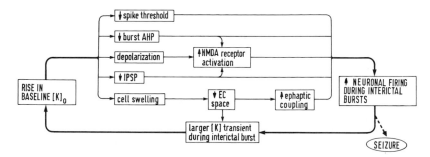

Fig. 14.8. Proposed positive feedback scheme for the initiation of electrographic seizures in CA1. This scheme illustrates possible events occurring in the CA1 region given CA3 interictal input of constant frequency and intensity. With each cycle, $[K^+]_o$ rises incrementally and bursts in CA1 become more intense, until a threshold level of excitation enables the next burst to recruit a sufficient number of neurons to become the leading edge of the tonic phase of the seizure. Boxes connected with arrows show postulated causal relationships among a number of consequences of elevating $[K^+]_o$. (From Traynelis & Dingledine, 1988.)

(4) What consequences of glial cell swelling are involved in seizure initiation and do these mechanisms extend to the neuronal population, causing neurons to swell?

(5) Which of the differences between CA1 and CA3 are most critical for the precipitation of seizure activity?

(6) What mechanisms govern the appearance and removal of K^+ in the extracellular environment?

(7) What cellular properties are responsible for the duration and the ultimate termination of seizure activity?

Such information will need ultimately to be viewed in the light of the microscopic environment of the neurons, which will include not only information describing the distribution of glial processes and K^+ pumps and channels, but also a quantitative description of the extracellular space (e.g., McBain *et al.*, 1990). In this manner a clearer picture should emerge concerning the relationship between $[K^+]_o$ and its clearance, and the initiation, maintenance and termination of epileptiform activity. Future work to address these issues should advance understanding of the causes of seizures.

References

Aitken, P. G. & Schiff, S. J. (1986). Selective neuronal vulnerability to hypoxia *in vitro. Neuroscience Letters*, **67**: 92–6.

Alger, B. E., McCarren, M. & Fisher, R. S. (1983). On the possibility of simultaneously recording from two cells with a single microelectrode in the hippocampal slice. *Brain Research*, **270**: 137–41.

Alger, B. E. & Nicoll, R. A. (1983). Ammonia does not selectively block IPSPs in rat hippocampal pyramidal cells. *Journal of Neurophysiology*, **49**: 1381–91.

Alger, B. E. & Williamson, A. (1988). A transient calcium-dependent potassium component of the epileptiform burst after-hyperpolarization in rat hippocampus. *Journal of Physiology*, **399**: 191–205.

Aram, J. A. & Lodge, D. (1987). Epileptiform activity induced by alkalosis in rat neocortical slices: block by antagonists of N-methyl-D-aspartate. *Neuroscience Letters*, **83**: 345–50.

Ayala, G. F., Dichter, M., Gummit, R. J., Matsumoto, H. & Spencer, W. A. (1973). Genesis of epileptic interictal spikes. New knowledge of cortical feedback systems suggests a neurophysiological explanation of brief paroxysms. *Brain Research*, **52**: 1–17.

Ballanyi, K., Grafe, K. B. & ten Bruggencate, G. (1987). Ion activities and potassium uptake mechanisms of glial cells in guinea-pig olfactory cortex slices. *Journal of Physiology*, **382**: 159–74.

Bekkers, J. M. & Stevens, C. F. (1989). NMDA and non-NMDA receptors are co-localized at individual excitatory synapses in cultured rat hippocampus. *Nature*, **341**: 230–3.

Benveniste, H., Drejer, J., Schousboe, A. & Diemer, N. H. (1984). Elevation of the extracellular concentrations of glutamate and aspartate in rat hippocampus during transient cerebral ischemia monitored by intracerebral microdialysis. *Journal of Neurochemistry*, **43**: 1369–74.

Bilkey, D. K. & Schwartzkroin, P. A. (1990). Variation in electrophysiology and morphology of hippocampal CA3 pyramidal cells. *Brain Research*, **514**: 77–83.

Bourke, R. S. & Nelson, K. M. (1972). Further studies on the K^+-dependent swelling of primate cerebral cortex *in vivo*: the enzymatic basis of the K^+-dependent transport of chloride. *Journal of Neurochemistry*, **19**: 663–85.

Brierly, J. B. & Graham, D. I. (1984). Hypoxia and vascular disorders of the central nervous system. In *Greenfield's Neuropathology*, ed. J. H. Adams, J. A. N. Corsellis & L. W. Duchen, pp. 125–209. New York: Wiley.

Brown, T. H., Wong, R. K. S. & Prince, D. A. (1979). Spontaneous miniature synaptic potentials in hippocampal neurones. *Brain Research*, **175**: 194–9.

Carlini, W. G. & Ransom, B. R. (1986). Regional variation in stimulated extracellular pH transients in the mammalian CNS. *Society for Neuroscience Abstracts*, **12**: 452.

Chamberlin, N. L. & Dingledine, R. (1988). GABAergic inhibition and the induction of spontaneous epileptiform activity by low chloride and high potassium in the hippocampal slice. *Brain Research*, **445**: 12–18.

Chamberlin, N. L., Traub, R. D. & Dingledine, R. (1990). Role of epsps in initiation of spontaneous synchronized burst-firing in rat hippocampal neurons bathed in high potassium. *Journal of Neurophysiology*, **64**: 1000–8.

Chesler, M. (1990). The regulation and modulation of pH in the nervous system. *Progress in Neurobiology*, **34**: 401–27.

Christian, E. P. & Dudek, F. E. (1988). Electrophysiological evidence from glutamate microapplications for local excitatory circuits in the CA1 area of rat hippocampal slices. *Journal of Neurophysiology*, **59**: 110–23.

Cotman, C. W., Monaghan, D. T., Ottersen, O. P. & Storm-Mathisen, J. (1987). Anatomical organization of excitatory amino acid receptors and their pathways. *Trends in Neurosciences*, **10**: 273–80.

Dam, A. M. (1980). Epilepsy and neuronal loss in the hippocampus. *Epilepsia*, **21**: 617–29.

Dichter, M. A., Herman, C. J. & Selzer, M. (1972). Silent cells during interictal discharges and seizures in hippocampal penicillin foci. Evidence for the role of extracellular K^+ in the transition from the interictal state to seizures. *Brain Research*, **48**: 173–83.

Dietzel, I., Heinemann, U. & Lux, H. D. (1989). Relations between slow extracellular potential changes, glial potassium buffering, and electrolyte and cellular volume changes during neuronal hyperactivity in cat brain. *Glia*, **2**: 25–44.

Dudek, F. E., Snow, R. W. & Taylor, C. P. (1986). Role of electrical interactions in synchronization of epileptiform bursts. In *Advances in Neurology*, vol. 44, ed. A. V. Delgado-Escueta, A. A. Ward Jr, D. M. Woodbury & R. J. Porter, pp. 593–617. New York: Raven Press.

Feldberg, W. & Sherwood, S. L. (1957). Effects of Ca^{2+} and K^+ injected into the cerebral ventricle of the cat. *Journal of Physiology*, **139**: 408–16.

Fertziger, A. P. & Ranck, J. B., Jr (1970). Potassium accumulation in interstitial space during epileptiform seizures. *Experimental Neurology*, **26**: 571–85.

Fisher, R. S., Pedley, T. A., Moody, W. J., Jr & Prince, D. A. (1976). The role of extracellular potassium in hippocampal epilepsy. *Archives of Neurology*, **33**: 76–83.

Forsythe, I. & Westbrook, G. L. (1987). Slow excitatory postsynaptic currents mediated by N-methyl-D-aspartate receptors on cultured mouse hippocampal neurones. *Journal of Physiology*, **396**: 515–33.

Gilles, R. (1987). Volume regulation in cells of euryhaline invertebrates. In *Current Topics in Membranes and Transport*, vol. 30, ed. R. Gilles, A. Kleinzeller, & L. Bolis, pp. 205–47. New York: Academic Press.

Green, J. D. (1964). The hippocampus. *Physiological Review*, **44**: 561–608.

Hablitz, J. J. (1987). Spontaneous ictal-like discharges and sustained potential shifts in the developing rat neocortex. *Journal of Neurophysiology*, **58**: 1052–65.

Haglund, M. M. & Schwartzkroin, P. A. (1990). Role of Na–K pump potassium regulation and IPSPs in seizures and spreading depression in immature rabbit hippocampal slices. *Journal of Neurophysiology*, **63**: 225–39.

Haglund, M. M., Stahl, W. L., Kunkel, D. D. & Schwartzkroin, P. A. (1985). Developmental and regional differences in the localization of Na,K-ATPase activity in the rabbit hippocampus. *Brain Research*, **343**: 198–203.

Halliwell, J. V. & Adams, P. R. (1982). Voltage-clamp analysis of muscarinic excitation in hippocampal neurons. *Brain Research*, **250**: 71–92.

Hansen, A. J. (1977). Extracellular potassium concentration in juvenile and adult brain cortex during anoxia. *Acta Physiologica Scandinavica*, **99**: 412–20.

Heinemann, U. & Lux, H. D. (1977). Ceiling of stimulus induced rises in extracellular potassium concentration in the cerebral cortex of cat. *Brain Research*, **120**: 231–49.

Holsheimer, J. (1987). Electrical conductivity of the hippocampal CA1 layers and application to current-source-density analysis. *Experimental Brain Research*, **67**: 402–10.

Hounsgaard, J. & Nicholson, C. (1983). Potassium accumulation around individual Purkinje cells in cerebellar slices from the guinea pig. *Journal of Physiology*, **340**: 359–88.

Ives, A. E. & Jefferys, J. G. R. (1990). Synchronization of epileptiform bursts induced by 4-aminopyridine in the in vitro hippocampal slice preparation. *Neuroscience Letters*, **112**: 239–44.

Jefferys, J. G. R. & Haas, H. L. (1982). Synchronized bursting of CA1 hippocampal pyramidal cells in the absence of synaptic transmission. *Nature*, **300**: 448–50.

Kawasaki, K., Traynelis, S. F. & Dingledine, R. (1990). Different responses of CA1 and CA3 regions to hypoxia in rat hippocampal slice. *Journal of Neurophysiology*, **63**: 385–94.

Kimelberg, H. K. & Frangakis, M. V. (1985). Furosemide- and bumetanide-sensitive ion transport and volume control in primary astrocyte cultures from rat brain. *Brain Research*, **361**: 125–34.

Kimelberg, H. K., Goderie, S. K., Higman, S., Pang, S. & Waniewski, R. A. (1990). Swelling-induced release of glutamate, aspartate and taurine from astrocyte cultures. *Journal of Neuroscience*, **10**: 1583–91.

Knowles, W. D., Traub, R. D. & Strowbridge, B. W. (1987). The initiation and spread of epileptiform bursts in the in vitro hippocampal slice. *Neuroscience*, **21**: 441–55.

Korn, S. J., Giacchino, J. L., Chamberlin, N. L. & Dingledine, R. (1987). Epileptiform burst activity induced by potassium in the hippocampus and its regulation by GABA-mediated inhibition. *Journal of Neurophysiology*, **57**: 325–40.

Lancaster, B. & Adams, P. R. (1986). Calcium-dependent current generating the afterhyperpolarization of hippocampal neurons. *Journal of Neurophysiology*, **55**: 1268–82.

Matsumoto, H. & Ajmone-Marsan, C. (1964*a*). Cortical cellular phenomena in experimental epilepsy: interictal manifestations. *Experimental Neurology*, **9**: 286–304.

Matsumoto, H. & Ajmone-Marsan, C. (1964*b*). Cortical cellular phenomena in experimental epilepsy: ictal manifestations. *Experimental Neurology*, **9**: 305–26.

McBain, C. J., Traynelis, S. F. & Dingledine, R. (1990). Regional variation of extracellular space in hippocampus under physiological and pathological conditions. *Science*, **249**: 674–7.

McBain, C. J. & Dingledine, R. (1992). Dual-component miniature excitatory synaptic currents in rat hippocampal CA3 pyramidal neurons. *Journal of Neurophysiology*, **68**: 16–27.

Meldrum, B. S., Horton, R. W. & Brierly, J. B. (1974). Epileptic brain damage in adolescent baboons following seizures induced by allylglycine. *Brain*, **97**: 407–18.

Miles, R. & Wong, R. K. S. (1986). Excitatory synaptic connections between CA3 neurones in guinea-pig hippocampus. *Journal of Physiology*, **373**: 397–418.

Miles, R. & Wong, R. K. S. (1987). Inhibitory control of local excitatory circuits in the guinea-pig hippocampus. *Journal of Physiology*, **388**: 611–29.

Miles, R., Traub, R. D. & Wong, R. K. S. (1988). Spread of synchronous firing in longitudinal slices from the CA3 region of the hippocampus. *Journal of Neurophysiology*, **60**: 1481–96.

Misgeld, U., Deisz, R. A., Dodt, H. U. & Lux, H. D. (1986). The role of chloride transport in postsynaptic inhibition of hippocampal neurons. *Science*, **232**: 1413–15.

Moody, W. J., Jr, Futamatchi, K. J. & Prince, D. A. (1974). Extracellular potassium activity during epileptogenesis. *Experimental Neurology*, **42**: 248–63.

Newberry, N. R. & Nicoll, R. A. (1984). A bicuculline-resistant inhibitory post-synaptic potential in rat hippocampal pyramidal cells in vitro. *Journal of Physiology*, **348**: 239–54.

Nicholson, C. & Phillips, J. M. (1981). Ion diffusion modified by tortuosity and volume fraction in the extracellular microenvironment of the cat cerebellum. *Journal of Physiology*, **321**: 225–57.

Nowak, L., Bregestovski, P., Ascher, P., Herbet, A. & Prochiantz, A. (1984). Magnesium gates glutamate-activated channels in mouse central neurones. *Nature*, **307**: 462–5.

Onodera, H., Sato, G. & Kogure, K. (1986). Lesions to Schaffer collaterals prevent ischemic death of CA1 pyramidal cells. *Neuroscience Letters*, **68**: 169–74.

Pennefather, P., Lancaster, B., Adams, P. R. & Nicoll, R. A. (1985). Two distinct Ca-dependent K currents in bullfrog sympathetic ganglion cells. *Proceedings of the National Academy of Sciences, USA*, **82**: 3040–4.

Perreault, P. & Avoli, M. (1989). Effects of low concentrations of 4-aminopyridine on CA1 pyramidal cells of the hippocampus. *Journal of Neurophysiology*, **61**: 953–70.

Ransom, B. R., Yamate, C. L. & Conners, B. W. (1985). Activity-dependent shrinkage of extracellular space in rat optic nerve: a developmental study. *Journal of Neuroscience*, **5**: 532–5.

Rapport, R. L., Harris, A. B., Friel, P. N. & Ojemann, G. A. (1985). Human epileptic brain Na⁺,K⁺-ATPase activity and phenytoin concentration. *Archives of Neurology*, **32**: 549–55.

Rutecki, P. A., Lebeda, F. J. & Johnston, D. (1985). Epileptiform activity induced by changes in extracellular potassium in the hippocampus. *Journal of Neurophysiology*, **57**: 1911–1924.

Sah, P., Hestrin, S. & Nicoll, R. A. (1989). Tonic activation of NMDA receptors by ambient glycine enhances excitability of neurons. *Science*, **246**: 815–18.

Snow, R. W. & Dudek, F. E. (1984). Synchronous epileptiform bursts without chemical synaptic transmission in CA2 and CA3 and dentate areas of the hippocampus. *Brain Research*, **298**: 382–5.

Solomon, G. E., Kutt, H. & Plum, F. (1983). *Clinical Management of Seizures*. Philadelphia, PA: Saunders.

Somjen, G. G. & Giacchino, J. L. (1985). Potassium and calcium concentrations in the interstitial fluid of the hippocampal formation during paroxysmal responses. *Journal of Neurophysiology*, **53**: 1079–97.

Storm, J. F. (1987). Action potential repolarization and a fast afterhyperpolarization in rat hippocampal pyramidal cells. *Journal of Physiology*, **385**: 733–59.

Swann, J. W. & Brady, R. J. (1984). Penicillin-induced epileptogenesis in immature rat CA3 hippocampal pyramidal cells. *Developmental Brain Research*, **12**: 243–54.

Taylor, C. P. & Dudek, F. E. (1982). Synchronous neural afterdischarges in rat hippocampal slices without active chemical synapses. *Science*, **218**: 810–12.

Traub, R. D. & Dingledine, R. (1990). Model of synchronized epileptiform bursts induced by high potassium in the CA3 region of the rat hippocampal slice: role of spontaneous epsps in initiation. *Journal of Neurophysiology*, **64**: 1009–18.

Traynelis, S. F. & Cull-Candy, S. G. (1990). Proton inhibition of N-methyl-D-aspartate receptors in cerebellar neurons. *Nature*, **345**: 347–50.

Traynelis, S. F. & Dingledine, R. (1988). Potassium-induced spontaneous electrographic seizures in the rat hippocampal slice. *Journal of Neurophysiology*, **59**: 259–76.

Traynelis, S. F. & Dingledine, R. (1989a). Role of extracellular space in hyperosmotic suppression of potassium-induced electrographic seizures. *Journal of Neurophysiology*, **61**: 927–38.

Traynelis, S. F. & Dingledine, R. (1989b). Modification of potassium-induced interictal bursts and electrographic seizures by divalent cations. *Neuroscience Letters*, **98**: 194–9.

Walz, W. (1989). Role of glial cells in the regulation of the brain ion microenvironment. *Progress in Neurobiology*, **33**: 309–33.

Walz, W. & Mukerji, S. (1988). KCl movements during potassium-induced cytotoxic swelling of cultured astrocytes. *Experimental Neurology*, **99**: 17–29.

Wong, R. K. S., Prince, D. A. & Bausbaum, A. L. (1979). Intradendritic recordings from hippocampal neurones. *Proceedings of the National Academy of Sciences, USA*, **76**: 986–90.

Yaari, Y., Konnerth, A. & Heinemann, U. (1986). Nonsynaptic epileptogenesis in the mammalian hippocampus in vitro. II. Role of extracellular potassium. *Journal of Neurophysiology*, **56**: 424–38.

Zuckermann, E. C. & Glaser, G. H. (1968). Hippocampal epileptic activity induced by localized ventricular perfusion with high-potassium cerebrospinal fluid. *Experimental Neurology*, **20**: 87–110.

15

Anti-epileptic effects of organic calcium channel blockers in animal experiments

ERWIN-JOSEF SPECKMANN and JÖRG WALDEN

Introduction

This chapter describes the anti-epileptic effects of calcium channel blockade. The first sections deal with the underlying hypothesis and the experimental animal epilepsy models. Further sections describe the anti-epileptic effects of organic calcium channel blockers in single neurons and in neuronal populations. The last section is devoted to control experiments showing the failure of effects of calcium channel blockers on non-epileptic neuronal activity.

The calcium mechanism underlying epileptic discharges

There are many observations that indicate that calcium ions are essentially involved in the generation of epileptic activity in the central nervous system (for reference, see Lux & Heinemann, 1983; Heinemann et al., 1986; Speckmann et al., 1986). At the level of single neurons, epileptic activity consists of a steep depolarization giving rise to a burst of action potentials, a plateau-like diminution of the membrane potential, and a steep repolarization that turns eventually into an afterdepolarization or an afterhyperpolarization (cf. Figs. 15.1–15.5)). This sequence of membrane potential changes has been described by Goldensohn & Purpura (1963), and called the paroxysmal depolarization shift (PDS) by Matsumoto & Ajmone Marsan (1964a,b).

Some landmarks leading to the 'calcium concept' of epileptic neuronal discharges are described in the following. First, the concentration of calcium ions in the extracellular space is diminished during seizure activity (Fig. 15.1(a); Heinemann et al., 1977; Caspers et al., 1980; Heinemann & Louvel, 1983). Second, the extracellular calcium concentration decreases steeply with the commencement of paroxysmal depolarization and then

462

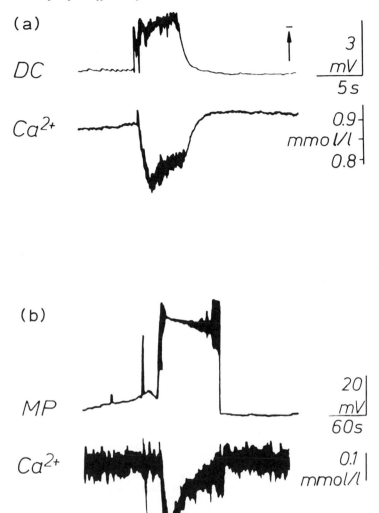

Fig. 15.1. Decrease of the concentration of calcium ions in the extraneuronal micromilieu during epileptic activity. (a) Negative shift of the epicortical DC potential and simultaneous decrease of the extracellular calcium concentration, in anesthetized, artificially ventilated rat motorcortex. Epileptic activity induced by systemic administration of pentylenetetrazol. (b) Paroxysmal depolarization shift (membrane potential, MP) and simultaneous decrease of the extracellular calcium concentration at the outer surface of a single neuron (*Helix pomatia*, buccal ganglion, neuron B3). MP shifts elicited by systemic administration of pentylenetetrazol. (Experiments in collaboration with U. Altrup, D. Bingmann, A. Lehmenkühler & A. Lücke.)

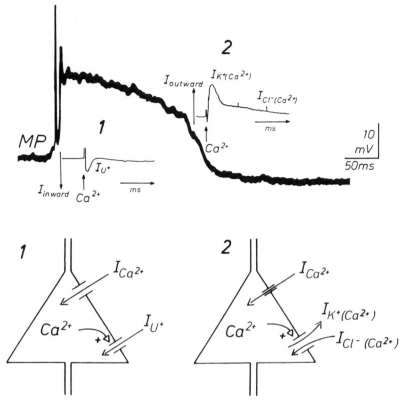

Fig. 15.2. Conceptual outline of the role played by calcium ions in the generation of epileptic discharges. Upper part: Typical paroxysmal depolarization shift. Insets: Transmembranous ion currents induced by intracellular injection of calcium ions into *Helix pomatia*, buccal ganglion, neuron B3. (1) Holding potential (V_h) = -50 mV; calcium ions elicit an inward current. (2) $V_h = -15$ mV; calcium ions elicit two outward currents. Lower part: Flow chart of opening of membrane channels (in relation to upper part). Due to an influx of calcium ions ($I_{Ca^{2+}}$) and to a calcium-induced non-specific inward current of cations (I_{U^+}) the neuron is depolarized (1). The repolarization of the neuron (2) is elicited by a calcium-dependent potassium current ($I_{K^+(Ca^{2+})}$) and a calcium-dependent chloride current ($I_{Cl^-(Ca^{2+})}$). (Experiments in collaboration with U. Altrup, D. Bingmann, A. Lehmenkühler & A. Lücke.)

increases as the paroxysmal depolarization reaches its plateau level (Fig. 15.1(b); Lücke *et al.*, 1990). Third, intracellular injection of calcium ions leads to an inward current when the membrane potential is relatively negative (Fig. 15.2(1)) and to a sequence of outward currents when the membrane potential is relatively positive (Fig. 15.2(2)). The calcium-dependent currents represent a specific cation current triggered at negative membrane potential (Colquhoun *et al.*, 1981; Yellen, 1982; Kramer & Zucker, 1985; Swandulla & Lux, 1985; Walden *et al.*, 1987) and a potassium and chloride current triggered at more positive potentials (Meech, 1974; Gorman & Hermann, 1979; Walden & Speckmann, 1981; Walden *et al.*, 1988; Müller *et al.*, 1989*b*).

From the above-mentioned results the following hypothesis has been proposed (Speckmann, 1986; Speckmann *et al.*, 1989). As shown by the flow chart in Fig. 15.2 the steep depolarization of the neuron is due to an inward calcium current. The transmembranous calcium flux induces a non-specific cation current that supports the neuronal depolarization. The persistence of the plateau-like diminution of the membrane potential is based on the rectifying characteristic of neuronal membrane resistance (Gola, 1974). The repolarization of the membrane potential that terminates the paroxysmal depolarization shift is induced by an outward potassium current and an inward chloride current, both being switched on by the increase in the intracellular calcium concentration. Thus, the first step in the sequence of events is an inward calcium current that leads to an increase in the intracellular calcium concentration and to calcium-dependent ion fluxes. In this context it should be mentioned that, depending (a) on the degree of increase of the intracellular calcium concentration and (b) on the actual membrane potential, a cation influx predominates in the negative range of the membrane potential and a cation efflux and an anion influx in the positive potential range.

Taking all observations in the literature concerning the elementary mechanisms of neuronal epileptic discharges together, the hypothesis presented is assumed to pertain to all nerve cells in molluscan, vertebrate, and mammalian nervous systems. There is, as yet, no crucial finding inconsistent with this hypothesis. In detail, however, there may be differences in the cascade of individual processes. Nevertheless, calcium influx seems to be the primary event of the epileptic phenomenon. Whether it represents also the primary cause of abnormality or an epiphenomenon of another abnormality remains obscure (see below).

Experimental animal epilepsy models for testing anti-epileptic calcium antagonism

For testing the anti-epileptic effects of calcium channel blockade, differing in-vivo and in-vitro experimental epilepsy models have been applied.

In the in-vivo investigations partial and generalized tonic–clonic seizure activity was elicited. These experiments were carried out on anesthetized, artificially ventilated rats and cats. Artificial ventilation and anesthesia were controlled by monitoring the cortical DC potential (cf. Speckmann & Caspers, 1969; Caspers *et al.*, 1987). Body temperature was kept constant at 37 °C. The motor and/or somatosensory cortex was exposed and covered by agar–agar dissolved in artificial cerebrospinal fluid (ACSF) or was superfused with thermostabilized ACSF (cf. Fertziger & Ranck, 1970; Meyers, 1972).

EEG and DC potential were recorded from the surface and from different laminae of the cortex (Elger & Speckmann, 1983). The epicortical recordings were performed by means of a glass capillary and laminar recordings by a micropipette. The reference electrode consisted of a Perspex tube placed on the frontal nasal bone. All these electrodes were filled with agar-agar dissolved in ACSF. The membrane potential (MP) of cortical neurons was recorded by microelectrodes filled with potassium methylsulfate or KCl. The electrical signals were amplified by conventional techniques and stored on magnetic tape. Graphical evaluations were performed by hand or with a computer.

Partial seizure activity was elicited by local application of penicillin (Elger & Speckmann, 1980; Speckmann *et al.*, 1983). As shown in Fig. 15.3(a1) this led to the development of single epileptiform potentials in the superficial DC recording. This process was associated with the following changes in neuronal activity in the upper cortical laminae. A few minutes after the penicillin application, slowly rising depolarizations of small amplitudes, followed by steep de- and hyperpolarizations, coincided with developing epileptiform spikes in the surface DC potential. The depolarizations grew in amplitude and thus gave rise to burst activity.

Fig. 15.3. Animal experimental epilepsy models for testing the anti-epileptic effects of organic calcium channel blockers. (a) In-vivo preparations. (1) Motorcortex of anesthetized, artificially ventilated rat. Focal epileptic activity was elicited by local application of penicillin. Development of epileptic spikes in the epicortical DC potential and of paroxysmal depolarization shifts (membrane potential, MP) in a cortical neuron. Time after penicillin application (PEN-Appl.) is indicated. (2) Motorcortex of anesthetized, artificially ventilated cat. Generalized tonic–clonic seizure activity elicited by repeated intraperitoneal injections of pentylenetetrazol (PTZ). Graphic superimposition of changes in the epicortical DC potential and of MP of a cortical neuron. (b) In-vitro recording from a CA3 neuron in a hippocampal slice from guinea pig. Epileptic activity was induced by superfusion of (1) bicuculline and (2) PTZ (seventh application). The MP is recorded by an inkwriter (MP2) and by a storage oscilloscope (MP1). The tracings are related to each other by lines. (c) In-vitro preparation of a single neuron (B3 cell) from buccal ganglion of *Helix pomatia*. Paroxysmal depolarization shifts (MP) were elicited by superfusion of PTZ. (Experiments in collaboration with U. Altrup, D. Bingmann, C. E. Elger, R. W. C. Janzen & H. Straub.)

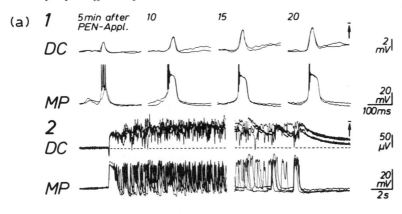

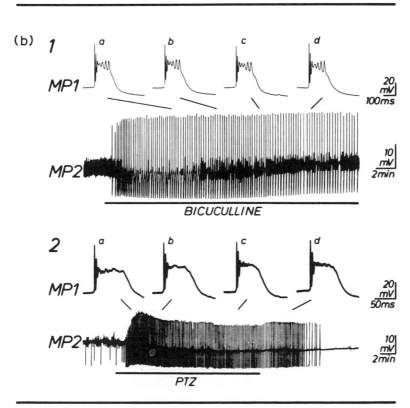

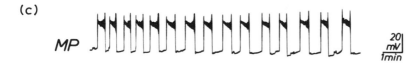

Eventually, they became rectangular and represented typical PDSs. The duration of the PDS then increased until the epileptic focus was fully established (Elger & Speckmann, 1980, 1983; cf. Klee et al., 1982; Speckmann et al., 1986; Wieser et al., 1987).

Generalized tonic–clonic seizures were elicited by repeated administrations of pentylenetetrazol (PTZ; Caspers & Simmich, 1966; Caspers & Speckmann, 1969; Speckmann et al., 1978). The development of recurrent tonic–clonic seizures could be facilitated by single weak electrical stimuli applied to the cortical surface. The effect of PTZ is reflected in characteristic shifts and fluctuations in the cortical DC potential (Caspers et al., 1987). Typical tracings are displayed in Figs. 15.3(a2) and 15.5(b). The first injection of PTZ displaced the DC potential to the negative side of its initial value (Fig. 15.6(b2). Single and sometimes grouped EEG spikes occurred with this negative DC shift. Negative deviations of the DC potential were observed also following the second and third PTZ injections. They were as a rule smaller than the first one (Fig. 15.6(b2)). With repeated injections of PTZ, recurrent convulsions appeared that represented typical tonic–clonic seizures. During these events additional negative DC fluctuations occurred (Figs. 15.3(a2) and 15.6(b1)). They were superimposed by the fast waves of the conventional EEG. The bioelectrical potentials allowed a clear distinction between a tonic phase and a clonic phase during a seizure (Fig. 15.3(a2)). The fluctuations of the cortical DC potential were associated with a series of typical neuronal PDSs (Fig. 15.3(a2); cf. Speckmann, 1986).

Negative DC shifts comparable to those after the first administrations of PTZ occur during arousal reactions accompanied by orienting motor activity (Caspers & Schulze, 1959), during direct electrical and sensory stimulation (cf. O'Leary & Goldring, 1964; cf. Goldring, 1974), and during application of excitatory amino acids (Hamon & Heinemann, 1986; Walden et al., 1989). From these observations, the negative DC displacement after PTZ administration is interpreted as being due to an increase in mean cortical activity level (Caspers et al., 1987).

In the in-vitro investigations epileptic activity was elicited by superfusion of PTZ or bicuculline in organotypic neocortical tissue cultures, hippocampal slice preparations, and in snail buccal ganglia. Neocortical organotypic tissue cultures were prepared from 6 day old rats. The excised tissue was positioned on plastic grids in Petri dishes and superfused by a defined nutrient medium (Romijn et al., 1987, 1988). After three weeks in culture, explants retained their organotypic neuronal and glial arrangement (Romijn et al., 1988). The explants were transferred to a Perspex chamber and positioned on the bottom of optically plane glass through which they could be observed by means of an inverted microscope. The cultures were superfused by a 2 mm deep layer of a 32 °C warm saline solution (Bingmann *et al.*, 1988). Hippocampal slice preparations were taken from guinea pigs. Under ether anesthesia the hippocampus was exposed and transverse slices (*ca* 400 μm thick) were cut. After a preincubation period of 2 h the slices were positioned on the bottom of a recording chamber, which was mounted on an inverted microscope and superfused by a 32 °C warm saline (Bingmann & Speckmann, 1986, 1989). Buccal ganglia were derived from the land snail *Helix pomatia*. They were excised from the animal under ether anesthesia, transferred to a recording chamber, and superfused with a 20 °C warm snail saline solution (Schulze *et al.*, 1975; Altrup, 1987; Altrup *et al.*, 1990).

Organotypic neocortical tissue cultures were superfused by a 5 mmol/l PTZ saline medium. After latencies of 2–3 min, PDSs were initiated in all tested neurons. These PDSs occurred typically at a rate of 2–6/min (Bingmann *et al.*, 1988). In hippocampal slice preparations administration of 10 μmol/l bicuculline elicited typical PDSs in all CA3 neurons. The frequency of occurrence of PDS was in the range 2–9/min (Fig. 15.3(b1); Straub *et al.*, 1990a). PDSs could be elicited in this preparation also with repeated exposures to 3–10 mmol/l PTZ (Fig. 15.3(b2)). They developed from spontaneous and typically aperiodic activity (Bingmann & Speckmann, 1986). Periodical paroxysmal hyperpolarizations occurred at first. They were replaced by burst activity and eventually by PDSs, the frequency of occurrence of which was in the range of 8–12/min. In buccal ganglia of *H. pomatia*, PDSs were elicited by superfusion of 40 mmol/l PTZ (Fig. 15.3(c)). The inter-depolarization interval ranged from 0.5 to 6/min (Speckmann & Caspers, 1973, 1978).

Epileptic activity of single neurons: anti-epileptic effects of organic calcium channel blockers

In motor cortex cells in vivo, repeated intracellular injections of the organic calcium channel blocker D890 reduced the amplitude of penicillin-induced PDSs (Fig. 15.4(a)). In a few experiments, the first injection of D890 led to an increase of PDS amplitude; further injections descreased the PDSs in all cases (Witte *et al.*, 1987a,b; Walden *et al.*, 1984). In contrast to the D890 effect, an intracellular injection of the calcium channel agonist BAY K8644 augmented amplitude and afterdepolarization of PDSs (Walden *et al.*, 1986). In organotypic neocortical tissue cultures (Fig.

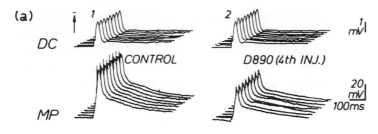

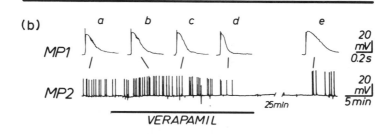

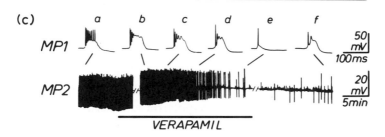

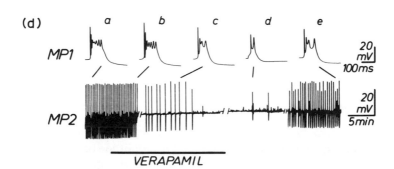

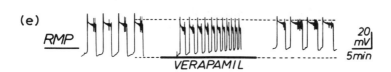

15.4(b)) and in hippocampal slice preparations (Fig. 15.4(c) and (d)), PDSs elicited by PTZ (Fig. 15.4(b) and (c)) and bicuculline (Fig. 15.4(d)) were depressed when the organic calcium channel blocker verapamil was added to the bath fluid (Fig. 15.4(b)–(d); Bingmann & Speckmann, 1989; Bingmann *et al.*, 1988; Straub *et al.*, 1990*b,c*). In buccal ganglia of *H. pomatia*, verapamil added to the superfusate reduced maximal depolarizations and afterhyperpolarizations associated with the PDSs (Fig. 15.4(e); Speckmann *et al.*, 1988).

The results demonstrate that verapamil is able to depress not only PDSs elicited by the epileptogenic agents penicillin and PTZ but also PDSs induced by bicuculline. This shows: (a) that a calcium current is essentially involved in the generation of bicuculline PDSs; and (b) that the generation of a bicuculline PDS is not due only to a block of GABAergic inhibition, since verapamil has been shown to have no effect on normal postsynaptic potentials (Jones & Heinemann, 1987; Bingmann & Speckmann 1989). These interpretations are in line with the observations in the literature that (a) the bicuculline concentration used is not sufficient for complete abolition of inhibitory postsynaptic potentials (Müller *et al.*, 1989*a*) and (b) GABA is assumed to exert calcium channel blocking effects that might be released by its antagonist bicuculline (cf. Deisz & Lux, 1985).

Different anti-epileptic effects of organic calcium channel blockers could be observed in neocortical and archicortical neurons. Thus, both the papaverine derivative verapamil and the piperazine derivative flunarizine were able to suppress epileptic depolarizations in archicortical neurons,

Fig. 15.4. Anti-epileptic effects of organic calcium antagonists demonstrated in single neurons. (a) Motor cortex of anesthetized, artificially ventilated rat. Focal epileptic activity was elicited by local application of penicillin. Simultaneous recordings of epileptic spikes in the epicortical DC potential and of paroxysmal depolarization shifts (membrane potential, MP) in a cortical neuron (1) before and (2) after the fourth intracellular injection (4th INJ.) of the organic calcium channel blocker D890 through the recording microelectrode. (b) Organotypic neocortical tissue culture from newborn rat. Epileptic activity elicited by administration of pentylenetetrazol (PTZ). The MP is recorded by an inkwriter (MP2) and by a storage oscilloscope (MP1). The tracings are related to each other by lines. Superfusion of the organic calcium antagonist verapamil is indicated by the horizontal bar. (c) and (d) CA3 neuron from a hippocampal slice preparation from guinea pig. Epileptic activity was induced by superfusion of PTZ (c) and of bicuculline (d). Recording technique as in (b). Superfusion of verapamil is indicated. (e) B3 neuron from buccal ganglion of *Helix pomatia*. Paroxysmal depolarization shifts elicited by systemic administration of PTZ. Inkwriter tracing. RMP, resting membrane potential (before drug application). Superfusion of verapamil is indicated. Horizontal broken lines are to aid comparison. (Experiments in collaboration with U. Altrup, D. Bingmann, H. Straub & O. W. Witte.)

whereas only verapamil was effective in neocortical neurons (Bingmann et al., 1988). This is evident in the inkwriter recordings of Fig. 15.5(a) and (b). The dihydropyridine derivative nifedipine has been found to depress PDS in neocortical preparations in about 50% of the neurons recorded (Fig. 15.5(c) and (d); Bingmann et al., 1991). Since all cells produced bursts of the same shape and in the same manner, it can be concluded that their calcium channels have different sensitivities to this group of drugs. As the cells in question are otherwise electrically indistinguishable, this may be of special interest.

Focal and generalized tonic–clonic epileptic activity in neuronal populations: anti-epileptic effects of organic calcium channel blockers

In the light of the findings described above, the effects of the organic calcium channel blocker verapamil on focal and generalized tonic–clonic epileptic activity in neuronal populations was studied. This calcium channel blocker of the papaverine group was chosen in our experiments, as the calcium channel blockers of the dihydropyridine and piperazine group may have minor effects on neuronal membranes and exert other effects, e.g., on the cerebral circulatory system.

Verapamil was found to cross the blood–brain barrier to only a small extent (Hamann et al., 1983). Therefore, the drug was administered intracerebroventricularly. With this technique it could be expected that relatively high concentrations of the drug are reached in brain tissue, and that effects on the systemic circulatory system are simultaneously avoided (cf. Speckmann et al., 1990; Walden et al., 1985).

For intracerebroventricular perfusion a stainless steel cannula (concentric configuration; outer diameter 1.05 mm) was inserted into a lateral ventricle according to standard stereotaxic coordinates (cf. Koenig & Klippel, 1973; Paxinos & Watson, 1982). The location of the cannula was controlled after each experiment by injection of dye and/or by cutting the brain. Verapamil was dissolved in ACSF, giving a concentration of 1 or

Fig. 15.5. Presence ((a) and (c)) and failure ((b) and (d)) of an anti-epileptic effect of different calcium antagonists in neocortical neurons. Organotypic neocortical tissue culture from newborn rat. Epileptic activity was elicited by superfusion of pentylenetetrazol. The membrane potential (MP) is recorded by an inkwriter (MP2) and by a storage oscilloscope (MP1). The tracings are related to each other by lines. Superfusion of a calcium antagonist of the papaverine group (verapamil (a)), of the piperazine group (flunarizine (b)) and of the dihydropyridine group (nifedipine, (c) and (d)). Administration of calcium antagonists is indicated by horizontal bars. (Experiments in collaboration with R. Baker, D. Bingmann, J. Ruijter & H. Straub. Modified after Bingmann et al., 1991.)

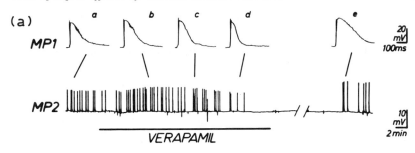

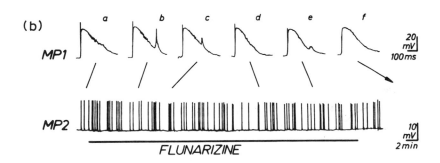

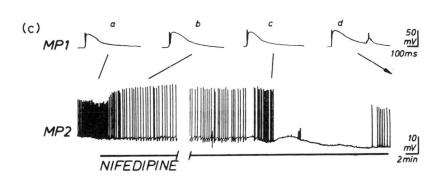

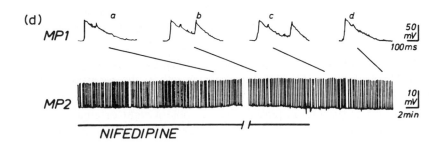

10 mmol/l. The pH of the solution ranged from 6.72 to 7.10. The solutions were perfused continuously (push–pull technique) for 30–90 min, with the final volume circulated being 4–10 ml. From the difference in the drug concentrations of the pushed and pulled solutions, a total uptake of verapamil of between 10 and 40 μmol was determined (gas chromatographic analysis). An occasionally occurring increase in intracranial pressure due to an imbalance in the push–pull system was immediately indicated by a negative shift of the cortical DC potential and by abolition of the conventional EEG (cf. Dill et al., 1979; Walden et al., 1985; Caspers et al., 1987). In these cases the experiments were stopped.

When the epileptic focus was fully developed after topical penicillin application (Fig. 15.3(a1)), verapamil was administered into the lateral ventricle of the focal side. As can be seen in Fig. 15.6(a), verapamil perfusion abolished the epileptic EEG potential at the cortical surface. This holds true also for laminar field potentials. The depression of seizure discharges was sometimes preceded by a transient enhancement. Focal seizure activity reappeared on termination of intracerebroventricular application of verapamil (cf. Walden et al., 1985). Intracerebroventricular perfusion of verapamil did not change the action of the heart in frequency and rhythm. Moreover, the shape of the electrocardiogram did not change with verapamil administration (cf. Walden et al., 1985; Walden & Speckmann, 1988).

When recurrent stereotyped tonic–clonic seizures occurred after intraperitoneal injections of PTZ, verapamil was perfused intracerebroventricularly. During this perfusion the amplitudes of the negative DC fluctuations appearing during tonic–clonic seizures decreased and the interval between the seizures increased. A typical experiment is presented in Fig. 15.6(b1). In about 30% of the experiments tonic–clonic seizure activity ceased within a perfusion time of 15 min, and in about 40% of the experiments seizure intensity, as determined from the negative DC fluctuation, diminished below 10% of its initial value within a perfusion time of 30 min. When tonic–clonic seizure activity was abolished, only single EEG spikes persisted (cf. Fig. 15.6(b1)). In the postperfusion period generalized tonic–clonic seizures reappeared only in some experiments. In all of these cases the seizures were shorter and the amplitude of the accompanying DC shifts was significantly smaller (Walden & Speckmann, 1988). The depression of tonic–clonic seizure activity during intracerebroventricular verapamil perfusion occurred in parallel with a positive displacement of the DC potential. Evaluations of eight original tracings are displayed as mean values in Fig. 15.6(b2). It can be seen that the

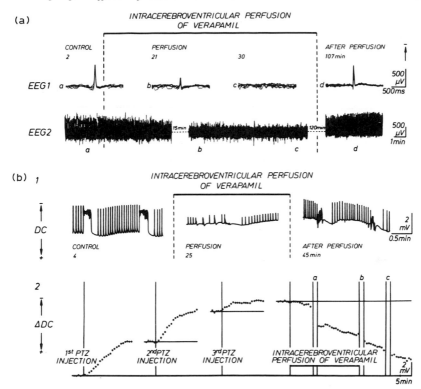

Fig. 15.6. Anti-epileptic effects of organic calcium antagonists demonstrated in neuronal populations with (a) focal and (b) generalized tonic–clonic epileptic activity; anesthetized, artificially ventilated rat. Intracerebroventricular perfusion of verapamil (lateral cerebral ventricle). Time of recordings before and after commencement as well as after termination of perfusion are indicated in minutes. (a) Epileptic activity induced by local application of penicillin. Focal epileptic discharges in the EEG at the motor cortex surface. The potentials are recorded by an inkwriter (EEG2) and by a storage oscilloscope (EEG1). The recordings are related to each other by letters. (b) Generalized tonic–clonic activity elicited by repeated intraperitoneal injections of pentylenetetrazol (PTZ). (b1) DC potential led from the surface of the motor cortex. (b2) Displacements of the epicortical DC potentials (ΔDC) after the first, second and third PTZ injection and during intracerebroventricular perfusion of verapamil. Mean value of eight original tracings. Interruptions of curve: (a) 45 min; (b) and (c) 20 min. (Experiments in collaboration with O. W. Witte.)

positive DC shift was not completely reversed after the end of the perfusion within 60 min. With the positive displacement of the DC potential occurring during the administration of verapamil, the DC potential level recorded before the first administration of PTZ was nearly re-established.

Positive DC shifts comparable to those induced by perfusion of verapamil during an established ictal state appear during transition from wakefulness to sleep (Caspers & Schulze, 1959; cf. Bechtereva, 1974), during application of anesthetic and depressive neurotropic drugs (Caspers *et al.*, 1963), during hypercapnia (Caspers & Speckmann, 1972, 1974; Speckmann & Caspers, 1974) and during application of inhibitory transmitter substances (Walden *et al.*, 1989). The findings indicate that the positive DC displacements reflect a decrease of the mean cortical activity level (Caspers *et al.*, 1987). Combining the observations described, the positive shift of the DC cortical potential occurring during verapamil perfusion may be interpreted as reflecting a decrease of the mean cortical activity level, which had been elevated by the injections of PTZ before the application of the calcium channel blocker.

Non-epileptic activity of neuronal populations and of single neurons: failure of effects of organic calcium channel blockers

From the investigations in which the drug was administered intracerebro-ventricularly, the following questions arise. First, does the perfusion per se influence epileptic activity? Second, does verapamil exert a general depressive effect on cortical activity that is not exclusive to seizure discharges? The following series of control experiments was designed to answer these questions.

In a first series of control experiments, ACSF without an organic calcium channel blocker was perfused intracerebroventricularly during fully established focal and generalized tonic–clonic epileptic activity. A typical experiment with focal activity after local penicillin application is presented in Fig. 15.7(a). The rate and duration of perfusion were the same as in the experiments in which verapamil was administered. Under these conditions the perfusion had no significant effect on partial and generalized seizure activity (Walden *et al.*, 1985; Walden & Speckmann, 1988).

In a second series of control experiments, we examined whether the intracerebroventricular perfusion of verapamil exerted an effect on somato-sensory evoked potentials, the power of the spontaneous EEG waves and on the cortical DC potential under non-epileptic conditions. The rate and duration of intracerebroventricular perfusion and the concentration of the calcium channel blocker in the perfusate were the same as in the experiments with seizure activity. From Fig. 15.7(b1) and (b2) it is apparent that the evoked potentials and the power of the EEG waves were either not changed or tended to increase. Figure 15.7(b3) shows

(a)

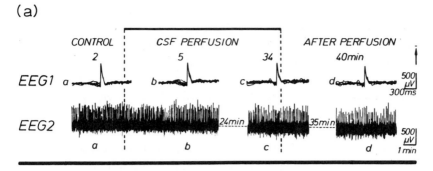

(b)

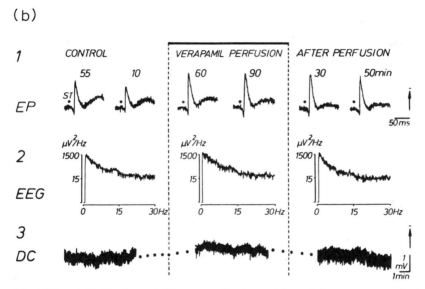

Fig. 15.7. (a) Epileptic and (b) non-epileptic activity of the neocortex during intracerebroventricular perfusion of cerebrospinal fluid (CSF) (a) without and (b) with the organic calcium antagonist verapamil. Perfusion of a lateral ventricle. Times of recordings before and after commencement as well as after termination of perfusion are indicated in minutes. (a) Epileptic activity elicited by local application of penicillin. Focal epileptic discharges in the EEG are at the cortical surface. The potentials are recorded by an inkwriter (EEG2) and by a storage oscilloscope (EEG1). The recordings are related to each other by letters. Perfusion of artificial cerebrospinal fluid (CSF) without an organic calcium antagonist. Duration of perfusion: 35 min. (b) Non-epileptic activity. (1) Somatosensory evoked potentials at the cortical surface (EP). The potentials were elicited by stimulation (ST) of the sciatic nerve. Duration of perfusion: 50 min. (2) Power spectra of the spontaneous EEG at the cortical surface. Analysis time: 2 min. Duration of perfusion: 90 min. (3) DC potential led from the cortical surface. Duration of perfusion: 90 min. (Experiments in collaboration with O. W. Witte.)

moreover that the positive shift of the cortical DC potential occurring in epileptic animals during verapamil perfusion was missing and replaced by a slight negative displacement in some experiments (Walden *et al.,* 1985; Walden & Speckmann, 1988).

Lack of action of calcium channel blockers on non-epileptic activity was also apparent at the level of single neurons. In the in-vivo preparations, the calcium channel blocker D890, a derivative of verapamil, was injected intracellularly together with KCl. The chloride injection shifted the equilibrium potential of the inhibitory postsynaptic potentials (IPSPs) towards the positive. This was used as an indication of a successful intracellular injection. Typical recordings of motorcortical neurons are presented in Fig. 15.8(a) and (b). From Fig. 15.8(a) it can be seen that neither amplitude nor steepness of action potentials were changed with the drug injection, but the recurrent IPSP were reversed in polarity. The failure of the effect of the calcium antagonist on action potentials shows that normal information processing is unaffected (Witte *et al.,* 1987*a,b*). Figure 15.8(b1–3) presents excitatory postsynaptic potentials elicited by a low intensity stimulation of the nucleus ventralis lateralis of the thalamus. In these experiments, Cl^--dependent inhibitory postsynaptic potentials induced by stimulation of the cortical surface alternated with the excitatory postsynaptic potentials (Fig. 15.8(b4–6)). Intracellular injection of D890 together with KCl changed the amplitude of the IPSPs by shifting the chloride equilibrium potential but did not affect the excitatory postsynaptic potentials (EPSPs). In the in-vitro preparations, verapamil was added to the superfusate, which contained no epileptogenic agent. Experiments in which IPSPs and EPSPs were elicited in hippo-campal slices by single electrical stimuli are presented in Fig. 15.8(c1–3) and (c4–6), respectively. As in neocortical neurons in vivo, no significant

Fig. 15.8. Failure of effects of organic calcium antagonists on action potentials and postsynaptic potentials in preparations without epileptic activity. (a) Motor cortex of anesthetized, artificially ventilated rat. Action potentials and their derivative (dU/dt) before (CONTROL) and after intracellular injection (INJ.) of the organic calcium antagonist D890 and KCl by pressure pulses from the recording microelectrode. Ten spontaneously occurring action potentials super-imposed each displayed at two different time scales ((a) and (b)). Depth of neuron: 1300 μm. Resting membrane potential (MP): -65 mV. Immediately following intracellular injection, spontaneously occurring chloride-dependent inhibitory postsynaptic potentials were inverted, indicating a successful intracellular injection. (b) Same preparation as in (a). Excitatory (1–3) and inhibitory (4–6) postsynaptic potentials of a cortical neuron before (CONTROL) and after intracellular injection of the organic calcium antagonist D890 and KCl by pressure pulses from

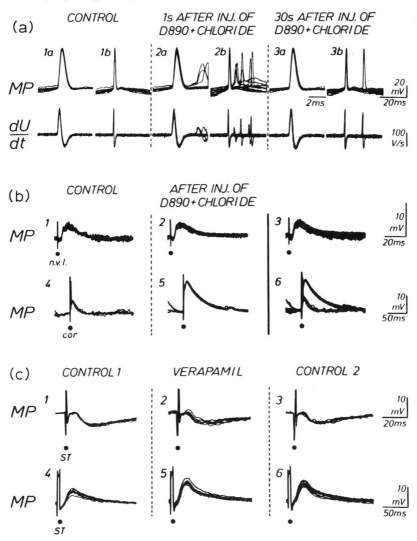

the recording microelectrode. Superimposition of three recordings each (1, 2, 4, 5). Depth of neuron: 1000 μm. MP: −65 mV. Excitatory (1–3) and inhibitory (4–6) potentials were elicited by stimulation of the thalamic nucleus ventralis lateralis (n.v.l.) and of the cortical surface (cor), respectively. The inhibitory postsynaptic potentials (4) are already inverted by a preceding injection of a hyperpolarizing retaining current for D890. (3 and 6) Superimposition of the recordings in 1, 2 and 4, 5, respectively. (c) CA3 neuron (1–3) and CA1 neuron (4–6) from hippocampal slice preparations from guinea pig. Postsynaptic potentials evoked by stimulation (ST) of afferent fibers before (CONTROL 1), during and after (CONTROL 2) exposure of the preparation to the organic calcium antagonist verapamil. Superimposition of six recordings each. (Experiments in collaboration with D. Bingmann and O. W. Witte.)

effect of the organic calcium antagonist on synaptic potentials could be detected.

Interpretations and conclusion

Anti-epileptic calcium channel blockade has been found to exist in all models of epileptogenesis so far tested. Thus, organic calcium channel blockers inhibit epileptic activity induced by: (a) drugs, e.g., pentylene-tetrazol (Bingmann & Speckmann, 1986; Walden & Speckmann, 1988), penicillin (Walden *et al.*, 1985; Witte *et al.*, 1987*a*), etomidate (Altrup *et al.*, 1991), bicuculline (Aicardi & Schwartzkroin, 1990; Straub *et al.*, 1990*b,c*), kainic acid (Paczynski *et al.*, 1990) and cefazolin (Morocutti *et al.*, 1986); (b) electrical stimulation (Ashton & Wauquier, 1979; Meyer *et al.*, 1986*b*); (c) changes in the extracellular ionic environment, e.g., low magnesium epilepsy (Pohl *et al.*, 1992); as well as (d) spontaneously occurring epileptic activity (i.e., occurring without epileptogenic manipulations) (Straub *et al.*, 1990*a*). The anti-epileptic calcium channel blockade was independent of whether ictal or interictal activities were present. The anti-epileptic effect was found: (a) in different animal species, e.g., rabbits, rats, guinea pigs and snails; (b) in different types of neuron, e.g., neocortical and archicortical neurons, and (c) with different preparation techniques, e.g. whole animal preparations (anesthetized and artificially ventilated animals), slice preparations, tissue cultures and isolated cells. It is unclear yet whether the organic calcium antagonists exert more pronounced anti-epileptic effects during the development of epileptic activity or after epileptic activity had already been established. It is also unclear whether the calcium channel blockers act particularly when cells depolarize as would be suggested by the voltage-dependency of their binding.

The anti-epileptic effects exerted by calcium channel blockers point to the fact that transmembranous calcium fluxes play an essential role in the generation of epileptic discharges. What, therefore, is the nature of calcium conductances involved in epileptic activity? In this context it can be speculated that, with epileptogenesis, pre-existing calcium channels may be disinhibited, calcium channels may be newly expressed or ion conductances counteracting the effect of calcium influx may be depressed (O. Pongs, personal communication). It could be claimed, therefore, that there is a change or an abnormality of calcium conductances in those neurons producing epileptic activity. The 'epileptic calcium influx' may represent either the initial and primary cause of epileptic activity and/or a reflection of some other abnormality leading via the epileptic calcium influx to epileptic activity.

On the basis of the hypothesis that a transmembranous calcium flux plays an essential role in epileptic activity, the action of organic calcium channel blockers was tested and found to exert a specific anti-epileptic effect in animal experiments. Considering other observations (Desmedt *et al.*, 1975; Ashton & Wauquier, 1979; Meyer *et al.*, 1986*a,b*; Morocutti *et al.*, 1986; Pockberger *et al.*, 1986; De Sarro *et al.*, 1988; Dolin *et al.*, 1988), the findings presented justify the hope that organic calcium channel blockers might be useful in the treatment of human epilepsies. A prerequisite for that is the development of new drugs that (a) exert their calcium channel blocking effects on neurons of the central nervous system, (b) are able to pass the blood–brain barrier, and (c) have no or only minimal effects on the cardiovascular system. The great advantage of this type of therapy would be that only abnormal activity is suppressed while the normal activity remains unaffected.

References

Aicardi, G. & Schwartzkroin, P. A. (1990). Suppression of epileptiform burst discharges in CA3 neurons of rat hippocampal slices by the organic calcium channel blocker verapamil. *Experimental Brain Research*, **81**: 288–96.

Altrup, U. (1987). Inputs and outputs of giant neurons B1 and B2 in the buccal ganglia of *Helix pomatia*: an electrophysiological and morphological study. *Brain Research*, **414**: 271–84.

Altrup, U., Lehmenkuehler, A., Madeja, M. & Speckmann, E.-J. (1990). Morphology and function of the identified neuron B3 in the buccal ganglia of *Helix pomatia*. *Comparative Biochemistry and Physiology* **97A**: 65–74.

Altrup, U., Lehmenkühler, A. & Speckmann, E.-J. (1991). Effects of the hypnotic drug etomidate in a model nervous system (buccal ganglia, *Helix pomatia*). *Comparative Biochemistry and Physiology* **99C**: 579–87.

Ashton, D. & Wauquier, A. (1979). Behavioral analysis of the effects of 15 anticonvulsants in the amygdaloid kindled rat. *Psychopharmacology*, **65**: 7–13.

Bechtereva, N. P. (1974). DC changes associated with the sleep–wakefulness cycle. In *Handbook of Electroencephalography and Clinical Neurophysiology*, vol. 10, part A, ed.-in-chief A. Remond, pp. 25–32. Amsterdam: Elsevier.

Bingmann, D. & Speckmann, E.-J. (1986). Actions of pentylenetetrazol (PTZ) on CA3 neurons in hippocampal slices of guinea pigs. *Experimental Brain Research*, **64**: 94–104.

Bingmann, D. & Speckmann, E.-J. (1989). Specific suppression of pentylenetetrazol-induced epileptiform discharges in CA3 neurons (hippocampal slice, guinea pig) by the organic calcium antagonists flunarizine and verapamil. *Experimental Brain Research*, **74**: 239–48.

Bingmann, D., Speckmann, E.-J., Baker, R. E., Ruijter, J. & de Jong, B. M. (1988). Differential antiepileptic effects of the organic calcium antagonists verapamil and flunarizine in neurons of organotypic neocortical explants from newborn rats. *Experimental Brain Research*, **72**: 439–42.

Bingmann, D., Speckmann, E.-J., Walden, J., Straub, H., Baker, R. E. & Ruijter, J. (1991). Differential antiepileptic effects of organic calcium antagonists in CA3 neurons of hippocampal slices and in neurons of organotypic neuronal explants. In *Physiology, Pharmacology and Development of Epileptogenic Phenomena*. Experimental Brain Research Series 20, ed. M. R. Klee, H. D. Lux & E.-J. Speckmann, pp. 232–6. Heidelberg: Springer-Verlag.

Caspers, H. & Schulze, H. (1959). Die Veränderungen der corticalen Gleichspannung während der natürlichen Schlaf-Wach-Perioden beim freibeweglichen Tier. *Pflügers Archiv*, **270**: 103–20.

Caspers, H., Schütz, E. & Speckmann, E.-J. (1963). Gleichspannungsänderungen an der Hirnrinde bei Sauerstoffmangel. *Zeitschrift für Biologie*, **114**: 112–26.

Caspers, H. & Simmich, W. (1966). Cortical DC shifts associated with seizure activity. In *Comparative and Cellular Pathophysiology of Epilepsy*, ed. Z. Servit, pp. 151–63. Amsterdam: Excerpta Medica Foundation.

Caspers, H. & Speckmann, E.-J. (1969). DC potential shifts in paroxysmal states. In *Basic Mechanisms of the Epilepsies*, ed. H. H. Jasper, A. A. Ward & A. Pope, pp. 375–95. Boston, MA: Little, Brown.

Caspers, H. & Speckmann, E.-J. (1972). Cerebral pO_2, pCO_2 and pH: changes during convulsive activity and their significance for spontaneous arrest of seizures. *Epilepsia*, **13**: 699–725.

Caspers, H. & Speckmann, E.-J. (1974). Cortical DC shifts associated with changes of gas tensions in blood and tissue. In *Handbook of Electroencephalography and Clinical Neurophysiology*, vol. 10, part A, ed.-in-chief A. Remond, pp. 41–65. Amsterdam: Elsevier.

Caspers, H., Speckmann, E.-J. & Lehmenkuehler, A. (1980). Electrogenesis of cortical DC potentials. In *Motivation, Motor and Sensory Processes of the Brain: Electrical Potentials, Behavior and Clinical Use*. Progress in Brain Research, vol. 54, ed. H. H. Kornhuber & L. Deecke. pp. 3–15. Amsterdam: Elsevier Biomedical Press.

Caspers, H., Speckmann, E.-J. & Lehmenkuehler, A. (1987). DC potentials of the cerebral cortex. Seizure activity and changes in gas pressure. *Reviews of Physiology, Biochemistry and Pharmacology*, **106**: 127–78.

Colquhoun, D., Neher, E., Reuter, H. & Stevens, C. F. (1981). Inward current channels activated by intracellular Ca in cultured cardiac cells. *Nature*, **294**: 752–4.

De Sarro, G. B., Meldrum, B. S. & Nistico, G. (1988). Anticonvulsant effects of some calcium entry blockers in DBA/2 mice. *British Journal of Pharmacology*, **93**: 247–56.

Deisz, R. A. & Lux, H. D. (1985). Gamma-aminobutyric acid-induced depression of calcium currents of chick sensory neurons. *Neuroscience Letters*, **56**: 205–10.

Desmedt, L. K. C., Niemegeers, C. J. E. & Janssen, P. A. J. (1975). Anticonvulsive properties of cimarizine and flunarizine in rats and mice. *Drug Research*, **25**: 1408–13.

Dill, R. C., Romet, J. A. & Porter, R. W. (1979). Suppression of epileptiform activity by increased intracranial pressure in cat. *Experimental Neurology*, **66**: 186–99.

Dolin, S. J., Hunter, A. B., Halsey, M. J. & Little, H. J. (1988). Anticonvulsant profile of the dihydropyridine calcium channel antagonists, nitrendipine and nimodipine. *European Journal of Pharmacology*, **152**: 19–27.

Elger, C. E. & Speckmann, E.-J. (1980). Focal interictal epileptiform discharges (FIED) in the epicortical EEG and their relations to spinal field potentials in the rat. *Electroencephalography and Clinical Neurophysiology*, **48**: 447–60.

Elger, C. E. & Speckmann, E.-J. (1983). Penicillin-induced epileptic foci in the motor cortex: vertical inhibition. *Electroencephalography and Clinical Neurophysiology*, **56**: 604–22.

Fertziger, A. P. & Ranck, J. B. (1970). Potassium accumulation in interstitial space during epileptiform seizures. *Experimental Neurology*, **26**: 741–9.

Gola, M. (1974). Neurones à ondes-salves des mollusques. Variation cycliques lentes des conductances ioniques. *Pflügers Archiv*, **352**: 17–36.

Goldensohn, E. S. & Purpura, D. P. (1963). Intracellular potentials of cortical neurons during focal epileptogenic discharges. *Science*, **139**: 840–2.

Goldring, S. (1974). DC shifts released by direct and afferent stimulation. In *Handbook of Electroencephalography and Clinical Neurophysiology*, vol. 10, part A, ed.-in-chief A. Remond, pp. 12–24. Amsterdam: Elsevier.

Gorman, A. L. F. & Hermann, A. (1979). Internal effects of divalent cations on potassium permeability in molluscan neurones. *Journal of Physiology*, **296**: 393–410.

Hamann, S. R., Todd, G. D. & McAllister, R. G. (1983). The pharmacology of verapamil. V. Tissue distribution of verapamil and norverapamil in rat and dog. *Pharmacology*, **27**: 1–8.

Hamon, B. & Heinemann, U. (1986). Effects of GABA and bicuculline on N-methyl- D-aspartate and quisqualate-induced reductions in extracellular free calcium in area CA1 of the hippocampal slice. *Experimental Brain Research*, **64**: 27–36.

Heinemann, U., Klee, M. R., Neher, E. & Singer, W. (eds.) (1986). Calcium electrogenesis and neuronal functioning. *Experimental Brain Research Supplement*, **14**.

Heinemann, U. & Louvel, J. (1983). Changes in $(Ca^{2+})_o$ and $(K^+)_o$ during repetitive electrical stimulation and during pentetrazol induced seizure activity in the sensorimotor cortex of cats. *Pflügers Archiv*, **398**: 310–17.

Heinemann, U., Lux, H. D. & Gutnick, M. J. (1977). Extracellular free calcium and potassium during paroxysmal activity in cerebral cortex of the cat. *Experimental Brain Research*, **27**: 237–43.

Jones, R. S. G. & Heinemann, U. H. (1987). Differential effects of calcium entry blockers on pre- and postsynaptic influx of calcium in the rat hippocampus in vitro. *Brain Research*, **416**: 257–66.

Klee, M. R., Lux, H.-D. & Speckmann, E.-J. (eds.) (1982) *Physiology and Pharmacology of Epileptogenic Phenomena*. New York: Raven Press.

Koenig, J. F. R. & Klippel, R. A. (1973). *The Rat Brain: A Stereotaxic Atlas of the Forebrain and Lower Parts of the Brain Stem*. Baltimore, MD: Williams & Wilkins.

Kramer, R. H. & Zucker, R. S. (1985). Calcium-dependent inward current in *Aplysia* bursting pace-maker neurones. *Journal of Physiology*, **362**: 107–30.

Lücke, A., Speckmann, E.-J., Altrup, U., Lehmenkühler, A. & Walden, J. (1990). Decrease of free calcium concentration at the outer surface of identified snail neurons during paroxysmal depolarization shifts. *Neuroscience Letters*, **112**: 190–3.

Lux, H. D. & Heinemann, U. (1983). Consequences of calcium-electrogenesis for the generation of paroxysmal depolarization shift. In *Epilepsy and*

Motor System, ed. E.-J. Speckmann & C. E. Elger, pp. 100–19, Munich: Urban & Schwarzenberg.

Matsumoto, H. & Ajmone Marsan, C. (1964*a*). Cortical cellular phenomena in experimental epilepsy: interictal manifestations. *Experimental Neurology*, **9**: 286–304.

Matsumoto, H. & Ajmone Marsan, C. (1964*b*). Cortical cellular phenomena in experimental epilepsy: ictal manifestations. *Experimental Neurology*, **9**: 305–26.

Meech, R. W. (1974). The sensitivity of *Helix aspersa* neurones to injected calcium ions. *Journal of Physiology*, **237**: 259–77.

Meyer, F. B., Anderson, R. E., Sundt, T. M. & Sharbrough, F. W. (1986*a*). Selective central nervous system calcium channel blockers. A new class of anticonvulsant agents. *Mayo Clinic Proceedings*, **61**: 239–47.

Meyer, F. B., Tally, P. W., Anderson, R. E., Sundt, T. M., Yaksh, T. L. & Sharbrough, F. W. (1986*b*). Inhibition of electrically induced seizures by a dihydropyridine calcium channel blocker. *Brain Research*, **384**: 180–3.

Meyers, R. D. (1972). Methods for perfusing different structures of the brain. In *Methods in Psychobiology*, ed. R. D. Meyers, pp. 169–211. New York: Academic Press.

Morocutti, C., Pierelli, F., Sanarelli, L., Stefano, E., Peppe, A. & Mattioli, G. L. (1986). Antiepileptic effects of a calcium antagonist (Nimodipine) on cefazolin-induced epileptogenic foci in rabbits. *Epilepsia*, **27**: 498–503.

Müller, W., Misgeld, U. & Lux, H. D. (1989*a*). Gamma-aminobutyric acid-induced ion movements in the guinea pig hippocampal slice. *Brain Research*, **484**: 184–91.

Müller, T. H., Swandulla, D. & Lux, H. D. (1989*b*). Activation of three types of membrane currents by various divalent cations in identified molluscan pacemaker neurons. *Journal of General Physiology*, **94**: 997–1014.

O'Leary, J. L. & Goldring, S. (1964). D-C potentials of the brain. *Physiological Reviews*, **4**: 91–125.

Paczynski, R. P., Meyer, F. B. & Anderson, R. E. (1990). Effects of the dihydropyridine Ca^{2+} channel antagonist nimodipine on kainic acid-induced limbic seizures. *Epilepsy Research*, **6**: 33–8.

Paxinos, G. & Watson, C. (1982). *The Rat Brain in Stereotaxic Coordinates*. London: Academic Press.

Pockberger, H., Rappelsberger, P. & Petsche, H. (1986). Calcium antagonists and their effects on generation of interictal spikes: a field potential analysis in the neocortex of the rabbit. In *Epilepsy and Calcium*, ed. E.-J. Speckmann, H. Schulze & J. Walden, pp. 357–78. Munich: Urban & Schwarzenberg.

Pohl, M., Straub, H. & Speckmann, E.-J. (1992). Low magnesium-induced epileptiform discharges in guinea pig hippocampal slices: depression by the organic calcium antagonist verapamil. *Brain Research*, **577**: 29–35.

Romijn, H. J., de Jong, B. M. & Ruijter, J. M. (1988). A procedure for culturing rat neocortex explants in a serum-free nutrient medium. *Journal of Neuroscience Methods*, **23**: 75–83.

Romijn, H. J., van Huizen, F. & Wolters, P. S. (1987). Towards an improved serum-free chemically defined medium for longterm culturing of cerebral cortex tissue. *Neuroscience and Biobehavior Reviews*, **8**: 301–34.

Schulze, H., Speckmann, E.-J., Kuhlmann, D. & Caspers, H. (1975). Topography and bioelectrical properties of identifiable neurons in the buccal ganglion of *Helix pomatia*. *Neuroscience Letters*, **1**: 277–81.

Speckmann, E.-J. (1986). *Experimentelle Epilepsieforschung.* Darmstadt: Wissenschaftliche Buchgesellschaft.

Speckmann, E.-J. & Caspers, H. (1969). Verschiebungen des corticalen Bestandpotentials bei Veränderungen der Ventilationsgröße. *Pflügers Archiv,* **310**: 235–50.

Speckmann, E.-J. & Caspers, H. (1973). Paroxysmal depolarization and changes in action potentials induced by pentylenetetrazol in isolated neurons of *Helix pomatia. Epilepsia,* **14**: 397–408.

Speckmann, E.-J. & Caspers, H. (1974). The effects of O_2 and CO_2 tensions in the nervous tissue on neuronal activity and DC potentials. In *Handbook of Electroencephalography and Clinical Neurophysiology,* vol. 10, part A, ed.-in-chief A. Remond, pp. 71–89. Amsterdam: Elsevier.

Speckmann, E.-J. & Caspers, H. (1978). Effects of pentylenetetrazol on isolated snail and mammalian neurons. In *Abnormal Neuronal Discharges,* ed. N. Chalazonitis & M. Boisson, pp. 165–76. New York: Raven Press.

Speckmann, E.-J., Caspers, H. & Janzen, R. W. C. (1978). Laminar distribution of cortical field potentials in relation to neuronal activities during seizure discharges. In *Architectonics of the Cerebral Cortex,* ed. M. A. B. Brazier & H. Petsche, IBRO Monograph Series, vol. 3, pp. 191–209. New York: Raven Press.

Speckmann, E.-J., Elger, C. E. & Lehmenkühler, A. (1983). Penicillin activity in brain tissue: a method for continuous measurements. *Electroencephalography and Clinical Neurophysiology,* **56**: 664–7.

Speckmann, E.-J., Schulze, H. & Walden, J. (eds.) (1986). *Epilepsy and Calcium.* Munich: Urban & Schwarzenberg.

Speckmann, E.-J., Walden, J. & Bingmann, D. (1989). Die funktionelle Bedeutung von Calciumionen bei epileptischen Anfällen. *Drug Research,* **39**: 149–56.

Speckmann, E.-J., Walden, J., Bingmann, D., Lehmenkühler, A. & Altrup, U. (1990). Mechanism underlying generalized tonic–clonic seizures in the rat: functional significance of calcium ions. In *Generalized Epilepsy,* ed. M. Avoli, P. Gloor, G. Kostopoulos & R. Naquet, pp. 344–54. Boston: Birkhäuser.

Speckmann, E.-J., Walden, J., Pockberger, H., Altrup, U. & Bingmann, D. (1988). Action of the organic calcium antagonist verapamil on paroxysmal depolarization shifts of identified neurons of the snail *Helix pomatia. Pflügers Archiv,* **411**: R145.

Straub, H., Baker, R. E., Bingmann, D. & Speckmann, E.-J. (1990*a*). Suppression of spontaneous occurring burst discharges by verapamil in archicortical and neocortical neurons (in vitro). *European Journal of Neuroscience, Supplement* **3**, 124.

Straub, H., Speckmann, E.-J., Bingmann, D. & Walden, J. (1990*b*). Paroxysmal depolarization shifts induced by bicuculline in CA3 neurons of hippocampal slices: suppression by the organic calcium antagonist verapamil. *Neuroscience Letters,* **111**: 99–101.

Straub, H., Baker, R. E., Walden, J., Bingmann, D. & Speckmann, E.-J. (1990*c*) Depressive effects of verapamil on bicuculline-induced epileptic activity in hippocampal and neocortical neurons (in vitro). *European Journal of Neuroscience, Supplement,* **3**: 124.

Swandulla, D. & Lux, H. D. (1985). Activation of a nonspecific cation conductance by intracellular Ca^{2+} elevation in bursting pacemaker neurons of *Helix pomatia. Journal of Neurophysiology,* **54**: 1430–43.

Walden, J., Dietrich, L. H. & Speckmann, E.-J. (1987). A long-lasting inward current induced by intracellular injection of calcium ions in identified neurons of *Helix pomatia*. *Neuroscience Letters*, **76**: 53–7.

Walden, J., Pockberger, H., Speckmann, E.-J. & Petsche, H. (1986). Paroxysmal neuronal depolarizations in the rat motorcortex in vivo: intracellular injection of the calcium agonist BAY K 8644. *Experimental Brain Research*, **64**: 607–9.

Walden, J. & Speckmann, E.-J. (1981). Effects of quinine on membrane potential and membrane currents in identified neurons of *Helix pomatia*. *Neuroscience Letters*, **27**: 139–43.

Walden, J. & Speckmann, E.-J. (1988). Suppression of recurrent generalized tonic–clonic seizure discharges by intracerebroventricular perfusion of a calcium antagonist. *Electroencephalography and Clinical Neurophysiology*, **69**: 353–62.

Walden, J., Speckmann, E.-J. & Bingmann, D. (1989). Augmentation of glutamate responses by GABA in the rat's motorcortex in vivo. *Neuroscience Letters*, **101**: 209–13.

Walden, J., Speckmann, E.-J. & Witte, O. W. (1985). Suppression of focal epileptiform discharges by intraventricular perfusion of a calcium antagonist. *Electroencephalography and Clinical Neurophysiology*, **61**: 299–309.

Walden, J., Speckmann, E.-J. & Witte, O. W. (1988). Membrane currents induced by pentylenetetrazol in identified neurons of *Helix pomatia*. *Brain Research*, **473**: 294–305.

Walden, J., Witte, O. W., Speckmann, E.-J. & Elger, C. E. (1984). Reduction of calcium currents in identified neurons of *Helix pomatia*: Intracellular injection of D890. *Comparative Biochemistry and Physiology*, **77C**: 211–17.

Wieser, H. G., Speckmann, E.-J. & Engel, J. (eds.) (1987). *The Epileptic Focus*. London: John Libbey Eurotext.

Witte, O. W., Speckmann, E.-J. & Walden, J. (1987*a*). Motorcortical epileptic foci in vivo: actions of a calcium channel blocker on paroxysmal neuronal depolarizations. *Electroencephalography and Clinical Neurophysiology*, **66**: 43–55.

Witte, O. W., Walden, J. & Speckmann, E.-J. (1987*b*). Antiepileptic effects of calcium antagonists in animal experiments. In *The Epileptic Focus*, ed. H. G. Wieser, E.-J. Speckmann & J. Engel, pp. 191–205. London: John Libbey Eurotext.

Yellen, G. (1982). Single Ca-activated non-selective cation channels in neuroblastoma. *Nature*, **296**: 357–9.

Recent advances

1 The kindling model of epilepsy

James O. McNamara, Douglas W. Bonhaus, and Cheolsu Shin

Morphologic rearrangements of kindled animals

Identification of neuronal rearrangements in the brain of kindled animals has provided a potential structural explanation for the hyperexcitability of the kindled brain. Sutula and colleagues were the first to demonstrate the sprouting and permanent reorganization of the mossy fiber axons of the dentate granule cells of the hippocampus of kindled animals (Sutula et al., 1988; Cavazos et al., 1991). They subsequently demonstrated a 40% loss of neurons in the dentate hilus of animals in which 30 kindled seizures had been evoked (Cavazos & Sutula, 1990). This latter observation is important for two reasons. It demonstrates that periodic seizures without overt cyanosis are sufficient to induce neuronal loss and at least part of the picture of Ammon's horn sclerosis; this, in turn, suggests that recurrent isolated complex partial seizures, not merely status epilepticus, may be sufficient to kill neurons in humans. It also suggests that part of the mechanism of the mossy fiber sprouting involves a denervation or loss of synaptic input into the inner third of the granule cell dendrites.

The functional consequences of the mossy fiber rearrangements in the kindled brain and in other models remain controversial. Whether the net effect of the synaptic rearrangements is an elevated or reduced seizure threshold has generated intense arguments. Another observation from Sutula et al. (1992) provided circumstantial evidence suggesting that the mossy fiber rearrangement contributes to the hyperexcitability. A single systemic treatment with the limbic convulsant kainic acid produces hippocampal seizures, neuronal death in some of the pyramidal cell fields and the dentate hilus, and mossy fiber sprouting. This treatment is associated with a marked and lasting facilitation of subsequent kindling development. Treatment of additional animals with a single dose of kainic acid and the anticonvulsant phenobarbital, for several days, suppressed seizure activity and protected. The dentate hilar neurons (but not the pyramidal neurons) from death. Mossy fiber sprouting was also markedly attenuated in the phenobarbital-treated animals. Interestingly, animals receiving both kainic acid and phenobarbital did *not* exhibit the expected facilitation of kindling development. Thus, an additional correlation between the presence of mossy fiber sprouting and epileptogenesis was established. A detailed understanding of the synaptic targets of the sprouted axons together with correlative electrophysiological analyses of the synaptic consequences of the rearrangements are required to elucidate the functional significance of this rearrangement.

Enhanced sensitivity of CA3 pyramidal neurons to NMDA agonists

Enhanced sensitivity of hippocampal neurons to synaptically released glutamate provides an attractive explanation for the lowered seizure threshold and enhanced seizure propagation characteristic of kindled animals. Biochemical evidence of a selective and long-lasting enhanced sensitivity of hippocampal neurons to NMDA-evoked depolarization was previously identified in slices isolated from kindled animals (Morrisett *et al.*, 1989). To pinpoint the hippocampal neuronal population exhibiting the enhanced sensitivity, Martin *et al.* (1992) utilized the grease gap preparation in analyses of slices from kindled animals. These authors found a strikingly selective increase in sensitivity to NMDA receptor agonists of CA3, but not CA1, pyramidal neurons. The increased sensitivity was found in the presence or nominal absence of extracellular magnesium; thus a reduction of a γ-aminobutyric acid-mediated inhibition, with resultant partial depolarization of the CA3 neurons, cannot account for this observation. The increased sensitivity was detected in slices isolated from animals either one day or one month after the last seizure. Our unpublished investigations based on previous observations (Yeh *et al.*, 1989) indicate that a molecular correlate of the enhanced sensivitiy to NMDA may have been identified. The intrinsic propensity to exhibit bursting, together with robust recurrent excitatory synapses among CA3 pyramidal cells, explain the striking propensity of these cells to exhibit seizures in the normal hippocampus. The enduring increased sensitivity of CA3 pyramidal cells of the kindled hippocampus to NMDA might enhance their responsiveness to synaptically released glutamate and trigger initiation and/or propagation of a seizure.

References

Cavazos, J., Golarai, G. & Sutula, T. (1991). Mossy fiber synaptic reorganization induced by kindling: time course of development, progression, and permanence. *Journal of Neuroscience*, **11**: 2795–803.

Cavazos, J. & Sutula, T. P. (1990). Progressive neuronal loss induced by kindling: a possible mechanism for mossy fiber synaptic reorganization and hippocampal sclerosis. *Brain Research*, **527**: 1–6.

Martin, D., McNamara, J. O. & Nadler, J. V. (1992). Kindling enhances sensitivity of CA3 hippocampal pyramidal cells to NMDA. *Journal of Neuroscience*, **12**: 1928–35.

Morrisett, R. A., Chow, C., Nadler, J. V. & McNamara, J. O. (1989). Biochemical evidence for enhanced sensitivity to N-methyl-D-aspartate in the hippocampal formation of kindled rats. *Brain Research*, **496**: 25–8.

Sutula, T., Cavazos, J. & Golarai, G. (1992). Alteration of long-lasting structural and functional effects of kainic acid in the hippocampus by brief treatment with phenobarbital. *Journal of Neuroscience*, **12**: 4173–87.

Sutula, T., He, X. X., Cavazos, J. & Scott, G. (1988). Synaptic reorganization in the hippocampus induced by abnormal functional activity. *Science*, **239**: 1147–50.

Yeh, G. C., Bonhaus, D. W., Nadler, J. V. & McNamara, J. O. (1989). N-methyl-D-aspartate receptor plasticity in kindling: quantitative and qualitative alterations in the N-methyl-D-aspartate receptor–channel complex. *Proceedings of the National Academy of Sciences, USA*, **86**: 8157–60.

2 Focal trigger zones and pathways of propagation in seizure generation

Karen Gale

Focally evoked limbic seizures in monkeys

Recent studies (in progress) by K. Gale and M. Dubach at the University of Washington Regional Primate Center have identified a site equivalent to the rat area tempestas (AT) in the monkey. Unilateral focal administration of bicuculline methiodide into this site, located within a restricted region of the rostral piriform cortex, evoked seizures with motor manifestations strikingly similar to human complex partial seizures. These observations indicate that an AT-type of epileptogenic trigger zone exists also in the primate brain and provide strong support for the proposal that limbic motor seizures in rats (facial and forelimb clonus with rearing) are analogous to complex partial seizures in humans.

^{14}C-labeled 2-deoxyglucose (2DG) autoradiography and prolonged limbic seizures in rats

McIntyre *et al.* (1991) studied the regional pattern of 2DG accumulation in brain during amygdala-kindled seizures which were triggered by stimulus parameters that induced long durations of continuous seizure activity (status epilepticus). Unlike typical amygdala-kindled seizures, which occupy a very small percentage ($<5\%$) of the time during which the 2DG uptake occurs, these prolonged seizures ensure that seizure activity occupies the entire period of 2DG uptake. In this condition, highly contrasting regions of marked 2DG accumulation were observed, comparable to that observed with AT-evoked repetitive seizures. It is especially interesting that the pattern evoked by the amygdala-kindled status epilepticus which most closely resembled that evoked by AT-induced seizures was associated with seizures having little or no motor manifestations (i.e., the least severe motor seizure score). In contrast, AT-evoked increases in 2DG uptake were associated with motor seizures of at least moderate severity. Because AT-evoked seizures are intermittent, occupying not more than 10% to 25% of the 2DG uptake period, it would appear that both seizure severity and total time spent in seizure activity interact in determining the degree of 2DG accumulation in specific brain areas.

Lesions of the area tempestas and seizure sensitivity

A study by Wahnschaffe & Löscher (1990) that examined the effect of bilateral neurotoxin-induced lesions of the region containing the AT on seizure susceptibility to systemic bicuculline concluded that the deep prepiriform cortex is not a crucial site of convulsant action of bicuculline. However, these investigators did not verify functionally whether their lesions effectively destroyed the epileptogenic substrate in the prepiriform cortex. As discussed in Chapter 2 (p. 58), following focal lesions directed at AT, intact tissue immediately adjacent to the lesion appears to increase epileptogenic responsivity, thereby restoring the seizure-evoking capacity of the deep prepiriform cortex.

Forebrain–hindbrain seizure interactions in animals with chronic seizures

McCown & Breese (1991) recently demonstrated that under conditions in which repeated electrical stimulation has been applied to the rat inferior colliculus to 'kindle' seizures that come to engage forebrain circuits, focal inhibition of the AT can exert a suppressive effect on these seizures. This is in contrast to the lack of effect of AT inhibition on inferior colliculus-evoked seizures in the non-kindled rat (in the latter the seizures evoked from the inferior colliculus do not induce discharge in the forebrain). These observations provide further support for the proposal (see p. 83) that the chronic recurrence of seizures can modify the extent to which multiple seizure circuits may be engaged by the epileptogenic process. Further they indicate that the extent to which forebrain and hindbrain seizure mechanisms operate in an independent fashion can be modified as a consequence of repeated seizure experience. The observations that repeated audiogenic seizures (daily for 15–20 days) lead to seizures that display electrographic and behavioral concomitants of a forebrain seizure (Marescaux *et al.*, 1987; Naritoku *et al.*, 1992; features that are not observed under acute conditions) further support this notion.

Perirhinal and posterior piriform cortex as crucial relays of seizure propagation evoked from the area tempestas

Recent studies in our laboratory (A. Tortorella, T. Halonen, H. Zrebeet, F. Fornai and K. Gale) have identified the posterior piriform and perirhinal cortex region as being required for the induction of seizures triggered from AT. These regions were selected for study on the basis of their marked increases in c-*fos* mRNA and 2DG accumulation in response to AT-evoked seizures (see pp. 63–70). Inhibition of excitatory amino acid transmission in either of these regions by the unilateral focal application of non-NMDA (*N*-methyl-D-aspartate) receptor antagonists prevents seizures triggered from the ipsilateral AT. Focal application of muscimol is also anticonvulsant in these same regions. In contrast, unilateral inhibition of the adjacent amygdala or the entorhinal cortex did not attenuate seizures evoked from the ipsilateral AT (Halonen *et al.*, 1991; Tortorella *et al.*, 1992).

Anticonvulsant role of serotonergic transmission in the substantia nigra

Because previous studies have indicated that drugs which enhance serotonergic transmission can exert anticonvulsant effects, and in view of the high serotonin content of the substantia nigra (SN), Pasini *et al.* (1992) examined the effect of intranigral fluoxetine on seizures evoked from the AT. Bilateral intranigral fluoxetine produced dose-dependent anticonvulsant effects that were site-specific; unilateral application was ineffective. Moreover, the anticonvulsant action of intranigral fluoxetine was not altered by the blockade of GABA receptors in the SN, indicating that the fluoxetine action was not dependent upon nigral GABA transmission. Subsequently, it was determined that depletion of serotonin prevented the anticonvulsant effect of intranigral fluoxetine. These data indicate a role for endogenous serotonin in the SN in controlling seizure suceptibility and suggest that this action is exerted independently of GABA transmission in the SN. This raises the possibility that changes in nigral serotonin release could compensate for deficiencies in GABA transmission in the SN. If so, this would provide another explanation for why GABA depletion in the SN fails to exert proconvulsant effects in several seizure models (see p. 78).

Area tempestas evoked seizures, seizure-induced brain damage, and trophic factors

There is a large literature documenting the ability of prolonged seizures to cause neuronal injury. In cases in which the stimulation of the brain has been focally applied, the resulting neuronal damage is most evident in the regions that are targets of the stimulated site. Recently, Shimosaka *et al.* (1992) examined neuronal damage following prolonged repeated seizure activity evoked from the AT. To prolong the duration of seizure activity, these investigators reapplied bicuculline to the AT at 30 min intervals over a period of 1 to 3 h while monitoring EEG activity. By calculating the total time spent in continuous high voltage spiking, they were able to correlate this seizure activity with neuronal injury. Only when more than 20 min of total time was spent in high voltage spike trains (after three to six repeated doses of bicuculline in the AT) was there evidence of irreversible necrotic neuronal injury; this injury was located in a restricted region of the posterior piriform cortex ipsilateral to the stimulated AT, and in the mediodorsal thalamus. Increasing the cumulative time spent in high voltage spike trains resulted in greater cell damage in the same regions as well as the appearance of damage in the amygdala and posterior piriform cortex of the contralateral hemisphere. It is interesting that the region of the posterior piriform cortex in which damage was detected corresponds to the region that we have identified as a crucial relay station for AT-evoked seizures (see above).

With seizure activity that is not sufficiently prolonged to induce irreversible neuronal damage, other changes can be detected which may have long-term influences on neuronal survival. Shimosaka *et al.* (1992) observed increases in the expression of the 72 000 M_r heat shock protein (hsp72) in neurons located in the same brain regions in which necrotic injury occurred following AT-evoked seizures. However, as little as 12 min of cumulative time spent in high voltage spike trains was required for increasing the expression of hsp72 in the posterior piriform cortex ipsilateral to the stimulated AT. It therefore appears that increased expression of hsp72 anticipates neuronal injury, perhaps as an adaptive response to the 'stress' of prolonged seizure discharge.

There is evidence that other proteins that serve as trophic factors for neurons also increase their expression in response to non-injurious seizure activity triggered from the AT. Thus, following a single infusion of bicuculline into the AT (which produced recurrent intermittent seizure activity equivalent to approximately 6 min of cumulative time spent in high voltage spike trains), marked increases in mRNA for basic fibroblast growth factor (bFGF) and for nerve growth factor were observed in selected limbic system regions, including posterior piriform cortex and entorhinal cortex (Riva *et al.*, 1992). These increases were maximal by 6 h after seizure induction. Again, it is possible that the increased synthesis of neurotrophic factors may be an adaptive response to compensate for the potentially injurious actions of prolonged seizure discharge. The fact that bFGF is capable of protecting against glutamate-induced neurotoxicity in an in vitro model (Mattson *et al.*, 1989) supports this proposal.

References

Halonen, T., Zrebeet, H. & Gale, K. (1991). Glutamate receptors in piriform cortex regulate susceptibility to seizures evoked from prepiriform cortex. *Society for Neuroscience Abstracts*, **17**: 509.

Marescaux, C., Vergnes, M., Kiesmann, M., Depaulis, A., Michelletti, G. & Warter, J. M. (1987). Kindling of audiogenic seizures in Wistar rats: an EEG study. *Experimental Neurology*, **97**: 160–8.

Mattson, M. P., Murrain, M., Guthrie, P. B. & Kater, S. B. (1989). Fibroblast growth factor and glutamate: opposing roles in the generation and degeneration of hippocampal neuroarchitecture. *Journal of Neuroscience*, **9**: 3728–40.

McCown, T. J. & Breese, G. R. (1991). Seizure interactions between the inferior collicular cortex and the deep prepiriform cortex. *Epilepsy Research*, **8**: 21–9.

McIntyre, D. C., Don, J. C. & Edson, N. (1991). Distribution of ^{14}C-2-deoxyglucose after various forms and durations of status epilepticus induced by stimulation of a kindled amygdala focus in rats. *Epilepsy Research*, **10**: 119–33.

Naritoku, D. K., Mecozzi, L. B., Aiello, M. T. & Faingold, C. L. (1992). Repetition of audiogenic seizures in genetically epilepsy-prone rats induces cortical epileptiform activity and additional seizure behaviors. *Experimental Neurology*, **115**: 317–24.

Pasini, A., Tortorella, A. & Gale, K. (1992). Anticonvulsant effect of intranigral fluoxetine. *Brain Research*, **593**: 287–90.

Riva, M. A., Gale, K. & Mocchetti, I. (1992). Basic fibroblast growth factor mRNA increases in specific brain regions following convulsive seizures. *Molecular Brain Research*, **15**: 311–18.

Shimosaka, S., So, Y. T. & Simon, R. P. (1992). Distribution of HSP72 induction and neuronal death following limbic seizures. *Neuroscience Letters*, **138**: 202–6.

Tortorella, A., Hu, L. & Gale, K. (1992). The role of the perirhinal cortex in limbic motor seizures. *Society for Neuroscience Abstracts*, **18**: 910.

Wahnschaffe, U. & Löscher, W. (1990). Lesions of the deep prepiriform cortex ('area tempestas') in rats do not affect the convulsant action of systemically administered bicuculline. *Neuroscience Letters*, **108**: 161–6.

3 Genetic models of the epilepsies

Phillip C. Jobe, Pravin K. Mishra, Nandor Ludvig, and John W. Dailey

The recent literature on the genetic models of the epilepsies has expanded notably. Additional documentation of the overt characteristics of seizure predisposition in genetically epilepsy prone rats (GEPRs) has been reported by De Sarro & De Sarro (1991), Millan *et al.* (1991), Thompson *et al.* (1991) and Naritoku *et al.* (1992). Vergnes *et al.* (1991) found that the interrelationships between spike-and-wave discharges and certain non-seizure behavioral indices in generally absence epilepsy rats (GAERs) are similar to those of humans with absence seizures. The induction of seizures in different parts of the *quaking* mouse brain was studied by Gioanni *et al.* (1991). Seizures induced by sound and by a benzodiazepine receptor inverse agonist in recombinant congenic mouse strains were studied by Martin *et al.* (1992). Recombinant inbred mouse strains were also used in a study of high pressure seizure susceptibility by Plomin *et al.* (1991). A genetic analysis of audiogenic seizures in DBA/2J and C57BL/6J crosses was reported by Neumann & Collins (1991). Green & Seyfried (1991) compared olfactory bulb kindling rates in DBA/2 and *el* mice with those of non-epileptic inbred strains.

Insights into the electrophysiology of seizure mechanisms continue to accrue. Evans *et al.* (1991) and Pencek *et al.* (1991) have provided new information pertaining to excessive population spike facilitation in CA1 hippocampal slices from GEPRs. Hippocampal excitability in *tottering* mice was evaluated by Helekar & Noebels (1991, 1992) and Kostopoulos & Antoniadis (1991). Hyperexcitability in the dentate gyrus of epileptic gerbils was evaluated by Buckmaster & Schwartzkroin (1992).

Biochemical mechanisms of seizures and of seizure prediposition have been the subject of increasing experimental scrutiny. Postsynaptic noradrenergic deficits as determinants of seizure predisposition in GEPRs have been further documented by Yourick *et al.* (1991). Experiments with intracerebral microdialysis and with other experimental approaches have contributed to a clearer understanding of the role of serotonergic determinants of seizure predisposition and of anticonvulsant drug effectiveness in GEPRs (Dailey *et al.*, 1992*a, b*; Yan *et al.*, 1992). The roles of glutamine synthetase (Carl *et al.*, 1992), adenosine (De Sarro *et al.*, 1991*a*), excitatory amino acids (De Sarro & De Sarro, 1992), Ca^{2+} (De Sarro *et al.*, 1991*b*; Montpied *et al.*, 1991), GABAergic deficiencies (Doretto *et al.*, 1991; Faingold & Boersma Anderson, 1991; Gould *et al.*, 1991; Lasley, 1991) and deficient glucose utilization (Saija *et al.*, 1992) in epileptic mechanisms in GEPRs have also been examined and reported.

New GABAergic studies in the GAER have been undertaken by Snead *et al.* (1992) and Liu *et al.* (1991, 1992). Cerebral metabolic abnormalities (Nehlig *et al.*, 1991) and noradrenergic contributions to absence seizures (Lannes *et al.*, 1991) have also been examined.

Several studies have focused on the biochemistry of seizure processes in genetically epileptic mice. Noradrenergic mechanisms were targeted in an investigation of *tottering* and *stargazer* mice (Qiao & Noebels, 1991). Elevated methionine-enkephalin levels were noted in the *tottering* mouse (Patel *et al.*, 1991). A multiplicity of biochemical factors was examined in the *el* mouse (Mita *et al.*, 1991). Brigande *et al.* (1992) studied gliosis in adult *el* mice. Aspartate release was examined in hippocampal slices of *el* mice by Flavin *et al.* (1991). The roles of synaptosomal amino acid neurotransmitters in seizure mechanisms in the epileptic *Rb* mouse have been investigated by Simier *et al.* (1992). Genetic mapping for epilepsy in the *el* mouse has been reported by Rise *et al.* (1991).

Epileptic gerbils were used to demonstrate the effects of an NMDA receptor antagonist on seizures induced by bilateral carotid occlusion (Marciani *et al.*, 1991). Farias *et al.* (1992) examined the morphology of GABAergic organization in the hippocampus of the epileptic gerbil.

New data have also been obtained using genetically epileptic baboons as experimental subjects. Sakai *et al.* (1991) assessed the effects of an analog of thyrotropin-releasing hormone on photomyoclonus and on cortically kindled seizures.

New insights into the neuroanatomy of seizure predisposition have also been forthcoming. Partial success in obtaining an anti-epileptic effect with intracerebral grafting of locus coeruleus noradrenergic cells in GEPRs was reported by Clough *et al.* (1991). These observations provided evidence that noradrenergic determinants of seizure predisposition in GEPRs may reside in near-ventricular terminal fields. A more refined localization of the noradrenergic determinants of seizure predisposition has been achieved through a combination of biochemical, lesion, and intracerebral microdialysis studies. Accordingly, a growing data base implicates the superior colliculus as a site wherein noradrenergic deficits contribute to forebrain and brainstem seizure predisposition in GEPRs (Jobe *et al.*, 1991, 1992; Mishra *et al.*, 1991; Wang *et al.*, 1992).

In addition to the present review, two other recent reviews on genetic models of the epilepsies have been published. An assessment of convulsive and absence seizure models (Jobe *et al.*, 1991) provides a greater level of detail than the current review. Another recent review targets the genetic models of absence epilepsy with an emphasis on WAG/Rij rats (Coenen *et al.*, 1992). This emphasis on the WAG/Rij strain differs from that of the current review which focuses on the GAER to exemplify concepts pertaining to the genetic models of absence epilepsy.

References

Brigande, J. V., Wieraszko, A., Albert, M. D., Balkema, G. W. & Seyfried, T. N. (1992). Biochemical correlates of epilepsy in the El mouse – analysis of glial fibrillary acidic protein and gangliosides. *Journal of Neurochemistry*, **58**: 752–60.

Buckmaster, P. S. & Schwartzkroin, P. A. (1992). Hyperexcitability of the dentate gyrus in seizure-sensitive mongolian gerbils. *Society for Neuroscience Abstracts*, **18**: 159.

Carl, G. F., Thompson, L. A., Williams, J. T., Wallace, V. C. & Gallagher, B. B. (1992). Comparison of glutamine synthetases from brains of genetically epilepsy prone and genetically epilepsy resistant rats. *Neurochemical Research*, **17**: 1015–19.

Clough, R. W., Browning, R. A., Maring, M. L. & Jobe, P. C. (1991). Intracerebral grafting of fetal dorsal pons in genetically epilepsy-prone rats: effects of audiogenic-induced seizures. *Experimental Neurology*, **112**: 195–9.

Coenen, A. M. L., Drinkenburg, W. H. I. M., Inoue, M. & van Luijtelaar, E. L. J. M. (1992). Genetic models of absence epilepsy, with emphasis on the WAG/Rij strain of rats. *Epilepsy Research*, **12**: 75–86.

Dailey, J. W., Mishra, P. K., Ko, K. H., Penny, J. E. & Jobe, P. C. (1992a). Serotonergic abnormalities in the central nervous system of seizure-naive genetically epilepsy-prone rats. *Life Sciences*, **50**: 319–26.

Dailey, J. W., Yan, Q. S., Mishra, P. K., Burger, R. L. & Jobe, P. C. (1992*b*). Effects of fluoxetine on convulsions and on brain serotonin as detected by microdialysis in genetically epilepsy-prone rats. *Journal of Pharmacology and Experimental Therapeutics*, **260**: 533–40.

De Sarro, A. & De Sarro, G. B. (1991). Responsiveness of genetically epilepsy-prone rats to aminophylline-induced seizures and interactions with quinolone. *Neuropharmacology*, **30**: 169–176.

De Sarro, G. & De Sarro, A. (1992). Anticonvulsant activity of competitive antagonists of NMDA receptor in genetically epilepsy-prone rats. *European Journal of Pharmacology*, **215**: 321–30.

De Sarro, G., De Sarro, A. & Meldrum, B. S. (1991*a*). Anticonvulsant action of 2-chloroadenosine injected focally into the inferior colliculus and substantia nigra. *European Journal of Pharmacology*, **194**: 145–52.

De Sarro, G., Trimarchi, G. R. Federico, F. & De Sarro, A. (1991*b*). Anticonvulsant activity of some calcium antagonists in genetically epilepsy prone rats. *Epilepsy Research, Supplement*, **3**: 49–55.

Doretto, M. C., Burger, R., Garcia-Cairasco, N. & Jobe, P. C. (1991). Amino acids in substantia nigra intracerebral microdialysis in genetically epilepsy-prone rats. *Society for Neuroscience Abstracts*, **17**: 171.

Evans, S., McCabe, K. E., Faingold, C. L. & Caspary, D. M. (1991). Repetitive synaptic stimulation evokes increased excitatory responses in genetically epilepsy-prone rat hippocampus. *Epilepsia*, **32**: 41.

Faingold, C. L. & Boersma Anderson, C. A. (1991). Loss of intensity-induced inhibition in inferior colliculus neurons leads to audiogenic seizure susceptibility in behaving genetically epilepsy-prone rats. *Experimental Neurology*, **113**: 354–63.

Farias, P. A., Low, S. Q., Peterson, G. M. & Ribak, C. E. (1992). Morphological evidence for altered synaptic organization and structure in the hippocampal formation of seizure-sensitive gerbils. *Hippocampus*, **2**: 229–45.

Flavin, H. J., Wieraszko, A. & Seyfried, T. N. (1991). Enhanced aspartate release from hippocampal slices of epileptic (El) mice. *Journal of Neurochemistry*, **56**: 1007–11.

Gioanni, Y., Gioanni, H. & Mitrovic, N. (1991). Seizures can be triggered by stimulating non-cortical structures in the quaking mutant mouse. *Epilepsy Research*, **9**: 19–31.

Gould, E. M., Craig, C. R., Fleming, W. W. & Taylor, D. A. (1991). Sensitivity of cerebellar Purkinje neurons to neurotransmitters in genetically epileptic rats. *Journal of Pharmacology and Experimental Therapeutics*, **259**: 1008–12.

Green, R. C., & Seyfried, T. N. (1991). Kindling susceptibility and genetic seizure predisposition in inbred mice. *Epilepsia*, **32**: 22–6.

Helekar, S. A. & Noebels, J. L. (1991). Synchronous hippocampal bursting reveals network excitability defects in an epilepsy gene mutation. *Proceedings of the National Academy of Sciences, USA*, **88**: 4736–40.

Helekar, S. A. & Noebels, J. L. (1992). A burst-dependent hippocampal excitability defect elicited by potassium at the developmental onset of spike–wave seizures in the *tottering* mutant. *Developmental Brain Research*, **65**: 205–10.

Jobe, P. C., Mishra, P. K., Ludvig, N. & Dailey, J. W. (1991). Scope and contribution of genetic models to an understanding of the epilepsies. *CRC Critical Reviews in Neurobiology*, **6**: 183–220.

Jobe, P. C., Burger, R. L., Dailey, J. W., Wang, C., Browning, R. A. & Mishra, P. K. (1992). Is the noradrenergic site for brainstem seizure regulation located within midbrain? Studies with desipramine infused via microdialysis in the GEPR. *Epilepsia*, **33**: 35.

Kostopoulos, G. & Antoniadis, G. (1991). A comparison of recurrent inhibition and of paired-pulse facilitation in hippocampal slices from normal and genetically epileptic mice. *Epilepsy Research*, **9**: 184–94.

Lannes, B., Vergnes, M., Marescaux, C., Depaulis, A., Micheletti, G., Warter, J. M. & Kempf, E. (1991). Lesions of noradrenergic neurons in rats with spontaneous generalized non-convulsive epilepsy. *Epilepsy Research*, **9**: 79–85.

Lasley, S. M. (1991). Roles of neurotransmitter amino acids in seizure severity and experience in the genetically epilepsy-prone rat. *Brain Research*, **560**: 63–70.

Liu, Z., Snead, O. C., Vergnes, M., Depaulis, A. & Marescaux, C. (1991). Intrathalamic injections of gamma-hydroxybutyric acid increase genetic absence seizures in rats. *Neuroscience Letters*, **125**: 19–21.

Liu, Z., Vergnes, M., Depaulis, A. & Marescaux, C. (1992). Involvement of intrathalamic GABA(B) neurotransmission in the control of absence seizures in the rat. *Neuroscience*, **48**: 87–93.

Marciani, M. G., Santone, G., Sancesario, G., Massa, R., Stanzione, P. & Bernardi, G. (1991). Epileptic activity following cerebral ischemia in mongolian gerbils is depressed by CPP, a competitive antagonist of the *N*-methyl-D-aspartate receptor. *Neuroscience Letters*, **129**: 306–10.

Martin, B., Chapouthier, G. & Motta, R. (1992). Analysis of B10.D2 recombinant congenic mouse strains shows that audiogenic and beta-CCM-induced seizures depend on different genetic mechanisms. *Epilepsia*, **33**: 11–13.

Millan, M. H., Wardley-Smith, B., Durmuller, N. & Meldrum, B. S. (1991). The high pressure neurological syndrome in genetically epilepsy prone rats: protective effect of 2-amino-7-phosphono heptanoate. *Experimental Neurology*, **112**: 317–20.

Mishra, P. K., Browning, R. A., Dailey, J. W., Wang, C., Burger, R. L., Bettendorf, A. F. & Jobe, P. C. (1991). The role of locus ceruleus noradrenergic neurons in regulation of forebrain and brainstem seizures. *Third IBRO World Congress of Neuroscience*, no. 32.26.

Mita, T., Sashihara, S., Aramaki, I., Fueta, Y. & Hirano, H. (1991). Unusual biochemical development of genetically seizure-susceptible El mice. *Developmental Brain Research*, **64**: 27–35.

Montpied, P., Winsky, L. & Jacobowitz, D. M. (1991). Alteration in calbindin expression in the caudate putamen and nucleus accumbens of genetically epileptic prone rats GEPR 3 and 9. *Society for Neuroscience Abstracts*, **17**: 972.

Naritoku, D. K., Mecozzi, L. B., Aiello, M. T. & Faingold, C. L. (1992). Repetition of audiogenic seizures in genetically epilepsy-prone rats induces cortical epileptiform activity and additional seizure behaviors. *Experimental Neurology*, **115**: 317–24.

Nehlig, A., Vergnes, M., Marescaux, C., Boyet, S. & Lannes, B. (1991). Local cerebral glucose utilization in rats with petit mal-like seizures. *Annals of Neurology*, **29**: 72–7.

Neumann, P. E. & Collins, R. L. (1991). Genetic dissection of susceptibility to audiogenic seizures in inbred mice. *Proceedings of the National Academy of Sciences, USA*, **88**: 5408–12.

Patel, V. K., Abbott, L. C., Rattan, A. K. & Tejwani, G. A. (1991). Increased methionine-enkephalin levels in genetically epileptic (tg/tg) mice. *Brain Research Bulletin*, **27**: 849–52.

Pencek, T. L., Elmore, T., Evans, M. S. & Moran, M. (1991). Hippocampus paired pulse facilitation in genetically epilepsy-prone rats. *Epilepsia*, **32**: 41–2.

Plomin, R., McClearn, G. E., Gora-Maslak, G. & Neiderhiser, J. M. (1991). Use of recombinant inbred strains to detect quantitative trait loci associated with behavior. *Behavior Genetics*, **21**: 99–116.

Qiao, X. & Noebels, J. L. (1991). Genetic and phenotypic heterogeneity of inherited spike–wave epilepsy. 2. Mutant gene loci with independent cerebral excitability defects. *Brain Research*, **555**: 43–50.

Rise, M. L., Frankel, W. N., Coffin, J. M. & Seyfried, T. N. (1991). Genes for epilepsy mapped in the mouse. *Science*, **253**: 669–73.

Saija, A., Princi, P., DePasquale, R., Costa, G. & De Sarro, G. B. (1992). Evaluation of local cerebral glucose utilization and the permeability of the blood–brain barrier in the genetically epilepsy-prone rat. *Experimental Brain Research*, **88**: 151–57.

Sakai, S., Baba, H., Sato, M. & Wada, J. A. (1991). Effect of DN-1417 on photosensitivity and cortically kindled seizure in Senegalese baboons, *Papio papio*. *Epilepsia*, **32**: 16–21.

Simier, S., Ciesielski, L., Clement, J., Rastegar, A. & Mandel, P. (1992). Involvement of synaptosomal neurotransmitter amino acids in audiogenic seizure-susceptibility and -severity of Rb mice. *Neurochemical Research*, **17**: 953–9.

Snead, O. C., Depaulis, A., Banerjee, P. K., Hechler, V. & Vergenes, M. (1992). The GABA(A)-receptor complex in experimental absence seizures in rat – an autoradiographic study. *Neuroscience Letters*, **140**: 9–12.

Thompson, J. L., Carl, F. G. & Holmes, G. L. (1991). Effects of age on seizure susceptibility in genetically epilepsy-prone rats (GEPR-9s). *Epilepsia*, **32**: 161–7.

Vergnes, M., Marescaux, C., Boehrer, A. & Depaulis, A. (1991). Are rats with genetic absence epilepsy behaviorally impaired? *Epilepsy Research*, **9**: 97–104.

Wang, C., Mishra, P. K., Jobe, P. C. & Browning, R. A. (1992). Noradrenergic regulation of electroshock-induced forebrain and brainstem seizures in rats. *Society for Neuroscience Abstracts*, **18**: 907.

Yan, Q. S., Mishra, P. K., Burger, R. L., Bettendorf, A. F., Jobe, P. C. & Dailey, J. W. (1992). Evidence that carbamazepine and antiepilespirine may produce a component of their anticonvulsant effects by activating serotonergic neurons in genetically epilepsy-prone rats. *Journal of Pharmacology and Experimental Therapeutics*, **261**: 652–9.

Yourick, D. L., Laplaca, M. C. & Meyerhoff, J. L. (1991). Norepinephrine-stimulated phosphatidylinositol metabolism in genetically epilepsy-prone and kindled rats. *Brain Research*, **551**: 315–18.

4 Noradrenergic modulation of excitability: transplantation approaches to epilepsy research
Olle Lindvall

In the experiments of Barry *et al.* (1987, 1989), the influence of the locus coeruleus grafts was anti-epileptogenic, i.e., they counteracted the development of hyperexcitability in response to stimulations in previously non-kindled rats. In a recent study (Bengzon *et al.*, 1993), no effect on the duration and severity of seizures was observed when locus coeruleus neurons were implanted bilaterally into the hippocampus in 6-hydroxy-dopamine-denervated animals *after* kindling had been established. These findings argue against an anticonvulsant action of grafted locus coeruleus neurons in kindling epilepsy. However, such an effect cannot yet be totally excluded, as it may require graft-derived innervations in widespread areas outside the hippocampus and/or in regions critical for seizure generalization.

Not least from the clinical point of view, it seems highly warranted to address the question of whether norepinephrine-rich grafts can reduce neuronal excitability after implantation into a region without prior lesion-induced denervation of the intrinsic noradrenergic input. However, grafting of locus coeruleus neurons into the non-denervated hippocampus, which gave rise to a noradrenergic hyperinnervation, did not influence seizure development in kindling, i.e., the 'extra' norepinephrine input had no anti-epileptogenic effect (Bengzon *et al.*, 1993). When implanted into intact, *kindled* animals, the grafts increased both basal and seizure-evoked norepinephrine release in the stimulated hippocampus (Bengzon *et al.*, 1993), but whether this increase led to any change in neuronal excitability within the area of the hippocampus innervated by the graft is unknown. This experimental situation is in some respects comparable to that when locus coeruleus neurons are grafted to genetically epilepsy prone animals. In this case the intrinsic noradrenergic system is present, although there are functional impairments. Genetically epilepsy prone rats (GEPRs) have lower levels and turnover rates of norepinephrine and reduced high affinity norepinephrine uptake, dopamine-β-hydroxylase activity and number of nerve terminals in the forebrain and some other central nervous system regions compared to controls (Jobe *et al.*, 1982; Laird *et al.*, 1984; Browning *et al.*, 1989; Lauterhorn & Ribak, 1989). Fetal norepinephrine-rich locus coeruleus tissue has, in preliminary study (Clough *et al.*, 1991), been implanted into GEPRs to elucidate whether restoration of norepinephrine transmission by grafts may have a suppressant effect on the severity of audiogenic seizures (evoked by a bell tone). The locus coeruleus grafts were implanted either in the hippocampus or in the third ventricle of GEPRs. No effect was observed in any of the animals with hippocampal implants, whereas some of the rats with grafts in the third ventricle displayed decreased seizure severity. However, there were no significant group effects and no correlation between seizure suppression and number of surviving noradrenergic neurons. Furthermore, no attempts were made to clarify the distribution and density of the graft-derived noradrenergic reinnervation.

In comparison with the studies using kindling and the subcortically denervated hippocampus, this experiment with the GEPR model was not based on prior lesioning in the brain but on a naturally occurring deficit. In that way, the transplantation in GEPR more closely resembles the situation in which grafts might be tested in a human epileptic disorder. Whether locus coeruleus grafts can change seizure susceptibility in GEPR must, however, be further analyzed.

References

Barry, D. I., Kikvadze, I., Brundin, P., Bolwig, T. G., Björklund, A. & Lindvall, O. (1987). Grafted noradrenergic neurons suppress seizure development in kindling-induced epilepsy. *Proceedings of the National Academy of Sciences, USA*, **84**: 8712–15.

Barry, D. I., Wanscher, B., Kragh, J., Bolwig, T. G., Kokaia, M., Brundin, P., Björklund, A. & Lindvall, O. (1989). Grafts of fetal locus coeruleus neurons in rat amygdala–piriform cortex suppress seizure development in hippocampal kindling. *Experimental Neurology*, **106**: 125–32.

Bengzon, J., Kokaia, Z. & Lindvall, O. (1993). Specific functions of grafted locus coeruleus neurons in the kindling model of epilepsy. *Experimental Neurology*, in press.

Browning, R. A., Wade, D. R., Marcinczyk, M., Long, G. L. & Jobe, P. C. (1989). Regional brain abnormalities in norepinephrine uptake and dopamine beta-hydroxylase activity in the genetically epilepsy-prone rat. *Journal of Pharmacology and Experimental Therapeutics*, **249**: 229–35.

Clough, R. W., Browning, R. A., Maring, M. L. & Jobe, P. C. (1991). Intracerebral grafting of fetal dorsal pons in genetically epilepsy-prone rats: effects on audiogenic-induced seizures. *Experimental Neurology*, **112**: 195–9.

Jobe, P. C., Laird, H. E., Ko, K., Ray, T. & Dailey, J. W. (1982). Abnormalities in monoamine levels in the central nervous system of the genetically epilepsy-prone rat. *Epilepsia*, **23**: 359–66.

Laird, H. E., II, Dailey, J. W. & Jobe, P. C. (1984). Neurotransmitter abnormalities in genetically epileptic rodents. *Federation Proceedings*, **43**: 2505–9.

Lauterhorn, J. C. & Ribak, C. E. (1989). Differences in dopamine beta-hydroxylase immunoreactivity between the brains of genetically epilepsy-prone and Sprague-Dawley rats. *Epilepsy Research*, **4**: 161–76.

5 Sensitivity of the immature central nervous system to epileptogenic stimuli

Solomon L. Moshé, Patric K. Stanton, and Ellen F. Sperber

Some of our recent studies further highlight the different sensitivities between the adult and immature CNS to seizures. We have observed that kainic acid seizures result in age-related changes in neuronal organization in the hippocampus; these changes are associated with alterations in synaptic circuitry (Sperber *et al.*, 1991*a*). We have shown that kainic acid seizures in adult rats result in cell loss in the CA3/CA4 hippocampal area, and in synaptic reorganization of the mossy fibers projecting to the supragranular layer of the dentate gyrus. In-vitro hippocampal slices from these same adult rats showed alteratons in the pattern of excitation/ inhibition of the dentate granule cells. By the use of paired-pulse orthodromic stimulation of the perforant path and concomitant recording from dentate granule cells, adult slices were shown to have a pronounced enhancement of late inhibition. In contrast, immature rats (16–17 days old) exposed to kainic acid did not show neuronal loss, synaptic reorganization of mossy fibers or changes in paired-pulse inhibition in hippocampal slices.

To examine further the differences in sensitivity of immature animals to pharmacologically induced seizures, we have also studied developmental differences in $GABA_B$ receptor binding (Garant *et al.*, 1992) and maturation of $GABA_A$ receptor subunits in the substantia nigra (Sperber *et al.*, 1991*b*). Results of these studies may partially explain the differences in sensitivity of immature rats to pharmacological seizures. We have demonstrated that there is a selective increase in the density of $GABA_B$ receptor binding in the developing rat (14–17 days old) substantia nigra in comparison with adults. This maturational difference in $GABA_B$ receptors may underlie the age-related differences in GABA-mediated responses to seizures. Furthermore, using in situ hybridization techniques, we have examined developmental changes in the $GABA_A$ $\alpha 1$ receptor subunit in the substantia nigra. In these studies, we have demonstrated that the density of $GABA_A$ $\alpha 1$ mRNA expression was much greater in adult substantia nigra reticulata than in substantia nigra compacta. In the

14 day old rat pup, there was a similar *pattern* of gene expression within the substantia nigra; however, the overall *density* of mRNA expression was significantly less in immature rats. These results suggest that maturation of the GABAergic system in the substantia nigra may also contribute to age-related differences in sensitivity to epileptogenic stimuli.

References

Garant, D., Sperber, E. F. & Moshé, S. L. (1992). The density of GABA_B binding sites in the substantia nigra is greater in rat pups than in adults. *European Journal of Pharmacology*, **214**: 75–8.

Sperber, E. F., Haas, K. Z., Stanton, P. K. & Moshé, S. L. (1991a). Resistance of the immature hippocampus to seizure-induced synaptic reorganization. *Developmental Brain Research*, **60**: 88–93.

Sperber, E. F., Pellegrini-Giampietro, D. E., Friedman, L. K., Zukin, R. S. & Moshé, S. L. (1991b). Maturational differences in gene expression of GABA_A α1 receptor subunit in rat substantia nigra. *Society for Neuroscience Abstracts*, **17**: 171.

6 Neurophysiological studies of alterations in seizure susceptibility during brain development

John W. Swann, Karen L. Smith, Robert J. Brady, and Martha G. Pierson

Since Chapter 6 (this volume) was written, advances have been made in our understanding of the ontogeny of excitatory amino acid receptors and synaptogenesis in the brain. These findings will undoubtedly have a major impact on basic epilepsy research in the coming years. Late in 1991, Moriyoshi *et al.* cloned an *N*-methyl-D-aspartate (NMDA) receptor subunit, which has been since termed NMDAR1 or NR1. Thereafter, other groups (e.g., Burnashev *et al.*, 1992) identified additional NMDA subunits (e.g., NR2A and NR2B). It is likely that other NMDA receptor subunits will be isolated in the very near future (see e.g., Henneberry, 1992).

Like other neurotransmitter receptors, NMDA receptors appear to be composed of combinations of subunits. In-situ hybridization and immunohistochemical studies have shown subunits to be differentially expressed in various areas of the central nervous system. A recent communication (Monver & Seeberg, 1992) reported alterations in expression of NMDA receptor subunits in different areas of rat brain during postnatal development.

Related to this, two recent electrophysiological studies have shown that, in the developing visual system, NMDA receptor-mediated excitatory postsynaptic currents (EPSCs) are unusually prolonged (Carmignoto & Vioini, 1992; Hestrin, 1992). This appears to be due to age-dependent alterations in the kinetics of the NMDA channel. Interestingly, Carmignoto & Vicini (1992) also showed that the maturational changes in the NMDA EPSCs could be prevented by experimental interventions in early life. Rearing rats in the dark or intracortical injections of tetrodotoxin appeared to prevent age-dependent changes in NMDA receptor-mediated EPSCs in visual cortex. These results parallel those of Constantine-Paton et al. (1990) in that maturational changes in the NMDA receptor and network remodeling both depend on activity within participating neurons.

Burnashev et al. (1992) reported that single asparagine residues in the putative channel-forming segment, TM2, of the NMDA receptor subunits NR1 and NR2A regulate Mg^{2+} blockade and Ca^{2+} permeability. Thus, channel blockade by Mg^{2+} appears to be controlled by RNA editing. In terms of the demonstrated ability of extracellular Ca^{2+} to modulate voltage dependency of the NMDA receptor and electrographic seizures (Brady et al., 1991), Burnashev et al. (1992) have shown that single amino acid substitutions could produce responses to NMDA that were blocked by extracellular Ca^{2+}. Thus, the possibility exists that in the near future, age-dependent alterations in excitatory synaptic physiology and plasticity will be explained by rather subtle alterations of receptor molecular biology.

Results of our most recent anatomical studies support the notion that remodeling of CA3 pyramidal cell recurrent collaterals takes place during early postnatal life (Swann et al., 1991). During the first postnatal week, few axon collaterals have been produced by CA3 pyramidal cells. However, by week 2, a substantial growth of axons has taken place. Results suggest that with further maturation there is a remodeling of recurrent excitatory collaterals. Axon collaterals appear to be pruned and synapses are eliminated. Whether this remodeling is activity dependent and how it may be modified by abnormal activity (e.g. hippocampal seizures) are avenues for future study.

In related studies, Pierson & Snyder-Keller (1992) have demonstrated the cortical origin of audiogenic seizure initiation within inferior colliculus. These studies have focused on the model of noise-exposure-induced susceptibility in rats. The mapping studies have employed Fos immunohistochemistry. These investigators have also found that the tonotopic organization of afferent projections to inferior colliculus is abnormal in susceptible rats (Snyder-Keller & Pierson, 1992). Instead of

Fos-immunoreactive cells restricted to narrow bands as occurs in non-susceptible rats, the pure tone response in susceptible rats is non-selective; i.e., pure tones induce c-*fos* gene expression within massive regions of central nucleus and dorsal cortex of inferior colliculus of susceptible animals. The authors have shown that inferior colliculus of young 14 day old rats is not yet organized into segregated frequency domains. Since it is at that age when susceptibility is initiated, it appears that the maintenance of a diffuse neonatal pattern of ascending auditory projection may contribute in an important way to seizure susceptibility in this model of developmental epilepsy.

In summary, understanding of the biology of normal brain development is advancing at an ever-increasing pace. Knowledge gained from molecular biology studies is likely to influence our thinking about age-dependent differences in nervous system functioning. The challenge to experimental epilepsy researchers will be to capitalize on newly emerging neurobiological concepts in order to understand better the origins of intractable forms of developmental epilepsy.

References

Brady, R. J., Smith, K. L. & Swann, J. W. (1991). Calcium modulation of the NMDA response and electrographic seizures in immature hippocampus. *Neuroscience Letters*, **124**: 92–6.

Burnashev, N., Schoepfer, R., Monyer, H., Ruppersberg, J. P., Gunther, W., Seeberg, P. H. &Sakmann, B. (1992). Control by asparagine residues of calcium permeability and magnesium blockade in the NMDA receptor. *Science*, **257**: 1415–19.

Carmignoto, G. & Vicini, S. (1992). Activity-dependent decrease in NMDA receptor responses during development of the visual cortex. *Science*, **258**: 1007–11.

Constantine-Paton, M., Cline, H. T. & Debski (1990). Patterned activity, synaptic convergence, and the NMDA receptor in developing visual pathways. *Annual Review of Neuroscience*, **13**: 129–54.

Henneberry, R. C. (1992). Cloning of the genes for excitatory amino acid receptors. *Bioessays*, **14**: 465–71.

Hestrin, S. (1992). Developmental regulation of NMDA receptor-mediated synaptic currents at a central synapse. *Nature*, **357**: 686–9.

Monver, H. & Seeberg, P. (1992). Developmental expression of NMDA receptor subtypes. *Society for Neuroscience Abstracts*, **18**: 395.

Moriyoshi, K., Masu, M., Ishii, T., Shigemoto, R., Mizuno, M. & Nakanishi, S. (1991). Molecular cloning and characterization of the rat NMDA receptor. *Nature*, **354**: 31–7.

Pierson, M. & Snyder-Keller, A. (1992). Dysgenesis of frequency representation in inferior colliculus of audiogenic seizure susceptible rats. *Epilepsia*, **33**: 23.

Snyder-Keller, A. M. & Pierson, M. G. (1992). Audiogenic seizures induce c-*fos* in a model of developmental epilepsy. *Neuroscience Letter*, **135**: 108–12.
Swann, J. W., Gomez, C. M., Rice, F. L., Smith, K. L. & Turner, J. N. (1991). Anatomical studies of CA_3 hippocampal neurons during postnatal development. *Society of Neuroscience Abstracts*, **17**: 1131.

7 Electrophysiology and pharmacology of human neocortex and hippocampus in vitro

Massimo Avoli and Philip A. Schwartzkroin

Many epilepsy surgery centers have initiated research programs to study tissue resected during surgery for medically intractable seizures (for a review, see Schwartzkroin, 1993). Recent reports relevant to tissue excitability focus primarily on the following areas.

Sprouting and synaptic reorganization

Several studies have indicated that sprouting and synaptic reorganization of mossy fibers orginating from dentate granule cells occur in the hippocampal formation of patients suffering from temporal lobe epilepsy (TLE) (see also Chapter 9, this volume). These changes have been assessed by the Timm histochemical method (Sutula *et al.*, 1989) and by dynorphin immunoreactivity (Houser *et al.*, 1990), and it has been proposed that they might contribute to the abnormal excitability that characterizes mesial structures in TLE. In keeping with this view, histochemical and ultrastructural data have indicated that in damaged hippocampus of TLE patients, mossy fiber reactive synaptogenesis may result in monosynaptic recurrent excitation of granule cells that could contribute to onset of focal seizures (Babb *et al.*, 1991). Furthermore, a recent in-vitro electrophysiological study has shown an increase in N-methyl-D-aspartate (NMDA) responses and dendritic degeneration in human epileptic hippocampal neurons (Isokawa & Levesque, 1991). Houser (1990) has also found dispersion of granule cells (i.e., they occur in ectopic positions) in the dentate gyrus of TLE patients. Interestingly, the patients assessed in this latter study had most often suffered from febrile seizures and/or brain infections during the first four years of life. Reorganization of the hippocampus in TLE appears to involve both the selective loss of interneurons immunoreactive to somatostatin and neuropeptide Y and the axonal sprouting of other neuropeptide Y neurons and dynorphin A immunoreactive granule cells (de Lanerolle *et al.*, 1989). Efforts to correlate these histological changes with electrophysiological hyper-excitability have provided promising results. Masukawa *et al.* (1992) and Pokorný *et al.* (1991) have reported that the degree of sprouting (assessed with Timm staining) correlated positively with the burst discharge propensity of dentate granule cells. The study by Pokorný (1991) further demonstrated, via intracellular staining, that individual granule cells elaborated axon collaterals within the inner molecular layer of many (but not all) tissue samples from TLE patients.

Electrophysiological properties

Correlative analysis of the morphological and physiological characteristics of neurons in the human neocortex has confirmed the presence of regular spiking (i.e., spiny pyramidal) and fast spiking (i.e., aspiny non-pyramidal) neurons (Foehring *et al.*, 1991). This study also confirmed the absence of intrinsic burst-firing neurons, although an initial, phasic-firing behavior, presumably caused by a low threshold spike mechanism, was observed. Similar findings have been obtained by Avoli *et al.* (1993) in the superficial–middle layers of epileptogenic temporal neocortex. Lorenzon & Foehring (1992) have characterized both the electrophysiological and the pharmacological properties of the after-hyperpolarizations generated by human neocortical cells. Finally, Sayer *et al.* (1990), using the acutely dissociated preparation and whole-cell patch-clamp techniques, have characterized voltage-dependent calcium channels from human epileptogenic neocortex; this study identified low threshold (transient or T-type) and high threshold (L- and N-type) calcium channels with characteristics similar to those of cat cortex.

Excitatory amino acid receptors

Pharmacological characterization of stimulus-induced excitatory post-synaptic potentials (EPSPs) has been obtained by Wuarin *et al.* (1990) in slices of neocortex resected from infants and children undergoing surgical treatment for intractable epilepsy. Wuarin *et al.* have shown that these excitatory synaptic responses are depressed by the broad spectrum excitatory amino acid antagonist kynurenic acid. Furthermore, they have used voltage-clamp recordings to establish the participation of an NMDA-mediated component to synaptic potentials in disinhibited neocortical slices (Wuarin *et al.*, 1992). Finally this group of investigators has provided evidence for local inhibitory and excitatory circuits in human neocortex from children as young as eight months (Tasker *et al.*, 1992). The participation of NMDA and non-NMDA receptors in excitatory synaptic responses has also been assessed in the superficial and middle layer neurons of temporal lobe neocortex (Hwa & Avoli, 1992). The response characteristics of NMDA receptor/channels in epileptic human cortex appear to be similar to receptor properties described from normal animal cortex (Wuarin *et al.*, 1992). However, Louvel & Pumain (1992) have suggested that the distribution of NMDA-induced responses is much broader in epileptogenic neocortex than would be expected in normal cortex.

Receptor binding analyses of hippocampal tissue resected from TLE patients has resulted in apparently inconsistent data across laboratories. Hosford *et al.* (1991) have reported increased α-amino-3-hydroxy-5-methylisoxazole-4-propionic acid (AMPA) and decreased NMDA receptor binding. McDonald *et al.* (1991), however, have found an increase in NMDA binding in epileptic hippocampus. Represa *et al.* (1989) have reported an increase in kainate binding in the hippocampus of children with epilepsy.

A recent study has also revealed the presence of a metabotropic receptor in the human cerebral cortex. Its function was found to be negatively modulated by the NMDA receptor (Morari *et al.*, 1991).

GABA-mediated transmission and cell burst discharge

Knowles *et al.* (1992) have reported that presumed pyramidal cells from sclerotic hippocampus are less likely to display stimulus-induced inhibitory postsynaptic potential and are more likely to fire spontaneous bursts of action potentials than are cells from patients with structural lesions. Strowbridge *et al.* (1992) have found abnormal burst discharge associated with cortical lesions, and Williamson *et al.* (1991) reported spontaneous burst discharge in epileptic cortical samples; in these experiments it was shown that bursting was modulated by NMDA, but not non-NMDA, antagonists.

References

Avoli, M., Hwa, G. G. C. & Lacaille, J. C. (1993). Electrophysiological and repetitive firing properties of neurons in the superficial/middle layers of the human neocortex. *Experimental Brain Research*, in press.

Babb, T. L., Kupfer, W. R., Pretorius, J. K., Crandall, P. H. & Levesque, M. F. (1991). Synaptic reorganization by mossy fibers in human epileptic fascia dentata. *Neuroscience*, **42**: 351–63.

de Lanerolle, N. C., Kim, J. H., Robbins, R. J. & Spencer, D. D. (1989). Hippocampal interneuron loss and plasticity in human temporal lobe epilepsy. *Brain Research*, **495**: 387–95.

Foehring, R. C., Lorenzon, N. M., Herron, P. & Wilson, C. J. (1991). Correlation of physiologically and morphologically identified neuronal types in human association cortex *in vitro*. *Journal of Neurophysiology*, **66**: 1825–37.

Hosford, D. A., Crain, B. J., Cao, Z., Bonhaus, D. W., Friedman, A. H., Okazaki, M. M., Nadler, J. V. & McNamara, J. O. (1991). Increased AMPA-sensitive quisqualate receptor binding and reduced NMDA receptor binding in epileptic human hippocampus. *Journal of Neuroscience*, **11**: 428–34.

Houser, C. R. (1990). Granule cell dispersion in the dentate gyrus of humans with temporal lobe epilepsy. *Brain Research*, **535**: 195–204.

Houser, C. R., Miyashiro, J. E., Swartz, B. E., Rich, J. R. & Delgado-Escueta, A. V. (1990). Altered patterns of dynorphin immunoreactivity suggest mossy fiber reorganization in human hippocampal epilepsy. *Journal of Neuroscience*, **10**: 267–82.

Hwa, G. G. C. & Avoli, M. (1992). Excitatory synaptic transmission mediated by NMDA and non-NMDA receptors in the superficial/middle layers of the epileptogenic human neocortex maintained *in vitro*. *Neuroscience Letters*, **143**: 83–6.

Isokawa, M. & Levesque, M. F. (1991). Increased NMDA responses and dendritic degeneration in human epileptic hippocampal neurons in slices. *Neuroscience Letters*, **132**: 212–16.

Knowles, W. D., Awad, I. A. & Nayel, M. H. (1992). Differences of *in vitro* electrophysiology of hippocampal neurons from epileptic patients with mesiotemporal sclerosis versus structural lesions. *Epilepsia*, **33**: 601–9.

Lorenzon, N. M. & Foehring, R. C. (1992). Relationship between repetitive firing and afterhyperpolarizations in human neocortical neurons. *Journal of Neurophysiology*, **67**: 350–63.

Louvel, J. & Pumain, R. (1992). *N*-methyl-D-aspartate-mediated responses in epileptic cortex in humans: an in-vitro study. In *Neurotransmitters in Epilepsy (Epilepsy Research Supplement 8)*, ed. G. Avanzini, J. Engel, Jr., R. Fariello & U. Heinemann, pp. 361–7. Amsterdam: Elsevier.

Masukawa, L. M., Urono, K., Sperling, M., O'Connor, M. J. & Burdette, L. J. (1992). The functional relationship between antidromically evoked field responses of the dentate gyrus and mossy fiber reorganization in temporal lobe epileptic patients. *Brain Research*, **579**: 119–27.

McDonald, J. W., Garofalo, E. A., Hood, T., Sackellares, J. C., Gilman, S., McKeever, P. E., Troncoso, J. C. & Johnston, M. V. (1991). Altered excitatory and inhibitory amino acid receptor binding in hippocampus of patients with temporal lobe epilepsy. *Annals of Neurology*, **29**: 529–41.

Morari, M., Calo, G., Antonelli, T., Gaist, G., Acciarri, N., Fabrizi, A., Bianchi, C. & Beani, L. (1991). Inhibitory effect of NMDA receptor activation on quisqualate-stimulated phosphatidylinositol turnover in the human cerebral cortex. *Brain Research*, 553: 14–17.

Pokorný, J., Schwartzkroin, P. A. & Franck, J. E. (1991). Physiologic and morphologic characteristics of granule cells from human epileptic hippocampus. *Epilepsia*, **32** (Suppl. 3): 46.

Represa, A., Robain, O., Tremblay, E. & Ben-Ari, Y. (1989). Hippocampal plasticity in childhood epilepsy. *Neuroscience Letters*, **99**: 351–5.

Sayer, R. J., Schwindt, P. C. & Crill, W. E. (1990). High- and low-threshold calcium currents in rat sensorimotor cortical neurons. *Society for Neuroscience Abstracts*, **16**: 677.

Schwartzkroin, P. E. (1993). Basic research in the setting of an epilepsy surgery center. In *Surgical Treatment of the Epilepsies*, ed. J. Engel Jr, pp. 755–73. New York: Raven Press.

Strowbridge, B. W., Masukawa, L. M., Spencer, D. D. & Shepherd, G. M. (1992). Hyperexcitability associated with localizable lesions in epileptic patients. *Brain Research*, **587**: 158–63.

Sutula, T., Cascino, G., Cavazos, J., Parada, I. & Ramirez, L. (1989). Mossy fiber synaptic reorganization in the epileptic human temporal lobe. *Annals of Neurology*, **26**: 321–30.

Tasker, J. G., Peacock, W. J. & Dudek, F. E. (1992). Local synaptic circuits and epileptiform activity in slices of neocortex from children with intractable epilepsy. *Journal of Neurophysiology*, **67**: 496–507.

Williamson, A., Shepherd, G. M. & Spencer, D. D. (1991). Evidence for hyperexcitability near neocortical lesions in epileptic patients. *Epilepsia*, **32** (Suppl. 3): 40.

Wuarin, J. P., Kim, Y. I., Cepeda, C., Tasker, J. G., Walsh, J. P., Peacock, W. J., Buchward, N. A. & Dudek, F. E. (1990). Synaptic transmission in human neocortex removed for treatment of intractable epilepsy in children. *Annals of Neurology*, **28**: 503–11.

Wuarin, J. P., Peacock, W. J. & Dudek, F. E. (1992). Single-electrode voltage-clamp analysis of the N-methyl-D-aspartate component of synaptic responses in neocortical slices from children with intractable epilepsy. *Journal of Neurophysiology*, **67**: 84–93.

9 Sprouting as an underlying cause of hyperexcitability in experimental models and the human epileptic temporal lobe

Thomas P. Sutula

The possible functional effects of mossy fiber sprouting have been considered in several recent papers. Using ultrastructural and light level analysis, Ribak & Peterson (1991) have demonstrated that some mossy fiber terminals identified by the Timm method form asymmetric, and thus putatively excitatory, synapses with neurons which have morphological features characteristic of inhibitory interneurons or basket cells. As previous studies have demonstrated that sprouted mossy fiber terminals also form synapses with dendrites of granule cells (Frotscher & Zimmer,

1983), these studies support the possibility that sprouting of the mossy fiber pathway reorganizes synaptic connections in a manner that could enhance both excitation and inhibition. Difficult quantitative analyses would be necessary to assess the relative frequency of these patterns of circuit reorganization, and would not obviate the need for additional physiological experiments to assess the functional capabilities of reorganized pathways and the net effect on synaptic transmission in the hippocampal circuits.

Recent studies and work in progress from several laboratories using both anatomical and physiological techniques have provided additional evidence that assessment of the functional effects of mossy fiber reorganization remains a complex and unresolved issue. In the hippocampus of rats treated with kainate, Sloviter (1991) has used in-vivo recording methods to demonstrate evidence of decreased inhibition and increased granule cell excitability in the dentate gyrus before the development of extensive mossy fiber synaptic reorganization. These physiological alterations were restored toward normal as more extensive mossy fiber reorganization was observed, and the results were interpreted as evidence that sprouting could restore inhibition.

Two additional studies have provided evidence that the physiological properties of reorganized circuitry are not static, but may be expressed conditionally as a function of the state of inhibition. Using in-vitro recording methods, Cronin et al. (1991) demonstrated that synaptic responses of granule cells in the dentate gyrus of kainate-treated rats with mossy fiber sprouting appeared normal in slices perfused with normal bathing media. However, when $GABA_A$ inhibition was blocked with bicucullines, spontaneous and synaptically evoked bursts were observed in 25% to 33% of slices. This finding is of interest as granule cells in slices from normal rats without sprouting do not generate bursts when inhibition is blocked. Golarai & Sutula (1991) have also observed population bursts in granule cells under conditions of decreased inhibition in slices from kindled rats with mossy fiber sprouting, and in slices from normal rats without sprouting after enhancement of N-methyl-D-aspartate-dependent conductances by brief exposure to low Mg^{2+} solutions. These observations are consistent with the possibility that the sprouted pathway could form recurrent excitatory circuits, and illustrate the potential complexity of physiological assessment of recurrent circuitry. As in the CA3 region (Miles & Wong, 1983), the expression of possible recurrent excitation in the dentate gyrus may be dynamically altered by the state of inhibition.

Recent studies therefore support the need for continuing investigation to characterize the functional effects of sprouting in the dentate gyrus under a variety of physiological conditions, and to assess the contribution of seizure-induced sprouting and synaptic reorganization to epileptic phenomena in hippocampal circuitry.

References

Cronin, J., Obenaus, A., Houser, C. & Dudek, F. E. (1991). Electrophysiology of dentate granule cells after kainate-induced synaptic reorganization of the mossy fibers. *Brain Research*, **573**: 305–10.
Frotscher, M. & Zimmer, J. (1983). Lesion-induced mossy fibers to the inner molecular layer of the rat fascia dentata: identification of post synaptic granule cells by the Golgi–EM technique. *Journal of Comparative Neurology*, **215**: 299–311.
Golarai, G. & Sutula, T. (1991). Local generation of burst discharges in dentate granule cells associated with NMDA mediated transmission and mossy fiber sprouting. *Society for Neuroscience Abstracts*, **17**: 169.
Miles, R. & Wong, R. K. S. (1983). Single neurones can initiate synchronized population discharge in the hippocampus. *Nature*, **306**: 371–3.
Ribak, C. & Peterson, G. (1991). Intragranular mossy fibers in rats and gerbils form synapses with the somata and proximal dendrites of basket cells in the dentate gyrus. *Hippocampus*, **1**: 355–64.
Sloviter, R. (1991). Possible functional consequences of synaptic reorganization in the dentate gyrus of kainate-treated rats. *Neuroscience Letters*, **137**: 91–6.

10 Rapidly recurring seizures and status epilepticus: ictal density as a factor in epileptogenesis

Eric W. Lothman, Janet L. Stringer, and Edward H. Bertram

Since the text of Chapter 10 (this volume) was submitted, several studies have been completed that add insight into the issues introduced there. The work can be grouped into four areas: (a) structural brain changes in models of chronic epilepsy; (b) alterations in γ-aminobutyric acid (GABA)-ergic inhibition in the rapidly recurring hippocampal stimulation (RRHS) and continuous hippocampal stimulation (CHS) models; (c) functional anatomy of the RRHS and CHS models; and (d) response of rats of various ages to the RRHS and CHS models.

Neuropathological experiments were carried out on brains from three groups of rats: (a) those that had experienced up to 1500 seizures in the RRHS protocol; (b) those that experienced an episode of CHS-induced self-sustaining limbic status epilepticus; and (c) age-matched electrode-implanted controls not experiencing seizures. Quantitative morphometric studies were done one month or more after the last seizure. The findings were that after the status epilepticus there was significant neuronal loss and atrophy in the neuropil of Ammon's horn, an experimental counterpart of mesial temporal sclerosis (Bertram *et al.*, 1990), and in the dentate gyrus stratum granulosum and hilus (Bertram & Lothman, 1993), whereas with widely spaced intermittent seizures (RRHS protocol) these changes did not occur. With both the RRHS and CHS groups there was profound sprouting of mossy fibers of dentate granule cells. Clearly more work needs to be done on whether there is a loss of particular types of neurons. These data indicate that sprouting may occur in response to loss of target cells normally reached by mossy fibers but may also arise in response to seizure activity per se or some biochemical signal that is triggered after seizures.

As mentioned in Chapter 10, several findings indicate alterations in GABAergic inhibition in association with the RRHS and CHS protocols. Additional studies on this point are as follows. Administration of the non-competitive NMDA receptor antagonist MK-801 blocked rapid kindling and changes in paired-pulse inhibition normally associated with the RRHS protocol (Kapur & Lothman, 1990). This observation indicates that activation of NMDA receptors is involved in the acute deterioration of GABAergic inhibition with RRHS, which, in turn, participates in the pathophysiology of rapid kindling. Once the self-sustaining limbic status epilepticus that is elicited with CHS has become established, it is resistant to phenytoin but attenuated by anti-epileptic agents such as phenobarbital and benzodiazepines that interact with the $GABA_A$ receptor complex; it is also attenuated by NMDA receptor antagonists (Bertram & Lothman, 1990). These findings support the concept that GABAergic inhibition deteriorates with CHS-induced seizures (see p. 343) and also indicate that such seizures activate NMDA receptors. In fact, it is possible to hypothesize an interplay between these two processes that may provide additional clinical strategies for treating status epilepticus (Lothman, 1990).

The electrophysiological findings indicating a disturbance of GABAergic inhibition that were presented in the main text of the chapter were obtained with a paired-pulse protocol that delivered two stimuli to the same set of afferents. This homosynaptic paired-pulse protocol has the potential confound of changes of inhibition, as measured by suppression of population spikes, arising from factors other than alterations in

GABAergic inhibition. To deal with this issue, further studies were done with a heterosynaptic paired-pulse protocol (Bekenstein *et al.*, 1992). Three groups of animals were examined: (a) rats one month after CHS that induced self-sustaining limbic status epilepticus; (b) rats one month after CHS that failed to trigger status epilepticus; and (c) age-matched electrode implanted controls. There were decreases in paired-pulse inhibition evoked by the heterosynaptic protocol in the first group, but the second was not different from controls. The decrements in paired-pulse inhibition were in the early (interpulse interval < 50 ms) and late (interpulse intervals > 300 ms) phases of paired-pulse inhibition that can be linked to $GABA_A$ and to $GABA_B$ receptors, respectively. The lack of changes in the second group of rats establishes that it is the seizure activity and not the stimulation that causes the changes of inhibition after CHS-induced status epilepticus.

A direct test of the potency of GABA-mediated inhibition has been done using intracellular recordings from CA1 pyramidal cells in hippocampal slices taken from rats that had experienced CHS-induced self-sustaining limbic status epilepticus two to five months before (Bekenstein & Lothman, 1993). The findings were a virtual abolition of inhibitory postsynaptic potentials (IPSPs) evoked by antidromic activation of pyramidal cells from the stimulation of alveus and orthodromically from stimulation of the Schaeffer collaterals. The alvear stimulation selectively activates $GABA_A$ receptor-mediated IPSPs, whereas the other stimulus paradigm activates both $GABA_A$ and $GABA_B$ receptors. Thus, the observations from the slices from animals after CHS-induced self-sustaining limbic status epilepticus indicate a loss of both $GABA_A$- and $GABA_B$-receptor-mediated inhibition. Additional studies, using a procedure to activate GABAergic interneurons selectively and directly, then showed that the problem was not an inability of pyramidal cells to generate GABA-mediated IPSPs nor a loss of GABAergic interneurons, but rather a deafferentation of the inhibitory interneurons in accord with the dormant cell hypothesis proposed by Sloviter (1991).

Work on mapping the functional anatomy of CHS-induced self-sustaining limbic status epilepticus using a combination of 2-deoxyglucose autoradiography and depth electrodes has been published (VanLandingham & Lothman, 1991*a*). Animals were examined at the peak of status epilepticus or one week or one month after it had resolved. Acutely there were dramatic bilateral, symmetrical increases in glucose utilization in the hippocampus, parahippocampal structures, and associated limbic and subcortical non-limbic regions, particularly certain thalamic nuclei;

hypometabolism was found in several neocortical structures. Chronically, glucose utilization was elevated in certain limbic areas one week after status epilepticus had resolved, but returned to control values at one month. These experiments show involvement of the hippocampal–parahippocampal loop in CHS-induced self-sustaining limbic status epilepticus, in accord with discussion above. In addition, the findings of hypometabolism suggest that seizure activity in subcortical structures can influence the physiological operation of the neocortex. Additional studies of this type, done in animals with transections of the hippocampal commissures (VanLandingham & Lothman, 1991*b*), showed status epilepticus confined to the side of stimulation; i.e., activation of the hippocampal–parahippocampal loop occurred only on that side. These results show that the hippocampal commissures are not necessary for the establishment of self-sustaining limbic status epilepticus. VanLandingham & Lothman (1991*b*) also discuss further points indicating functional differences in the commissures connecting rostral versus those connecting ventral hippocampi. The material is beyond the scope of this review, but has implications for human epilepsy when viewed against the fact that the rat dorsal hippocampus is similar to the human posterior hippocampus and the rat ventral hippocampus to the human anterior hippocampus.

Additional studies have been completed using the RRHS protocol. Removal of the entorhinal cortex from the hippocampal–parahippocampal loop, either via electrolytic lesions or via 'pharmacological' lesions with tetrodotoxin, blocked maximal dentate activation (MDA) on the side of the lesion but not on the opposte side where the loop was intact (Stringer & Lothman, 1991). This observation further supports the view that the hippocampal–parahippocampal loop behaves as a unit in epileptogenesis and that the dentate gyrus is a critical control point in this unit. In the intact brain, bilateral MDA is critical for the development of afterdischarges in the dentate gyrus (Stringer & Lothman, 1992). However, after transections of the hippocampal commissures, MDA could be readily elicited on the side of stimulation and rapid kindling took place with the RRHS protocol, whereas afterdischarges did not occur in the dentate gyrus on the unstimulated side. This corroborates the results from the functional anatomy mapping experiments presented above showing that the commissures are not needed to elicit the epileptic phenomenon evoked by the RRHS and CHS protocols and that the hippocampal commissures exert a complex effect on epileptogenesis. It is of interest to note (Stringer *et al.*, 1991) that MDA, and the associated reverberatory activity in the hippocampal–parahippocampal loop, can be activated from a site extrinsic to the loop, the amygdala in this study, as well as as sites in the loop (entorhinal cortex or hippocampus proper).

Since epilepsy preferentially strikes the younger brain and since epilepsy displays such a wide array of age-dependent phenomena it is important to study epileptogenesis and the pathophysiology of seizures at various points in ontogeny (for a review, see Lothman, 1993). Thus, the RRHS and CHS protocols were examined in rats of various postnatal ages. Rats of postnatal ages 7, 14, 21, and 28 days after birth were found to show rapid kindling, like that in adults (Michelson & Lothman, 1991). Animals of age 14 days postnatal kindled the fastest, indicating an ontogenic profile for the processes involved in kindling. Another finding was that day 7 postnatal rats showed behavioral seizures different from those of older rats. This age-dependent difference in seizure expression is in keeping with observations made clinically in humans. Of particular interest was the finding that the rapid kindling of rats on day 7 postnatal developed promptly during the stimulation on a particular day but was not retained to the next day of stimulation. This indicates that not only is seizure manifestation markedly age dependent, but so also may be the sequela to seizures. This topic is further discussed elsewhere (Lothman, 1993). Other work has shown that young rats of various ages develop self-sustaining limbic status epilepticus in response to the CHS protocol (H. B. Michelson & E. W. Lothman, unpublished results).

References

Bekenstein, J. W. & Lothman, E. W. (1993). Dormancy of inhibitory interneurons in a model of temporal lobe epilepsy. *Science*, **259**: 97–100.

Bekenstein, J. W., Rempe, D. & Lothman, E. W. (1992). Decreased heterosynaptic and homosynaptic paired pulse inhibition in the rat hippocampus as a chronic sequela to limbic status epilepticus. *Brain Research*, in press.

Bertram, E. H., Lothman, E. W. & Lenn, N. J. (1990). The hippocampus in experimental chronic epilepsy: a morphometric analysis. *Annals of Neurology*, **27**: 43–8.

Bertram, E. H. & Lothman, E. W. (1990). NMDA receptor antagonists and limbic status epilepticus: a comparison with standard anticonvulsants. *Epilepsy Research*, **5**: 177–84.

Bertram, E. H. & Lothman, E. W. (1993). The morphometric effects of intermittent kindled seizures and limbic status epilepticus in the dentate gyrus. *Brain Research*, in press.

Kapur, J. & Lothman, E. W. (1990). NMDA receptor activation mediates the loss of GABAergic inhibition induced by recurrent seizures. *Epilepsy Research*, **5**: 103–11.

Lothman, E. W. (1990). The biochemical basis and pathophysiology of status epilepticus. *Neurology*, **40** (Suppl. 2): 47–51.

Lothman, E. W. (1992). Pathophysiology of seizures and epilepsy in the mature and immature brain: cells, synapses, and circuits. In *Epilepsy in Childhood*, ed. W. E. Dodson & J. M. Pellock. New York: Demos Press, in press.

Michelson, H. B. & Lothman, E. W. (1991). An ontogenetic study of kindling using rapidly recurring seizures. *Developmental Brain Research*, **61**: 79–85.

Sloviter, R. S. (1991). Permanently altered hippocampal structure, excitability and inhibition after experimental status epilepticus in the rat: the 'dormant basket cell' hypothesis and its possible relevance to temporal lobe epilepsy. *Hippocampus*, **1**, 41–66.

Stringer, J. L. & Lothman, E. W. (1991). Maximal dentate activation is a marker for reverberatory seizure activity in hippocampal–parahippocampal circuits. *Experimental Neurology*, **116**: 198–203.

Stringer, J. L. & Lothman, E. W. (1992). Bilateral maximal dentate activation is critical for the appearance of an afterdischarge in the dentate gyrus. *Neuroscience*, **46**: 309–14.

Stringer, J. L., Williamson, J. M. & Lothman, E. W. (1991). Maximal dentate activation is produced by amygdala stimulation in unanesthetized rats. *Brain Research*, **542**: 336–42.

VanLandingham, K. E. & Lothman, E. W. (1991a). Self-sustaining limbic status epilepticus. I. Acute and chronic metabolic studies-limbic hypermetabolism and neocortical hypometabolism. *Neurology*, **41**: 1942–9.

VanLandingham, K. E. & Lothman, E. W. (1991b). Self-sustaining limbic status epilepticus. II. Role of hippocampal commissures in metabolic responses. *Neurology*, **41**: 1950–7.

11 Brain slice models for the study of seizures and interictal spikes

Wilkie A. Wilson and Andrew Bragdon

One of the most valuable improvements to slice models of seizures would be to have the slices develop secondary seizure foci as well as the ability to express spontaneous seizures without ionic or pharmacological alterations. Since Chapter 11 (this volume) was prepared there has been significant movement toward this goal.

As reviewed in Chapter 11, we were able to use low magnesium artificial cerebrospinal fluid (ACSF) to study the relationship between epileptiform events in CA3 and in the entorhinal cortex. Heinemann and his colleagues have now reported far more extensive studies of an extended slice model of the hippocampal–parahippocampal structures; this slice includes the hippocampus, the neocortical temporal area 3, the entorhinal cortex, the dentate gyrus, and the subiculum (Dreier & Heinemann, 1991).

In this slice preparation, Dreier & Heinemann have demonstrated the preservation of subicular connections to entorhinal cortex and connections from entorhinal cortex to the dentate gyrus. The entorhinal cortex, the temporal cortex, or the subiculum could represent the focus for electrographic seizures, but the hippocampus did not express full seizures until the slices were treated with baclofen. This suggests that baclofen inhibits inhibitory interneurons and allows the dentate granule cells to transmit activity from the entorhinal cortex to the hippocampus. The authors did not see signs that the hippocampus could initiate seizures in their model.

Our experience was slightly different, using thicker slices in which the connections may have been better preserved (Wilson *et al.*, 1988). We found that CA3 bursting could project to the entorhinal cortex and trigger activity which developed into a seizure and then projected back to the hippocampus. Thus, in our hands, CA3 was the 'focus'. This is one of many subtle differences that can be seen between models, and illustrates the point that slice models may be especially vulnerable to different outcomes, depending on the amount of circuitry involved.

Most important, a remarkable finding has been reported by Rafiq *et al.* (1992). They have been able to obtain the electrical equivalent of status epilepticus in a slice model without alterations to the ionic media or the addition of drugs. In young rats (aged 21–30 days), they used the extended slice preparation described by Dreier & Heinemann, but modified the slice plane to increase connections from the entorhinal cortex to the hippocampus. They subjected this preparation, in normal ACSF, to repeated electrical stimulation, similar to that which we used for hippocampal seizure induction.

After a number of stimulations (7–9 stimulus trains), a secondary, delayed discharge developed several minutes after the primary electrographic seizure. The secondary discharge showed gradual lengthening with repeated stimulation and involved the entire hippocampal–parahippocampal loop. In some slices this secondary discharge continued unabated for 20–60 min, mimicking status epilepticus.

The development of this preparation is an outstanding advance in the use of in-vitro models for studies of seizure genesis and expression. It has far more intact circuitry than most models, yet is amenable to rapid fluid perfusion and detailed electrophysiological study. Most importantly, the epileptiform activity occurs in a relatively 'normal' environment. The ability to induce the equivalent of status epilepticus in vitro will allow detailed analyses of the circuit components that support this activity, as well as an opportunity for studying different pharmacological approaches to this problem.

With this advance, slice models have evolved to the point that almost all of the important aspects of seizure genesis and expression can be seen in slices. This is not to say that all of our questions about epilepsy can be addressed through them, but that they offer a widening window onto this devastating disorder.

References

Dreier, J. P. & Heinemann, U. (1991). Regional and time dependent variations of low Mg^{++} induced epileptiform activity in rat temporal cortex slices. *Experimental Brain Research*, **84**: 581–96.

Rafiq, A., DeLorenzo, R. J. & Coulter, D. A. (1992). Seizure generation and propagation in combined entorhinal cortex/hippocampal slice. *Epilepsia*, **33** (Suppl. 3): 34.

Wilson, W. A., Swartzwelder, H. S., Anderson, W. W. & Lewis, D. V. (1988). Seizure activity in vitro: a dual focus model. *Epilepsy Research*, **2**: 289–93.

12 Generation of epileptiform discharge by local circuits of neocortex

Barry W. Connors and Yael Amitai

Research on the basic biology of neocortex has accelerated, and here we highlight only a few findings. Our view of the intrinsic physiology of cortical neurons is increasingly complex. Kawaguchi (1993) has demonstrated elegantly that some smooth non-pyramidal cells of the neocortex have fast-spiking properties, but that others clearly adapt and generate low threshold spikes. These two groups of cells are morphologically distinct. The work raises questions about the particular roles each inhibitory cell type might play in regulating cortical excitability. Among pyramidal cells of neocortex there is functional diversity at the subcellular level. Direct recordings from the apical dendrites of layer V pyramids reveal a spectacular array of electrogenic properties, including sodium- and calcium-dependent spiking (Kim & Connors, 1992; Amitai *et al.*, 1993). Although the apical dendrite does not strongly influence the spiking properties of the pyramidal cell soma (Telfeian *et al.*, 1991), its excitability is apparently essential for the efficacy of distal apical inputs (Cauller & Connors, 1992). The non-linear properties of apical dendrites (and perhaps other cortical dendrites) may facilitate the synchronizing effects of intracortical connections.

To understand the essence of epileptiform discharge in neocortex will require a formal mathematical model; to build the model requires a myriad of biological measurements. The strength, probability and time course of individual synaptic connections are now being determined by the direct, albeit laborious, method of paired intracellular recordings. Mason *et al.* (1991) have shown in layers II/III pyramidal cells that local excitatory connectivity is sparse ($P \approx 0.09$), and unitary excitatory post-synaptic potentials are small (ranging from 0.05 to 2.0 mV; most are less than 0.5 mV). Interestingly for the hypothesis presented in Chapter 12, similar measurements from pairs of pyramids in layer V (Thomson *et al.*, 1992; Nicoll & Blakemore, 1993) suggest that, although the probability of pyramidal interconnection may be lower than in layer II/III, the mean strength of the connections may be much stronger. The data are too sparse to allow reliable comparisons between regular-spiking and intrinsically bursting neurons of layer V, but such information will bear directly upon our central hypothesis.

Despite burgeoning interest in the synchronized activity of normal neocortex (see e.g., Gray *et al.*, 1992), there has been little progress in unraveling its cellular mechanisms. One novel observation is of a cortical system that may allow the selective synchronization of inhibitory interneurons (Aram *et al.*, 1991). The potassium channel blocker 4-aminopyridine causes large, spontaneous, γ-aminobutyric acid-(GABA)-ergic inhibitory postsynaptic potentials that do not appear to be synchronized by glutaminergic synapses, but may (in part) be coordinated by excitatory GABA responses (Michelson & Wong, 1991). Thus, both excitatory and inhibitory neurons of the cortex may have inherent tendencies to synchronize their activity; neocortical activity would then depend upon the simultaneous expression and interaction of these interwoven processes.

References

Amitai, Y., Friedman, A., Connors, B. W. & Gutnick, M. J. (1993). Regenerative activity in the apical dendrites of pyramidal cells in neocortex. *Cerebral Cortex*, in press.

Aram, J. A., Michelson, H. B. & Wong, R. K. S. (1991). Synchronized GABAergic IPSPs recorded in the neocortex after blockade of synaptic transmission mediated by excitatory amino acids. *Journal of Neurophysiology*, **65**: 1034–41.

Cauller, L. J. & Connors, B. W. (1992). Functions of very distal dendrites: experimental and computational studies of layer I inputs to layer V pyramidal neurons in neocortex. In *Single Neuron Computation*, ed. T. McKenna, J. Davis & S. F. Zornetzer, pp. 199–230. New York: Academic Press.

Gray, C. M., Engel, A. K., Konig, P. & Singer, W. (1992). Synchronization of oscillatory neuronal responses in cat striate cortex: temporal properties. *Visual Neuroscience*, **8**: 337–47.

Kawaguchi, Y. (1993). Groupings of non-pyramidal and pyramidal cells with specific physiological and morphological characteristics in rat frontal cortex. *Journal of Neurophysiology*, in press.

Kim, H. G. & Connors, B. W. (1992). Calcium currents in the apical dendrites of neocortical pyramidal neurons. *Society for Neuroscience Abstracts*, **18**: 217.

Mason, A., Nicoll, A. & Stratford, K. (1991). Synaptic transmission between individual pyramidal neurons of the rat visual cortex *in vitro*. *Journal of Neuroscience*, **11**: 72–84.

Michelson, H. B. & Wong, R. K. S. (1991). Excitatory synaptic responses mediated by GABA$_A$ receptors in hippocampus. *Science*, **253**: 1420–3.

Nicoll, A. & Blakemore, C. (1993). Single-fibre EPSPs in layer 5 of rat visual cortex *in vitro*. *NeuroReport*, in press.

Telfeian, A. E., Cauller, L. J. & Connors, B. W. (1991). Contribution of apical dendrites to somatic membrane properties of layer V pyramidal cells in neocortex. *Society for Neuroscience Abstracts*, **17**: 311.

Thomson, A., West, D. C. & Deuchars, J. (1992). Local circuit, single axon excitatory postsynaptic potentials (EPSPs) in deep layer neocortical pyramidal neurones. *Society for Neuroscience Abstracts*, **18**: 1340.

13 Study of GABAergic inhibition and GABA$_A$ receptor in experimental epilepsy

Robert K. S. Wong and Richard Miles

In Chapter 13 (this volume), we describe properties of inhibitory post-synaptic potentials (IPSPs) mediated by γ-aminobutyric acid-(GABA)-ergic neurons in the hippocampus. The possibility that use-dependent depression of such IPSPs may develop upon tetanization of afferent input is emphasized. Furthermore, we raise the possibility that the efficacy of postsynaptic GABA$_A$ receptors, functional only when phosphorylated, could be reduced upon repeated activation. The other plausible sites for the use-dependent depression of inhibition included (a) the presynaptic input to the GABA interneurons, (b) interneurons themselves, and (c) the presynaptic terminals of GABAergic neurons. This list of modifiable sites is not exhaustive and has to be lengthened in view of new unexpected findings regarding the interconnections between GABAergic neurons and the postsynaptic effects of GABA. These new findings are described briefly below.

On the basis of the existing information, we know that GABAergic neurons are activated by afferent fibers (feedforward inhibition) and by recurrent axons of pyramidal cells (feedback inhibition) during normal activity. Excitation through these pathways is mediated by glutamatergic synapses. However, recent studies in the cortex (Aram *et al.*, 1991; Michelson & Wong, 1991) suggest that another mechanism, independent of glutamate transmission, may be involved in the synchronized activation of GABAergic interneurons. This conclusion is based on studies using neocortical and hippocampal slice preparations in the presence of the convulsant compound 4-aminopyridine (4-AP) and glutamate receptor blockers 3-(2-carboxypiperazin-4-yl)propyl-1-phosphonic acid (CPP) and 6-cyano-7-nitroquinxaline-2,3-dione (CNQX). Under such conditions, rhythmic, synchronized IPSPs can be recorded in pyramidal and granule cells. The synchronized IPSPs are larger than unitary IPSPs (up to 15 mV in amplitude and 900 ms in duration) and occur at frequencies ranging from 0.1 to 0.3 Hz.

Direct intracellular recordings from GABAergic interneurons in the hilar region of the hippocampus revealed that, simultaneously with the synchronized IPSPs in the pyramidal cells, synchronized burst firing occurred. The burst firing in the inhibitory interneurons was sustained by large amplitude synchronized excitatory postsynaptic potentials (EPSPs). Since the recordings were made in the presence of glutamate receptor blockers, the synchronized EPSPs in the interneurons could not be accounted for by activation of glutamate receptors. Instead the data revealed that application of the GABA$_A$ receptor blockers picrotoxin and bicuculline blocked the synchronized EPSPs (Michelson & Wong, 1991).

The above results demonstrate unexpected features of the GABAergic inhibitory system. They suggest that GABA can function as an excitatory neurotransmitter onto inhibitory interneurons in the hippocampus. Thus, recurrent connections between GABAergic neurons can elicit excitation of the interneurons. Through the recurrent GABAergic synapses, synchronized firing of the GABAergic interneurons can be activated much in the same way as that depicted in Fig. 13.1 (which describes the synchronized firing of pyramidal cells). The consequences of the excitatory coupling between GABAergic cells is an enhanced output of the interneuron population, giving rise to synchronized IPSPs in the pyramidal cells. In this way the excitatory action of GABA on interneurons remains consistent with the role of GABA as an inhibitory transmitter in the signalling process.

Thus, as we attempt to identify modifiable sites in the GABAergic inhibitory pathway, we have realized that there is much more to learn about GABAergic inhibitory neurons and their circuit organizations. Continuing work at this basic level is required to enable us to under-

stand possible deficits in inhibition that may contribute to epileptogenesis.

References

Aram, J. A., Michelson, H. B. & Wong, R. K. S. (1991). Synchronized
    GABAergic IPSPs recorded in the neocortex after blockade of synaptic
    transmission mediated by excitatory amino acids. *Journal of
    Neurophysiology*, **65**: 1034–41.
Michelson, H. B. & Wong, R. K. S. (1991). Excitatory synaptic responses
    mediated by GABA$_A$ receptors in the hippocampus. *Science*, **253**: 1420–3.

14 High potassium-induced synchronized bursts and electrographic seizures

Christopher J. McBain, Stephen F. Traynelis, and
Raymond Dingledine

In the past two years several research groups have demonstrated novel
properties of the hippocampus, and of the central nervous system in
general, which are pertinent to some of the ideas discussed in Chapter 14
(this volume). Below is a non-exhaustive list of the most relevant of these
advances.

McBain & Dingledine (1992)

Whole cell recordings have revealed that the high frequency barrage of
excitatory postsynaptic currents (EPSCs) received by immature CA3
pyramidal neurons during interictal bursts comprise both N-methyl-D-
aspartate (NMDA) and non-NMDA receptor-mediated components.
These EPSCs are abolished by the addition of tetrodotoxin, indicating
that they are synaptically driven by spiking in nearby neurons. Since
mossy fibre synapses are thought to be devoid of NMDA receptors these
data strengthen the role for CA3 recurrent collaterals in initiating
interictal burst firing.

Westenbroek, Ahlijanian & Catterall (1990)

By using a monoclonal antibody raised against L-type calcium channels
the authors demonstrate that these channels are clustered in high density
at the base of major dendrites in both CA1 and CA3 pyramidal neurons.
This result suggests that these channels serve to mediate large influxes
of calcium ions in response to summed excitatory inputs to the

distal dendrites. Such a mechanism of calcium entry, while mediating intracellular modulatory mechanisms under physiological conditions, may also predispose neurons to bursting activity and cell damage under pathological conditions.

Bilkey & Schwartzkroin (1990)

This paper demonstrates that cells with somata located close to the stratum pyramidale/oriens border were more likely to generate bursts than cells located closer to the stratum radiatum. One notable morphological feature of these cells was the greater length of the initial portion of their apical dendrite. This observation is consistent with the hypothesis that burst-type activity arising in CA3 neurons is generated or modulated by ion channels on this section of the dendrite (Westenbroek *et al.*, 1990).

The expression cloning of the first glutamate receptor subunit cDNA (GluR1) in late 1989 triggered a predictable frenzy of activity that has subsequently led to the identification of more than 13 genes that encode structurally related proteins (for a review, see Dingledine, 1992). A significant feature of the glutamate receptors is that different subunit combinations produce functionally different receptors. The regional variation in distribution of these subunits and the presence of splice variants highlight the likely existence of a myriad of glutamate receptors with differing properties throughout the central nervous system.

Hume, Dingledine & Heinemann (1991)

A single amino acid site within a putative transmembrane domain was found to determine divalent ion permeability and the current–voltage relation within α-amino-3-hydroxy-5-methylisoxazole-4-propionic acid (AMPA) receptor subunits. This position (the Q/R site) is occupied by a glutamine (Q) in the subunits GluR1 and GluR3 but an arginine (R) in GluR2. The presence of an R in the Q/R-site substantially reduces the divalent permeability of the expressed subunit combinations.

Sommer, Kohler, Sprengel & Seeburg (1991)

Interestingly the genomic DNA sequence of the Q/R site in GluR1 through 3, as described by Hume *et al.* (1991) all have a glutamine codon in this position. In GluR2, RNA editing appears to control the amino acid encoded by this critical codon, i.e., an arginine is substituted for the glutamine. Pathological states that interfere with the correct RNA editing will probably result in significant alterations to calcium ion permeability in such cells, increasing the likelihood of neuronal damage.

Müller, Moller, Berger, Schnitzer & Kettenmann (1992)

Glutamate receptors on Bergmann glial cells have been demonstrated to have a high permeability to divalent cations. One functional consequence of calcium permeation through these channels is the consequent blockade of potassium channels on these cells. If this calcium-dependent blockade of potassium channels were to extend to neuronal glutamate receptors, the concommitant reduction of a potassium current would remove an important regulatory mechanism. Under conditions of intense neuronal firing, removal of this potassium current would counteract those mechanisms acting to dampen electrical excitability.

Tsaur, Sheng, Lowenstein, Jan & Jan (1992)

This paper demonstrates that differences in neuronal excitability within the central nervous system may arise from the differential expression of K^+-channel genes, regulated spatially in a cell type-specific manner, or temporally in response to neuronal activity. More importantly this paper shows that, following periods of intense seizure activity, expression of a likely delayed rectifier-type and an A-type potassium channel is repressed at the mRNA level, thus removing important inhibitory mechanisms.

MacVicar & Hochman (1991) and Rice & Nicholson (1991)

In the study of MacVicar & Hochman, image analysis techniques were used to monitor the intrinsic optical properties of hippocampal slices. Changes in extracellular space were observed in the dendritic region of CA1 pyramidal cells following high frequency stimulation of the Schaffer collaterals. Agents that blocked synaptic transmission or prevented postsynaptic receptor activation abolished changes in the optical density of the tissue, suggesting that postsynaptic receptor activation was essential for the changes in tissue volume observed.

In the paper by Rice & Nicholson, direct measurements of the extracellular volume fraction (EVF) were made in slices of neostriatum (see also McBain *et al.*, 1990). Under periods of hypoxia, the EVF of these slices was shown to be significantly reduced. These data suggest that periods of hypoxia cause glial cell swelling and a consequent reduction of the extracellular space similar to that reported by McBain *et al.* (1990) in hippocampal slices exposed to high K^+ (see Chapter 14 for details).

Traynelis & Cull-Candy (1991)

Further to the original report of Traynelis & Cull-Candy (see Chapter 14), this paper documents the effect of proton inhibition on whole cell currents evoked by NMDA, AMPA and kainate. The IC_{50} for proton inhibition of NMDA currents was 7.3, near to the physiological pH. AMPA and kainate whole cell currents were inhibited by protons, with IC_{50} values that corresponded to pH 6.3 and pH 5.7, respectively. The AMPA and kainate receptors were, however, insensitive to H^+ concentrations that inhibited NMDA receptor responses.

References

Bilkey, D. K. & Schwartzkroin, P. A. (1990). Variation in electrophysiology and morphology of hippocampal CA3 pyramidal cells. *Brain Research*, **514**: 77–83.

Dingledine, R. (1992). New wave of non-NMDA excitatory amino acid receptors. *Trends in Pharmacological Sciences*, **12**: 360–2.

Hume, R. I., Dingledine, R. & Heinemann, S. F. (1991). Identification of a site in glutamate receptor subunits that controls calcium permeability. *Science*, **253**: 1028–31.

MacVicar, B. A. & Hochman, D. (1991). Imaging of synaptically evoked intrinsic optical signals in hippocampal slices. *Journal of Neuroscience*, **11**: 1458–69.

McBain, C. J. & Dingledine, R. (1992). Dual component miniature excitatory synaptic currents in rat hippocampal CA3 pyramidal neurons. *Journal of Neurophysiology*, **68**: 16–27.

McBain, C. J., Traynelis, S. F. & Dingledine, R. (1990). Regional variation of extracellular space in the hippocampus. *Science*, **249**: 674–7.

Müller, T., Moller, T., Berger, T., Schnitzer, J. & Kettenmann, H. (1992). Calcium entry through kainate receptors and resulting potassium-channel blockade in Bergmann glial cells. *Science*, **256**: 1563–6.

Rice, M. E. & Nicholson, C. (1991). Diffusion characteristics and extracellular volume fraction during normoxia and hypoxia in slices of rat neostriatum. *Journal of Neurophysiology*, **65**: 264–72.

Sommer, B., Kohler, M., Sprengel, R. & Seeburg, P. H. (1991). RNA editing in brain controls a determinant of ion flow in glutamate-gated channels. *Cell*, **67**: 11–19.

Tsaur, M. L., Sheng, M., Lowenstein, D. H., Jan, Y. N. & Jan, L. Y. (1992). Differential expression of K^+ channel mRNAs in the rat brain and down-regulation in the hippocampus following seizures. *Neuron*, **8**: 1055–67.

Traynelis, S. F. & Cull-Candy, S. G. (1991). Pharmacological properties and H^+ sensitivity of excitatory amino acid receptor channels in rat cerebellar granule neurones. *Journal of Physiology*, **433**: 727–63.

Westenbroek, R. E., Ahlijanian, M. K. & Catterall, W. A. (1990). Clustering of L-type Ca^{2+} channels at the base of major dendrites in hippocampal pyramidal neurons. *Nature*, **347**: 281–4.

15 Anti-epileptic effects of organic calcium channel blockers in animal experiments

Erwin-Josef Speckmann, Jörg Walden, and Heidrum Straub

Epileptiform activity can be suppressed by calcium channel blockade in animal experiments. Thus, an anti-epileptic effect of the calcium channel blocker verapamil has been demonstrated in various animal models in which epileptiform activity is elicited by changes of the ionic microenvironment or by application of different epileptogenic agents (Speckmann & Walden, Chapter 15, this volume). The action of verapamil in depressing epileptiform activity in the human neocortex in vitro has also been investigated (Straub *et al.*, 1992).

The human neocortical tissue used was a small portion of that which is normally removed for the treatment of human brain tumor. Transverse slices (350–500 μm thick) were preincubated for at least 1 h in 28 °C artificial cerebrospinal fluid (ACSF), using a submersion chamber. After preincubation, slices were transferred to a recording submersion chamber, which was continuously perfused by ACSF at 32 °C. Field potentials were recorded from layer III or V using conventional electrophysiological techniques (glass micropipettes; ca 1 MΩ).

Epileptiform activity was induced by omission of Mg^{2+} from the bath solution, as this epilepsy model has been studied intensively in hippocampal and neocortical slices of animals as well as in human neocortex maintained in vitro (Avoli *et al.*, 1991). The induction of epileptic activity and the application of the calcium channel blocker was done with increased K^+ concentration (8 mmol/l), because under these conditions the anti-epileptic effect of verapamil is pronounced (Pohl *et al.*, 1992).

The experimental protocol consisted of five periods.

Period 1: Control 1; superfusion with ACSF.
Period 2: Induction of epileptiform activity; superfusion with ACSF without Mg^{2+}.
Period 3: Test of the anti-epileptic calcium channel blockade; addition of verapamil at a concentration of 40 or 60 μmol/l to the solution used in period 2.

Period 4: Washout of the organic calcium channel blocker with ACSF without Mg^{2+}.

Period 5: Control 2; superfusion with ACSF.

In the first control period, spontaneously occurring epileptiform activity of the type often found in animal preparations was not detected. During superfusion with Mg^{2+}-free ACSF, epileptiform field potentials (EFPs) were induced in the slices within 30 min. The EFPs occurred at a mean rate of 10/min. During administration of verapamil the frequency of occurrence of EFPs decreased down to zero level. With 40 µmol verapamil/l, 90% depression was reached within 2 h. With 60 µmol verapamil/l the latency of depression was markedly reduced to 1 h. Washout of the organic calcium channel blocker led to a reappearance of EFPs within a quarter of an hour. When Mg^{2+} was added again to the ACSF, the epileptiform discharges disappeared.

This observation, that the epileptic activity elicited in human neocortical slices with low Mg^{2+} could be abolished by verapamil, as has been shown for several animal epilepsy models, suggests that there is a general role for transmembranous calcium current in epileptogenesis in humans. This anti-epileptic calcium channel blockade may offer the chance of a new strategy in the treatment of the epilepsies.

References

Avoli, M., Drapeau, C., Louvel, J., Pumain, R., Olivier, A. & Villemure, J.-G. (1991). Epileptiform activity induced by low extracellular magnesium in the human cortex maintained in vitro. *Annals of Neurology*, **30**: 589–96.

Pohl, M., Straub, H. & Speckmann, E.-J. (1992). Low magnesium-induced epileptiform discharges in guinea pig hippocampal slices: depression by the organic calcium antagonist verapamil. *Brain Research*, **577**: 29–35.

Straub, H., Lücke, A., Köhling, R., Moskopp, D., Pohl, M., Wassmann, H. & Speckmann, E.-J. (1992). Low-magnesium-induced epileptiform activity in the human neocortex maintained in vitro: suppression by the organic calcium antagonist verapamil. *Journal of Epilepsy*, **5**: 166–70.

Index

529